Cognitive Informatics in Biomedicine and Healthcare

Series Editor
Vimla L. Patel, Ctr Cognitive Studies in Med & PH
New York Academy of Med, Suite 454, New York, NY, USA

T0234239

Enormous advances in information technology have permeated essentially all facets of life. Although these technologies are transforming the workplace as well as leisure time, formidable challenges remain in fostering tools that enhance productivity, are sensitive to work practices, and are intuitive to learn and to use effectively. Informatics is a discipline concerned with applied and basic science of information, the practices involved in information processing, and the engineering of information systems.

Cognitive Informatics (CI), a term that has been adopted and applied particularly in the fields of biomedicine and health care, is the multidisciplinary study of cognition, information, and computational sciences. It investigates all facets of computer applications in biomedicine and health care, including system design and computer-mediated intelligent action. The basic scientific discipline of CI is strongly grounded in methods and theories derived from cognitive science. The discipline provides a framework for the analysis and modeling of complex human performance in technology-mediated settings and contributes to the design and development of better information systems for biomedicine and health care.

Despite the significant growth of this discipline, there have been few systematic published volumes for reference or instruction, intended for working professionals, scientists, or graduate students in cognitive science and biomedical informatics, beyond those published in this series. Although information technologies are now in widespread use globally for promoting increased self-reliance in patients, there is often a disparity between the scientific and technological knowledge underlying healthcare practices and the lay beliefs, mental models, and cognitive representations of illness and disease. The topics covered in this book series address the key research gaps in biomedical informatics related to the applicability of theories, models, and evaluation frameworks of HCI and human factors as they apply to clinicians as well as to the lay public.

Pei-Yun Sabrina Hsueh • Thomas Wetter
Xinxin Zhu

Editors

Personal Health Informatics

Patient Participation in Precision Health

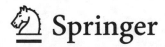

Editors
Pei-Yun Sabrina Hsueh
Bayesian Health
New York, NY, USA

Xinxin Zhu
Center for Biomedical Data Science
Yale University
New Haven, CT, USA

Thomas Wetter
Heidelberg University Hospital
Institute of Medical Informatics
Heidelberg, Germany

Biomedical Informatics and Medical
Education
University of Washington
Seattle, WA, USA

ISSN 2662-7280 ISSN 2662-7299 (electronic)
Cognitive Informatics in Biomedicine and Healthcare
ISBN 978-3-031-07698-5 ISBN 978-3-031-07696-1 (eBook)
https://doi.org/10.1007/978-3-031-07696-1

This Springer imprint is published by the registered company Springer Nature Switzerland AG
The registered company address is: Gewerbestrasse 11, 6330 Cham, Switzerland

Foreword

We live in turbulent times. The pace of technological innovation around us is relentless. Its impacts on society, some expected some not, are reshaping the way we engage with each other and with once trusted monoliths like the healthcare system. Washing over all this tumult are the far reaching and still unrevealed consequences of climate change and what may well be an age of pandemics. Society will not be the same, no matter how we struggle to engineer that it will.

It is no surprise then that as individuals we all want more control, and more understanding of the direction of our health care. Many expect to be equal partners with clinicians in healthcare decisions. We want to know how vaccines work, and the relative risk of one vaccine strategy over another, before we decide to follow public health recommendations. We want to know that our disease treatments are safe, and for major illness many want to leave no option unexplored. Some of us go one step further and want to be the decision-maker, relegating trained professionals to advisers.

The challenges we face as engaged patients however are formidable. If it is truly not possible for a clinician to be up to date with medical science because the pace of innovation is so frenetic, what chance is there for a patient? When in doubt, our human response is to speak to others and understand their own journey and decisions—but that strategy can be risky if we use social media to ask the questions. The promised bounty of the internet, connection to all people and all things, is increasingly tarnished by community polarization, lack of trust, and skepticism in science. Truth itself is often victim to disinformation campaigns created for unclear motive.

It is with this challenging context that we must try not just to understand the sweeping changes that are happening in health care, but to get ahead of them. We are tasked to imagine ways of rebalancing the new dynamic of the world by giving patients and clinicians new options to succeed. What skills and tools must we invent so that patients can both find the information they need and understand the underlying science behind it—itself ever mutating because of technological innovation? What new conceptions of communication and relationships will help patients and their professional carers work together with trust when the old options fall away?

Some of the answers are social and cultural, some are to be found in the embrace of new models of care, where one face-to-face interaction is replaced by a multitude of small digital touches. Some technological answers bring both revolution and their own burden of problems. Artificial intelligence will likely transform the way many patients manage their care. Personal AIs will be our first port of call, noticing health problems emerge before we do, suggesting pathways for care shaped by our past preferences, and coordinating that journey for us. AIs will not just be digital front-doors for us into the health system, they will be networked into it, creating what is known as a cyber-social system. These AIs will be connected into our clothes, our wearable devices and jewelry, our home, and our cars. AIs will negotiate, search, recommend, optimize, and disagree—all on our behalf and not always transparently or fairly. A new age with new opportunity, and a new bag of challenges and decisions for us to face.

In the pages of this book, you will find many of the elements of this next stage in our journey towards a dynamic health system that better fits the challenges ahead. New ways of interacting, new ways of behaving, and new tools for thinking are all part of the solution. The chapters in this book also make clear how early we are in our journey to truly embrace what is to come. The healthcare systems of different countries are all unique, but in one way are all the same—they are monolithic in behavior and slow to change. It is often said that revolution cannot come from within old large organizational structures. Revolution comes from the boundaries of the old hegemony and the wild borderlands. So maybe you need to read these chapters not as stories from the old healthcare empire, but as reports from the wild border country of patient-led change.

Australian Institute of Health Innovation   Enrico Coiera
Macquarie University
Sydney, NSW, Australia
enrico.coiera@mq.edu.au

Preface

Overview

The world of health informatics is constantly changing given the ever-increasing variety and volume of health data, care delivery models that shift from fee-for-service to value-based care, new entrants in the ecosystem, and the shifting regulatory decision landscape. In the area of cognitive informatics, the changes have increased the importance of the role of patients in research studies for understanding work processes and activities within the context of human cognition, as well as the design and implementation of health information systems (Haldar et al. 2020; Trevor Rohm 2010). Therefore, personal health informatics, in recent years, has risen up to provide research tools and protocols to zoom into individual health-related contexts when developing engineering, computing, and service solutions that can improve clinical practice, patient engagement, and public health (Hsueh et al. 2017a; Hsueh et al. 2017b; Lai et al. 2017; Patel and Kannanmpallil 2015; Reading and Merrill 2018). This is particularly important to bridge the previous gaps in patient-provider information (Tang and Lansky 2005).

The rise of personal health informatics is also in line with the emerging utilization of real-world evidence generated from real-world data. Here, "real-world data" (RWD) refers to data generated from the actual practice and delivery of health care (e.g., electronic health records, insurance claims, disease registries), while "real-world evidence" (RWE) refers to the inferences made from RWD. In some areas such as clinical trial design, RWE has been successfully applied to bring greater efficiency to the development of clinical programs (e.g., as its external control arm as indicated by the FDA's Real-World Evidence Framework (FDA, n.d.) and received regulatory approval (Berger et al. 2016; Miksad and Abernethy 2018; Shah et al. 2019). In many other areas, the development of personal health informatics has opened up new opportunities to generate RWE through integrating data science with the science of care (Bica et al. 2020; Hsueh et al. 2018).

Through this book, we intend to compile a collection of high-quality scholarly work that seeks to provide clarity, consistency, and reproducibility, with an updated and shared view of the status quo of consumer and pervasive health informatics and its relevance to precision medicine and healthcare applications. The new term "Personal Health Informatics" is being proposed to cover a broader definition of this emerging field. In one way or another, individuals are not just consuming health; they are active participants, researchers, and designers in the healthcare ecosystem. The book will offer a snapshot of this emerging field, supported by the method-ological, practical, and ethical perspectives from researchers and practitioners. In addition to being a research reader, this book will provide pragmatic insights for practitioners in designing, implementing, and evaluating personal health informat-ics in healthcare settings. The volume will also be an excellent reader for students in all clinical disciplines as well as in biomedical and health informatics to learn from case studies in this emerging field.

This is a starting point for us to show the direction where the whole field is going. The chapters include (1) case studies including reflections on implementation les-sons learned, (2) theoretical frameworks, (3) design methodologies, and (4) evalua-tion and critical appraisal.

These chapters will be organized under four main sections: (1) the state-of-the-art novel care delivery models (using case study examples), (2) methods for trans-lating biomedical research and RWE into patient-centric precision health application, (3) methods for patient-centric design, and (4) ethics, bias, privacy, and fairness. Chapter authors have been invited based on their reputation and fit with the topic, and all chapters have been reviewed independently.

This book is intended to appeal to a wide range of audiences including academic researchers, educators, professional informaticians, healthcare providers and administrators, healthcare consumers, and policymakers. Although this book is not considered a standard textbook, it will be of great value for graduate programs in which courses in applied informatics are relevant, such as courses that focus on behavioral, cognitive, and social aspects of health information technology.

Section I: The State-of-the-Art Novel Care Delivery Models

Since its inception—then by the name Consumer Health Informatics–about 25 years ago the field of Personal Health Informatics (PHI) has achieved worldwide reach across many health problems and clinical disciplines. The book presents ser-vices from approximately 20 countries and several methodological chapters with international reach. The authors provide us with a different lens to observe different target populations, learn about various methods of deployment, and how they fit with or transgress from present models of healthcare delivery.

Kuziemsky et al. in their Chap. 1, "E-enabled Patient-Provider Communication in Context," present examples of enhanced patient-provider communication from Denmark, Fiji, Columbia, and Canada. In Denmark, the emphasis is on overcom-ing the intermittent and fragmented practice of care for patients with Chronic Obstructive Pulmonary Disease. In the EHealth Care Model (ECM) patients receive basic measurement and problem staging equipment for their home environment that connects them continuously, 24/7, to the same care team. Adaptations of the treatment regime can be initiated through the distance before emerging problems exacerbate. The project from Fiji addresses mental health problems for which specialists are extremely rare and care is mostly provided through nurses. To lift the level and guideline adherence of treatments, an educational effort was launched which compared the presentation of guideline knowledge through different media. A smartphone-based study arm showed the best results. In Columbia, similar to many low and middle-income countries, perinatal mortality is still high. In addition, the involvement of stakeholders hinders timely intervention during pregnancy. The presented project aims to technically support interventions suggested to the gynecologist through AI-driven clinical decision support. The respective system needs to technically integrate with clinical workflows and is supposed to communicate with expecting mothers through their smartphones. The Canadian example studies collaboration through the macro, meso, and micro levels. It emphasizes the dynamic nature of collaboration which showed intensely in the transition of care with the onset of the COVID pandemic. New tools were spontaneously adopted by individual providers and patients, posing organizational and data security challenges at the meso level. The challenges thus call for the reform at the national level on data standards, new legislation, and billing codes, to name just a few.

In Chap. 2, "Direct Primary Care: A New Model for Patient-Centered Care," Snowdon et al. lay out one specific novel model of Direct Primary Care (DPC). The DPC model aims to improve the quality of primary care through better patient-provider relations and communication. The payment model of DPC is based on a per capita fee per time period to a provider or its provider organization. It can be either paid by the patients or by their employers. Compared to the fee-for-service payment model, the value-based model can help incentivize providers to spend more quality time with the patient and promote prevention. For patients, it also removes financial and organizational barriers to healthcare access, which in turn leads to rational and sustainable utilization of primary care services. This chapter also helps the readers learn to distinguish the implementation needed at different scales, and how the implementation of DPC improves utilization of designated preventive measures and decreases preventable emergency room visits.

In Chap. 3, "Smart Homes for Personal Health and Safety," Demiris et al. address how to make the home environment safer through controls, sensors, and algorithms that can interpret the clinical needs behind sensor signals. Smart home applications that can benefit from surveillance include physiological and functional indicators of health and their trajectory over time, protection against physical and intrusion hazards, and cognitive and social functioning. The authors illustrate the smart home-based delivery of care through the example of Mild Cognitive Impairment (MCI) and fall management in the Sense4Safety project. Fall risks increase slowly and are often unnoticeable, entailing tremendous cost and morbidity. Sense4Safety uses personalized configurations that include nursing assessment of the home situation and resident education and alerts to a trusted party to mitigate the risk. The authors also address an ethical framework to analyze the impact on privacy, the burden imposed on caregivers, and the validity of informed consent of cognitively impaired citizens.

In Chap. 4, "Health App by Prescription: The German Nation-Wide Model," Pobiruchin and Strotbaum introduce how Germany enables the development of digital health services via German DiGA (Digitale GesundheitsAnwendung— Digital Health Application) to enable self-care for a variety of medical problems. Medical problems presently addressed include migraine, multiple sclerosis, tinnitus, mental disorders (e.g., panic disorder), or coxarthrosis. Patients can access DiGA "by prescription," meaning that its access is as easy as getting a medication prescribed by a physician and would be covered by the Social Health Insurance (SHI) plan. Germany's 140 years old insurance system, first established by ex-chancellor Otto von Bismarck, is robust enough to incorporate such new services for insured patients and their kins, which means more than 90% of the German population. The efficacy of the DiGA assessments resembles those used in phase 3 clinical trials. If the services can be certified as a low-risk medical product, it can receive preliminary temporal approval including financial coverage. This allows developers to launch at an early stage and collect evidence of its therapeutical effectiveness from routine use. While this book is being produced, the number of DiGAs in the approval process counts in the hundreds.

In Chap. 5, "Patient Portal for Critical Response During Pandemic: A Case Study of COVID-19 in Taiwan," Lee et al. depict Taiwan's response to the pandemic and the role of ICT. COVID-19 poses a unique challenge where appropriate actions had to be taken in the interest of personal and population health at times when nobody really knew what "appropriate" meant. Taiwan with its regular flights to and from Wuhan PRC was hit by this challenge early. In this chapter, the authors first introduce what was concretely done in Taiwan and how ICT had to evolve to support data collection and action. The design goals include integration and interoperability of data, as well as barrier-free access for all with the need to know. Its data collection and exchange system include a web interface with full functionality for government authorities and healthcare professionals and another mobile interface with reduced e functionality for citizens. Different types of data are being governed with different levels of security/ privacy measures. For example, sensor data such as body temperature, GPS location, and behavioral instructions were at citizens' fingertips; symptoms and whereabouts were at the disposal of government authorities for contact tracing. The authors also discuss the balance between individual privacy and the public good, as well as the challenges incurred by culture, education, and other non-technical issues.

In Chap. 6, Collins Rossetti and Tiase discuss "The Integration of Patient-Generated Health Data to EHRs." They start by introducing how Patient-Generated Health Data (PGHD) are captured and shared among lay citizens and proceed to discuss the impact on healthcare professionals. They identify not only challenges but also facilitators that would enable the use of PGHD in clinical settings. They introduce the concept of Personal Health Record (PHR) to refer to privately held and shared health data. By contrast, patient portals are held by providers. The portals are designed to give patients access to their electronic records and allow the scheduling of appointments. Some portals also provide patients access points to upload their health history, answers to surveys and questionnaires, or sensor data and observations. Presently, a large number of health apps come with a wide range of user and technical interface idiosyncrasies. Therefore, it has not been easy for the users to use these apps productively, and the benefits are not clear. However, the continuous growth and ubiquity of apps have led to unprecedented innovation in the space. The participation from the providers and health systems, for example, the Remote Patient Monitoring (RPM) programs, has further fueled the field with organization resources for standardization. All of the abovementioned trends are expected to help collect data between visits so as to provide the physicians a longitudinal view of their patients' whole-person health.

Section II: Methods for Translating Biomedical Research and Real-World Evidence into Patient-Centric Precision Health Application

Active citizens create myriads of data meant to monitor their own health status and to share experiences and advice with peers. Behaviors of mutual support in self-care health groups as well as patterns that AI and ML methods may discover make crowd intelligence an invaluable source for medical and quality-of-life research and personalized guidance. In this section, examples of added value derived from citizen-created data will be presented. This ranges from robust signal analysis through geospatial tracing to natural language processing, from standards to health policies, privacy, and regulatory concerns, and many more. It also addresses questions of ownership of data and insights and liabilities incurred from being the holder of such insights. Last but not least, this section lays the theoretical foundation and framework for handling the questions of ownership and incurred liabilities discussed in section IV.

First in Chap. 7, "Role of Digital Healthcare Approaches in the Analysis of Personalized (N-of-1) Trials," Chandereng et al. elaborate on the role of health applications and other digital healthcare approaches in the design and analysis of an exemplar series of personalized trials in a chronic lower back pain study (CLBP). They share with readers how a series of personalized (N-of-1) trials were conducted and elaborate on the computing platform built to analyze the time-series trial data. They also emphasize the importance of personalized trials by displaying the heterogeneity of the treatment effect in the study participants. Readers could learn how to use health apps to analyze personalized trials, as well as how to compute and interpret patient-by-patient analysis from this study.

In Chap. 8, "Early Detection of Mental Decline via Mobile and Home Sensors," Jimison et al. discuss several important topics underlying approaches to cognitive assessments, focusing on self-motivating computer games. Fundamental concepts of measurements and their application to cognitive functionality are addressed.

Equipped with the extended notions of measurement and computational modeling, they describe ways that use streams of data from unobtrusive sensors and associated algorithms for inferring patient cognitive function. Readers can expect to compare a wide array of data acquisition techniques including sensors available for monitoring health and cognitive states and understand how computer games and interactions with technology can be used to assess cognitive functions.

Chapter 9 "The Role of Patient-Generated Data in Personalized Oncology Care and Research: Opportunities and Challenges for Real-World Implementation" by Fernandez-Luque et al. provides an overview of current practices on data collection for routine cancer care. It identifies current regulatory issues for a real-world implementation of using patient-generated data in personalized cancer care and ongoing actions to overcome them. The authors discuss in depth the different types of questions posed by policymakers and regulatory bodies for the real-world deployment and implementation of strategies to foster a patient-generated data grounding for care delivery. Readers will learn to identify the exogenous determinants of health-related quality of life (HRQoL) in cancer survivorship and understand how data science can be leveraged to accelerate real-world evidence (RWE) discovery.

Chapter 10 "Semantic Technologies for Clinically Relevant Personal Health Applications" by Chen et al. describes the motivation for, and illustrative applications of, semantic technologies for enabling clinically relevant personal health applications. Using nutrition behavior as a focus, the authors present two use cases that demonstrate how semantic web technologies, machine learning, and data mining methods can be used in combination to provide personalized insights to support behaviors that are consistent with nutritional guidelines. Readers will be able to provide a conceptual description of what a knowledge graph is, identify standards for semantic modeling, and learn the advantages of using semantic technologies in combination with machine learning for building personal health applications.

Chapter 11 "Privacy Predictive Models for Homecare Patient Sensing" by Sun et al. provides an overview of homecare sensing and assisted living technologies and discusses people's privacy attitudes towards healthcare monitoring and video surveillance systems. The authors share their findings from the preliminary study, which includes focus group discussions and questionnaires to collect people's privacy attitudes and test results from different methods to predict patients' privacy preferences. Readers will learn more about legal and ethical considerations of using camera monitoring for homecare patient sensing along with methodologies to predict privacy preferences.

Chapter 12 "Detecting Personal Health Mentions from Social Media Using Supervised Machine Learning" by Yin et al. investigates how people disclose their own or others' health status over a broad range of health issues on Twitter by applying both traditional and deep learning-based machine learning models to detect such online personal health status mentions. The authors show that health status mentions can be effectively detected from Twitter using machine learning, especially deep learning algorithms. Their findings set the stage for readers with similar interests to build a scalable system to efficiently extract such health mentions from online environments to make them useful in practice.

Chapter 13 "Common Data Models (CDMs): The Basic Building Blocks for Fostering Public Health Surveillance and Population Health Research Using Distributed Data Networks (DDNs)" by Podila provides a detailed and important introduction to CDMs and offers step-by-step guidance on the process by which potential participating sites or members of a DDN could build CDMs. It highlights the governance policies and their significance in fostering the public and population health efforts and shares specific examples from some most popular Distributed Health Data Networks (DHDNs). This easy read will enable the readers to define CDMs, outline key principles related to CDMs, and describe the levels of data models for their own clinical scenario.

Section III: Methods for Patient-Centric Design

Patients are recognized as both the least utilized and the most vulnerable resource in health care. To fully unleash the opportunities for patients to contribute as citizen scientists, health systems need to enable barrier-free access and design software that can directly meet the patients' needs.

To achieve this, the health system designers need to account for education, locality, ethnicity, values, beliefs, and many other considerations that would affect health equity. In addition, we would need support from a diverse, open, integrated healthcare ecosystem around patient-centered design. Many technological, organizational, and collaboration issues have emerged from the discussion before. Therefore, in this section, we address the emerging issues by first providing an overview of what is happening in the subfield and then showcasing studies that could provide exciting angles into how a patient-centered ecosystem is currently working in health care.

One significant barrier in this section is the lack of participatory design methods that would work well with patients in the loop directly in the health system and workflow redesign. In Chap. 14, "Person-Centered Design Methods for Citizen Science," Austin and Wang present an overview of citizen science and specific methodologies used in the person-centered design. Person-centered design is essential to support the ecosystem partners to know that they have accounted for the patient's needs. In addition, this co-design principle is essential for treating patients as a whole person and as an equal partner within the design team. This chapter introduces citizen science resources, design principles, design thinking methods, and the different phases while applying the design thinking method in actual practice. As a bonus point, this chapter also provides a checklist and a list of questions for practitioners applying the co-design principles to practice.

Another barrier that impedes the progress of patient-centered design and the growth of a patient-centered ecosystem is the lack of common terminologies for the ease of communication and integration. In Chap. 15, "Leveraging Library and Information Science to Discover Consumer Health Informatics Research," Martin et al. provide an overview of literature covering the subfield of consumer health informatics (CHI) in recent years' publications and a database-agnostic understanding of the structures and factors relevant to the retrieval of CHI literature. The authors start by designing a literature search and consider different ways to combine concepts and choose relevant databases to execute the search. The authors then discuss the difference between keywords and subject heading search queries and recommend strategies to retrieve CHI literature. This chapter presents a window of opportunity to navigate the ever-changing field of CHI.

In Chap. 16, "The Ecosystem of Patient-Centered Research and Information System Design," Hsueh provides an overview of the patient-centered healthcare ecosystem. This chapter starts by identifying the stakeholders and their roles and challenges in the ecosystem. The author then summarizes the common challenges in tackling emerging issues. One such important issue is how to regulate AI/ML algorithms to maintain fairness and equity in healthcare systems while curating real-world evidence from heterogeneous sources of patient-generated health data.

In Chap. 17, "Personalizing Research: Involving, Inviting, and Engaging Patient Researchers," Lewis provides examples of patient-involved research studies and offers tools to support traditional researchers who want to support patient-led research efforts and improve their ability to engage patient stakeholders in their research successfully. This chapter provides practitioners tips on how to invite and recruit patients in research as partners and the essential factors to know to prepare for productive collaboration. This chapter also summarizes the benefits and opportunities of engaging patients in traditional research. Finally, it provides practical suggestions for patient participation in research, whether or not there is an established patient and public involvement (PPI) program. The tips included in this chapter would be necessary for any researchers thinking about developing a productive working relationship and culture between researchers and the patients involved in research.

Finally, Chaps. 18 and 19 provide example case studies on different ways to tackle specific challenges facing the development of patient-centered design in the ecosystem.

In Chap. 18, "User-Centered Development and Evaluation of Patient-Facing Visualizations of Health Information," Turchioe and Creber incorporate the direct input from patient researchers to design patient-facing visualizations to support self-monitoring of symptoms for older adults with heart failure. The authors illustrate the best practice of user-centered design and depict the research framework, the key considerations during the requirement gathering phase, and the options of evaluation study designs. They also present their case study on designing a mobile app to support elderly routine symptom checking and summarize the activities related to defining the relevance, rigor, and design cycles.

In Chap. 19, "Social Determinants of Health During the COVID-19 Pandemic in the US: Precision Through Context," Camacho-Rivera et al. present the case study of the National COVID Cohort Collaborative (N3C), specifically around how the COVID-19 pandemic brought Social Health Determinants of Health (SDoH) to the forefront of informatics. In addition, the authors also provide a summary of crucial SDoH concepts and frameworks, with a focus on the social-ecological model and their impacts on a variety of infectious and chronic diseases. The summary would serve as a practical guide for healthcare professionals interested in assessing the impacts of SDOH on their practice. The case study would support researchers in translating research into practice.

In summary, fast technological progress in the methods of patient-centered design across all the discussions in this subsection calls for a societal debate and decision-making process on a multitude of challenges: how emerging or foreseeable results transform privacy; how to interpret novel patient-generated health data modalities in light of clinical data and vice versa; how the sheer mass and partially abstract mathematical properties of the achieved insights can be interpreted to a broad public and can consequently facilitate the development of patient-centered services; and how to evaluate the remaining risks and uncertainties against new benefits. This section summarizes the status quo of the challenges and emerging best practices that address these issues. The opportunities and barriers identified can serve as action items individuals can bring to their organizations when facing challenges to add value from the primary and secondary use of patient-generated health data and patient-centered design.

Section IV: Ethics, Bias, Privacy, and Fairness

The goal of this section is to identify and summarize ethical, legal, privacy, and social issues related to information technology in personal health.

In Wetter's Chap. 20, "Personal Health Informatics Services and the Different Types of Value They Create," he presents a variety of perspectives on how Personal Health Informatics (PersHI) services take effect in society. He distinguishes clinical effectiveness, which is typically shown through controlled experiments such as Randomized Controlled Trials (RCTs), from discoveries that emerge from data volunteered by citizens and are later aggregated to show some association or effect. He further distinguishes individual changes of mindset from group power. Individually, new knowledge may be learned, and propensity for healthy behavior may evolve. It is important to gain group power with the help of online interest groups, wherein public attention and resources can be solicited to understand how group members attenuate a medical problem. There exist both positive and negative examples to demonstrate the subtlety of the field: RCTs with clearly significant effects and others that were terminated prematurely due to the lack of participation and retention; knowledge gained with no behavioral consequences and behavior change without notable knowledge increase; and lobby groups with true benefits for their clientele but others that lead to the waste of resources due to the low efficacy of the therapy advocated.

Chapter 21 by Kluge on "Electronic Health Records: Ethical Considerations Touching Health Informatics Professionals" explores the nature of medical data, mainly Electronic Health Records (EHRs) and what roles and consequential duties individuals and institutions that handle EHRs have. The core proposition is that medical data function as patient analogs. Whenever used in clinical, research, or other situations they represent the patient and therefore deserve the same proactive diligence to foster legitimate and prevent illegitimate use. In other words: Health Information Professionals (HIPs) act as fiduciaries of patient data. While fiducial conduct is technically rooted in informatics and should be governed by applicable law several reasons require that, to fulfill their fiduciary duties, HIPs have to think and behave ahead of technology and legislation. The reasons include personalized medicine and its genetic roots, the pecuniary value of the data, the mobility of citizens across borders of national legislation, and cloud storage of data outside the country of residence.

International legislation is one of the topics in deMuro's and Norwood's Chap. 22 on "Healthcare Organizations as Health Data Fiduciaries: An International Analysis." Their analysis culminates in a comparison of 15 countries and regions worldwide. In this chapter, the authors outlined and contrasted the risk by threats of intrusions. These risks originate from legislation that should protect health data against include different forms of monetization, outsourcing of physical storage, new informatics technologies such as Artificial Intelligence and Big Data Analysis, and new forms of care delivery such as Telehealth. The authors also illustrate concrete legal assets to be protected. These threats are also enhanced by cybercrime that is incentivized by the monetary value of the data and the potential exposure of providers to ransomware. The obligation to protect the assets and to fend off the threats is rooted through a fiduciary relation of individual health professional and healthcare providers towards the patients and their data. This leads to the challenges to establish structures and procedures to safely share data and maintain data interoperability among providers.

Chapter 23 "Ethical, Legal, and Social Issues Pertaining to Virtual and Digital Representations of Patients" by Kaplan investigates into the fact that medical treatment increasingly means working with patient data instead of working with the person and the body. This depersonalization as an outgrowth of "data-ization" has several consequences that need to be controlled. For one, the data only imperfectly map the patient and subtle details and distinctions between patients blur. Decisions are made without full appreciation of the context and algorithmic decision support lacks transparency. The ambiguity of data and the over-abstraction of data for population-related assertions make it hard to predict what holds for the individual. The secondary and tertiary use through the network among stakeholders also raise concerns about privacy and about how informed an "informed consent" actually is. All of these concerns undermine trust on the part of the patients and result in biased assumptions in services. It is therefore essential to design an Ethical, Legal, and Social Issues (ELSI) bioethics framework to keep the negative consequences of the inevitable development at bay and to allow the benefits of personalized medicine to materialize.

References

1. Berger ML, Curtis MD, Smith G, Harnett J, Abernethy AP. Opportunities and challenges in leveraging electronic health record data in oncology. Future Oncol. 2016;12(10):1261–74. https://doi.org/10.2217/fon-2015-0043

2. Bica I, Alaa AM, Lambert C, van der Schaar M. From real-world patient data to individualized treatment effects using machine learning: current and future methods to address underlying challenges. Clin Pharmacol Ther. 2020. https://doi.org/10.1002/cpt.1907

3. FDA. Use of real-world evidence to support regulatory decision-making for medical devices. FDA. n.d. Retrieved September 5, 2020, from https://www.fda.gov/regulatory-information/search-fda-guidance-documents/use-real-world-evidence-support-regulatory-decision-making-medical-devices

4. Haldar S, Mishra SR, Pollack AH, Pratt W. Informatics opportunities to involve patients in hospital safety: a conceptual model. JAMIA. 2020;27(2):202–11. https://doi.org/10.1093/jamia/ocz167

5. Hsueh P-YS, Cheung Y-K, Dey S, Kim KK, Martin-Sanchez FJ, Petersen SK, Wetter T. Added value from secondary use of person generated health data in consumer health informatics. IMIA Yearbook. 2017a; 26(1). https://doi.org/10.15265/IY-2017-009

6. Hsueh P-YS, Dey S, Das S, Wetter T. Making sense of patient-generated health data for interpretable patient-centered care: the transition from "More" to "Better." In: Studies in health technology and informatics. vol 245. 2017b. https://doi.org/10.3233/978-1-61499-830-3-113

7. Hsueh P-YS, Das S, Maduri C, Kelly K. Learning to personalize from practice: a real world evidence approach of care plan personalization based on differential patient behavioral responses in care management records. AMIA ... Annual Symposium Proceedings. AMIA Symposium. 2018. p. 592–601. Retrieved from http://www.ncbi.nlm.nih.gov/pubmed/30815100

8. Lai AM, Hsueh P-YS, Choi YK, Austin RR. Present and future trends in consumer health informatics and patient-generated health data. Yearbook Med Inform. 2017. 26(01):152–9. https://doi.org/10.15265/IY-2017-016

9. Miksad RA, Abernethy AP. Harnessing the power of real-world evidence (RWE): a checklist to ensure regulatory-grade data quality. Clin Pharmacol Ther. 2018. 103(2):202–5. https://doi.org/10.1002/cpt.946

10. Patel VL, Kannampallil TG. Cognitive informatics in biomedicine and healthcare. J Biomed Inform. 2015;53:3–14. https://doi.org/10.1016/j.jbi.2014.12.007

11. Reading MJ, Merrill JA. Converging and diverging needs between patients and providers who are collecting and using patient-generated health data: an integrative review. J Am Med Inform Assoc. 2018; 25(6):759–771. https://doi.org/10.1093/jamia/ocy006

12. Shah P, Kendall F, Khozin S, Goosen R, Hu J, Laramie J et al. Artificial intelligence and machine learning in clinical development: a translational perspective. NPJ Digit Med. 2019;2(1):1–5. https://doi.org/10.1038/s41746-019-0148-3

13. Tang PC, Lansky D. The missing link: bridging the patient-provider health information gap. Health Aff. 2005;24(5):1290–1295. https://doi.org/10.1377/hlthaff.24.5.1290

14. Trevor Rohm BW. Personal health informatics: the evolving paradigm of patient self care. In: Communications of the IIMA. vol. 10. 2010. Retrieved from http://scholarworks.lib.csusb.edu/ciimaAvailableat:http://scholarworks.lib.csusb.edu/ciima/vol10/iss1/4
15. Wang Y. The theoretical framework of cognitive informatics. Int J Cogn Inform Nat Intell. 2007;1(1):1–27. https://doi.org/10.4018/jcini.2007010101

New York, NY   Pei-Yun Sabrina Hsueh
Heidelberg, Germany   Thomas Wetter
New Haven, CT   Xinxin Zhu

Acknowledgment

We thank the following reviewers for their invaluable contributions:
Andrew Nguyen
Anna Ostropolets
Anthony Solomonides
Arash Shaban-Nejad
Audie Atienza
Carlo Botrugno
Carolyn Petersen
Christie L. Martin
Christina Eldredge
Daniella Meeker
Erin MacLean
Georgios Raptis
John Sharp
Jorge Cancela
Josette Jones
Kiron Nair
Liz Salmi
May Wang
Marisa L. Conte
Matt Volansky
Najeeb Al-Shorbaji, Jordan
Pradeep S. B. Podila
Sara Riggare
Stephen Keating
Tamara Winden
Thomas Agresta
Tony Solomonides
Vickie Nguyen

Contents

About the Editors and Contributors

About the Editors

Pei-Yun Sabrina Hsueh, PhD is an elected Fellow of the American Medical Informatics Association (FAMIA), the co-Chair of AMIA AI Showcase 2023, the Vice Chair of AMIA SPC 2022, and the Past-Chair of the Consumer Health Informatics Work Group at AMIA. She is also currently serving on the Practitioner Board of ACM. She is a global health AI leader and innovator, specializing in translating real-world problems into data science formulations and developing AI/ML solutions to decode individual biology and behavior for precision healthcare delivery applications. She has a decade of experience leading cross-functional teams to productize and evaluate health AI applications in practice. Previously at IBM Research, she co-chaired the Health Informatics Professional Community and was elected as an IBM Academy of Technology Member. Dr. Hsueh has been a pioneer in Health AI, focusing on real-world evidence strategy and the development of platforms to deliver clinical studies and actionable insights at the point of care. Her achievements have won her a series of awards, including the AMIA Distinguished Paper Award, invention, research achievement, manager choice awards, Eminence and Excellence Award, and the Google Anita Borg Scholar Award. In addition, she authored 20+ patents and 60+ technical articles in computational linguistics and health informatics. Her expertise in the emerging areas and industry solutions makes her a sought-after speaker and consultant, a thought leader in real-world evidence, and chairs of applied data science events at major conferences such as AMIA, MEDINFO, MIE, and KDD. She is also an editor of Machine Learning for Medicine and Healthcare (Springer Nature), a guest editor of special issues in Sensors Journal, Public Health, Journal of American Medical Informatics Association [JAMIA OPEN], and the Frontier of Public Health.

Thomas Wetter is a Medical Informatics scholar with 12 years of experience in industry research and 30 years of experience in academic research and teaching in Biomedicine. He is a graduate and PhD in Mathematics from Aachen Technical

University; he worked most of his career on applying formal methods to biomedical problems. After 8 years of physiological research in Aachen, he joined the IBM Heidelberg Scientific Center. Here he researched and published on Human Computer Interface design, Artificial Intelligence, Natural Language Processing, Voice Recognition, and Software Quality. In 1997, he was appointed a full professor for Medical Informatics at Heidelberg University. Besides teaching in the curricula Medical Informatics and Medicine, his research interests were in clinical applications of Voice Recognition and Artificial Intelligence and later in Consumer Health Informatics. In the years till 2018, his assignments included the management of a CME academy, the Heidelberg part of an international student exchange program (IPHIE), associate editor of the International Journal of Medical Informatics, and deputy chair and later chair of the IMIA WG Consumer Health Informatics.

Besides various articles in scientific journals, he is the editor of conference proceedings in artificial intelligence and author of the Springer 2016 textbook "Consumer Health Informatics. New Services, Roles, and Responsibilities." During his active time, Dr. Wetter spent sabbaticals at the University of Utah and the University of Washington. After his retirement, he was engaged by Ben-Gurion-University of the Negev in Be'er Sheva, Israel, to help develop a curriculum in Medical Informatics.

Xinxin Zhu, MD, PhD is an elected Fellow of the American Medical Informatics Association (FAMIA) and Fellow of the International Academy of Health Sciences and Informatics (FIAHSI). She is currently the Executive Director for the Center for Biomedical Data Science at Yale University. Dr. Zhu is a clinician and healthcare informatics professional with more than a decade of experience in health management, health informatics, research, and advisory. In addition to her medical training and practice in anesthesiology, she also received her MS in Computer Science from Rensselaer Polytechnic Institute and PhD in Biomedical Informatics from Columbia University under the National Library of Medicine fellowship. Prior to joining the Yale faculty, Dr. Zhu served as an External Advisory Board member to the Center for Advanced Technology at Columbia University, physician scientist lead of pervasive health at the Center for Computational Health at IBM Watson Research, Chief Medical Information Officer at Kforce Government Solutions, associate medical director at Pfizer, clinical project manager at Philips, and healthcare subject matter expert at the U.S. Department of Veterans Affairs. She is the recipient of many excellence awards and author of dozens of scientific publications and 13 issued patents. She served as the Consumer Health Area Editor for the Health Systems Journal and co-editor of the book *Digital Health: Mobile and Wearable Devices for Participatory Health Applications*. Dr. Zhu has served several leadership roles at the American Medical Informatics Association, including Vice-President of Membership for the Consumer and Pervasive Health Informatics Working Group, Co-Chair of the Global Health Informatics Working Group, as well as Scientific Award Program and Women Leadership Committee members. She is also the Vice Chair for the International Medical Informatics Association's Organizational and Social Issues in Healthcare Working Group.

About the Contributors

Kristine M. Alpi is Associate Dean of Libraries & Information Sciences at Icahn School of Medicine at Mount Sinai in New York. She was previously University Librarian at Oregon Health and Science University (OHSU) and an Associate Professor in the OHSU Department of Medical Informatics and Clinical Epidemiology. Alpi holds a Masters in Library Science from Indiana University, a Master of Public Health from Hunter College, City University of New York, and a PhD in Educational Research and Policy Analysis from North Carolina State University (NCSU). Her expertise includes information retrieval, interprofessional education, data and health and technology literacy, consumer health, public health and veterinary informatics, and research methods in adult learning, informatics, and librarianship. Drawing on her prior experience at the New York City Department of Health and Mental Hygiene, Weill Cornell Medical Library, and as Adjunct Faculty in the Department of Population Health and Pathobiology at the College of Veterinary Medicine at NCSU, she facilitated team learning with students across schools and programs in the Interprofessional Education course and mentored graduate students on capstones and projects involving public health or consumer health informatics. She was the 2021–2022 President of the Medical Library Association and chairs the Education Working Group of the American Medical Informatics Association.

Robin R. Austin, PhD, DNP, RN-BC, FAMIA, FNAP is an Assistant Professor at the University of Minnesota, School of Nursing and Graduate Faculty in the Earl E. Bakken Center for Spirituality and Healing. Dr. Austin has over 20 years clinical healthcare experience and has translated this experience to focus on patient-centered research. Dr. Austin integrates her clinical background with informatics and data science methods to represent the patients' perspective across the healthcare continuum. Through her research, she seeks to empower individuals through the use of technology and include their voice in person-centered care.

Marion Jokl Ball is Professor Emerita at Johns Hopkins University in the School of Nursing and affiliate Professor in Health Sciences Informatics in the School of Medicine. She is a member of the National Academy of Medicine (NAM), served on the Board of Health on the Net (HON) in Geneva, Switzerland, Board of Regents, at the National Library of Medicine (NLM), HIMSS, and IMIA, is an elected member of the IBM Industry Academy, author/editor of over 25 books and 300 papers. Dr. Ball known nationally and internationally for her work on enabling technologies as they effect healthcare initiatives.

Sasha E. Ballen is the Chief Technology Officer for R-Health, Inc., an organization that is committed to delivering superior Primary Care. She graduated from Bowdoin College and completed a master's degree in Health Informatics at Drexel

University. Ms. Ballen is passionate about using data and technology to support clinical innovation.

Mark Butler, PhD is an investigator in the Institute of Health System Science at the Feinstein Institutes for Medical Research of Northwell Health. He is a clinical psychologist and quantitative researcher with experience studying the psychological and behavioral correlates of cardiovascular health. Previously, Dr. Butler worked as a research scientist in the Center for Healthful Behavior Change in the NYU School of Medicine. His work included community-level behavioral health interventions and analyses of large population datasets. Dr. Butler also has extensive experience with data analysis, data management, and statistics.

Marlene Camacho-Rivera, ScD, MPH, MS is an Assistant Professor of Community Health Sciences at SUNY Downstate School of Public Health. A social epidemiologist by training, Dr. Camacho-Rivera's research focuses on three main themes: (1) social and structural determinants of chronic disease disparities among urban racial and ethnic minority communities; (2) exploring patterns and determinants of within-group heterogeneity in chronic disease outcomes among Latinos; (3) design, implementation, and evaluation of multilevel and community-engaged interventions to improve chronic disease self-management among urban minority communities, with a focus on mHealth and new technologies.

Sergio Cervera-Torres got his PhD in Psychology at the Leibniz-Institut für Wissensmedien-Eberhard University of Tübingen, in Germany. He has a solid background in motivation and emotion processes. He has remarkable research publications within the clinical, health, and cognitive psychology fields. His research interests focus on psychological interventions through the use of the so-called information and communication technologies (ICTs), particularly by means of mobile devices (mHealth) and virtual/augmented reality. He is also part-time lecturer of Perception and Emotion at the Open University of Catalonia (UOC).

Thevaa Chandereng, PhD is a post-doctoral research scientist in the Dept. of Biostatistics at Columbia University. His research interests and professional activities focus on designing adaptive clinical trials and leveraging digital health for precision medicine.

Po-Lun Chang a tenure professor and Chief of the Health Informatics Competency, Leadership and Innovation Center of Excellence in the National YMCT University in Taiwan. He has successfully promoted the development of nursing informatics in both Taiwan and Mainland China since 2003. His team, led by Dr Jessie Ming Chuan Kuo, won the first Pi2 Provider Innovation in Informatics Award sponsored by the AMIA in 2014. He was the Chair of the local host of NI2014 and will lead to organize the Medinfo2025 in Taiwan. He is one of the founding fellows of International Academy of Health Sciences Informatics.

Ching-Hua Chen leads an interdisciplinary team of psychologists, data scientists, and medical informatics researchers, whose goal is to implement innovative computational approaches for supporting increased patient engagement. She has a PhD in Operations Research from Penn State University and BS in Nursing from the University of Alabama, Birmingham.

Ying Kuen Cheung, PhD is Professor of Biostatistics and Vice Dean for Faculty in the Mailman School of Public Health at Columbia University. His research interests and professional activities focus on advancing precision medicine and digital health using data science and biostatistical methods. He is a recipient of the IBM Faculty Award on Big Data and Analytics. He is a Fellow of the American Statistical Association and a Fellow of the New York Academy of Medicine.

Yi-Ru Chiu is currently a PhD student at the Institute of Biomedical Informatics, National Yang Ming Chiao Tung University, Taiwan. His major is medical informatics. He has developed dementia assessment and care system, chronic disease risk assessment system, and home care case management system. And in January 2020, he assisted Dr. Polun Chang to establish an epidemic monitoring mobile health platform for epidemic prevention management in communities, enterprises, and campuses.

Ruth Masterson Creber is an Associate Professor in the Department of Population Health Sciences at Weill Cornell Medicine in New York City. As a principal investigator of multiple NIH and PCORI-funded studies, her program of research focuses on improving quality of life for patients with cardiac conditions and pioneering innovative interventions for the delivery of health care. Dr. Masterson Creber earned a PhD from the University of Pennsylvania, MSc in Epidemiology from the London School of Hygiene and Tropical Medicine, and a BA and BSN from the University of Pennsylvania. She also completed her post-doc at Columbia University School of Nursing.

Stefani D'Angelo, CCRC, CHES® is a clinical research manager with the Institute of Health System Science at the Feinstein Institutes for Medical Research at Northwell Health. Her role centers on the implementation of virtual and N-of-1 research protocols that leverage mobile technology and wearable devices. She has a BS in Health Promotion and is currently a working towards an MS in Health.

Karina W. Davidson is Senior Vice-President of research, dean of academic affairs, and Institute Director at the Feinstein Institutes for Medical Research at Northwell Health. She is the Endowed Donald and Barbara Zucker Professor in Health Outcomes in the Department of Medicine at the Zucker School of Medicine at Hofstra University/Northwell Health. Her research focuses on innovations in personalized trials and healthcare systems to manage chronic disease and patient symptoms that incorporate patient preferences and values. She currently serves as Chair of the U.S. Preventive Services Task Force. She has a PhD in Clinical Health Psychology and an MA.c in Industrial/Organizational Psychology.

George Demiris, PhD, FACMI is a Professor at the University of Pennsylvania. He is exploring innovative ways to utilize technology and support patients and their families in various settings including home and hospice care. He has conducted numerous federally funded studies and his work has been funded consistently over the years both by the National Institutes of Health (NIH) and the National Science Foundation (NSF). His expertise is also in designing and evaluating "smart home" solutions for aging, and in understanding the potential of wearable devices, robotics, or digitally augmented residential settings to facilitate passive monitoring and support independence and quality of life for community dwelling older adults. He has examined the challenges of privacy and obtrusiveness in the context of technology use, and he has provided a comprehensive examination of technical, ethical, and practical challenges associated with the use of technology to support aging.

Paul R. DeMuro is the Data Science/Data Analytics Advisor to Protoqual Learning Systems, LLC, of Reno, Nevada, that delivers targeted learning to physician practices based on real-time patient feedback to elevate the patient experience and value of care, working on evidence-based content technology solutions to improve population health. He served as "legal architect" for the joint venture transaction to lease and operate a 120,000 square-foot health and well-being facility in Miami, merging the best practices of hospitality and health care. An economist by education, Paul holds an MBA in Finance, is a licensed CPA (Maryland), with a law degree, and a PhD in Biomedical Informatics. He is a former Associate Professor at a College of Pharmacy. He is chair of the American Medical Informatics Association Conflict of Interest Committee, and a member of its Finance Committee. He is an author of over 200 publications and has delivered over 400 presentations around the world.

Juan Espinoza, MD, FAAP is an Assistant Professor of Clinical Pediatrics at Children's Hospital Los Angeles and the USC Keck School of Medicine. Dr. Espinoza's research interests include digital media and technology and their role in medicine and medical education, with a special focus on patient (user) generated health data.

Daniel Fabbri, PhD, FAMIA is an Assistant Professor of Biomedical Informatics in the School of Medicine at Vanderbilt University Medical Center. He is also an Assistant Professor of Computer Science in the School of Engineering. His research focuses on database systems and machine learning applied to electronic medical records and clinical data. He developed the Explanation-Based Auditing System, which uses data mining techniques to help hospital compliance officers monitor accesses to electronic medical records in order to identify inappropriate use.

Luis Fernandez-Luque has been involved in medical informatics research for over 15 years. He has published more than 120 scientific publications, and he has been a reviewer and editor for leading journals and conferences in the field. Dr. Fernandez-Luque has been involved in real-world digital health initiatives in Europe, Asia, Americas, and Africa. In particular, he has been studying how to use web, mobile, and wearable technologies to support patient self-management. He is currently Chief Scientific Officer at Adhera Health Inc.

José F. Florez-Arango Health Informatician with broad experience, ranging from human–computer interaction and human factors research to policymaking and service implementation. Former co-chair of the Global Health Informatics working group at the American Medical Informatics Association and former chair for the Latin American and Caribbean Chapter at the American Telemedicine Association.

Thomas A. Gagliardi is a second-year medical student at New York Medical College in Valhalla, NY. After graduating Union College in 2019 as Valedictorian, Mr. Gagliardi joined IBM Watson Health, working under the Chief Health Officer. Here, he collaborated with research teams of IBM Watson Health, IBM Research, and outside organizations to conduct meaningful research regarding the future of artificial intelligence and health informatics. Mr. Gagliardi's current research interests are in the microbiome as well as graft versus host disease following hematopoietic stem cell transplant. He is interested in a career as a medical oncologist and physician scientist.

Panagis Galiatsatos, MD, MHS is an Assistant Professor at the Johns Hopkins School of Medicine in the Division of Pulmonary and Critical Care Medicine. Dr. Galiatsatos is an expert in the diagnosis and treatment of obstructive lung disease, tobacco cessation, and in the care of critically ill patients. He is co-chair of the Johns Hopkins Health Equity Steering Committee and is the co-director and co-founder of the novel medical initiative, Medicine for the Greater Good.

Judy George is a data scientist at the Center for AI, Research, and Evaluation within Watson Health. In this role, she works with data to evaluate Watson Health offerings and provides the scientific evidence for those applications. Prior to joining IBM, Dr. George conducted data analysis and program evaluations across the public and private healthcare settings at the Department of Veterans Affairs, Department of Defense, Booz Allen, and the Cleveland Clinic Foundation. Dr. George earned her PhD in Health Services Research from Boston University and MPH from the University of Michigan.

Daniel Gruen is the Founder and Principal Consultant of Gruen Design Research LLC and a Senior Scientist at Rensselaer Polytechnic Institute. Dr. Gruen is an experienced design researcher with a proven track record driving innovation in high-stakes domains. Dr. Gruen's experience includes over 20 years as a scientist and strategic research designer at IBM, exploratory work funded by Apple and the National Science Foundation, and user experience consulting and mentoring in business and academic settings. Dr. Gruen received a PhD in Cognitive Science from the University of California at San Diego and holds over 50 US and international patents is a Cognitive Scientist and Design Researcher in RPI's HEALS (Health Empowerment by Analytics, Learning, and Semantics) group. He joined RPI after a career in IBM Research where he served in multiple scientific and leadership roles and led IBM's Cognitive Experience Invention Development Team. Dan is an inventor on over 50 US and international patents in UX, Visualization, Social Software, and related areas. He consults on Design and UX Strategy to companies in a variety of industries. Dan has a PhD in Cognitive Science from UCSD and a BA from the University of Pennsylvania

Jonathan Harris is a fourth-year PhD student studying Computer Science at Rensselaer Polytechnic Institute. His thesis work mainly focuses on mining temporal personal health data for behavioral insights and translating them into comprehensive natural language for non-expert individuals. After graduating, he hopes to continue working on research that focuses on improving the everyday lives of others.

James Hendler is the Director of the Institute for Data Exploration and Applications and the Tetherless World Professor of Computer, Web, and Cognitive Sciences at RPI. He also is acting director of the RPI-IBM Artificial Intelligence Research Collaboration and serves as a member of the Board of the UK's charitable Web Science Trust. Hendler has published over 400 books and articles on AI and in 2021 became chair of the Association for Computing Machinery's (ACM) global Technology Policy Council. Hendler is a Fellow of the AAAI, AAAS, ACM, BCS, IEEE, and the US National Academy of Public Administration.

Nancy A. Hodgson, RN, PhD, FAAN is a professor in the Department of Biobehavioral Health and Anthony Buividas Term Chair in Gerontology at the University of Pennsylvania School of Nursing. A nationally recognized nurse researcher, Dr. Hodgson's career has been focused on the development, testing, and dissemination of person-centered and family-centered interventions for persons living with dementia. This work has helped to inform care practices for persons living with dementia and their caregivers through the development of palliative care protocols that address the leading symptoms in dementia that cause distress or impair quality of life. As a clinician and educator, Dr. Hodgson seeks out innovative ways to foster academic-community partnership by linking research and practice in order to move evidence-based findings into dementia care practice. She is a Fellow in the American Academy of Nursing and the Gerontological Society of America.

Jessica Y. Islam, PhD, MPH is an Assistant Member in the Cancer Epidemiology Program at H. Lee Moffitt Cancer Center and Research Institute. Dr. Islam's research focuses on describing and intervening on cancer care disparities across the continuum, at the intersection of infections and cancer. Through her research program, Dr. Islam aims to improve cancer outcomes among vulnerable populations, including racial/ethnic minorities and people living with HIV, using multilevel approaches, epidemiological methods, and an equity-focused lens.

Holly B. Jimison is a research professor in the Khoury College of Computer Sciences and directs the Consortium on Technology for Proactive Care. Prior to joining Northeastern, she was Technology Advisor for the Office of Behavioral & Social Science Research at NIH. Her earlier work as medical informatics faculty at Oregon Health & Sciences University focused on technology for successful aging and scalable remote care. She served on the Executive Board of the Oregon Center for Aging & Technology and was past president of Oregon's Health Information Management Systems Society chapter. As a fellow of the American College of Medical Informatics, Professor Jimison has made significant and sustained contributions to the field of biomedical informatics in the areas of pattern recognition, decision support, and consumer health informatics. She continues to deepen her influence in the field through her research on technology for successful aging and scalable remote care for older adults and patients with chronic conditions. As the director of the Consortium on Technology for Proactive Care at Northeastern University, she leads a multidisciplinary, multi-institutional effort to facilitate research in the area of home monitoring of health behaviors, including helping researchers address the challenges of big data related to large amounts of complex and noisy streaming data from multiple sources used to infer clinically relevant health behaviors. Dr. Jimison is currently also a visiting professor at UC Davis working on their Healthy Aging in a Digital World Initiative.

Bonnie Kaplan, PhD, FACMI serves on the faculty of the Yale University School of Medicine at the Yale Center for Medical Informatics, Program for Biomedical Ethics, and the Center for Biomedical Data Science. She is a Yale Interdisciplinary Bioethics Center Scholar, a Faculty Affiliate Fellow of the Yale Law School's Information Society Project, and Faculty Affiliate of the Yale Solomon Center for Health Law and Policy. Dr. Kaplan researches and consults on ethical, legal, social, and organizational issues; user perspectives and experiences; and evaluation. She twice chaired the American Medical Informatics Association (AMIA) Working Groups on Ethical, Legal, and Social Issues and People and Organizational Issues and the International Medical Informatics Association Organizational and Social Issues Working Group. Dr. Kaplan graduated from Cornell University (BA) and the University of Chicago (PhD). She received the AMIA President's Award and is an elected Fellow of the American College of Medical Informatics.

George Kim is a co-editor of Health Information Management Systems, Ed 5. He is a Research Associate in Biomedical Informatics and Data Science in the Division of General Internal Medicine/Department of Medicine at the Johns Hopkins University School of Medicine in Baltimore, MD, USA.

Eike-Henner W. Kluge was the first expert witness in medical ethics recognized by Canadian courts, has acted in that capacity at various levels, and acts as an ethics consultant to various levels of government. He established and was the first director of the Canadian Medical Association Department of Ethics and Legal Affairs, and currently is a professor at the University of Victoria, Canada, specializing in biomedical ethics, privacy, and medical informatics. He was the author of the International Medical Informatics Association's *Code of Ethics* and the accompanying *Handbook of Ethics for Health Informatics Professionals*. Other publications include *The Electronic Health Records: Ethical Considerations*. In 2007, he was awarded the Abbyann Lynch Medal in Bioethics by the Royal Society of Canada and was made Fellow of the Royal Society in 2018.

Maciej Kos is a PhD candidate at Northeastern University's Khoury College of Computer Sciences and Bouvé College of Health Sciences. Before joining Khoury's Personal Health Informatics doctoral program, Kos graduated with master's degrees in Economics from Barcelona Graduate School of Economics and in Information Science from the University of Michigan.

Kos's research focuses on extending healthspan and amplifying cognition through individualized technology-enabled health interventions, computational modeling, and scientific discovery. He has also led research projects in behavioral economics and user experience.

Currently, Kos works on developing digital biomarkers of cognitive health for supporting interventions aimed at preventing or postponing the onset of neurodegeneration. In his research, Kos applies his interdisciplinary background in behavioral, computer, and health sciences to creating individualized novel health technologies, specifically targeting marginalized and underrepresented populations.

Kos's work is supported by the NIH National Institute of Aging's Transition to Aging Research training fellowship.

Craig E. Kuziemsky is Associate Vice-President, Research at MacEwan University in Edmonton, Canada. Dr. Kuziemsky's research focuses on developing innovative approaches for modeling collaborative healthcare delivery so we can better design information and communication technology (ICT) to support different contexts of collaborative healthcare delivery. His studies of collaboration have used concepts such as complexity theory to understand the nature of collaborative interactions in different healthcare settings (clinical healthcare and public health for disaster management).

Siang Hao Lee Chief of Staff of Taiwan Association for Medical Informatics and COO of KenKone Medical Co., Ltd. He was responsible for the EMR and related PACS/LIS/NIS/CIS system construction of more than 40 hospitals in Taiwan. He was elected as the second Technical Committee of IHE-China in 2014. In January 2020, he assisted Dr. Polun Chang in establishing an epidemic surveillance mHealth Platform before the first wave of the COVID-19 epidemic in both China and Taiwan.

In 2020 Q3, participated in organizing the first Taiwan Medical Information Interoperability Standards Connectathon, mainly tested HL7 FHIR® and DICOMWeb standards in local scenarios.

Dana Lewis After building her own DIY "artificial pancreas," Dana Lewis helped found the open source artificial pancreas movement (known as "OpenAPS"), making safe and effective artificial pancreas technology available (sooner) for people with diabetes around the world. She has been a Principal Investigator for multiple Robert Wood Johnson Foundation-funded grant projects to scale patient-led innovation and scientific discovery in more patient communities, as well as co-PI on numerous other research projects. She authored the book, *Automated Insulin Delivery: How artificial pancreas "closed loop" systems can aid you in living with diabetes*, to help more people understand automated insulin delivery systems.

Zhongxing Liao is full professor with term tenure in the Department of Radiation Oncology, the University of Texas MD Anderson Cancer Center. She is currently the Deputy Chair of Clinical Research and Director for Clinical Research in the Department. She has a broad background in thoracic radiation oncology, with specific expertise in prospective comparative clinical trials, predictive model using radiation dosimetric metrics and biomarkers. She has pioneered in implementing advanced radiation delivery technologies to enhance the therapeutic ratio by significantly reducing lung toxicity. She has NIH funding translational research project investigating mechanism and methods for mitigation in TRAE in heart. There are 363 peer-reviewed publications and many remarkable awards in her CV.

Ziwei Liao is a researcher in the Department of Biostatistics at Columbia University. His research interest lies in the design and analysis of clinical trials, Bayesian statistics, and applications of statistical methods in N-of-1 trials. He received his doctoral degree from the Department of Biostatistics at Columbia University.

José Luis López-Guerra PhD in Radiation Oncology (University of Barcelona). Radiation Oncologist in the Department of Radiation Oncology at the Virgen del Rocio University Hospital. Radiation Oncology Research Coordinator in the Physical and biological predictors of tumor and normal tissue response laboratory (The Sevilla Biomedicine Institute). Visiting Scientist at the MD Anderson Cancer Center, Houston, Texas (USA) in 2010–2011. He has more than 70 publications, with an accumulated impact factor of 211.802. He is reviewer and editor in 11 and 5 journals, respectively. He has participated in 33 research projects, in 7 as principal investigator. He has obtained 10 international research awards.

Hao Luo received the BS, MS, and PhD degrees from Harbin Institute of Technology, Harbin, China, in 2002, 2004, and 2008, respectively. He is currently an Associate Professor with the School of Aeronautics and Astronautics, Zhejiang

University, Hangzhou, China. His research interests include deep learning, embedded systems, information security, and signal processing.

Charisse Madlock-Brown, PhD, MLS is an Assistant Professor in Health Informatics and Information Management at the University of Tennessee Health Science Center. Dr. Madlock-Brown received her master's in Library Science and PhD in Health Informatics from the University of Iowa. She has expertise in data management, data mining, and visualization. She has a broad background in health informatics, with a current focus on obesity trends, multimorbidity, and COVID-19. Other areas of interest are network analysis and emerging topic detection in biomedicine.

Bradley Malin, PhD is the Accenture Professor of Biomedical Informatics, Biostatistics, and Computer Science at Vanderbilt University Medical Center. His research is funded through various grants from the National Science Foundation (NSF), National Institutes of Health (NIH), and Patient-Centered Outcomes Research Institute (PCORI) to construct technologies that enable artificial intelligence and machine learning applications (AI/ML) in the context of real-world organizational, political, and health information architectures. He is an elected Fellow of the National Academy of Medicine (NAM), the American College of Medical Informatics (ACMI), the International Academy of Health Sciences Informatics (IAHSI), and the American Institute for Medical and Biological Engineering (AIMBE).

Christie L. Martin is an Assistant Professor at the University of Minnesota School of Nursing and works as a medical-surgical nurse at Abbott Northwestern in Minneapolis. Martin completed a PhD in Nursing, a Master of Nursing, and a certificate in Leadership in Health Information Technology for Health Professionals from the University of Minnesota School of Nursing, and she received a Master of Public Health from the University of Minnesota School of Public Health. Martin's research interests include health equity, health promotion, and informatics, specifically consumer health informatics and mobile health technologies. Martin is the VP of Membership of the American Medical Informatics Association (AMIA) Consumer Health Informatics working group.

Deborah L. McGuinness is the Tetherless World Senior Constellation Chair and Professor of Computer, Cognitive, and Web Sciences and the founding director of the RPI Web Science Research Center. Deborah has been recognized as a Fellow of the American Association for Advancement of Science (AAAS) for contributions to the Semantic Web, knowledge representation, and reasoning environments and as the recipient of the Robert Engelmore Award from the Association for the Advancement of Artificial Intelligence (AAAI) for leadership in Semantic Web research and in bridging Artificial Intelligence and eScience, significant contributions to deployed AI applications, and extensive service to the AI community.

Marco Monti is a senior consultant and a research scientist at IBM Cognitive and Advanced Analytics Group. He is also an adjunct professor at Catholic University of Milan where he teaches Data Mining and Pattern Recognition. He previously worked as a researcher at the Max Planck Institute for Human Development of Berlin within the Adaptive Behavior and Cognition group led by Prof. Gerd Gigerenzer. Dr. Monti's interests lie in decision theory, ecological rationality, and cognitive sciences applied to explainable AI in the financial and medical domains. Marco holds a PhD in Economics from the Bocconi University of Milan, Italy.

Congning Ni, ME is a PhD student of Computer Science at Vanderbilt University. Her research focuses on machine learning, nautical language processing and their applications in health and well-being. She is currently working on learning online support for Alzheimer's caregivers, prediction of medication discontinuation using electronic health records, as well as stance analysis and prediction for public controversial events on multiple social media platforms.

Christian Nohr, MSc, PhD, FACMI, FIAHSI Professor of health informatics at the research group Techno-Anthropology and Participation at Aalborg University, Denmark; Adjunct Professor at the University of Tasmania, Australia; and the University of Victoria, BC, Canada; Research Professor at Jacobs School of Medicine and Biomedical Sciences University at Buffalo, State University of New York, Director for Danish Centre for Health Informatics.

Dr. Nøhr is Vice-President of the Danish Society for Digital Health, Chair of IMIA working group of organizational and social issues, and Associate Editor of Applied Clinical Informatics.

Henry E. Norwood is an attorney with the law office of Kaufman, Dolowich, and Voluck, practicing law primarily in the areas of healthcare compliance and corporate litigation. Mr. Norwood is a graduate of the University of Maine (BA) and of the Nova Southeastern University Shepard Broad College of Law (JD) and is licensed to practice law in the States of Florida, Maine, and Massachusetts. He and his wife live in Orlando, Florida.

Francisco J. Núñez-Benjumea currently works as innovation manager at the Hospital Universitario Virgen Macarena (Spain). He was Director of R&D in Adhera Health, Inc., member of the Research Data Alliance, and member of AENOR CTN139 on Information Technologies and Communications for Health. He has coordinated several international collaborative research initiatives in the field of Digital Health, Telecommunications Engineer, MSc in Electronics, Signal Processing and Communications, and PhD candidate in Learning Healthcare Systems at the University of Seville.

José A. Pagán, PhD is Professor and Chair of the Department of Public Health Policy and Management in the School of Global Public Health at New York University. He is also Chair of the Board of Directors of New York City Health +

Hospitals, the largest public healthcare delivery system in the United States. He is a health economist and health services researcher who has led research, implementation, and evaluation projects on the redesign of healthcare delivery and payment systems.

Yoonyoung Park is a Research Staff Member in the Center for Computational Health, IBM Research. She applies various statistical and analytic methods to observational health data to find answers for problems in health care. Her research interest lies in the areas of algorithmic fairness in artificial intelligence/machine learning (AI/ML) and social determinants of health. She is a pharmacist by training and received both a master's degree in Biostatistics and a doctoral degree in Epidemiology from Harvard.

Vimla L. Patel is a Senior Research Scientist and Director of the *Center for Cognitive Studies in Medicine and Public Health* at the New York Academy of Medicine and an adjunct Professor of Biomedical Informatics at Columbia University. As a past associate editor of the *Journal of Biomedical Informatics* and editor of the Springer book series on *Cognitive Informatics in Biomedicine and Healthcare*, her research focuses on medical decision-making and the impact of technology on human cognition for safer clinical practice. She is an elected Fellow of the Royal Society of Canada, the American College of Medical Informatics, and the International Academy of Health Sciences Informatics.

Misha Pavel, PhD holds a joint faculty appointment in Northeastern University's Khoury College of Computer Sciences and Bouvé College of Health Sciences and visiting faculty at UC Davis. His background comprises electrical engineering, computer science, and experimental psychology. His research includes multi-scale dynamic computational modeling of behaviors and psychological states, with applications ranging from elder care to augmentation of human performance. Pavel uses these model-based approaches to develop algorithms transforming unobtrusive monitoring from smart homes and mobile devices to practical and actionable knowledge for diagnosis and intervention. Under the auspices of the Northeastern-based Consortium on Technology for Proactive Care, Pavel and his colleagues target technological innovations to support the development of economically feasible, proactive, distributed, and individual-centered health care. In addition, Pavel is investigating approaches to inferring and augmenting human cognition using computer games, EEG, gait characteristics, and transcranial electrical stimulation. Before his current positions, he was a program director at the National Science Foundation, faculty at NYU, OHSU, and Stanford University, and Member of Technical Staff at Bell Laboratories.

Monika Pobiruchin works as research associate at the GECKO Institute at Heilbronn University. She received her diploma in Medical Informatics in 2010 and finished her doctoral degree in 2017. Since 2014, she has been (co-)chair of the working group "Consumer Health Informatics" within the GMDS e.V (German Association for Medical Informatics, Biometry and Epidemiology). Her research topics focus on the analysis of clinical care data (secondary use of data) as well as consumers' data generated by smartphone apps or via social media applications.

Pradeep S. B. Podila, PhD, MHA, MS, FACHE, CPHIMS is a Health Services Researcher with over **15** years of combined multisectoral experience in health/public health informatics, EHR-based health and research data analytics, health services/population health research and advanced research/operational data analytics. He received Masters degrees in electrical/biomedical engineering and healthcare administration; and PhD in public health (epidemiology) from the University of Memphis. He graduated from Massachusetts Institute of Technology's (MIT) Applied Data Science Program (ADSP) jointly offered by the Institute for Data, Systems, and Society (IDSS), Great Learning, and MIT's Professional Educational Programs. He is a fellow of American College of Healthcare Executives (ACHE) and Healthcare Financial Management Association (HFMA). He is a Board Member of the National Association for Healthcare Quality's (NAHQ) Education Commission, American Medical Informatics Association's (AMIA) Workgroup on Global Health Informatics and Healthcare Information and Management Systems Society's (HIMSS)—Professional Certification **Board.**

Nidhi Rastogi is an Assistant Professor at GCCIS, Rochester Institute of Technology. Her research is at the intersection of cybersecurity, artificial intelligence, autonomous vehicles, graph analytics, and data privacy. Prior to this, she was a Research Scientist at RPI. For her contributions to cybersecurity and encouraging women in STEM, Dr. Rastogi was recognized in 2020 as an International Women in Cybersecurity by the Cyber Risk Research Institute. She is an invited speaker at Aspen Cyber Summit ('21), SANS cybersecurity summit ('19), and the Grace Hopper Conference ('14), FADEx laureate for the first French-American Program on Cyber-Physical Systems'16.

Therese S. Richmond, PhD, RN, FAAN is the Andrea B Laporte Professor at the University of Pennsylvania, School of Nursing and serves as its Associate Dean for Research and Innovation. Dr. Richmond has an extensive program of research aimed at improving recovery from serious injury by addressing the interaction between physical injury and its psychological repercussions. Her science also focuses on prevention of violence and firearm violence. Dr. Richmond serves on the Executive Committee of the CDC-funded Penn Injury Science Center, where she directs the Research Core. She is a Fellow in the American Academy of Nursing and an elected member of the National Academy of Medicine. Dr. Richmond was appointed to the Board of Population Health for the National Academies of Sciences, Engineering, and Medicine in 2021.

Bedda Rosario is a Senior Biostatistician for the Center for AI, Research and Evaluation within IBM Watson Health. In this role, she supports the center by providing statistical expertise to support research and provide scientific evidence for Watson Health offerings. Dr. Rosario received her PhD degree in Biostatistics from the University of Pittsburgh, and an MPH degree in Biostatistics from the University of Puerto Rico. Dr. Rosario is passionate about scientific research, public health, and the power of using data and technology to improve health care and population health.

S. Trent Rosenbloom, MD, MPH, FACMI is the Vice Chair for Faculty Affairs, the Director of Patient Engagement. and a Professor of Biomedical Informatics with secondary appointments in Medicine, Pediatrics and the School of Nursing at Vanderbilt University. He is a board-certified internist and pediatrician and is a nationally recognized investigator in the field of health information technology evaluation. His research has focused on studying how healthcare providers interact with health information technologies when documenting patient care and when making clinical decisions.

Sarah Collins Rossetti, RN, PhD is an Assistant Professor of Biomedical Informatics and Nursing at Columbia University. Her research is focused on identifying and intervening on patient risk for harm by applying computational tools to mine and extract value from EHR data and leveraging user-centered design for patient-centered technologies. Dr. Rossetti is an experienced critical care nurse, received her PhD from Columbia University School of Nursing, and completed a Post-Doctoral Research Fellowship at Columbia University's Department of Biomedical Informatics. She was selected as a 2019 recipient of the Presidential Early Career Award for Scientists and Engineers (PECASE).

Oshani Seneviratne is the Director of Health Data Research at Rensselaer Polytechnic Institute. She has co-organized health and semantic-focused events such as the Personal Health Knowledge Graph Workshops in 2020 and 2021, AAAI Fall Symposiums on AI for Social Good in 2019 and 2020, and served in the ISWC organizing committees 2012, 2019, 2020, and 2021. Oshani is a guest editor of Semantic Technologies for Data and Algorithmic Governance and actively reviews for the Journal of Web Semantics, Medical Internet Research, Journal of Biomedical and Health Informatics, and many conferences, including ISWC and the Web Conference.

Scott Sittig is an Associate Professor at the College of Nursing and Allied Health at the University of Louisiana at Lafayette. Sittig received a master's in Health Informatics from Louisiana Tech University and a PhD in Biomedical Informatics from the School of Biomedical Informatics at the University of Texas Health Science Center—Houston. His expertise is in the area of consumer health informatics with a particular focus on the development of digital health interventions to improve patient engagement and self-management. He has developed courses in consumer health informatics, is actively sought out to review journal articles for publication, is a frequent NSF panel reviewer in the area of healthcare workflow, and an active conference program committee member (recently for the Behavior Change Support Systems Workshop).

Jane L. Snowdon is the Deputy Chief Science Officer, Science Operations, of the Center for AI, Research and Evaluation at IBM Watson Health and an IBM Industry Academy Member. Dr. Snowdon assists the Chief Science Officer in developing scientific strategy and integrating scientific expertise and evaluation into the product design and development process from innovation through post-market evaluation and surveillance. She leads a multidisciplinary team of physicians, data scientists, biostatisticians, researchers, and program managers in executing the strategy. Dr. Snowdon received her PhD from the Georgia Institute of Technology in Industrial and Systems Engineering and has published more than 100 papers and book chapters.

Veronika Strotbaum BA Gerontology, MA Healthcare Management, has been working at ZTG Zentrum für Telematik und Telemedizin GmbH in Bochum/Hagen as a consultant for telemedicine and mobile applications since 2013. Her work focuses on the evaluation and acceptance analysis of digital health applications, health reporting as well as the conception and implementation of advanced training courses in eHealth. She has written a wide range of articles in books and journals and is a member of the DGGÖ e.V. (German Association for Health Economics) and GMDS e.V. (German Association for Medical Informatics, Biometry and Epidemiology).

Luyi Sun received the BS degree from Huazhong University of Science and Technology, Wuhan, China, in 2019. She took part in the joint program between Huazhong University of Science and Technology and KTH Royal Institute of Technology in 2018 and received the MS degree in KTH Royal Institute of Technology, Stockholm, Sweden, in 2020. After that she joint the PriMa (Privacy Matters)-ITN under EU-Horizon-2020 Framework and was admitted to the Department of Information Security and Communication Technology at the Norwegian University of Science and Technology. Her research interests include data protection and privacy, information security, and machine learning.

Issa Sylla is a Research Engineer in the Center for Computational Health, where he focuses on healthcare research leveraging electronic health records and medical claims datasets. His areas of interest are algorithmic fairness, event prediction, and simulation. Mr. Sylla is an MBA and Health Policy MS candidate at the Darden School of Business and Stanford University, respectively, and he is interested in exploring the intersection of health economics, policy, and outcomes.

Victoria Tiase is the Director of Research Science at NewYork-Presbyterian Hospital and Assistant Professor at Weill Cornell Medicine. Her expertise ranges from leading EHR implementations, leveraging patient-generated health data, to mentoring digital health startups. Dr. Tiase serves on the boards of the Alliance for Nursing Informatics, AMIA, NODE.Health, and chairs the HIMSS Nursing Informatics Committee. She was the informatics expert for the National Academy of Medicine's Future of Nursing 2030 Committee to envision the use of technology to promote health equity and create healthier communities. She received degrees from the University of Virginia, Columbia University, and the University of Utah.

Meghan Reading Turchioe studies ways to use consumer health technology like mobile applications, wearable devices, and telehealth to support patient and clinician decision-making around chronic condition management. Her program of research involves applying data science methods to generate insights from patient-generated health data and electronic health records and returning data-driven insights to patients and clinicians. Dr. Turchioe earned a PhD from Columbia University, MPH from George Washington University, and BSN from Boston College. She completed a post-doc in Health Informatics in the Department of Population Health Sciences at Weill Cornell Medicine, where she is currently an Instructor.

Egil Utheim is an entrepreneur with 25 years of experience as engineer and manager within the field of robotics, automation, and health technology. Specialties: Automation systems, Entrepreneurship, Gamification, Health technology, Innovation, and Robotics.

Denise C. Vidot, PhD is an Assistant Professor in the School of Nursing and Health Sciences at the University of Miami. Dr. Vidot's research interest is centered upon physical health outcomes of substance use and abuse across the life span among racial/ethnic minority populations. Specifically, she examines cardiovascular and metabolic outcomes among cannabis users from an epidemiological perspective. Dr. Vidot is also interested in the cardiovascular and metabolic health outcomes among HIV patients (and those at risk for HIV) who use cannabis.

Cecilia X. Wang, PhD is an Assistant Professor in the University of Minnesota, College of Design. Dr. Wang's primary research interests lie in the overlap of design philosophy, user experience design, healthcare design, service design, visual communication design, and multidisciplinary design. Dr. Wang's philosophy includes with the underlying of an increasingly complex and dynamic social and culture, we must rethink the value of design. The critical near-term challenge is understanding how better design thinking can help achieve an organic flow of experience in concrete situations, making such experiences more intelligent, meaningful, and sustainable.

Elizabeth V. Weinfurter is an Associate Librarian and liaison to the School of Nursing at the Health Sciences Library of the University of Minnesota—Twin Cities. Weinfurter holds an MLIS from Dominican University in River Forest, Illinois, and her expertise includes information retrieval, curriculum-integrated library instruction, and open access publishing. She works closely with students, staff, and faculty in the

School of Nursing and is a partner in their research and education missions. She is the Production Editor for the Interdisciplinary Journal of Partnership Studies, has served as President of the Midwest Chapter of the Medical Library Association, and was part of the 2012–2013 Medical Library Association Rising Stars cohort.

Thomas Wetter is Professor emeritus at Heidelberg University, Heidelberg (Germany) and Affiliate Professor at University of Washington, Seattle (WA). He received Diploma (aka MSc) and PhD degrees from Aachen Technical University, Aachen (Germany). After working for the IBM Scientific Center Heidelberg for 12 years, he joined Heidelberg University and taught classes to BSc and MSc Medical Informatics students and students of medicine. His research first focused on knowledge-based decision support and later on personal health informatics. From 2007 to 2018 he served as the chairperson of the IMIA WG Consumer Health Informatics and is author of the textbook *Consumer Health Informatics. New Services, Roles and Responsibilities*. He spent sabbaticals at the University of Utah, the University of Washington, and the Ben-Gurion-University of the Negev and also taught classes at the Universidad de Chile, Santiago de Chile, and the Universidad Peruana Cayetano Heredia, Lima.

Bian Yang (BS 2000, MS 2002, PhD 2006) has been an Associate Professor with the Department of Information Security and Communication Technology at the Norwegian University of Science and Technology since year 2015. He founded and has been coordinating the eHealth and Welfare Security group at the Center for Cyber and Information Security since 2016. Before that he worked as a lecture and researcher at the Harbin Institute of Technology (2005–2007), research engineer at Thomson Corporate Research Beijing (2007–2008), post-doctoral researcher and EU project manager at the Gjøvik University College (2008–2015). His research interests include eHealth and welfare technology, information security and privacy enhancing technologies, security practice and human factors, biometric data protection, identity and access management, and multimedia security. He has also experience from ISO SC27/37 and CEN TC224 on standardizing identity management, biometrics, and ID proofing projects. He has patents and innovation commercialization experience since 2015 on privacy-preserving biometrics with international and Norwegian market leaders in border control security and healthcare sectors.

Zhijun Yin, PhD is an Assistant Professor of Biomedical Informatics and Computer Science at Vanderbilt University Medical Center, where he teaches the Machine Learning in Healthcare course. His research is motivated by large-scale health-related datasets generated by human beings in either online or offline environments. His research focuses on applying data mining, machine learning, and statistical inference for modeling, analyzing, and predicting health-related behaviors and their associated health outcomes.

Mohammed J. Zaki is a Professor of Computer Science at RPI. He received his PhD in Computer Science from the University of Rochester in 1998. His research interests focus on novel data mining and machine learning techniques, especially for applications in text mining, knowledge graphs, and personal health. He has over 250 publications (and 6 patents), including the Data Mining and Machine Learning textbook (Second Edition, Cambridge University Press, 2020). He was a recipient of the NSF and DOE CAREER Awards, and he is an ACM Distinguished Scientist and a Fellow of the IEEE.

Francisco Zambrana is a Medical Oncologist in Madrid and an Assistant Professor in the European University of Madrid (UEM). He is dedicated to gastrointestinal and genitourinary cancers and is the Principal Investigator of industry and investigator-initiated trials. He obtained his MD and specialization at the University of Seville. He has worked as Clinical Research Fellow at the University College London Hospital and Cancer Institute, in projects of translational oncology. His other areas of interest involve patient-physician communication strategies and the process of advance care planning in patients with advanced cancer.

Part I
The State-of-the-Art Novel Care Delivery Models

Chapter 1
E-enabled Patient-Provider Communication in Context

Craig E. Kuziemsky, Christian Nohr, José F. Florez-Arango, and Vimla L. Patel

Abstract With continued focus on the move to value-based care payment models, one major challenge is how to enable effective critical response for patient-centered care delivery. Several alternative care delivery models have emerged to support asynchronous, non-traditional communication modalities between patients and providers beyond in-person clinical visits. These new models are pertinent not only to chronic and preventive care, but also to other care scenarios that require critical responses, such as the situation we are currently experiencing during the COVID-19 pandemic. However, our understanding of new care delivery models to support critical response is still under-investigated. This chapter explores informatics approaches for designing and implementing E-enabled novel care delivery models to support patient-provider communication. Our work goes beyond the usual social determinants of health, such as age, gender and socio-economic status, to include communication-related factors such as e-health literacy, regional and individual differences in communication preferences and styles, ethics and regulatory issues, and different modalities for care delivery.

Keywords E-enabled · Patient · Provider · Communication collaboration

C. E. Kuziemsky (✉)
MacEwan University, Edmonton, AB, Canada
e-mail: KuziemskyC@macewan.ca

C. Nohr
Maersk McKinney Møller Institute, University of Southern Denmark, Odense, Denmark

J. F. Florez-Arango
Texas A&M University, College Station, TX, USA

V. L. Patel
The New York Academy of Medicine, New York, NY, USA

P.-Y. S. Hsueh et al. (eds.), *Personal Health Informatics*, Cognitive Informatics in Biomedicine and Healthcare, https://doi.org/10.1007/978-3-031-07696-1_1

Introduction

In the global healthcare arena, our aim has been to improve care experiences, improve population health, and reduce costs. An equally important initiative coming into focus is the emphasis on patient-centered care enabled by a combination of technologies, innovative care design, and aligned incentives towards a patient-empowered environment. This has deep implications on care scenarios that require critical responses, such as the situation we are currently experiencing with the COVID-19 pandemic (Legido-Quigley et al. 2020). Past research studies have shown the key to effective management for patients to handle critical responses is to maintain regular communication between patients and health care providers not only during in-person clinical visits, but also, critically, between visits (Stewart 1995). However, in practice, traditional care delivery models do not support patient-provider communication outside clinical visits effectively. For lower-middle income countries, besides technological support, socio cultural values of trust in an artificial system and traditional practices play important roles in successful e-enabled care delivery process.

To resolve this, alternative care delivery models via asynchronous, non-traditional communication modalities have emerged. Take behavioral health services for example. Globally, we have observed adoption of integrated behavioral health services using various e-enabled communication modalities, which aim to maintain regular communication between providers, and patients to increase patient understanding and adherence to behavioral health goals. However, to bring out the full potential of patient-provider communication beyond clinical visits, we need further investigation on the gaps in the use of different communication modalities to influence patient behavior. Moreover, electronic, and mobile communication technologies can further facilitate patient-provider relationships between clinical visits. Yet the adoption rate has been low to date due to barriers such as physician time, compensation, and factors such as lack of access to internet or technology (Niazkhani et al. 2020; Palacholla et al. 2019; Scott et al. 2018). While novel delivery models like bundled care can potentially remove such barriers to improve physician adoption, the caveat is that the providers need to first overcome technology-related adoption barriers, such as those introduced by the closed nature of healthcare systems on integrating communication technologies with EHRs.

The COVID-19 pandemic ramped up the need to deliver virtual care to limit face-to-face encounters as part of supporting public health guidelines (Bhatia et al. 2021). The increase in virtual care has raised questions about how we configure e-enabled patient-provider communication (Wittenberg et al. 2021). We have known for some time that patient-provider communication is challenging and while macro level models of it are needed to help us understand how it works. The healthcare communication space comprises all the activities that take place within a communication system and we need to understand the micro and macro aspects of how communication systems work in different contexts (Coiera 2000).

Our approach looks at communication from the perspective of systems thinking. Systems thinking starts with a recognition that healthcare delivery does not occur in isolated entities but rather through several integrated systems (Champion et al. 2019; Clarkson et al. 2018). Health systems include financial, technological, human resource and governance components and while it is not reasonable for a study to address all aspects of a health system, it is important to recognize that changing one part of a health system will impact other parts of it. While our focus is on e-enabled models of patient-provider communication we do provide insight on how other health system components influence communication.

In this chapter we provide four global perspectives on e-enabled patient-provider communication. Our perspectives differ by resource availability and country. We offer one high resource country case example (Denmark) and two low-resource country case examples (Fiji, Brazil). We then have a summative section that presents a systems model for e-enabled collaborative care delivery developed by our co-author from Canada. We first present the three global case examples from each country followed by the systems model on collaborative care delivery. We conclude the chapter with overall lessons learned from our chapter to inform future design and evaluation of e-enabled patient provider communication systems.

Case Example #1: Development of the E-Health Care Model and Implementation in the PreClinic in Denmark

Innovation is a positive term. It denotes something we all want to see and be part of. However, innovation also creates dilemmas because it introduces changes. On an aggregate level we talk about innovations as "add-ons" or "transformations" (Wessel et al. 2021).

Add-ons is where activities remain within the same paradigm, work within old and well-known structures, and stick to the familiar organization. We only see small surface changes and no fundamental alterations. Add-ons will use the same models for financing and regulation. Digitization can introduce add-ons as we have seen it within healthcare in many countries. Healthcare systems are often characterized as a silo system defined as the set of individual or group mindsets that creates divisions inside an organization. This division results in the creation of barriers to communication and the development of disjointed work processes with negative consequences to the organization, employees, and patients (Alves and Meneses 2018).

The experience from introducing fundamental changes to silo organizations indicate that changes are temporary and long-term effects are absent. When introducing real transformations potential conflicts will easily be expose and there will be impendent danger to light devastating fires. Many things in the Danish health care sector work well with the General practitioners as the anchor point and other institutions to follow up. Citizens live longer and specific groups in society can add quality life years. The hospitals are getting more and more specialized and have reduced time of admission dramatically. At the same time older patients (+65 years) experience more short-term hospital admissions and there is a significant inequity in health status in the population.

In Denmark and in many other countries more than 60% of citizens over the age of 65 have more than one chronic disease which in the current organization of the health care system a significant societal and financial burden. Care for chronic patients is divided between hospitals and municipalities as well as general practitioners who take care of citizens in their everyday life with chronic conditions. If they need follow-up or treatment of their disease, the hospital takes over and the municipalities support after discharge with rehabilitation and home care. It is however frequently seen that patients gets lost in the siloed triangle: Hospitals, GPs and municipal rehabilitation. There is a need for a new model of care that can prevent citizens with chronic diseases to end up being acute admitted to hospitals. Such a model is the Ehealth Care Model (ECM). The model was developed with a special focus on caring for citizens with severe Chronic Obstructive Pulmonary Disease (COPD) (Phanareth et al. 2017).

The model introduces a shift in paradigm from the profession dominated health care system where the citizens turn to the health care institutions when they decide they need acute attention by health professionals; to a citizen centred paradigm where the citizens monitor themselves on vital parameters and share the measurements and information with health care professionals.

To make this work the citizens must go through an inclusion process to join the ECM network. The citizens must be capable of monitoring four quantitative measures (FEV1, Heart Rate, O2 saturation, and temperature), and three qualitative parameters (breathing difficulties, cough, and secretion). The measures are transmitted to a Response Coordination Centre (RCC) where the health professionals can triage the patients. The RCC is staffed with a trained e-nurse who proactively can initiate treatments rather than allowing the conditions to exacerbate to a level, which requires more severe intervention. The e-nurse can instruct the citizen to adjust their medication or refer to an e-physician who can initiate new medication from the medical first aid box located at the citizens home or pay a visit to the citizen's home in acute severe cases.

The ECM model consists of six stages (ECM 1–6) characterizing the citizens state of health and with varying degrees of intervention (see Fig. 1.1). The key feature of the model is to bring the citizen back to their habitual condition (ECM 1) as quick as possibly to live an active and independent life.

The first stage—ECM0—of the model encompass citizens with unknown long-term conditions—this segment is invisible and therefore not included in the ECM service network. If citizens qualify for inclusion, they enter stage ECM1 and get connected to the ECM services in accordance with personal needs and values. They are supported in self-management of their life with COPD, and once they enroll, they will also get a medical first aid box with prescribed medication for acute exacerbations that the e-physician can initiate for urgent treatment at home.

At stage 2 the citizen makes use of the virtual support through one point of contact—the Response Coordination Centre—with immediate response 24/7

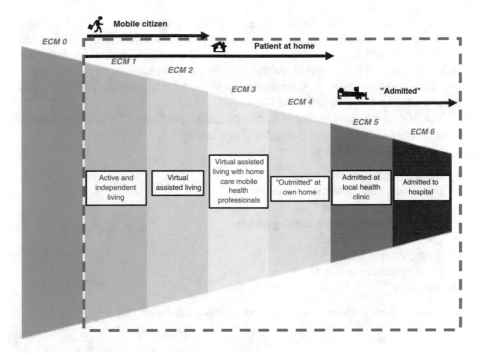

Fig. 1.1 The Ehealth Care Model. (Phanareth et al. 2017)

availability of the RCC nurse and if needed also contact to the e-physician. Proactive medication may be initiated using the acute medicine box.

If the citizen's condition gets worse, they will enter ECM3—called virtual assisted living with assistance from home care mobile health professionals. It means added support in their home, with regular physical visits from the mobile acute team. The goal is to enable the citizen to stay in their home as long as possible without compromising safety. In ECM4 the treatment, monitoring and follow up in their home is intensified corresponding to an inpatient setting—hence the term "outmitted".

In the case of further exacerbations, the citizen moves into ECM5 where the e-physician can admit the citizen to a sub-acute bed in a municipal institution, which is staffed 24 h. Here it is possible to give oxygen and more advanced treatment. This is the last decentralized step.

If more advanced care is needed the citizen will be admitted to a specialized respiratory department at a larger hospital where adequate services are available—ECM6. In the first two stages ECM1 and ECM2 the citizen is mobile and can move around as needed. In the stages ECM1 to 4 the citizen is cared for at their own home, and in ECM5 and 6 they are admitted to an institution outside their own home. The technology it takes to run the COPD care system following the ECM model is not so complicated. The citizens have a few devices: Tablet computer, and devices to measure FEV1, Heart Rate, O2 saturation, and temperature—and of course an internet connection.

The response and coordination centre and the e-physician have computers or smartphones for communication and displaying citizen self-monitoring. The software for easy communication of the monitoring values is specifically developed for this project. There is a simple algorithm using the self-measurements for triaging to prioritize the home visits. To integrate the ECM model in an existing national health care system is a more complicated issue.

The RCC is the most critical as it must be staffed 24/7 with COPD trained nurses to ensure rapid response and one point of contact.

Furthermore, there has to be an:

• E-mobile clinical acute team
• E-technical service team
• E-clinical service team
• E-observation and home nursing service
• Local rehabilitation unit
• Empowerment network
• Local in-bed health clinic
• Pharmacy

To make all these different interests work together is the real challenge.

Evaluation of ECM Accomplishments

The ECM model has been the framework for a local COPD clinic in Region Zealand in Denmark called the PreClinic. The first patients were enrolled late 2018, and the accomplishments have been evaluated (Data og udviklingsstøtte 2020) with respect to a number of activity parameters, and patient satisfaction. 115 citizens with COPD had been enrolled in 2019. 15 of these died and two left the clinic.

Figure 1.2 shows the average annual number of visits to hospital outpatient clinics for COPD patients in four different risk groups for citizens before and after being enrolled in the ECM clinic. The column to the far right shows the average for all the risk groups.

It appears that the number of outpatient contacts to the hospital decreases by an average of 1.7 contacts per year after inclusion in the ECM program, when looking at the total group of citizens. This corresponds to a decrease of 27%.

It is also seen that all risk groups (high risk, medium risk, rising risk and low risk group) experience a decrease in the number of outpatient contacts after inclusion. The high risk group has the largest decline in number of contacts of an average of 3.5 fewer outpatient contacts per year after inclusion corresponding to a decrease of 41%.

The patient satisfaction was evaluated in a survey in February 2020 among the 44 citizens in the PreClinic who had been treated for a light to severe exacerbation during the last quarter of 2019 (Data og udviklingsstøtte 2020). 38 individuals responded to the survey.

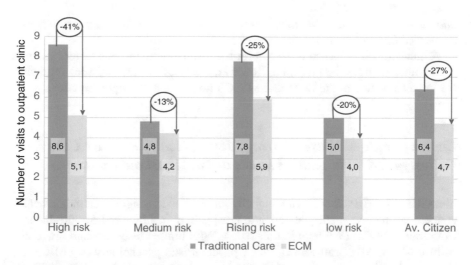

Fig. 1.2 Average annual number of outpatient contacts before and after enrolment in the ECM program (Data og udviklingsstøtte 2020)

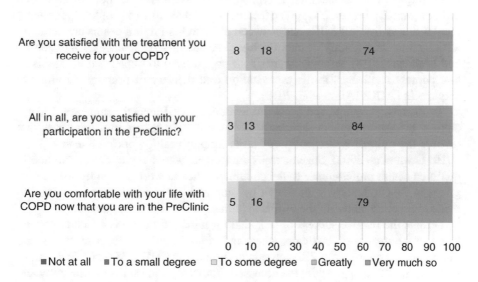

Fig. 1.3 The citizens overall impression of participation in the PreClinic

Figure 1.3 shows the citizens satisfaction with the treatment they receive, their overall satisfaction with their participation, and whether they are comfortable with their life with COPD. The majority indicate that they are very satisfied and comfortable.

The citizens enrolled in the PreClinic were interviewed individually to let them express their opinion about their experience. One of the citizens stated *"It is super cool that there is a prompt response if something is not ok with the measurements, and that one can always call no matter what. You are in treatment immediately and thus avoid hospitalization, which in itself provides security".*

A much longer timespan is needed for the evaluation to provide better evidence of the outcome from the PreClinic. However, the results of the activities following the implementation of the ECM in the PreClinic points in the right direction.

Case Example #2: Task-Sharing Mental Health Primary Care Delivery Model Via Smart Phones in Pacific Island Countries

Mental health (MH) disorders are globally recognized as a significant public health concern yet receive inadequate attention, especially in Low- and Middle-Income Countries (LMICs) (Whiteford et al. 2013). With limited resources and few clinically qualified MH professionals (e.g., psychiatrists, psychologists), LMICs are challenged with meeting the needs of those who have mental illness. For instance, there is a 90% treatment gap in LMICs (Alloh et al. 2018; Singh et al. 2013). which is not surprising given that there is typically one psychiatrist per population of one million (McKenzie et al. 2004). The fact that more than 80% of people experiencing mental illness live in LMICs and between 5.7 and 8.4 million deaths are annually attributed to poor quality of care (National Academies of Sciences, Engineering, and Medicine 2018), strongly suggests an urgent need to implement mechanisms that address challenges in the organization and delivery of primary care quality services in LMICs (Alloh et al. 2018).

To increase coverage and access to evidence based mental healthcare, LMICs employ task shifting or task sharing, as it commonly referred to, initiatives that involve the rational redistribution of tasks among health workforce teams (Patel 2019; Lawn et al. 2008). Specific tasks are moved, where appropriate, from highly qualified health professionals to the community health workers, the front-line care givers in the community, with shorter training and fewer qualifications, in order to make more efficient use of the available human resources for healthcare.

Despite the relative success of task sharing initiatives, there is a lack of consistency in the quality of MH care, where individuals suffering from severe mental illness are not appropriately diagnosed and treated by CHWs. Most CHWs believe that they are ill-equipped with the necessary knowledge and skills to efficiently and effectively identify and safely manage patients suffering from severe mental illness (Larkins et al. 2018; Patel et al. 2004).

Modern mHealth systems have great promise to aid in this task-sharing and to improve the health care nurses' performance with the use of Smart mobile phones, which are readily available in the community. However, such interventions are most often ad hoc and lack a sound empirical basis for providing adequate evidence for successful delivery of efficient, but safe care. Our study was conducted in the Pacific Island Countries [PICS], where there is a high risk a severe burden of suicide and severe depression Furthermore, approximately 15 psychiatrists are available to

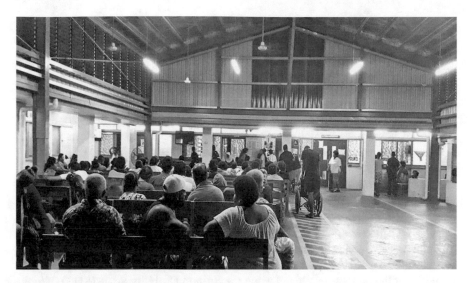

Fig. 1.4 A community health center in Fiji

deliver MH care needs of 11 million people living in the PICs. Research reports in the past decade illustrate the dire consequences of the current MH crisis in Fiji, the largest of the PICs, where 36 people every hour either attempt or commit suicide (Zeitvogel 2018). Primary and community care (e.g., health centers, nursing stations, and village clinics) are the formal first step for patients in the health care system (Fig. 1.4).

Leveraging e-enabled technological tools via mobile phones programmed with evidence-based clinical guidelines can support the community health nurses (CHNs) with clinical problem-solving and patient care decision-making through task sharing process.

The Study

The study was conducted in collaboration with Drs. Odille Chang and William May from Fiji National University in Suva, Fiji, and Sriram Iyengar from The University of Arizona Medical School, in Phoenix, AZ. The objectives of the study was to evaluate the CHNs performance under three conditions, current practices as the baseline, and using culturally-validated guidelines (screening tools) on paper, and on mHealth technology in view to

- to characterize cognitive (thinking) processes underlying diagnosis for depression and suicide risk patients
- to measure the time taken to process the information
- to assess the accuracy of diagnostic and recommendation decisions, andto evaluate the usability of mobile smart phones by the CHNs.

The nurses in the control condition were tasked with four clinical problem-solving activities: (1) Think aloud while reading through each case, providing tentative diagnoses (referred to as the "think aloud" task) (Ericsson and Simon 1980), (2) summarize each case (referred to as the "summary problem" task) (3) provide a final diagnosis (referred to as "final diagnosis" task), and (4) provide recommendation(s) for treatment (referred to as "recommendation(s) for treatment" task). After completion of all four activities, only the CHNs in the two treatment conditions were given guidelines and asked to engage in the same four activities mentioned above using the respective guideline, as illustrated in Fig. 1.5.

Two clinical scenarios reflecting severe depression and suicide risk were developed by psychiatrists and primary care physicians based on what would be expected in real community clinics in Fiji. The Center for Epidemiologic Studies Depression Scale (CES-D) (Radloff 1997) and the Suicide Behaviours Questionnaire-Revised (SBQ-R) (Osman et al. 2001) tool were the assessment tools used as the respective guidelines. The Suicide Risk and Depression Assessment mHealth tool (ASRaDA) was developed on an Android smartphone app and using iterative design principles. Usability of the app was evaluated using the System Usability Scale (SUS) (Brooke 2013). To deliver the intervention, ASRaDA was loaded on Samsung J3 smartphones. CHNs logged with the patient's name into the ASRaDA application before administering the assessment. Once logged in, the CES-D and SBQ-R guidelines were displayed as selection choices.

In response from the patient for each of the guideline-prompted question, nurses had to provide a quantitative score on a provided scale, which had be manually added to provide a total final score, based on which treatment recommendations had

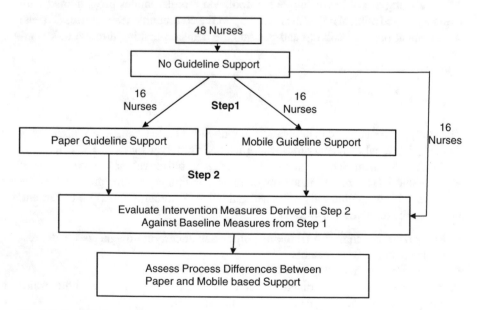

Fig. 1.5 Empirical evaluation process

Evaluation of two local **patient scenarios**

• Time on task automatic recording: **Efficiency**

• "Think aloud" while reading the case: **Reasoning**

• Summarize the case: **Comprehension [Understanding]**

• Provide diagnosis and patient management plan: **Accuracy**

With and without ecologically-valid clinical guideline support for severe depression and suicide risks

Fig. 1.6 Tasks and cognitive measures

to be made. However, in ASRaDA, the scores were automatically added and the treatment recommendation calculated. The mobile phone also recorded the time taken to complete the tasks, automatically. Forty-eight CHNs were recruited, following the inclusive and exclusive criteria from an available pool of 5000 female participants. Only women traditionally train as nurses in the Pacific Islands. Data were audio recorded through the mobile phone and transcribed for analysis. Using mixed methods approach that closely aligned with the tasks and the corresponding cognitive measures were used for gathering data and analyses. (given in Fig. 1.6).

Summary of Results

Nurses using smart phone took less time on task than with paper-based or no guideline support, showing the use of smart phones to be most efficient. There were no errors of calculation and interpretation with the smart phone, as opposed to paper-based version. The nurses thinking was more organized, showing patterns of improved reasoning process (Patel et al. 2021). The results show that the use of ASRaDA was relatively safe (Chang et al. 2021). Identified usability problems were corrected (Iyengar et al. 2021). These results are valid in simulated conditions. The use of smart phone to communicate with patients work well for both patients and the health care provider for to allow for quick and accurate screening for depression and suicide risk in the community, mostly through decreased cognitive load. Our studies show that this method is efficient, effective and relatively safe in care delivery in the community by the nurses, although we found some errors in translation of patient narrative into quantitative scores were generated. However, these errors did not alter the final decision accuracy in this case.

Challenges and Opportunities

One of the biggest challenges with just providing mobile support to the community nurses without checking the prior knowledge of the discipline was that prior training in mental health was shown to be related to diagnostic accuracy, as shown on

Table 1.1 Diagnosis provided by nurses during the "think aloud" task

		Severe depression N (%)	High risk for suicide N (%)
Correct	MH training	4 (100)	0 (0)
	No MH training	0 (0)	0 (0)
	Total	4 (8)	0 (0)
Partially correct	MH training	8 (26)	12 (40)
	No MH training	22 (73)	18 (60)
	Total	30 (63)	30 (63)
Incorrect	MH training	3 (60)	0 (0)
	No MH training	2 (40)	7 (100)
	Total	5 (13)	7 (15)
Missing		9 (24)	11 (23)
Total		48	48

Table 1.1. Thus, training the health provider in the required content domain and the use of mobile app, are necessary. Furthermore, our results are true in the laboratory studies, and a pilot study of implementation in the community clinics is much needed, before large scale implementation and dissemination are carried out, since real world practice raise some additional challenges, which need to be evaluated and corrected, iteratively.

Besides challenges, there are the opportunities in moving forward with the use of e-enabled health care program in this community. This model could be generalized to another communities provided it is ecologically validated in that community. This model of e-enabled mental health care through task-sharing community nurses could be applied to rural community areas where access to healthcare is not readily available.

Finally, the Mobile app requires face to face communication between the provider and the patient, and this will create a challenge during a pandemic, such as Covid-19. However, the nurses could use telehealth, if there was some infrastructure support with a good internet bandwidth. Then, the use of the mobile health app will be extremely useful to provide a much-needed assessment and comfort given the long social isolation period. We expect the depression, PTSD and Suicide issues will be more pronounced during post pandemic period and mobile health support via smart phones will be useful in quick identification and treatment recommendation.

Future Directions

As the next step, we developed a concept model of information flow during nurse-patient communication in community clinic to the overall healthcare system in Fiji. In this model the nurse uses the mobile app for patient evaluation and records the diagnosis and management recommendation in the paper chart (as it is currently used) and then sends the encrypted data to the servers at College of Medicine (CoM)

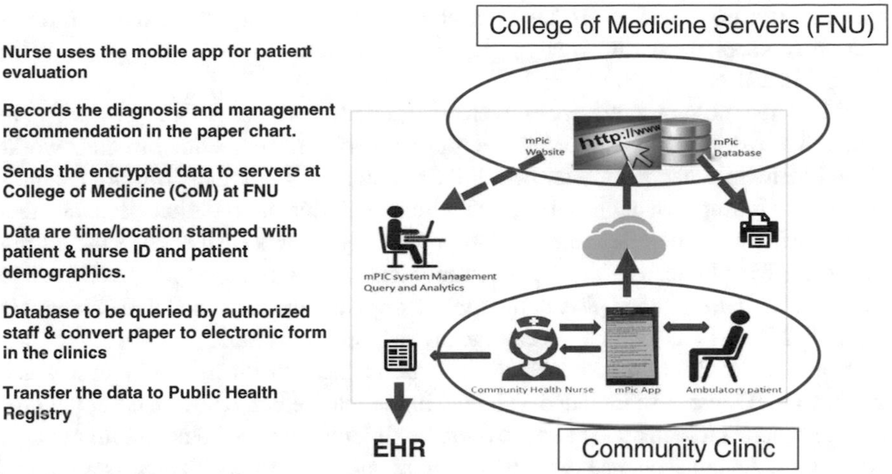

Nurse uses the mobile app for patient evaluation

Records the diagnosis and management recommendation in the paper chart.

Sends the encrypted data to servers at College of Medicine (CoM) at FNU

Data are time/location stamped with patient & nurse ID and patient demographics.

Database to be queried by authorized staff & convert paper to electronic form in the clinics

Transfer the data to Public Health Registry

Fig. 1.7 Information flow during nurse-patient communication

at FNU. The data are time/location stamped with patient and nurse ID and patient demographics. A long term goal is to have the database to be queried by authorized staff and convert paper to electronic form in the clinics, and have the transferred to Public Health Registry for public health decision makers, given in Fig. 1.7.

A nurse can use the app to retrieve patient's past record, and the record can be printed out locally. For this model, steps will have to be taken to preserve the provider-patient privacy and patient confidentiality. The long run sustainability of this e-enabled program: will be in building a strong local research capacity.

Case Example #3: Colombia: Prenatal Care and Early Risk Identification

Colombia, as many lower-middle income countries (LMIC) faces a lowering but still high maternal mortality rate (ranges from 20 to 132 maternal deaths/100,000 live births) (OMS 2015), presents big health disparities regardless of almost universal health coverage, it has a non-equative resource allocation (Restrepo-Zea et al. 2018), with high concentration of healthcare providers in the cities and presents communication and connectivity challenges gives the geography (Hoyos-Vertel and Muñoz de Rodríguez 2019).

Health care system in Colombia, and its information workflow, is complex, involving providers, payers, regulators, patients, and many other stakeholders. The case study explores a multilayer prenatal control model that aims to empower patients and caregivers in the active surveillance of health conditions. The model is a patient-centered model with a tailored AI-driven clinical decision support system for primary care providers (Torres Silva et al. 2020), that triggers telemedicine contact when specialized care is suggested by the system (Luna Gómez et al. 2015; Colombia 2013).

When technology preferences were evaluated, we found that providers are inclined to use desktop web-based interoperable systems embedded in their workflow. Meanwhile patients prefer cellphone centered technologies. Mobile technology allows to implement persuasive behaviors. With this intervention clinicians feel more confident in their decisions, and supported by experts easily, while increasing coverage. We still need to work in a communication channel to answer questions to patients, further than the Q&A in the mobile app, and during scheduled encounters with clinicians, in addition to an emergency response channel.

Colombia's adoption of telehealth in general has growth in steady pace since 2003. COVID response included a change in the telemedicine law, making the process to enable a telemedicine service more flexible, totaling 3750 across all medical specialties. As consequence there was an explosion of services. There is a total of 249 (around 7% of all telemedicine services) Ob/Gyn related services registered in the country (12 obstetrics, 185 ob/gyn, 48 of prenatal control, and 4 for delivery assistance), with at least 33 (13.2%) of them registered in 2020. This creates a favorable scenario for future growth of model like the one presented in Fig. 1.8.

We need to improve the Sustainability model, that so far is grant lead. Our system is proved with an in-house development, that requires additional development to warranty Interoperability with other vendors in the health information system ecosystem. The most needed patients still the underserved that already have a Digital Gap that need to be explored and covered.

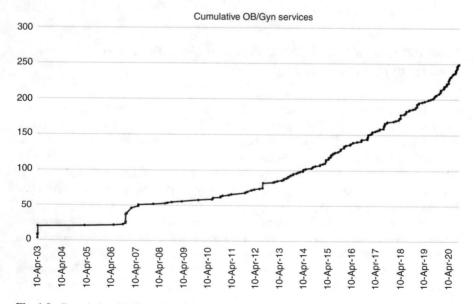

Fig. 1.8 Cumulative Ob/Gyn related telemedicine services in Colombia

A Systems Model for E-Health Enabled Collaborative Care Delivery

Collaborative care delivery has increased in importance in recent years as patient care has become more complex due to an aging population and increased prevalence of co-morbidities. While studies of collaboration and health IT (HIT) design to support it have increased in recent years, it remains an understudied phenomenon (Eikey et al. 2015). To properly design HIT to support collaboration we first must understand the nature of how collaboration works. Collaboration as a care delivery model is not a single process or event but rather a dynamic system of activities (Kuziemsky 2018). This system of activities includes clinical processes such as assessments and diagnoses but also tasks specific to collaboration such as the development of awareness and common ground to enable shared understanding across team members (Eikey et al. 2015).

To date there is a lack of explicit studies on collaboration and little insight on how to design HIT to support it. Systems design for collaborative care delivery is an entirely new phenomenon that goes beyond just adapting the interface on existing HIT (Karsh et al. 2010). New models of collaboration are an essential first step to understanding and designing for collaboration as workflow models for individual providers are often unsatisfactory when scaled up to collaborative teamwork (Ozkaynak et al. 2013). Collaborative systems are dynamic, and we need to understand the connectivity factor for how the system components integrate during care delivery (Kuziemsky et al. 2016). Models of collaborative care delivery must also be based on the clinical, social and governance reality where care delivery occurs, recognizing that different local and global contexts will impact how collaborative care delivery is operationalized and implemented. Studying collaboration starts with understanding individual workflows, terminologies etc. and then understanding how they scale up and are reconciled into collaborative competencies and processes (Kuziemsky et al. 2019).

Figure 1.9 shows a systems model of collaborative care delivery and how it connects across micro, meso and macro levels. The micro level begins with care for an

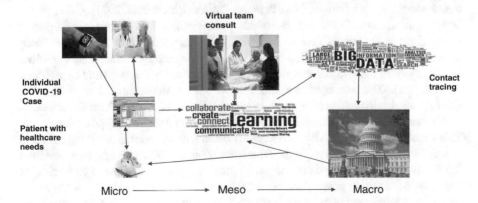

Fig. 1.9 Systems model of collaborative care delivery across micro, meso and macro levels

individual patient. This could be a patient with COVID-19 or a chronic medical condition that is currently well managed by a family physician. Over time the patient's condition could get more complicated and they are referred to the team based "meso" level where other team members such as medical specialists, a dietician, social worker, or a pharmacist become involved in care delivery. The meso level data then rolls up to the macro level where artificial intelligence and other data analysis approaches are used to develop evidence to shape programs and policy and to inform informatics research such as on data standards and system interoperability. The macro level outputs form the evidence that enables the micro and meso delivery models to learn and evolve going forward. While the micro, meso and macro levels are distinct from each other, they feed into other as an integrated system.

While Fig. 1.9 shows an ideal systems model of collaboration, putting the model into action is where the challenges arise. A collaborative system is defined by both the structure and behavior of the system (Kuziemsky et al. 2019) and it only works if all the system concepts across all levels work in unison. Team-based models may describe the structure of a team (Kuziemsky and Harris 2019), but collaboration goes beyond the structure where it is delivered. Collaboration is about how individual workflows, terminologies etc. are reconciled into collaborative behaviors and protocols (Kuziemsky et al. 2019). Below we use Fig. 1.9 as a basis to discuss some of the lessons learned from COVID-19 and how they can help shape collaborative care delivery moving forward.

Collaborative Care Delivery in the Time of COVID-19

The COVID-19 pandemic brought a rapid uptake of digital communication and collaboration tools to support patient care delivery (Webster 2020; Liaw et al. 2021). At the micro level this involved a shift in patient care delivery as countries worldwide transitioned from face-to-face to virtual care delivery (Snoswell et al. 2020; Bhatia et al. 2021). COVID-19 was credited with eroding some of the historical barriers to virtual care delivery including reimbursement issues and clinicians being mandated to use certain digital health technologies (Bhatia et al. 2021). Other micro level implications of COVID-19 included a positive impact on patient satisfaction in comparison to traditional face-to-face visits (Ramaswamy et al. 2020). However, micro level challenges have also been identified including interface and workflow complexity and inability for marginalized communities to access virtual care (Shaw et al. 2021). The scope of communication and collaboration tools when the COVID-19 pandemic forced a move to virtual care used ranged from formal electronic medical record or telehealth tools to informal ones such as Skype or FaceTime. This created extra complexity as clinicians often had freedom in what digital tools to use for communication with their patients (Glauser 2020). While this provided flexibility, it also introduced challenges by creating a vast landscape of technologies being used leading to privacy and security issues as well as scalability issues at the meso level when additional care team members are engaged through meso level collaborations (Liaw et al. 2021).

At the meso level, collaborative across disciplines and settings has been identified as essential to help us successfully navigate the challenges imposed by the COVID-19 pandemic (Xyrichis and Williams 2020). Care delivery via interdisciplinary teamwork played a big role in the early response to COVID-19 as mental health and other complex issues became more prevalent (Donnelly et al. 2021). The pandemic has also highlighted challenges to delivering collaborative care delivery including how teamwork is perceived and how formal and informal collaborative networks develop (El-Awaisi et al. 2020). How teams develop and create integrated work routines was also cited as a challenge, with virtual care posing unique challenges to delivering teamwork due to some team members struggling to transition their teams from face-to-face to virtual delivery (Tannenbaum et al. 2021). An overarching meso level challenge was that many of the known barriers to collaborative care delivery such as the need for shared mental models and common ground across team members and settings were difficult to do using digital modalities (Donnelly et al. 2021).

At a macro level, COVID forced governments to act quickly to address barriers to virtual care delivery such as the creation of virtual billing codes (Liaw et al. 2021). It has also been highlighted how governments may need to use emergency powers to create frameworks that enable data sharing to support clinical and public health needs from the pandemic (Bakken 2020). These macro level initiatives have trickled down to support collaboration at meso and micro levels by addressing some of the historical connectivity problems that have long impaired the delivery of collaborative care delivery. Macro level challenges included data standard issues and inequality (Nguyen et al. 2020). While governments worldwide quickly advocated for data sharing as part of managing the COVID-19 pandemic, a lack of congruent standards was a significant impediment to effective data management. Informatics infrastructure issues such as bandwidth for both audio and video connections created an uneven landscape for virtual care as service availability varied across urban and rural areas (Liaw et al. 2021). Access and cost of technology and internet access also created inequality with respect to access to virtual care (Shaw et al. 2021).

Lessons on Collaborative Care Delivery from COVID-19

The COVID-19 pandemic provided a case study of how Fig. 1.9 would be operationalized, and it offered some good insights on how we can design and evaluate HIT to support collaborative care delivery moving forward. The move to virtual care delivery emphasized the importance of collaborative competencies such as awareness and common ground as the basis for collaborative care delivery (Reddy and Spence 2008). It also highlighted the need for the development of these competencies prior to engaging in collaborative care delivery and the challenges to developing them through virtual means. It is easier to develop common ground or awareness in face-to-face settings, but the reality is virtual care delivery will be a big part of care delivery going forward and we need to we design HIT to support and nurture collaborative competencies such as common ground.

The pandemic also remined us that technology is only one part of a collaborative system and all underlying or adjacent system concepts (e.g. funding, organizational, workflow, human resource) involved in collaboration need to be co-designed with technology (Clarkson et al. 2018). Many of the challenges to collaborative care delivery from COVID-19 were governance, social or workflow related and not direct technological issues.

Finally, the pandemic emphasized that designing HIT to support collaborative care delivery is as much about understanding individual work practices and routines as it is about designing systems to support collaboration. Collaboration is the outcome we want to achieve and managing the individual-collaborative exchange by which individual workflows and domain specific terminologies are reconciled into collaborative ones is an essential first task (Kuziemsky 2015). Teamwork can be difficult to deliver in face-to-face settings and it is even more challenging to deliver virtually. As individuals engage in collaborative activities, they are changing the space of work into collaborative spaces and our inability to account for these changes is what leads to unintended consequences post HIT implementation (Kuziemsky et al. 2019).

Discussion

This chapter has provided insight into e-enabled patient-provider communication from four case examples highlighting different contexts of patient-provider communication. A common message in all the case examples was that technology is only one aspect of an e-enabled communication system. It is often non-technologically-related concepts such as data governance, workflow, socio-cultural factors, or cross-disciplinary integration that lead to communication difficulties. The automation of patient-provider communication cannot stray from the fundamental principles of quality and patient-centered care to avoid the plethora of HIT failures from the past. We cannot separate patient-provider communication from the contexts within which it occurs or the underlying clinical and social complexity that define modern health systems.

While the COVID-19 pandemic provided an excellent case study to evaluate the current HIT, we are not trying to solve COVID-19 as it is only the challenge of the moment. Instead, we need to use COVID-19 and the lessons learned from it to help us design resilient health systems for critical response. As highlighted in the section on e-enabled collaborative care delivery, an informatics infrastructure that spans micro, meso and macro levels must be in place as the basis for effective patient-provider collaboration before another pandemic occurs. After the COVID-19 pandemic forced health systems to move to virtual care delivery and the need arose for public health data sharing to support contact tracing, health systems worldwide realized they did have a sufficient informatics infrastructure to support critical response during a pandemic. Furthermore, in underdeveloped countries, where the burden of disease, including mental health with depression and suicide, is already high, Covid-19 has exacerbated this situation with no infrastructure to help the community. Such e-enabled infrastructure plus resilience-building strategies should be in place in preparedness for future disasters, either natural or artificial.

COVID-19 also provided other insight for system design to support critical response such as in a pandemic. The flexibility in digital tools used to deliver health services in the pandemic included formal tools like telehealth and EHRs and informal tools like Skype or WhatsApp. While this flexibility was beneficial for enabling expedited access to meet the needed demand, it also raised privacy and security concerns and presented scalability challenges when care delivery moved from micro to meso to macro levels. These concerns are even more severe for low-to-middle income countries, where infrastructure support for privacy and security is already the bare minimum, and the concept of privacy is not always a part of the culture.

Our chapter provided insight on how such an informatics infrastructure can be configured. E-enabled collaborative care delivery requires technology to be designed that can be used by all users. Successful design and implementation of a collaborative digital care delivery model for patients and providers requires the roles of health professionals to be refined from individual into collaborative competencies. A collaborative digital health model must include the involvement of patients as an essential partner in designing digital health systems. We need to work with patients, providers, and policy makers to address the non-technical issues of system interoperability including providing necessary training and education to ensure people have the necessary digital and health literacy. While technology is often the focus of digital health systems, implementing and managing these systems are true socio-technical endeavors with social, political, organizational, and economic implications. Digital health systems must be a driver of health equity for everyone. We must ensure that increased digital health capacity improves healthcare delivery and access to services for everyone and does not increase access for some while decreasing it for others.

In summary, technology alone will not solve ongoing health system issues around data interoperability, workflows, or equitable access to health services. E-enabled Patient-Provider Communication requires an informatics infrastructure that should be designed using principles of systems thinking to account for the technological, social, cultural, and policy contexts that contribute to equitable, efficient and safe healthcare delivery.

Acknowledgements Dr. Patel wishes to acknowledge that her study was supported by the National Institute of Mental Health of the National Institutes of Health under Award Number R21MH114621.

Dr. Kuziemsky acknowledges funding from a Discovery Grant from the Natural Sciences and Engineering Research Council of Canada.

References

Alloh FT, Regmi P, Onche I, van Teijlingen E, Trenoweth S. Mental health in low-and-middle income countries (LMICs): going beyond the need for funding. Heath Prospect: J Public Health. 2018;2018(17):12–7.

Alves J, Meneses R. Silos mentality in healthcare services. 11th Annual Conference of the EuroMed Academy of Business. EuroMed Press 2018. ISBN: 978-9963-711-67-3.

Bakken S. Informatics is a critical strategy in combating the COVID-19 pandemic. J Am Med Inform Assoc. 2020;27(6):843–4.

Bhatia RS, Chu C, Pang A, Tadrous M, Stamenova V, Cram P. Virtual care use before and during the COVID-19 pandemic: a repeated cross-sectional study. CMAJ Open. 2021;9(1):E107–14.

Brooke J. SUS: a retrospective. J Usability Stud. 2013;8(2):29–40.

Champion C, Kuziemsky C, Affleck E, Alvarez GG. A systems approach for modelling health information complexity. Int J Inf Manag. 2019;49:343–54.

Chang O, Patel VL, Iyengar S, May W. Impact of mhealth tool supporting community health nurses in early identification of depression and suicide risk in Pacific Island countries. Australas Psychiatry. 2021;29(2):200–3.

Clarkson J, Dean J, Ward J, Komashie A, Bashford T. A systems approach to healthcare: from thinking to -practice. Future Healthc J. 2018;5(3):151–5. https://doi.org/10.7861/futurehosp.5-3-151.

Coiera E. When conversation is better than computation. J Am Med Inf Assoc. 2000;7(3):277–86.

Colombia Ministerio de Salud y de la Protección Social República de. Procedimientos Estandarizados en Telesalud Colombia. Florez-Arango JF, Lopez JI, Pineda Gaviria M, Munera C, editors. Medellin: Canal U; 2013. 500 p.

Data og udviklingsstøtte, 2020: NærKlinikken – resultater efter 1 år. Data og udviklingsstøtte - Region Sjælland Alléen 15, 4180 Sorø (in Danish language). Title in English: "PreClinic – results after 1 year".

Donnelly C, Ashcroft R, Bobbette N, et al. Interprofessional primary care during COVID-19: a survey of the provider perspective. BMC Fam Pract. 2021;22:31.

Eikey EV, Reddy MC, Kuziemsky CE. Examining the role of collaboration in studies of health information technologies in biomedical informatics: a systematic review of 25 years of research. J Biomed Inform. 2015;57:263–77.

El-Awaisi A, O'Carroll V, Koraysh S, Koummich S, Huber M. Perceptions of who is in the health-care team? A content analysis of social media posts during COVID-19 pandemic. J Interprof Care. 2020;34(5):622–32.

Ericsson K, Simon H. Verbal reports as data. Psychol Rev. 1980;87:215–51.

Glauser W. Virtual care is here to stay, but major challenges remain. CMAJ. 2020;192(30):E868–9.

Hoyos-Vertel LM, Muñoz de Rodríguez L. Barreras de acceso a controles prenatales en mujeres con morbilidad materna extrema en Antioquia. Colombia Rev Salud Pública [Internet]. 2019;21(1):17–21.

Iyengar MS, Chang O, Florez-Arango JF, et al. Development and usability of a mobile tool for identification of depression and suicide risk in Fiji. Technol Health Care. 2021;29(1):143–53.

Karsh BT, Weinger MB, Abbott PA, Wears RL. Health information technology: fallacies and sober realities. J Am Med Inform Assoc. 2010;17(6):617–23.

Kuziemsky CE. Review of social and organizational issues in health information technology. Healthc Inform Res. 2015;21(3):152–60.

Kuziemsky C. A systems perspective on collaborative care delivery. Health Manage. 18(4):2018. Accessed from A systems perspective on collaborative care delivery - HealthManagement.org.

Kuziemsky CE, Harris A. An agent based framework for healthcare teamwork. In: Proceedings of the 2019 2nd international conference on information science and systems; 2019. p. 271–5. https://doi.org/10.1145/3322645.3322660.

Kuziemsky CE, Andreev P, Benyoucef M, O'Sullivan T, Jamaly S. A connectivity framework for social information systems design in healthcare. AMIA Annu Symp Proc. 2016;2016:734–42.

Kuziemsky CE, Abraham J, Reddy MC. Characterizing collaborative workflow and health information technology. In: Zheng K, Westbrook J, Kannampallil T, Patel V, editors. Cognitive
informatics. Health informatics. Cham: Springer; 2019.

Larkins S, Tuni SSM, Kowalenko N, Allen M, Gadai S. Strengthening mental health care in
primary care in low- and middle-income countries: the Fiji experience. J Fiji Public Health.
2018;7(1):35–7.

Lawn JE, Rohde J, Rifkin S, Were M, Paul VK, Chopra M. Alma-Ata 30 years on: revolutionary,
relevant, and time to revitalise. Lancet. 2008;372(9642):917–27.

Legido-Quigley H, Asgari N, Teo YY, Leung GM, Oshitani H, Fukuda K, et al. Are high-performing
health systems resilient against the COVID-19 epidemic? Lancet. 2020;395:848–50.

Liaw ST, Kuziemsky C, Schreiber R, Jonnagaddala J, Liyanage H, Chittalia A, Bahniwal R, He
JW, Ryan BL, Lizotte DJ, Kueper JK, Terry AL, de Lusignan S. Primary care informatics
response to Covid-19 pandemic: adaptation, progress, and lessons from four countries with
high ICT development. Yearb Med Inform. 2021; https://doi.org/10.1055/s-0041-1726489.

Luna Gómez IF, Torres Silva EA, Tamayo Correa C, Vélez S, Ramírez Morales MM,
González Serna C, et al. Uso de las tecnologías de información y comunicación para
el cuidado del binomio materno-fetal: revisión de tema. Medicina (B Aires) [Internet].
2015;34(2):138–47.

McKenzie K, Patel V, Araya R. Learning from low income countries: mental health. Br Med
J. 2004;7475:1148–0.

National Academies of Sciences, Engineering, and Medicine; Health and Medicine Division; Board
on Health Care Services; Board on Global Health; Committee on Improving the Quality of
Health Care Globally. Crossing the Global Quality Chasm: Improving Health Care Worldwide.
Washington (DC): National Academies Press (US); 2018.

Nguyen MH, Gruber J, Fuchs J, Marler W, Hunsaker A, Hargittai E. Changes in digital communication during the COVID-19 global pandemic: implications for digital inequality and future
research. Social Media + Society. July 2020. https://doi.org/10.1177/2056305120948255.

Niazkhani Z, Toni E, Cheshmekaboodi M, et al. Barriers to patient, provider, and caregiver adoption and use of electronic personal health records in chronic care: a systematic review. BMC
Med Inform Decis Mak. 2020;20:153.

OMS | Mortalidad materna. WHO 2015.

Osman A, Bagge CL, Gutierrez PM, Konick LC, Kopper BA, Barrios FX. The suicidal behaviour
questionnaire-revised (SBQ-R): validation with clinical and nonclinical samples. Assessment.
2001;8(4):443–54.

Ozkaynak M, Brennan PF, Hanauer DA, Johnson S, Aarts J, Zheng K, Haque SN. Patient-
centered care requires a patient-oriented workflow model. J Am Med Inform Assoc.
2013;20(e1):e14–6.

Palacholla RS, Fischer N, Coleman A, Agboola S, Kirley K, Felsted J, Katz C, Lloyd S, Jethwani
K. Provider- and patient-related barriers to and facilitators of digital health technology adoption for hypertension management: scoping review. JMIR Cardio. 2019;3(1):e11951.

Patel V. The lancet psychiatry. Task sharing: stopgap or end goal? Lancet Psychiatry. 2019;6(2):81.

Patel VL, Branch T, Mottur-Pilson C, Pinard G. Public awareness about depression: the effectiveness of a patient guideline. Int J Psychiatry Med. 2004;34(1):1–20.

Patel VL, Halpern M, Vijayalakshmi N, Chang O, Iyengar S, May W. Information processing by
community health nurses using mobile health (mHealth) tools for early identification of suicide
and depression risks in Fiji Islands [Under review, June, 2021].

Phanareth K, Vingtoft S, Christensen AS, Nielsen JS, Svenstrup J, Berntsen GK, Newman SP,
Kayser L. The epital care model: a new person-centered model of technology-enabled integrated care for people with long term conditions. JMIR Res Protoc. 2017;6(1):e6.

Radloff LS. The CES-D scale: a self-report depression scale for research in the general population.
Appl Psychol Meas. 1997;1(3):385–401.

Ramaswamy A, Yu M, Drangsholt S, Ng E, Culligan PJ, Schlegel PN, Hu JC. Patient satisfaction
with telemedicine during the COVID-19 pandemic: retrospective cohort study. J Med Internet
Res. 2020;22(9):e20786.

Reddy MC, Spence PR. Collaborative information seeking: a field study of a multidisciplinary patient care team. Inf Process Manag. 2008;44(1):242–55.

Restrepo-Zea JH, Casas-Bustamante LP, Espinal-Piedrahita JJ. Cobertura universal y acceso efectivo a los servicios de salud: ¿Qué ha pasado en Colombia después de diez años de la Sentencia T-760? Rev Salud Pública [Internet]. 2018;20(6):670–6.

Scott KC, Karem P, Shifflett K, Vegi L, Ravi K, Brooks M. Evaluating barriers to adopting telemedicine worldwide: a systematic review. J Telemed Telecare. 2018;24(1):4–12.

Shaw J, Brewer LC, Veinot T. Recommendations for health equity and virtual care arising from the COVID-19 pandemic: narrative review. JMIR Form Res. 2021;5(4):e23233.

Singh S, Chang O, Funk M, Shields L, Andrews A, Hughes F, Drew N. WHO Profile on mental health in development (WHO proMIND). 2013.

Snoswell CL, Caffery LJ, Haydon HM, Thomas EE, Smith AC. Telehealth uptake in general practice as a result of the coronavirus (COVID-19) pandemic. Aust Health Rev. 2020;44(05):737–40.

Stewart MA. Effective physician-patient communication and health outcomes: a review. CMAJ Can Med Assoc J Assoc Medicale Can. 1995;152(9):1423–33.

Tannenbaum SI, Traylor AM, Thomas EJ, et al. Managing teamwork in the face of pandemic: evidence-based tips. BMJ Quality Safety. 2021;30:59–63.

Torres Silva A, Uribe S, Smith J, Felipe I, Gomez L, Fernando Florez-Arango J, et al. XML data and knowledge-encoding structure for a web-based and mobile antenatal clinical decision support system: development study. JMIR [Internet] 2020 [cited 2021 Apr 16];4(10).

Webster P. Virtual health care in the era of COVID-19. Lancet. 2020;395(10231):1180–1.

Wessel L, Baiyere A, Ologeanu-Taddei R, Cha J, Blegind JT. Unpacking the difference between digital transformation and IT-enabled organizational transformation. J Assoc Inf Syst. 2021;22(1):6.

Whiteford HA, Degenhardt L, Rehm J, et al. Global burden of disease attributable to mental and substance use disorders: findings from the Global Burden of Disease Study 2010. Lancet. 2013;382:1575–86.

Wittenberg E, Goldsmith JV, Chen C, Prince-Paul M, Johnson RR. Opportunities to improve COVID-19 provider communication resources: a systematic review. Patient Educ Couns. 2021;104(3):438–51.

Xyrichis A, Williams U. Strengthening health systems response to COVID-19: interprofessional science rising to the challenge. J Interprof Care. 2020;34(5):577–79.

Zeitvogel K. Focus on suicide: research boosts mental health task-shifting, innovative approaches. NIH Fogarty Foundation Newsletter; 2018.

Chapter 2
Direct Primary Care: A New Model for Patient-Centered Care

Jane L. Snowdon, Sasha E. Ballen, Daniel Gruen, Thomas A. Gagliardi, Judy George, Yoonyoung Park, Issa Sylla, Bedda Rosario, George Kim, Ching-Hua Chen, and Marion Ball

J. L. Snowdon (✉) · J. George · B. Rosario
Center for AI, Research and Evaluation, IBM Watson Health, Cambridge, MA, USA
e-mail: snowdonj@us.ibm.com; judy.george@ibm.com; brosario@ibm.com;
https://www.linkedin.com/in/snowdonjane/;
https://www.linkedin.com/in/judy-george-62897122/;
https://www.linkedin.com/in/bedda-rosario-6439b41/

S. E. Ballen
Information Technology, R-Health Inc., Elkins Park, PA, USA
e-mail: sasha.ballen@eversidehealth.com; https://www.linkedin.com/in/sasha-ballen-448a378/

D. Gruen
Gruen Design Research LLC, Newton, MA, USA
e-mail: dan@grudr.com; https://www.grudr.com

T. A. Gagliardi
School of Medicine, New York Medical College, Valhalla, NY, USA
e-mail: tgagliar@student.nymc.edu;
https://www.linkedin.com/in/thomas-gagliardi-748393142/

Y. Park · I. Sylla
Center for Computational Health, IBM Research, Cambridge, MA, USA
e-mail: yoonyoung.park@ibm.com; issa.sylla@ibm.com; https://www.linkedin.com/in/
yoonyoung-park-48a1591b/; https://www.linkedin.com/in/issa-sylla13/

G. Kim
Division of Health Sciences Informatics, The Johns Hopkins School of Medicine,
Baltimore, MD, USA
e-mail: gkim9@jhmi.edu; https://www.linkedin.com/in/george-kim-58249131/

C.-H. Chen
Center for Computational Health, IBM T. J. Watson Research Center,
Yorktown Heights, NY, USA
e-mail: chinghua@us.ibm.com; https://www.linkedin.com/in/chinghuachen/

M. Ball
Multi-Interprofessional Center for Health Informatics, The University of Texas at Arlington,
Arlington, TX, USA
e-mail: marion.ball@uta.edu; https://www.linkedin.com/in/
marion-j-ball-edd-flhimss-fchime-faan-facmi-08322b131/

© The Author(s), under exclusive license to Springer Nature
Switzerland AG 2022
P.-Y. S. Hsueh et al. (eds.), *Personal Health Informatics*, Cognitive Informatics
in Biomedicine and Healthcare, https://doi.org/10.1007/978-3-031-07696-1_2

Abstract The goal of Primary Care is the optimization of individual and population health through timely, evidence-based care and prevention at the lowest cost. Direct Primary Care (DPC) is a compelling ambulatory practice model that aims to remove patient barriers to access and provide timely and personalized preventive and first-line care for a fixed periodic fee per patient or as a no-additional-cost option in employer-based health insurance programs. DPC's success and sustainability in different patient populations, care/community settings and physician practice configurations is of growing clinical practice and business research interest, particularly with respect to understanding which features (disease, social determinants of health) increase patient engagement in preventive care services (PCS) when access barriers (enrollment costs, co-pays, communication, distance) are removed. This chapter reviews literature about DPC and describes the shift occurring between patients-providers-payers and the associated impact on healthcare's future. Mixed-methods scientific qualitative (interviews, surveys) and quantitative (descriptive, predictive, and prescriptive analytics) techniques are described. The role of information and communications technologies (ICT) in improving care and its quality for both patients and practitioners are explored. Select results from R-Health Inc., a DPC practice, illustrate the major advantages of timely access, effectiveness (e.g. care coordination, preventive care), patient-centered, and efficiency/affordability.

Keywords Primary health care · Health informatics · Mathematical computing · Machine learning · Information technology · Evaluation studies · Data science

Learning Objectives
1. Define Direct Primary Care (DPC) as a practice and payment model and list characteristics that distinguish it from a Patient Centered Medical Home (PCMH) and other forms of primary care.
2. State the Quadruple Aim of Healthcare Improvement and how DPC attempts to address it for different healthcare stakeholders (patients, physicians, employers).
3. Describe the distinctions between qualitative and quantitative clinical data in terms of availability, quality (completeness, correctness, currency) study, and insights that may be gained with respect to assessing the quality and value of healthcare.
4. Describe benefits and limitations of qualitative methodologies. Explain how a semi-structured interview can be created and used to obtain information on physician motivations, processes, and satisfaction with DPC and other care models.
5. Describe benefits and limitations of quantitative methodologies. Explain how descriptive, predictive, and prescriptive analytics can be used to obtain insights into influential factors for engaging and retaining patients in a DPC care model.

Primary Care, the Patient-Centered Medical Home, and Direct Primary Care

Primary Care

Primary Care (PC) is comprehensive first contact and continuity medical care for patients. PC is performed by a personal physician or team that works in collaboration with other health professionals to address and optimize patient health through prevention and cost-effective management and coordination, in partnership with patients and caregivers. PC services include health promotion, disease prevention, health maintenance, counseling, patient education and advocacy, diagnosis, and treatment of acute and chronic illness.

A Primary Care Practice (PCP) is a patient's traditional entry point into healthcare (American Academy of Family Practice 2020a). Tasks of PC include care coordination, disease prevention and management, health maintenance, and patient education of patients, families and related stakeholders. PC is principally ambulatory, but may include urgent, emergency and/or inpatient care. PC is typically provided by family practitioners, internists, pediatricians, obstetricians/gynecologists and/or geriatricians, but may be provided by specialists where a patient's care may be complex (such as in cancer care) (Howley 2020).

A key component of assuring the quality of primary care is through regular measurement of its safety, effectiveness, timeliness, efficiency, equity, and patient-centeredness. The Quadruple Aim of improving healthcare quality is the continuous effort to: (a) improve the patient experience of care, (b) reduce per capita costs, (c) improve population health, and (d) improve the work experience of providers (Berwick et al. 2008; Bodenheimer and Sinsky 2014).

Patient Centered Medical Home

The Patient Centered Medical Home (PCMH) is a healthcare organization that provides, organizes, and delivers PC that is comprehensive, patient-centered, coordinated, accessible, and of the highest quality and safety (AHRQ, HHS 2021). The PCMH is based on a foundation of the use of certified health information technology, a strong primary care workforce, and adequate payment for services. PCMHs are accredited by the Health Resources and Services Administration ((HRSA) and its contractors) of the US Department of Health and Human Services (HHS) through a program of periodic evaluation and (electronic) clinical quality metrics of patient outcomes (The Joint Commission 2021; HRSA 2018). Payment for PCMH services is linked through Medicare and other insurances. Rosenthal et al. (2016) assessed the quality, utilization, and cost of 15 small and medium-sized PCMHs in a multi-payer pilot in Colorado.

Payment for health care has traditionally been based on fee-for-service (FFS), where remuneration is based on specific services and encounters (Healthcare.gov

2021a). Recent transition has been to value-based-payments (VBP), where remuneration is based on overall performance (pay-for-performance, utilization, and outcomes) of a healthcare provider for a given population of patients over time (Healthcare.gov 2021b). Other forms of payment for health services include capitation/managed care (Alexander et al. 2005) and subscription services (Alguire 2021).

Direct Primary Care

Direct Primary Care (DPC) is a practice and payment model for ambulatory care where patients/consumers pay a periodic retainer fee for access to a defined set of PC and administrative services (American Academy of Family Physicians 2018). It replaces third-party insurance and fee-for-service billing. Patients/consumers carry other insurance for non-covered services, such as specialty care, emergency, and hospital services (American Academy of Family Practice 2020b). Covered DPC services include but are not limited to routine care, regular checkups, preventive care, and care coordination (Roberts-Grey 2020).

DPC payments are a flat monthly or annual fee per patient, paid *directly* to the practice, which may come from a group (such as an employer) that has contracted for DPC (as part of a menu of health insurance products) for its constituents. This revenue model marked reducing uncompensated administrative burdens and costs, stabilizing practice finances, and freeing physicians and staff from coding and billing tasks.

DPC practice affords physicians more time for tasks *directly* related to patient care. In contrast to fee-for-service, which incentivizes large patient panels and shorter visits, DPC reverses this paradigm, allowing smaller patient panels and encouraging continuous, personalized, and comprehensive care. Because DPC fees cover the direct cost of services, patient access barriers to physicians are removed.

DPC arose from a collective effort to (a) improving patient experience of care, (b) reducing its per capita cost, and (c) improving the work life of healthcare providers (Mutter et al. 2018). Decoupling the assigned value of single interactions from the overall value of longitudinal primary care enables providers to support long-term health goals and quality improvement for individuals and populations. The DPC model can provide benefits to the many stakeholders involved.

DPC is not a single model. One version (1) consists of individual and family memberships, paid by the individuals directly to the practice on a monthly or annual basis. Another (2) consists of contracts between an employer who typically provides a self-funded insurance product to its employees and a DPC provider organization, giving access to DPC services for the employee population (and their families). In either case, the practice must charge a periodic fee and not participate in third-party fee-for-service (FFS) billing (Eskew and Klink 2015). A DPC provider may practice embodying either model or a combination of the two. The third implementation of DPC not explored here involves a "hybrid" approach, wherein a practice sees one subset of patients under a traditional FFS arrangement and another subset in a DPC capacity.

- Example of (1): An independent practice with extremely low overhead may effectively provide primary care services to a small panel of patients. The primary indicator of quality and value is member retention.
- Example of (2): In an employer-contracted membership, the employer is the purchaser on behalf of its enrolled workforce (the members). An employer with a large or geographically diverse population will usually work with a larger DPC organization to provide local service to its employees.

In an employer-contracted membership, the healthcare consumer is separate from the entity paying for the service. The employer may be providing the DPC membership for a variety of reasons, including valuing the role of primary care in lowering costs and improving outcomes, seeking to improve the long-term prognosis of employees with chronic conditions, or wanting to lower absenteeism by providing frictionless and timely access to a DPC physician. In this scenario, the employer naturally wants a precise evaluation of their return on investment. Metrics that indicate quality (effectiveness of care and utilization) are typically derived from claims data (Patient-Centered Primary Care Collaborative 2019). A DPC practice is, by definition, not billing third-parties on a fee-for-service basis, so the incentive to maintain the considerable overhead of a billing staff is diminished.

Herein lies a fundamental conundrum of changing paradigms in a large, complex, and bureaucratic system. In order to be a viable option for meeting the Quadruple Aim on a national scale, DPC must demonstrate its ability to deliver superior care and save money compared to traditional FFS care. Realistically, it will be the larger DPC organizations that have the organizational infrastructure to meet traditional expectations of coding and claims submission while still maintaining the philosophical intent behind the program. Submitting claims for quality purposes, without payment expectations, is a well-worn path in other capitated models. It will enable a fair and risk-adjusted comparison of a DPC population with a cohort receiving primary care in the FFS world. Documenting, coding, and submitting claims continue to divert healthcare dollars from clinical care to questionably valuable administrative work. This is a challenge in the DPC model. The many clinically oriented interactions between provider and patients facilitated in the DPC environment are not captured by the claims data. It will be up to the DPC community to determine how best to demonstrate the value and effect of these healthcare nudges.

Accreditation Process

DPC does not have a specified structure or accreditation process, such as the one that exists for the PCMH as summarized in Table 2.1. As DPC practices are outside of insurance payments (including Medicare/Medicaid), regulatory overhead and

Table 2.1 Patient centered medical home and direct primary care comparison

Aspect	PCMH	DPC
Name	Patient centered medical home	Direct primary care
Practice	Comprehensive	Primary care
Certification	HRSA and contractors	None
Insurance coverage	Comprehensive, through CMS and commercial	None required, but linked to comprehensive coverage
Clinical model	Team-based care with a defined network of practitioners and resources	Provider-led with supportive community and embedded resources
Practitioners	Internal medicine, pediatrics, family practice, Ob/Gyn, geriatrics, some specialty services	Principally family practice
Payment model	Value-based payment, flexible	Subscription, not fee-for-service
Use of health IT	Mandated; focus on EHR technology	Not mandated; not specified
Quality measures	Defined, including electronic clinical quality measures (eCQM)	Flexible to DPC structure

paperwork are much reduced. An area of interest is how to define and measure the quality and impact of DPC practices. Limitations include small sample sizes, lack of existing quality measures, data quality and variability in DPC practices and their patient populations (Busch et al. 2020).

Experience of the Patient and Provider

No matter the version of DPC in play, the model's core expects an enduring relationship between patient and provider. This relationship is built upon a foundation of three practice-side necessities: (1) Ample provider time for each patient, (2) Provider financial terms that incentivize long-term patient health and not volume of care, (3) Provider incentives to promote patient satisfaction and positive patient experience.

Ample provider time for direct patient care can be supported in two ways: reducing the overall number of patients in the panel and reducing the non-clinical burdens on providers. In a small independent DPC practice that focuses on individual memberships, the feedback loop is very efficient. Their membership will dwindle if a provider does not create an attentive, responsive, and clinically supportive environment. Larger DPC organizations with a less direct feedback loop are served by well-considered physician compensation structures and executing thoughtful contracts with customers.

Critics suggest that DPC will exacerbate the physician shortage by reducing the overall number of patients seen by a DPC provider (Weisbart 2016). The PCP shortage is driven by the extremely high burnout rates of PCPs practicing in an unreasonable FFS model of care coupled with a paucity of new doctors choosing primary care for fear of professional burnout (DeChant et al. 2019). There is no shortage of medical students interested in practicing primary care, so as career paths with a higher likelihood of professional satisfaction become available, more providers will choose primary care than currently do.

The experience of the patient is notable for the initial reconfiguration of expectations that must occur. Prior to joining a DPC practice, many patients have received their care in a traditional PCP office, or from urgent care, the emergency department, or specialists. Although the very definition of Primary Care includes continuity and prevention, the reality for many patients is minimal time with a PCP, and many barriers to direct access of that provider. Coordination between specialists is often fractured or non-existent. Without a PCP who has the time and incentive to "quarterback" complex chronic issues, patient care suffers. Once a patient is part of a DPC practice, there is often a need for significant education around the reasonable (and often heightened) expectations for primary care.

There is no single type of patient who most benefits from DPC. Providing DPC care to patients with chronic conditions supports the most prominent and immediate need. People with one or more poorly controlled chronic conditions often have looming health crises that may be averted by behavioral or lifestyle changes. DPC allows this category of patient to receive the focused attention of a provider trained to understand, educate, and motivate them. However, since an individual's interaction with the healthcare system is ultimately inevitable, long-term health and wellness can be effectively supported by the early adoption of regular preventive care. Providing everyone with access to effective primary care establishes the expectations and behaviors that will support people throughout their lives.

Direct primary care has been shown to reduce costs, increase health outcomes, support patient activation and health literacy and reduce provider burnout. Examples are given in (Huff 2015; Eskew and Klink 2015; Pofeldt 2016; Chappell 2017; Carlasare 2018; Breen et al. 2019; Pierce and Pierce 2020; Kauffman 2020; Busch et al. 2020).

The Patient-Provider-Payer Shift

Global forces and the COVID-19 pandemic have disrupted the status quo in healthcare. Four shifts are happening between patients, providers, and payers that will impact healthcare in the future.

First, a data explosion is taking place in healthcare amidst an industry-wide push for interoperability. The volume, velocity, and types of data (real-world, genomic, social, and patient-generated from wearables, etc.) are growing exponentially across the healthcare ecosystem. Rising patient and ecosystem expectations combined with new regulatory requirements are calling for better management and secure exchange of data while maintaining privacy governance.

Second, innovations in technology and patient-centricity are shifting care paradigms and driving digital transformation. Innovations in data and information technology (IT) are making care delivery more intelligent and autonomous through the use of artificial intelligence (AI), mobile devices and wearables, chatbots, and personalized clinical decision support. Virtual healthcare through telemedicine and remote patient monitoring is becoming more mainstream in response to the COVID-19 pandemic.

Third, consolidation and disruption are driving the transformation of business and operating models between payers and providers. A shift toward value-priced "payviders" is occurring with mega-mergers (e.g., CVS/Aetna, Optum/Davita, and Cigna/Express Scripts), the rise of retail clinics (e.g., CVS, Walmart), and nontraditional entrants (e.g., Amazon).

Finally, scarce resources and fluctuating demand are driving a relentless focus on cost reduction, quality, and access. Provider accountability is shifting from fee-for-service to outcomes improvement. Lower-cost care alternatives such as the direct primary care (DPC) model give family physicians an alternative to fee-for-service insurance billing, typically by charging patients a fixed fee that covers most primary care services and, in return, the patient receives improved access to and quality of care. Rising awareness of inequity of care across racial and socioeconomic groups is also pivoting focus to the quality of care for all.

The Implications for DPC in Practice

The implications of these shifts for DPC in practice are putting humanity back into medicine by taking a holistic, patient-focused approach with a focus on prevention and social determinants of health (SDoH). Hills-Briggs et al. (2020) show SDoH evidence supporting associations of socio-economic status, neighborhood and physical environment, nutrition, health care, and social context with diabetes-related outcomes in their scientific review. Nielsen (2019) and Tou et al. (2020) describe the needs and challenges for incorporating behavioral health and SDoH in DPC and other models. Zulman et al. (2020) and Davis et al. (2020) examine Veterans Affairs patients and the relationship of patient-reported social and behavioral determinants on health on estimated risk of hospitalization and emergency department utilization, respectively.

Superior human-to-human connections, or patient-provider communications (PPC), can lead to better outcomes and are especially important in pandemics to address isolation and mental health issues. Digital health innovation and technologies can reduce strain on physicians and help to ensure more timely, safe, and effective access for patients. The PCP and patient are free to communicate in the most effective manner for the individual situation. Sun et al. (2019a, b) model the personas of communication modality usage in a DPC practice. Okunrintemi et al. (2017) show a strong relationship between PPC and patient-reported outcomes, utilization of evidence-based therapies, healthcare resource utilization, and expenditures among those with established atherosclerotic cardiovascular disease. Laurance et al. (2014) report the positive impact of PPC in four global case studies: online mental health, follow-through on genetics screening, obstetrics, and a hospital-based patient engagement program. Finney Rutten et al. (2015) confirm the importance of PPC in shaping patients' ratings of care quality. Several studies describe the improvement PPC has in follow-through with cancer screenings and differences among various socio-cultural groups (Kindratt et al. 2020a, b; Jacob et al. 2012; Carcaise-Edinboro and Bradley 2008).

Mixed Methods Research Methodology

This section covers the topics of mixed methods research including qualitative and quantitative methods, data types, and data quality. Mixed methods research refers to a methodology that combines, or "mixes," quantitative and qualitative data in a scientific evaluation study (Tashakkori and Teddlie 1998, 2003). The integration of quantitative and qualitative approaches within a single evaluation can permit a more synergistic analysis of the data, suggest topics for further understanding and probing, confirm results, and unlock the value of the combined data compared with performing either approach independently. Evaluation of a DPC using mixed methods contributes to learning about best practices around effectiveness in achieving the quadruple aim outcomes of timely access, the effectiveness of care coordination and preventive care, patient experience of care, and efficiency.

Qualitative Methods

Qualitative research can serve a helpful purpose in evaluating primary care where important clinical messages may come from individuals of varying interprofessional backgrounds. Qualitative research investigates phenomena through an in-depth, holistic fashion, often involving a collection of rich narrative materials (Moser and Korstjens 2017, Korstjens and Moser 2018). Qualitative studies can give insights into the underlying factors—the "why"—behind statistical regularities seen in the data. The key to this approach is gaining a deep understanding of people's experiences, perceptions, and behaviors within the natural context of the phenomena being examined (Moser and Korstjens 2017; Thomas 2006; Britten et al. 1995).

Qualitative research questions tend to be broad to prompt reflection and preserve openness to unexpected findings (Korstjens and Moser 2017). Designs generally fall into the "big three" categories of qualitative research: ethnography—the study of culture within a society; phenomenology—a guided study of an experience; and grounded theory—the construction of theory from data collected (Korstjens and Moser 2017).

Participant observation, in-depth interviews, and focus group discussions are commonly used qualitative techniques (Moser and Korstjens 2018). Only certain techniques of observations, interviews, and focus groups are appropriate to use within each category. The data collected by those techniques have different weights and uses in analysis within each of those categories.

As an example, we conducted a series of semi-structured interviews with providers to understand their motivations for switching to a DPC practice and the extent to which they felt that their expectations had been realized, their patient facing goals, their overall work routines, what challenges they faced, their information needs, their perceptions of their patient panel and which patients benefit most from a DPC model of care. We also asked about their daily routines and the other people with whom they worked, and their impressions and relationship with their broader organization. A semi-structured interview aims to ensure that all desired topics are probed while allowing for a natural flow so topics can be pursued naturally as they arise, without artificially constraining the conversation to only the topics and ordering in the researcher's preconceived script. The ability for new and unanticipated themes to arise and be explored is an important feature of qualitative methodologies and can be especially valuable at early stages of an exploration (Braun and Clarke 2006, Campbell et al. 2013).

Interviews are typically recorded (after obtaining subjects' consent) and are often transcribed, either manually or with the assistance of speech-to-text software. Grounded theory methodologies can then be employed, providing a principled way for themes and insights to arise and be culled from the interview transcripts (Korstjens and Moser 2017).

Because of the commitment of time required, such studies typically involve a relatively small set of subjects and thus can lack the statistical significance of a large-scale data study or broadly cast survey. Nevertheless, what they lack in statistical significance is often more than made up for in the depth and breadth of understanding they provide, especially in new and complex settings. Direct primary care settings present an opportunity to research human and social phenomena that are unique to this novel model of care delivery.

Quantitative Methods

Quantitative methods for data analysis are commonly organized into the following four categories: (1) descriptive analyses, (2) predictive analyses, (3) diagnostic analyses, and (4) prescriptive analyses (Banerjee et al. 2013). Generally, these categories reflect the purpose of the analysis rather than the models or methods that may be used. Table 2.2 provides examples of the types of questions that each of these types of analyses intends to support.

Table 2.2 Examples of questions that different types of analysis could address

Analysis category	Exemplary questions
Descriptive	• What proportion of patients received their flu shot this month? • What are frequent patterns/modes of communication between patients and providers? • What is the distribution of wait-times for appointments?
Predictive	• What is the risk of complications for this diabetic patient? • How likely is it that this patient has asthma?
Diagnostic	• Could greater access to primary care lead to fewer visits to the emergency department? • Could greater access to primary care lead to increased use of colon cancer screening?
Prescriptive	• What medication(s) should I prescribe to this patient? • What is the ideal panel size for this population of patients?

Descriptive statistics describe the nature of quantitative data, and these statistics form the basis of descriptive analyses. Readers are referred to Spriestersbach et al. (2009) for a comprehensive overview of descriptive statistics.

The goal of predictive analytics in primary care is to forecast events in advance based on historical patterns to provide insights for patient triage, diagnostic or treatment decisions, resource allocation, and population health management (Lin et al. 2019, Rajkomar et al. 2019, Kang et al. 2021). Recent examples of predictive analytic applications in the primary care domain range from cardiovascular diseases risk prediction (Weng et al. 2017) to diabetes management (Dankwa-Mullan et al. 2019), asthma diagnosis (Daines et al. 2019), improving operating room efficiency (Bartek et al. 2019), and patient decision support, to name just a few (Wallace et al. 2016, Cabitza et al. 2017, Oude Nijeweme-d'Hollosy et al. 2018).

Diagnostic analyses are more narrowly focused on identifying causal relationships between data variables so that potential root cause issues can be targeted with an intervention. In section "Timely Access", we described how qualitative methods could be used to investigate "why" certain observed events may have occurred. If appropriate observational data are available, there are also quantitative methods for estimating whether certain events or factors could have caused certain other events. Listl et al. (2016), Mackay (2003), Cawley (2015), and Lechner (2011) provide accessible overviews of these causal inference methods, along with their limitations.

Finally, prescriptive analyses are used to produce specific recommended actions that a relevant stakeholder could take. In the primary care setting, prescriptive analyses are often used to address challenges related to improving patient access to care. Gupta and Wang (2008) and Qu et al. (2015) use Markov Decision Process (MDP) models to identify policies, or rules, that specify the circumstances under which to accept walk-ins and when to schedule or re-schedule appointments. For a systematic review of approaches used to determine provider panel sizes in primary care, the reader is referred to Shekelle et al. (2019). Examples of panel size optimization efforts include Balasubramanian et al. (2007), Murray et al. (2007), Green and Sergei (2008), and Raffoul et al. (2016). A recent, novel application of prescriptive analytics in primary care was proposed by Tang et al. (2021) for recommending more personalized treatment options for patients with chronic disease.

Qualitative and quantitative methods can complement each other to provide a complete and accurate understanding of real-world phenomena. The selection of subjects and topics to study can be informed by quantitative data, while insights gleaned from in-depth qualitative methods can often be informed or verified through quantitative analyses to see how consistent they are across a broader population.

Data Types

Data in a healthcare setting can refer to information about individual patients and population cohorts. Advanced data and analytic tools can help healthcare providers make more informed diagnoses and care plans, and allow administrators to more effectively allocate resources, control costs, and understand linkages to patient outcomes. Healthcare data can be categorized into the following types: electronic health records (EHR), administrative insurance claims and billing, communication (metadata about patient-provider communication, telehealth, surveys, interviews), and standardized clinical data for reporting, for example, to Medicare or other regulatory agencies.

Data Quality

The emergence of data environments with growing data volume, velocity, variety, veracity, and value creates a greater need for organizations to be supported by processes and technologies to produce and maintain high-quality data facilitating reuse, accessibility, analysis, validation of research findings, and long-term preservation. Organizations strive for complete, valid, accurate, timely, uniform, and organized data that is consistent. Higher quality data leads to better insights that can be used to make more informed decisions.

Data cleansing, or data cleaning, is the process of detecting and correcting (or removing) duplicate, conflicting, irrelevant, corrupt, inaccurate, or invalid observations from a database. The interested reader is referred to the following publications for an in-depth treatment of this topic (Cai and Zhu 2015; Ridzuan and Zainon 2019; Liu et al. 2015; Osborne and Overbay 2004; Kwak and Kim 2017; Kang 2013; Schafer and Graham 2002; Barnett 1983).

Data cleaning has several benefits and challenges. Benefits include improved decision making and increased productivity. Challenges include limited available information and knowledge about the cause of data anomalies, and data cleaning maintenance may be time-consuming and expensive.

Results can be corrupted if either actual outliers are not removed from the data set or if valid data is identified as an outlier and is removed in error. Additionally, bias may be introduced to skew the data to influence the outcome (this can go either way, i.e., lead to rejection of null hypothesis or overestimation of association).

Results

This section presents selected results from R-Health, an ambulatory care organization that offers preferred provider organization (PPO) plan subscribers the option to participate in DPC at no additional cost, to illustrate the four major advantages of DPC: timely access, effectiveness (care coordination, preventive care), patient-centered, and efficiency/affordability.

Timely Access

R-Health explored telehealth usage pre- and post- COVID-19 pandemic in their DPC practice. Prior to March 2020, before U.S. state governments began to declare states-of-emergencies due to the COVID-19 pandemic, a majority (62.58%) of patient interactions including encounters for regular visits, preventative care services, testing, and counseling, occurred in person; virtual interactions such as virtual visits, outreach, email, and phone calls accounted for 37.42% of all interactions. During the 12 months leading up to March 1, 2020, on average, 34.16% (standard deviation (SD) 1.99) of interactions per month were conducted virtually. During this period, 35.42% of all interactions/month were specifically office visits, whereas only 8.88% were virtual visits. The total number of office visits (11,568) was greater than the total number of virtual interactions (11,194). As the pandemic forced physicians to limit the types of services provided in person, patients and providers turned to virtual care. Immediately after March 2020, virtual interactions replaced physical, in-office interactions as the predominant mode of receiving care. From March 1, 2020 to October 29, 2020, virtual interactions accounted for 70.875% of all interactions (SD 13.67), with nearly 90% of interactions in April and May being virtual. During these 8 months, virtual visits made up 37.04% of interactions, whereas office visits made up only 11.8%. Figure 2.1 provides a distribution pre- and post-COVID-19 pandemic for six diagnoses, which occurred through both in-office and virtual visits. These six diagnoses include anxiety disorder, hyperlipidemia, examination, vitamin D deficiency, essential (primary) hypertension, and type 2 diabetes mellitus. In the 6 months post-March 1, 2020, a larger proportion of diagnoses were made virtually, reflecting a shift from the traditional source of diagnosis, in-office, prior to the pandemic. During the 6 months before the pandemic, 21% (n = 111) of anxiety disorder (F41.9), 14% (112) of

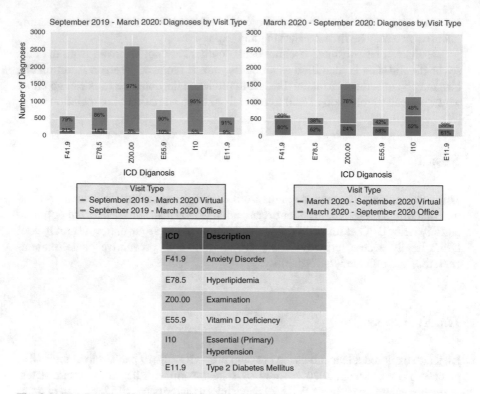

Fig. 2.1 Distribution of in-office and virtual visits 6 months pre-and post-COVID-19 pandemic for six prevalent diagnoses

hyperlipidemia (E78.5), 10% (74) of vitamin D deficiency (E55.9), 5% (68) of hypertension (I10), and 9% (47) of type 2 diabetes diagnoses (E11.9) were made virtually. During the pandemic, 80% (482) of anxiety disorder, 62% (329) of hyperlipidemia, 58% (303) of vitamin D Deficiency, 52% (610) of hypertension and 61% (225) of type 2 diabetes diagnoses were made virtually. R-Health's telemedicine service ensured providers could diagnose their patients and patients adapted quickly to this form of care.

Effectiveness

Sun et al. (2019a, b) explored patients' utilization of different direct and mediated communication modalities at R-Health and the patient characteristics that predict their communication behavior patterns. Based on this knowledge, they developed two patient personas that explicate the nuances of patients who tend to prefer visiting the clinic in person versus those who use mediated modalities more often. The results suggest that patients and their health team alike may be incentivized to adopt and utilize multi-modality communication in a DPC setting voluntarily.

Snowdon et al. (2020a) conducted a descriptive study to compare primary care quality (PCQ) metrics from EHR and claims data with similar populations benchmarked by the Agency for Healthcare Research and Quality's National Healthcare Quality and Disparities Reports (AHRQ-NHQDR) (Agency for Healthcare Research and Quality (AHRQ) (2015)), the Centers for Disease Control and Prevention's Behavioral Risk Factor Surveillance System (CDC-BRFSS) (Centers for Disease Control and Prevention (2017)), and the Office of Disease Prevention and Health Promotion's Healthy People 2020 (Centers for Disease Control and Prevention (2014)). A retrospective study of patients enrolled in R-Health's DPC practice from October 2016 to November 2019 was conducted to determine how well DPC patients met or exceeded state and national benchmark data. Data were stratified into three primary care cohorts: all patients, patients enrolled for 1 year or more, and engaged patients who were enrolled for at least 1 year and received care from R-Health. PCQ metrics were chosen based initially on National Quality Forum's validated measures and then mapped to benchmarks for comparisons. PCQ metrics were collected using CPT/ICD-9/ICD-10 codes from claims and EHR data for breast, cervical, and colorectal cancer screenings, cholesterol recordings, emergency department visits, and others. For the 7040 DPC patients retrospectively studied, analysis of nine adult PCQ metrics showed R-Health exceeded 55.5% of state and national benchmarks. Secondary analysis across all metrics indicated engaged patients had higher use of preventive services than patients in the other two categories, reflecting the desired aims of the R-Health DPC model. This study provided contemporary, real-word evidence on how DPC may serve as a viable model to support prevention goals set by select AHRQ, CDC, and Healthy People 2020 benchmarks.

Sylla et al. (2020) present an interactive, visual analytics tool for understanding the composition of a patient's network of providers and how these providers collaborate. The tool uses the power of network analytics to decrypt very complex and dynamic relationships between care delivery and outcomes. Network science offers both descriptive and prescriptive methods, enabling users to graph and analyze historical and real-time data to not only understand current system states, but also simulate different configurations. Networks can be optimized across various metrics and reconfigured to ensure every patient is paired with the necessary composition of caregivers based on the patient's conditions and health requirements. Users can employ the tool to automatically build, view, and analyze patient-sharing provider networks. Insights gleaned from R-Health's DPC practice included an understanding of referral patterns and specialty service utilization. Specialty services were utilized on average by 499 patients at approximately 12.2 visits per patient. Among the most strongly connected specialty pairs were Hospitalist-Radiology and Emergency Medicine-Radiology, indicating the types of providers who share the most patients and treat the same patients. The R-Health patient-provider has a low network density (0.08), meaning the network is not as connected as it can be. In the context of referrals, every patient is not seeing every specialist, which may suggest an added benefit of the DPC model—more efficient referrals.

Patient-Centered

Snowdon et al. (2020b) developed and tested six machine learning (Alpaydin 2021) models to predict patient and DPC practice features associated with utilization of preventive care visits (PCV) and preventive care screening (PCS) tests in a cohort of 3707 patients enrolled in DPC at R-Health for at least 1 year using electronic health record and administrative (claims/billing) data, and electronic provider-patient communication (e.g., secure email, phone, text messaging, mobile app) metadata. The Extreme Gradient Boost machine learning (Chen and Guestrin 2016) model had the highest performance for predicting ambulatory PCV (accuracy 0.86, F1 0.89), which is important for classifying which members would or would not obtain preventive care from R-Health providers using member and provider data as input features. Separate models were developed for predicting which members would receive preventive screening tests and then analyzed to identify members most likely to skip their recommended preventive visits and screening tests. Model accuracy for preventive screening tests were breast (0.92), colorectal (0.70), and cervical (0.66) cancers, and hemoglobin A1c (0.61). Explanatory factors extracted from models indicate PCS usage is most significantly associated with patient-provider communication, higher member age, and overall member health according to the Shapley additive explanation value (SHAP) (Lundberg and Lee 2017). DPC providers should consider increased and targeted communication efforts and targeting members in these categories to be more proactive with their preventive screenings.

Zhang et al. (2020) analyzed patient characteristics associated with preventable emergency department (ED) utilization among R-Health DPC enrollees. Practice EHR and external claims data were analyzed for diagnoses associated with ED visits for DPC patients. Chest pain was the most frequent principal diagnosis for DPC ED visits. A higher frequency of ED visits was associated with more extended DPC patient-provider interactions.

Efficiency/Affordability

Quantifying time demand for PCPs can help providers and health system managers optimize resource allocation. Park et al. (2020) used data from R-Health Inc. to estimate the future time demand and classify high-demand patients using machine learning. The predictive model could identify the top 20% patients in terms of time demand within the following year with >80% accuracy. This type of analysis can help hospitals plan and allocate resources for high demand patients, and also distribute burden across physicians and avoid physician burnout, which in turn positively affects patient-provider communication (Chung et al. 2020).

Conclusions, Implications, and Future Directions

Primary care can and should serve as a foundation for effective healthcare that spans an individual's lifetime and considers physical, mental, and social health and wellbeing (Zivin et al. 2010). In the United States, the intersection of technological advances, primary care shortages, and a global pandemic has highlighted the vast opportunity for improvement.

Healthcare must remake itself for the twenty-first century. The "new normal" includes information access, communication norms, and patient and provider expectations that were generally nonexistent in the last century. Information and data about health status, behaviors, and diagnostics are more readily available than ever before. The value of AI has come into focus, especially regarding patient outcomes and optimized experience for patients and healthcare workers alike. The COVID-19 pandemic has demonstrated that providers can deliver safe and effective primary care virtually. Combining an abundance of patient-generated data, ever more sophisticated clinically-oriented AI, and a wide variety of communication modalities will reshape the healthcare landscape. The healthcare industry must resist the urge to treat care delivery and primary care specifically as a business opportunity that can be endlessly optimized for maximum throughput and targeted referrals into the specialty care system.

Primary care occupies a significant and vital space in the healthcare arena. Over time, economic interests have unduly influenced this specific sector of the industry. While a fee-for-service approach is suitable for some types of healthcare, it is fundamentally at odds with the concept of supporting long-term health and prevention. The majority of a person's typical healthcare needs can be delivered in the primary care setting. Advancements in technology will undoubtedly bolster concurrent improvements in primary care. Still, care is ultimately provided by an individual capable of working with the patient on an ongoing basis to support the full spectrum of health and wellness-related needs.

In summary, in this chapter, the collective body of research studies described above employing both qualitative (interviews) and quantitative (descriptive, predictive, and prescriptive analytics) methods to uncover insights from complex healthcare delivery information (data and metadata from EHRs, claims and patient-provider communications) for R-Health has demonstrated that these enabling technologies are promising. Our results showed a DPC practice lowers patient access barriers to physicians and affords physicians more time for activities directly related to patient care. Our results also showed superior patient-provider communications can lead to better adherence to preventive screening test guidelines and outcomes. Our results showcased the importance of telemedicine and remote patient monitoring in traditional primary care and during acute events due to the COVID-19 pandemic. The future holds more opportunity for innovations in data and information technology to make care delivery more intelligent and autonomous through the use of artificial intelligence, mobile devices and wearables, multimodal communications including chatbots, and personalized clinical decision support.

Clinical Pearls
- A Direct Primary Care practice affords physicians more time for tasks <u>directly</u> related to patient care, in contrast to fee-for-service, which incentivizes large patient panels and shorter visits. DPC reverses this paradigm, allowing smaller patient panels and encouraging continuous, personalized, and comprehensive care, and because DPC fees cover the direct cost of services, patient access barriers to physicians are removed.
- Superior human-to-human connections, or patient-provider communications, can lead to better outcomes and are especially important in pandemics to address isolation and mental health issues.
- Telemedicine and remote patient monitoring are becoming more commonplace in traditional primary care, and not just for acute events, due to the COVID-19 pandemic, and these trends are expected to continue.
- Innovations in data and information technology are making care delivery more intelligent and autonomous through use of artificial intelligence, mobile devices and wearables, multimodal communications including chatbots, and personalized clinical decision support.

Chapter Review Questions
1. List characteristics of DPC that make it attractive to (a) individual patients and families, (b) practitioners, and (c) employer groups.
2. State the purpose of the Quadruple Aim and its four overarching goals.
3. How do aspects of direct primary care meet or not meet the Quadruple Aim for healthcare improvement for (a) providers and (b) patients?
4. What role do multi-modal communications (phone, email, text, video) play in patient outcomes?

Chapter Review Answers
1. Direct primary care is attractive to (a) individual patients and families for low (to no) cost and facilitated access to providers, personal relationship with practitioner; (b) practitioners for reduced patient panels and time to see patients and engage in knowing about patients; and (c) employer groups for low to fixed cost as a primary care/preventive service to employees.
2. The purpose of the Quadruple Aim is to guide the redesign and reform of healthcare systems and the transition to high-value care. The Quadruple aim has four overarching goals: improving the individual experience of care, improving the health of populations, reducing the per capita cost of healthcare, and improving the experience of providing care.
3. Direct primary care brings to (a) providers the time and incentive to focus on care and not administrative overhead and to (b) patients alternative modes of

access and timeliness and quality of care to meet the goals of the Quadruple Aim for healthcare improvement.
4. Superior patient-provider communications can lead to better outcomes and are especially important in pandemics to address isolation and mental health issues. Digital health innovation and technologies can reduce strain on physicians and help to ensure more timely, safe, effective, and alternative modes of access for patients. The primary care physician and patient are free to communicate in the most effective manner for the individual situation.

References

Agency for Healthcare Research and Quality (AHRQ). Measuring and Benchmarking Clinical Performance [Internet]. Rockville, MD; 2015, updated 2018. https://www.ahrq.gov/evidence-now/tools/primary-care-measuring.html. Accessed 26 Mar 2021.

AHRQ, HHS. Five key functions of a medical home, 2021. https://pcmh.ahrq.gov/page/5-key-functions-medical-home. Accessed 8 July 2021.

Alexander GC, Kurlander J, Wynia MK. Physicians in retainer ("concierge") practice. A national survey of physician, patient, and practice characteristics. J Gen Intern Med. 2005;20(12):1079–83.

Alguire PC. Residency career guidance: Understanding capitation 2021. https://www.acponline.org/about-acp/about-internal-medicine/career-paths/residency-career-counseling/guidance/understanding-capitation. Accessed 12 July 2021.

Alpaydin E. Machine learning, revised and updated edition. The MIT Press Essential Knowledge series. Cambridge, MA. 2021.

American Academy of Family Physicians. Data Brief. 2018 Direct Primary Care Study; 2018.

American Academy of Family Practice. Primary care; 2020a. https://www.aafp.org/about/policies/all/primary-care.html. Accessed 19 Mar 2021.

American Academy of Family Practice. Direct primary care. 2020b. https://www.aafp.org/about/policies/all/direct-primary-care.html. Accessed 19 Mar 2021.

Balasubramanian H, Banerjee R, Gregg M, Denton BT. Improving primary care access using simulation optimization. Winter Simulation Conference. 2007. Washington. p. 1494–500.

Banerjee A, Bandyopadhyay T, Acharya P. Data analytics: hyped up aspirations or true potential? Vikalpa. 2013;38(4):1–12.

Barnett V. Principles and methods for handling outliers in data sets. In: Wright T, editor. Statistical methods and the improvement of data quality. Academic; 1983. p. 131–66. https://doi.org/10.1016/B978-0-12-765480-5.50012-6.

Bartek MA, Saxena RC, Solomon S, Fong CT, Behara LD, Venigandla R, Velagapudi K, Lang JD, Nair BG. Improving operating room efficiency: machine learning approach to predict case-time duration. J Am Coll Surg. 2019;229(4):346–354.e3. https://doi.org/10.1016/j.jamcollsurg.2019.05.029.

Berwick DM, Nolan TW, Whittington J. The triple aim: care, health, and cost. Health Aff (Millwood). 2008;27(3):759–69. https://doi.org/10.1377/hlthaff.27.3.759

Bodenheimer T, Sinsky C. From triple to quadruple aim: care of the patient requires care of the provider. Ann Fam Med. 2014;12(6):573–6. https://doi.org/10.1370/afm.1713

Braun V, Clarke V. Using thematic analysis in psychology. Qual Res Psychol. 2006;3(2):77–101.

Breen JO, Blume GB, Adashi EY, Clodfelter RP, George P. Advantages and disadvantages of direct primary care. JAMA. 2019;321(2):207–8.

Britten N, Jones R, Murphy E, Stacy R. Qualitative research methods in general practice and primary care. Fam Pract. 1995;12(1):104–14. https://doi.org/10.1093/fampra/12.1.104.

Busch F, Grzeskowiak D, Huth E. Direct primary care: evaluating a new model of delivery and financing. Society of Actuaries, 2020. https://www.soa.org/globalassets/assets/files/resources/research-report/2020/direct-primary-care-eval-model.pdf. Accessed 12 July 2021.

Cabitza F, Rasoini R, Gensini GF. Unintended consequences of machine learning in medicine. JAMA. 2017;318(6):517–8. https://doi.org/10.1001/jama.2017.7797.

Cai L, Zhu Y. The challenges of data quality and data quality assessment in the big data era. Data Sci J. 2015;14(2):1–10. https://doi.org/10.5334/dsj-2015-002.

Campbell JL, Quincy C, Osserman J, Pedersen OK. Coding in-depth semistructured interviews: problems of unitization and intercoder reliability and agreement. Sociol Methods Res. 2013;42(3):294–320. https://doi.org/10.1177/0049124113500475.

Carcaise-Edinboro P, Bradley CJ. Influence of patient-provider communication on colorectal cancer screening. Med Care. 2008;46(7):738–45. https://doi.org/10.1097/MLR.0b013e318178935a.

Carlasare LE. Defining the place of direct primary care in a value-based care system. WMJ. 2018;17(3):106–10.

Cawley J. A selective review of the first 20 years of instrumental variables models in health-services research and medicine. J Med Econ. 2015;18(9):721–34. https://doi.org/10.311 1/13696998.2015.1043917.

Centers for Disease Control and Prevention. Healthy People 2020. March 13, 2014. https://wwwcdcgov/dhdsp/hp2020htm. Accessed 19 Mar 2021.

Centers for Disease Control and Prevention. Behavioral Risk Factor Surveillance System (CDC-BRFSS). Sept 22, 2017. https://www.cdc.gov/brfss/index.html. Accessed 19 Mar 2021.

Chappell GE. Healthcare's other big deal: direct primary care regulation in contemporary American health law. Duke Law J. 2017;66:1331–70.

Chen T, Guestrin C. XGBoost: a scalable tree boosting system. Proceedings of the 22nd ACM SIGKDD International Conference on Knowledge Discovery and Data Mining (KDD '16). 2016. p. 785–94.

Chung S, Dillon EC, Meehan AE, Nordgren R, Frosch DL. The relationship between primary care physician burnout and patient-reported care experiences: a cross-sectional study. J Gen Intern Med. 2020;35(8):2357–64.

Daines L, McLean S, Buelo A, Lewis S, Sheikh A, Pinnock H. Systematic review of clinical prediction models to support the diagnosis of asthma in primary care. NPJ Prim Care Respir Med. 2019;29(1):19. https://doi.org/10.1038/s41533-019-0132-z.

Dankwa-Mullan I, Rivo M, Sepulveda M, Park Y, Snowdon JL, Rhee K. Transforming diabetes care through artificial intelligence: the future is here. Popul Health Manag. 2019;22(3):229–42. https://doi.org/10.1089/pop.2018.0129.

Davis CI, Montgomery AE, Dichter ME, Taylor LD, Blosnich JR. Social determinants and emergency department utilization: findings from the veterans health administration. Am J Emerg Med. 2020;38(9):1904–9.

DeChant PF, Acs A, Rhee KB, Boulanger TS, Snowdon, JL, Tutty MA, Sinsky CA, Craig KJ. Effect of organization-directed workplace interventions on physician burnout: a systematic review. Mayo Clin Proc: Innov Qual Outcomes. 2019. https://doi.org/10.1016/j.mayocpiqo.2019.07.006

Eskew PM, Klink K. Direct primary care: practice distribution and cost across the nation. J Am Board Family Med. 2015;28(6):793–801.

Finney Rutten LJ, Agunwamba AA, Beckjord E, Hesse BW, Moser RP, Arora NK. The relation between having a usual source of care and ratings of care quality: does patient-centered communication play a role? J Health Commun. 2015;20(7):759–65. https://doi.org/10.108 0/10810730.2015.1018592.

Green LV, Sergei S. Reducing delays for medical appointments: a queueing approach. Oper Res. 2008;56(6):1526–38.

Gupta D, Wang L. Revenue management for a primary-care clinic in the presence of patient choice. Oper Res. 2008;56(3):576–92. https://doi.org/10.1287/opre.1080.0542.

Healthcare.gov. Glossary: Fee for service, 2021a. https://www.healthcare.gov/glossary/fee-for-service/. Accessed 12 July 2021.

Healthcare.gov. Glossary: Value-based purchasing, 2021b. https://www.healthcare.gov/glossary/value-based-purchasing-vbp/. Accessed 12 July 2021.

Hill-Briggs F, Adler NE, Berkowitz SA, Chin MH, Gary-Webb TL, Navas-Acien A, Thornton PL, Haire-Joshu D. Social determinants of health and diabetes: a scientific review. Diabetes Care. 2020;44(1):258–79. https://doi.org/10.2337/dci20-0053.

Howley EK. Types of primary care physicians: which doctor is right for you? US News and World Report, Nov 2020. https://health.usnews.com/health-care/top-doctors/articles/types-of-primary-care-doctors. Accessed 12 July 2021.

HRSA, HHS. HRSA Accreditation and patient-centered medical home recognition initiative, Aug 2018. https://bphc.hrsa.gov/qualityimprovement/clinicalquality/accreditation-pcmh/index.html. Accessed 8 July 2021.

Huff C. Direct primary care: concierge care for the masses. Health Aff. 2015:2016–2019.

Jacob BJ, Moineddin R, Sutradhar R, Baxter NN, Urbach DR. Effect of colonoscopy on colorectal cancer incidence and mortality: an instrumental variable analysis. Gastrointest Endosc. 2012;76(2):355–64.e1. https://doi.org/10.1016/j.gie.2012.03.247

Kang H. The prevention and handling of the missing data. Korean J Anesthesiol. 2013;64(5):402–6. https://doi.org/10.4097/kjae.2013.64.5.402.

Kang J, Hanif M, Mirza E, Khan MA, Malik M. Machine learning in primary care: potential to improve public health. J Med Eng Technol. 2021;45(1):75–80. https://doi.org/10.1080/03091902.2020.1853839.

Kauffman RD. Transitioning to direct primary care. Family Pract Manage. 2020:29–34.

Kindratt TB, Atem F, Dallo FJ, Allicock M, Balasubramanian BA. The influence of patient-provider communication on cancer screening. J Patient Exp. 2020a Dec;7(6):1648–57. https://doi.org/10.1177/2374373520924993.

Kindratt TB, Dallo FJ, Allicock M, Atem F, Balasubramanian BA. The influence of patient-provider communication on cancer screenings differs among racial and ethnic groups. Prev Med Rep. 2020b;2(18):101086. https://doi.org/10.1016/j.pmedr.2020.101086.

Korstjens I, Moser A. Series: practical guidance to qualitative research. Part 2: context, research questions and designs. Eur J Gen Pract. 2017;23(1):274–9. https://doi.org/10.1080/13814788.2017.1375090.

Korstjens I, Moser A. Series: practical guidance to qualitative research. Part 4: trustworthiness and publishing. Eur J Gen Pract. 2018;24(1):120–4. https://doi.org/10.1080/13814788.2017.1375092.

Kwak SK, Kim JH. Statistical data preparation: management of missing values and outliers. Korean J Anesthesiol. 2017;70(4):407–11. https://doi.org/10.4097/kjae.2017.70.4.407.

Laurance J, Henderson S, Howitt PJ, Matar M, Al Kuwari H, Edgman-Levitan S, Darzi A. Patient engagement: four case studies that highlight the potential for improved health outcomes and reduced costs. Health Aff (Millwood). 2014;33(9):1627–34. https://doi.org/10.1377/hlthaff.2014.0375.

Lechner M. The estimation of causal effects by difference-in-difference methods. Found Trends® Econometrics. 2011;4(3):165–224. https://doi.org/10.1561/0800000014.

Lin SY, Mahoney MR, Sinsky CA. Ten ways artificial intelligence will transform primary care. J Gen Intern Med. 2019;34:1626–30. https://doi.org/10.1007/s11606-019-05035-1.

Listl S, Jürges H, Watt RG. Causal inference from observational data. Community Dent Oral Epidemiol. 2016;44:409–15. https://doi.org/10.1111/cdoe.12231.

Liu J, Li J, Li W, Wu J. Rethinking big data: a review on the data quality and usage issues. ISPRS J. Photogrammetry Remote Sens. 2015;115. https://doi.org/10.1016/j.isprsjprs.2015.11.006

Lundberg SM, Lee SI. A unified approach to interpreting model predictions. 31st Conference on Neural Information Processing Systems (NIPS) 2017. Long Beach, CA.

Mackay DJC. Information theory, inference and learning algorithms. Cambridge: Cambridge University Press; 2003.

Moser A, Korstjens I. Series: practical guidance to qualitative research. Part 1: introduction. Eur J Gen Pract. 2017;23(1):271–3. https://doi.org/10.1080/13814788.2017.1375093.

Moser A, Korstjens I. Series: practical guidance to qualitative research. Part 3: sampling, data collection and analysis. Eur J Gen Pract. 2018;24(1):9–18. https://doi.org/10.1080/13814788.2017.1375091.

Murray M, Davies M, Boushon B. Panel size: how many patients can one doctor manage? Fam Pract Manag. 2007;14(4):44–51.

Mutter JB, Liaw W, Moore MA, Etz RS, Howe A, Bazemore A. Core principles to improve primary care quality management. J Am Board Fam Med. 2018;31(6):931–40. https://doi.org/10.3122/jabfm.2018.06.170172

Nielsen M. Direct primary care: where does integrated behavioral health fit? Fam Syst Health. 2019;37(3):255–9.

Okunrintemi V, Spatz ES, Di Capua P, Salami JA, Valero-Elizondo J, Warraich H, Virani SS, Blaha MJ, Blankstein R, Butt AA, Borden WB, Dharmarajan K, Ting II, Krumholz HM, Nasir K. Patient-provider communication and health outcomes among individuals with atherosclerotic cardiovascular disease in the United States: medical expenditure panel survey 2010 to 2013. Circ Cardiovasc Qual Outcomes. 2017;10(4):e003635. https://doi.org/10.1161/CIRCOUTCOMES.117.003635.

Osborne JW, Overbay A. The power of outliers (and why researchers should ALWAYS check for them). Pract Assess Res Eval. 2004;9:6. https://doi.org/10.7275/qf69-7k43

Oude Nijeweme-d'Hollosy W, van Velsen L, Poel M, Groothuis-Oudshoorn CGM, Soer R, Hermens H. Evaluation of three machine learning models for self-referral decision support on low back pain in primary care. Int J Med Inform. 2018;110:31–41. https://doi.org/10.1016/j.ijmedinf.2017.11.010.

Park Y, Sylla I, Ballen S, Das A. Estimating time demand for physicians in a direct primary care setting. American Medical Informatics Association (AMIA) 2020 Virtual Annual Symposium. November 14–18, 2020.

Patient-Centered Primary Care Collaborative. Investing in primary care 2019. https://www.pcpcc.org/sites/default/files/resources/pcmh_evidence_report_2019.pdf. Accessed 19 Mar 2021.

Pierce BR, Pierce C. Pandemic notes from a direct primary care practice. J Ambulatory Care Manage. 2020;43(4):290–3. https://doi.org/10.1097/JAC.0000000000000347

Pofeldt E. The rise of direct primary care. Med Econ. 2016:42–46.

Qu X, Peng Y, Shi J, LaGanga L. An MDP model for walk-in patient admission management in primary care clinics. Int J Prod Econ. 2015;168:303–20.

Raffoul M, Moore M, Kamerow D, Bazemore A. A primary care panel size of 2500 is neither accurate nor reasonable. Am J Am Board Family Med. 2016;29(4):496–9.

Rajkomar A, Dean J, Kohane I. Machine learning in medicine. N Engl J Med. 2019;380:1347–58. https://doi.org/10.1056/NEJMra1814259.

Ridzuan F, Zainon MNW. A review on data cleansing methods for big data. The Fifth Information Systems International Conference 2019. Procedia Computer Science. 2019;161:731–8. https://doi.org/10.1016/j.procs.2019.11.177

Roberts-Grey G. What Is direct primary care? A patient's guide to DPC. GoodRx, May 19, 2020. https://www.goodrx.com/insurance/direct-primary-care. Accessed 12 July 2021.

Rosenthal MB, Alidina S, Friedberg MW, Singer SJ, Eastman D, Li Z, Schneider EC. A difference-in-difference analysis of changes in quality, utilization and cost following the Colorado multipayer patient-centered medical home pilot. J Gen Intern Med. 2016;31(3):289–96. https://doi.org/10.1007/s11606-015-3521-1.

Schafer JL, Graham JW. Missing data: our view of the state of the art. Psychol Methods. 2002;7(2):147–77.

Shekelle PG, Paige NM, Apaydin EA, Goldhaber-Fiebert JD, Mak SS, Miake-Lye IM, Begashaw MM, Beroes-Severin JM. What is the optimal panel size in primary care? A systematic review. Washington: Department of Veterans Affairs (US); 2019. https://www.ncbi.nlm.nih.gov/books/NBK553674/

Snowdon JL, Bagchi S, George J, Jackson GP, Ballen S, Kim G, Ball M. Direct primary care: comparison of quality metrics to AHRQ, CDC, and Healthy People 2020 indicators. Values Health. 2020a;23(Suppl 1):S302–S303. https://doi.org/10.1016/j.jval.2020.04.1106

Snowdon JL, Chen CH, Kim G, George J, Gagliardi TA, Ball M, Ballen S, Bagchi S. Analysis of machine learning models and identification of factors for predicting care services usage in a direct primary care setting. 2020b. American Medical Informatics Association (AMIA) 2020 Virtual Annual Symposium. November 14–18, 2020.

Spriestersbach A, Röhrig B, du Prel JB, Gerhold-Ay A, Blettner M. Descriptive statistics: the specification of statistical measures and their presentation in tables and graphs. Part 7 of a series on evaluation of scientific publications. Dtsch Arztebl Int. 2009;106(36):578–83.

Sun S, Hsueh PY, Ballen S, Ball M. Modeling the personas of primary care communication modality usage: experiences from the R-health direct primary care model. In: Ohno-Machado L, Seroussi B, editors. 2019a. MEDINFO 2019: health and wellbeing e-networks for all. In: Proceedings of the 17th world congress on medical and health informatics. Lyon, France. 25–30 August 2019. Volume 264 of Studies in health technology and informatics. p. 818–23. IOS Press.

Sun S, Hsueh PS, Ballen S, Ball M. Modeling the personas of primary care communication modality usage: experiences from the R-Health direct primary care model. Stud Health Technol Inform. 2019b;21(264):818–23. https://doi.org/10.3233/SHTI190337.

Sylla I, Park Y, Ballen S, Das A. A visual analytics tool for understanding provider networks. American Medical Informatics Association (AMIA) 2020 Virtual Annual Symposium. November 14–18, 2020.

Tang PC, Miller S, Stavropoulos H, Kartoun U, Zambrano J, Ng K. Precision population analytics: population management at the point-of-care. J Am Med Inform Assoc. 2021;28(3):588–95.

Tashakkori A, Teddlie C. Mixed methodology: combining qualitative and quantitative approaches. Thousand Oaks, CA: Sage; 1998.

Tashakkori A, Teddlie C, editors. Handbook of mixed methods in social & behavioral research. Thousand Oaks, CA: Sage; 2003.

The Joint Commission. The accreditation Association for Ambulatory Health Care, the National Committee for quality assurance, 2021. https://www.jointcommission.org/accreditation-and-certification/. Accessed 8 July 2021.

Thomas DR. A general inductive approach for analyzing qualitative evaluation data. Am J Eval. 2006;27(2):237–46.

Tou LC, Prakash N, Jeyakumar SJ, Ravi S. Investigating social determinants of health in an urban direct primary care clinic. Cureus. 2020;2(10):e10791. doi:https://doi.org/10.7759/cureus.10791

Wallace E, Uijen MJ, Clyne B, Zarabzadeh A, Keogh C, Galvin R, Smith SM, Fahey T. Impact analysis studies of clinical prediction rules relevant to primary care: a systematic review. BMJ Open. 2016;6(3):e009957. https://doi.org/10.1136/bmjopen-2015-009957.

Weisbart ES. Is direct primary care the solution to our health care crisis? Family Pract Manage. 2016:10–11.

Weng SF, Reps J, Kai J, Garibaldi JM, Qureshi N. Can machine-learning improve cardiovascular risk prediction using routine clinical data? PLoS One. 2017;12(4):e0174944.

Zhang X, Kim G, Ballen S, Bagchi S, Hsueh PY, Ball M. Patient characteristics associated with preventable emergency department (ED) utilization among enrollees. American Medical Informatics Association (AMIA) 2020 Virtual Annual Symposium. November 14–18, 2020.

Zivin K, Pfeiffer PN, Szymanski BR, Valenstein M, Post EP, Miller EM, McCarthy JF. Initiation of primary care-mental health integration programs in the VA health system: associations with psychiatric diagnoses in primary care. Med Care. 2010;48(9):843–51. https://doi.org/10.1097/MLR.0b013e3181e5792b.

Zulman DM, Maciejewski ML, Grubber JM, Weidenbacher HJ, Blalock DV, Zullig LL, Greene L, Whitson HE, Hastings SN, Smith VA. Patient-reported social and behavioral determinants of health and estimated risk of hospitalization in high-risk veterans affairs patients. JAMA Netw Open. 2020;3(10):e2021457. https://doi.org/10.1001/jamanetworkopen.2020.21457.

Chapter 3
Smart Homes for Personal Health and Safety

George Demiris, Therese S. Richmond, and Nancy A. Hodgson

Abstract Passive monitoring technologies that can be embedded into the residential infrastructure have introduced new functionalities for "smart homes" that can facilitate health monitoring and promote well-being and safety of occupants. In this chapter we review emerging trends in smart home systems for health and safety and discuss clinical, technical and ethical implications. We present a case study of Sense4Safety, a technology supported nursing intervention targeting fall risk management among older adults with mild cognitive impairment (MCI) in low resource settings. More specifically, this system links at-risk older adults with a nurse telecoach who guides them in implementing evidence-based individualized plans to reduce fall risks. The system employs machine learning techniques to inform individualized plans to reduce fall risk and identify escalating risks for falls through real-time in-home passive monitoring. Using this system as an example, we highlight the potential of smart home technologies to facilitate health management and promote safety for various populations with diverse needs and cognitive and functional abilities. We discuss a framework to assess obtrusiveness of smart home

G. Demiris (✉)
Department of Biostatistics, Epidemiology and Informatics, Perelman School of Medicine, University of Pennsylvania, Philadelphia, PA, USA

Department of Biobehavioral Health Sciences, University of Pennsylvania School of Nursing, Philadelphia, PA, USA
e-mail: gdemiris@upenn.edu

T. S. Richmond · N. A. Hodgson
Department of Biobehavioral Health Sciences, University of Pennsylvania School of Nursing, Philadelphia, PA, USA
e-mail: terryr@nursing.upenn.edu; hodgsonn@nursing.upenn.edu

technologies and identify ethical implications, highlighting the role of behavioral sensing and passive monitoring in the design of personal health informatics tools.

Keywords Smart homes · Sensors · Passive monitoring · Falls · Patient safety · Home health · Internet of Things

Learning Objectives for the Chapter
Upon completion of this chapter, readers will be able to:

- Describe current and future trends in smart home technologies for health and safety
- Analyze technical, clinical and ethical challenges in the use of smart home technologies for health and safety
- Recognize the value of participatory design and stakeholder inclusion in all stages of design, implementation and evaluation of smart home systems
- Reflect on the role of behavioral sensing and passive monitoring in patient engagement and shared decision making

Introduction

The emergence of IoT (Internet of Things) devices has introduced new ways to create monitoring platforms in the home, ranging from sensors that detect motion and time spent in each room to fall detectors and sensors that measure environmental parameters such as humidity and luminosity. Internet of Things refers to the network of objects equipped in internet connectivity so that they can be controlled remotely and can also be interconnected as they exchange data. Current commercially available examples of IoT devices include home automation tools, such as the control of lighting, heating, and home appliances, and motion tracking. Users can control such systems by using smartphone applications (apps), web interfaces, or even with voice interaction via smart speakers. These features introduce ways to increase safety and convenience; for example, adults with limited mobility can control doors or light switches with voice commands.

A "smart home" is a residential setting with embedded technological features that enable passive monitoring of residents aiming to improve quality of life, detect or even prevent emergencies and adverse health events, and ultimately increase residents' independence. The technology becomes part of the residential infrastructure and does not require training of or major operation by the resident, making it a potentially desirable solution for residents with varying degrees of computer experience and cognitive and functional abilities.

Passive monitoring facilitated by smart home systems can provide insights into activities of daily living and facilitate health monitoring without reliance on human observers, in the natural real-world environment where people live their lives, and can support a proactive approach by which patterns and trends are identified before an actual adverse event occurs. This goal is not achieved by having humans review data points generated in real time but rather by developing appropriate algorithms that provide accurate inferences about activities of interest. The advancement of data analytics grounded in machine learning supports the early identification of potential changes in health, detecting anomalous activities based on vast amounts of sensor data, and prompting timely intervention to prevent adverse health events.

Many examples highlight the potential of data analytics to support smart home systems. Novel machine learning algorithms have been used to analyze data from multiple sensors to correctly classify and categorize older adults' activities of daily living to assess functional capacity (Ghayvat et al. 2015). Fall detection is another area of study especially for community dwelling older adults where different approaches have been tested such as acoustics (Salman Khan et al. 2015) or privacy preserving motion capture images (De Miguel et al. 2017). Smart monitoring systems have also been developed to increase medication adherence (Aldeer et al. 2018). Comprehensive solutions based on longitudinal studies such as the GatorTech project (Helal et al. 2005) or TigerPlace (Rantz et al. 2008) have demonstrated over the years how physiological and behavioral data collected through sensors can be used to assess both short-term and long-term health patterns, detect anomalous activities, and respond to emergencies (Helal et al. 2005).

The "smart home" functionalities can be grouped into the following categories:

- *Physiological monitoring:* Collection and processing of data that support physiological measurements ranging from basic measures of vital signs of pulse, respiration, temperature, weight, bladder and bowel output, to more complex measures such as electrocardiogram (ECG), continuous glucose monitoring, and anticoagulation testing devices.
- *Functional monitoring:* Collection and processing of data describing functional measurements such as general activity level, motion, gait, meal intake, medication monitoring and other activities-of-daily-living.
- *Security monitoring and assistance*: Measurements that detect human threats such as intruders. Assistance includes responses to identified threats.
- *Safety monitoring*: Collection and processing of data to detect environmental hazards such as fire or gas leak or emergencies such as falls or injury. Safety assistance includes functions such as automatic turning on of bathroom lights when getting out of bed, facilitating safety by reducing trips and falls. Location technologies aimed at safety also fit into this type.
- *Social interaction monitoring and assistance*: Collection and processing of data describing social interactions such as visits, phone calls, or other interactions. Social interaction assistance includes technologies that facilitate social interaction, such as video-based components that support video-mediated communication with friends and family, virtual participation in group activities etc.
- *Cognitive and sensory assistance*: provision of automated or self-initiated reminders and other cognitive aids such as medication reminders and management tools, or lost object locators, for persons with memory deficits. Cognitive assistance applications also include task instruction technologies, such as verbal instructions in using an appliance. Sensory assistance includes technologies that aid users with sensory deficits such as for sight, hearing, and touch.

Sense4Safety: Using Smart Home Technology to Reduce Fall Risk

Falls and MCI as Significant Public Health Problems

Falls and fall-related injuries are significant public health issues for adults 65 years of age and older. Over a third of older adults fall each year and 10–20% of falls result in serious injuries such as fractures and head trauma (Centers for Disease Control and Prevention 2005). Non-fatal fall-related injuries are associated with considerable morbidity including decreased functional status, increased dependence, and significant use of health care services. Fall-related injuries are among the most expensive medical conditions (Carroll et al. 2005). The annual direct medical costs in the US due to falls are estimated to exceed $50 billion (Florence et al. 2018; Carroll et al. 2005), and this estimate does not include the indirect costs of disability, dependence, and decreased quality of life (Burns et al. 2016).

Falls in older adults are not random events, but occur as a result of muscle weakness, slow reaction time, and cognitive changes (Holtzer et al. 2007). Cognitive impairment has been identified as a leading risk factor for falls in older adults. Over 60% of older adults living with mild cognitive impairment (MCI) fall annually— two to three times the rate of those without cognitive impairment (Gonçalves et al. 2018; Oliver et al. 2007). The physiologic mechanisms leading to falls in older adults with MCI include reduced gait speed and shortened stride length, which have been suggested as appropriate biomarkers of fall risk (Sterke et al. 2012). Yet, little research has focused on fall risk identification in older adults with MCI whom existing interventions could benefit. When implemented proactively, fall risk interventions (e.g., STEADI and other multicomponent interventions) can reduce fall rates by 20–30% (RAND Report 2003).

MCI in community-dwelling older adults may not be recognized due to its subtle onset and hesitancy of individuals and their families to acknowledge 'memory problems'. Yet, in addition to its significant contribution to falls, early cognitive impairment may have treatable components, and recent research supports a combination of medical and lifestyle interventions to delay and reduce further decline (Morley et al. 2015). The magnitude of fall-related costs underscores the need to evaluate cost effective and scalable strategies to proactively identify individuals at most risk.

Rationale for Passive In-Home Sensing

Depth sensing focuses on motor signs that may appear years before the onset of dementia (Buchman and Bennett 2011; Buracchio et al. 2010). An accumulating body of research has documented that changes in gait parameters precede cognitive decline and dementia (Best et al. 2016; Verghese et al. 2007). Slowed gait speed and greater stride-to-stride variability are associated with reduced cognitive function in non-demented older adults (McGough et al. 2011; Verghese et al. 2008), and slowed gait speed alone is predictive of cognitive decline and future onset of dementia (Mielke et al. 2012). Declining physical performance stemming from reduced health of sensory and motor systems contributes to progressive and catastrophic mobility disability in community-dwelling older adults (Guralnik et al. 2000), and adults with MCI are at even greater risk for gait instability and falls (Verghese et al. 2009). Assessment of physical function can provide clinically relevant information for identifying risk for accelerated functional decline leading to loss of independence in the home (Fried et al. 2000; Guralnik et al. 2001). A better understanding of functional mobility may shed light on the transition from functional independence to dependence, thus increasing identification of persons at greatest risk for falls and future decline (Di Carlo et al. 2016). Snapshot measures of functional mobility collected in standard clinical practice rely on a single evaluation to estimate a person's capacity. Rare events such as falls may go unreported and remain unassociated with an individual's change in, for example, gait or cognition (Whitney et al. 2012). Moreover, episodic evaluation of older adults does not lend itself to detecting events or syndromes that progress slowly (e.g., cognitive decline, frailty) between clinician visits (Kaye et al. 2011).

Use of Passive Monitoring Technology for Early Detection of Functional Changes

The capacity of in-home sensor technology to detect gait parameter changes suggestive of early illness in cognitively intact older adults has been established (Rantz et al. 2017). While passive monitoring has been used successfully in older adults, the correspondence between clinical assessments and sensor data that represent gait parameters, as well as decline in function and fall risk, has not been studied extensively in individuals with MCI. In a sample of 18 older adults, five of whom had cognitive impairment, researchers found moderate to strong correlations between clinical assessment of mobility and cognitive function and in-home activity patterns derived from machine learning algorithms applied to data collected from sensors (Dawadi et al. 2016). Another study using Passive Infrared (PIR) motion sensors to monitor gait demonstrated differential trajectories of gait speed and gait variability for cognitively intact participants compared to those with MCI, although over the 3-year data collection, those with MCI exhibited the most change (Dodge et al. 2012). Thus, passive monitoring technology is a promising tool for augmenting information obtained from clinical assessments, facilitating fall prevention and highlighting trends and challenges in a more proactive fashion (Boise et al. 2004). Prompt detection of an older adult's deviation from a sensor-recorded baseline provides the opportunity for early evaluation and treatment both of reversible problems, such as medication side effects or acute illness and of progression of chronic illnesses and conditions and the opportunity to institute evidence-based strategies to prevent falls (Hayes et al. 2008).

The Sense4Safety Intervention

We have developed Sense4Safety, a nursing-driven technology-enhanced intervention that includes multiple components (described below): (1) in-home assessment and action; (2) education; (3) passive monitoring and communication; and (4) alerts. The intervention is primarily via video-conferencing or phone, supplemented by in-home visits at intake, and 12 months to conduct in-person assessments.

In-home assessment and action An initial home visit is conducted by a nurse and a technician. The technician installs depth and motion sensors in the residence to facilitate the passive in-home sensing system. The nurse conducts an assessment of the older adult in the domains of socio-demographics, cognition, physical function, and activities of daily living. The nurse also conducts an evaluative direct observation to identify home fall hazards. This process identifies aspects of the physical environment (including objects, space and elements in and about the house) that pose a risk or danger of causing the older adult to fall. Upon completion of the assessments, the nurse will discuss findings and specific recommendations to reduce fall risk in the home environment with the individual and a family member or trusted other if the older adult chooses to identify such a care partner who is tasked to engage in and assist with the monitoring and decision making process. Identifying a trusted other is not required for participation.

Education Educational material is provided to the older adult/trusted other that describes resources for fall risk prevention strategies as well as instruction in the Otago Exercise Program (OEP) that can be performed at home to reduce fall risk. OEP is an evidenced-based, home-based, individually tailored strength and balance retraining program that improves strength and mobility and reduces falls and fall-related injuries in high-risk OA (Campbell et al. 1999; Thomas et al. 2010). The older adult is asked to keep a diary of their activities and debrief the nurse coach biweekly.

Passive Monitoring and Communication The nurse has access to a dashboard that summarizes functional mobility and gait information generated by the passive in-home sensing system that informs the tailored intervention recommendations. This information demonstrates potential changes in fall risk specific to the individual OA. During regularly scheduled bi-weekly video-conferencing calls (or phone calls) the nurse tele-coach discusses these findings with the individual/trusted other, identifies potential barriers to exercising, determines exercise progression, and addresses questions or concerns by the OA/trusted other.

Alerts When a fall or near-fall is identified by the passive in-home sensing system, an alert is generated and sent as text message and email message to the nurse and the trusted other. The nurse contacts the older adult/trusted other to examine the nature of the event and to capture the individual's narrative of the event and the perceived factors leading up to the event.

Ethical Implications

Smart home solutions introduce many challenges especially in terms of privacy and informed consent when targeting individuals with cognitive limitations. Investment in technology to support older adults with cognitive decline is growing as demand outpaces the supply of dedicated resources for supported care. The functions of these technological solutions range widely, including assistance with activities of daily living (ADL), physiological monitoring, cognitive assistance and monitoring, emotional and environmental support (Choi et al. 2019; Seelye et al. 2020). While ethical implications of the use of technologies for people living with cognitive impairment have not been fully examined (Ienca et al. 2018), issues such as autonomy, informed consent, dignity, and distributive justice, along with threats to values like privacy and identity, are beginning to receive increased attention (Meiland et al. 2017; Berridge 2016). Researchers have identified adoption barriers and user dissatisfaction that result when ethical reflections and conversations on social values are not considered in the development of devices (Robillard et al. 2019). The surveilling nature of some technologies can also place important values—and family members themselves—in tension with one another (Kenner 2008).

A recent study examining implications of Internet connected technologies in dementia care conducted in Europe (Wangmo et al. 2019) invited 20 clinicians, nursing home managers, and researchers in geriatrics and related fields to discuss ethical concerns about the use of intelligent assistive technology with older adults and people living with cognitive impairment. A range of concerns were described, including fair technology access, the possible replacement of human assistance, and the use of deception. The ethical importance of communicating risks and benefits to users of a given technology and consenting patients were core concerns. These concerns are amplified with emerging innovations in robotics, artificial intelligence (AI), sensor-based systems (Vallor 2016; Lindeman et al. 2020), including in-home sensors that monitor movement and behavior, and voice-activated systems that access information or remotely control appliances. A recent systematic review found that most (67%) technologies designed for older adults with cognitive impairment were developed without explicit consideration of any ethical principles (Ienca et al. 2018). These ethical concerns are amplified in our current period of rapid technological development, with marked growth of innovations in robotics, artificial intelligence (AI), sensor-based systems including in-home sensors that monitor movement and behavior, and voice-activated systems that access information or remotely control appliances. It is essential that all involved in the rapid expansion of these digital technologies follow accepted ethical principles and anticipate evolving issues that will arise (Nebeker et al. 2019).

A theoretical framework that can guide the formative and summative evaluation of smart homes is the obtrusiveness framework that defines obtrusiveness of smart home technology as "a summary evaluation by the user based on characteristics or effects associated with the technology that are perceived as undesirable and physically and/or psychologically prominent" (Hensel et al. 2006). The framework has four underlying assumptions: (a) obtrusiveness is a summary evaluation that may be based on the cumulative obtrusiveness of a number of characteristics or effects associated with the technology or on one characteristic or effect that is especially important or prominent to the user; (b) the obtrusiveness of a given technology is subjectively assigned by each person; (c) "user" refers to not only the patient, but also any other resident in the home; and (d) the framework focuses specifically on the home setting recognizing it as a person's private, personal space, with a very different psychological dynamic than in an institutional facility. Within this framework, 22 categories of what may be perceived as obtrusive in smart home technology are proposed based on a review of the literature. These categories are grouped into eight dimensions: physical aspects, usability, privacy, function, human interaction, self-concept, routine, sustainability.

Additional considerations include the potential burden that may be placed on family caregivers, issues of accessibility and informed consent. As we design new technological solutions for home monitoring especially for populations that require assistance with daily activities or health related processes and decisions, we may be introducing new challenges for family caregivers or trusted others who are often asked to assist with the gathering or interpretation of data leading to additional responsibilities that require further training and experience. The accessibility of smart homes needs to recognize factors affecting access including structural, financial and personal barriers. The operation of smart home technologies often requires infrastructure (such as broadband Internet) that may not be readily available, or retrofitting of home features that may be costly and time consuming.

Informed consent is a concept that requires careful consideration not only in the context of research projects but also for terms of agreement for use of smart home tools in the real world. Many argue that conventional ways of obtaining informed consent are not sufficient for systems of care using new technologies. Challenges emerge as a result of the the persistence and vastness of data created, stored, and transmitted by smart home technologies, which can lead to future reuse unspecified at the time of consent. Concerns specific to emerging technologies include the high level of digital literacy that may be needed to fully comprehend the mechanisms and purpose of the technology (Birchley et al. 2017). Even with traditional smart home systems patients may need to understand concepts of cloud storage, wireless data transfer and sensor data streams to fully appraise the risks associated with smart home systems. Individuals must understand how their data are collected, who may access them, and what the potential risks may be. This further stresses the importance of ongoing consent and the ability to rescind consent. Residents and their social network often experience the system and change their initial perceptions over time as they experience the system "in action." The degree of trust in the accuracy and overall performance of the system as well as an assessment of preferences of data sharing and others accessing smart home information are part of that "lived experience" that affects whether older adults and families will continue to approve and engage with the system.

Finally, health equity needs to be considered as technological advances designed to bridge geographic distance and increase access to care, may actually exacerbate inequities (Hong et al. 2020). Systems that place requirements on residential infrastructure or previous experience with specific hardware or software may become inaccessible to underserved populations. Some systems that include extensive software and hardware infrastructure based on extensive retrofitting of a home may introduce high equipment and/or maintenance costs. It is important to engage residents who are going to be introduced to smart home systems to co-design these solutions as they bring the wisdom of their lived experience and deep understanding of their circumstances and needs so that the design and implementation reflects their values rather than assumptions made by system developers.

Conclusion

Smart homes introduce new opportunities for health monitoring and improving safety for residents and their families in their home and many applications have been implemented targeting older adults who wish to remain independent for as long as possible, as well as individuals who may be experiencing cognitive or functional limitations. Behavioral sensing approaches can provide insights into activities of daily living and highlight trends or patterns in behavioral and social aspects of health in addition to physiological assessments that constitute a more comprehensive snapshot of one's well-being. Furthermore, specific smart home solutions can promote safety as they enable a more proactive approach that focuses on predicting adverse events rather than aiming to address their consequences after those have occurred. One such example is Sense4Safety where the use of depth sensors is supporting an educational and behavioral intervention with the goal to predict fall risk and proactively address changes of such risk scores in order to reduce the likelihood of a fall. While smart home systems introduce many new ways to promote home monitoring, they also introduce ethical challenges and privacy considerations that require a careful examination of design approaches to minimize obtrusiveness and empower individuals and families.

Question 1:
Smart home solutions can be appropriate monitoring tools for populations with functional or cognitive impairment because these tools:

(a) allow more intrusive solutions to monitor activities of daily living
(b) support passive monitoring that does not require training or operation by the user
(c) use wireless networks
(d) can be installed quickly

Correct Answer: *(b) support passive monitoring that does not require training or operation by the user.*

Smart home solutions that support passive monitoring are often more appropriate for populations with functional or cognitive impairments as the technology operates "in the background" without relying on a resident having to learn to operate new software or hardware. This approach eliminates the burden of data collection for the resident and the need to initiate data collection.

Question 2:
When it comes to ethical considerations, the design and deployment of smart home solutions for vulnerable populations need to be informed by:

(a) The preferences of system designers
(b) Issues of reimbursement
(c) Issues of privacy, autonomy, obtrusiveness of technology and informed consent
(d) Current technology trends

Correct Answer: *(c) Issues of privacy, autonomy, obtrusiveness of technology and informed consent.*

The design and deployment of smart home systems for vulnerable populations need to address how the technology may introduce risks and benefits for these populations and efforts to maximize protection of privacy and autonomy of residents as well as an understanding of the features of the technology that may be perceived as undesirable by the end users. Finally, engaging all stakeholders, assuring that there is transparency when it comes to identifying and communicating these risks and benefits and promoting informed consent as an ongoing process rather than a discrete event, are critical to the appropriate introduction of these systems into people's homes and daily lives.

Clinical Pearls
- As new home monitoring technologies emerge, clinicians are asked to help patients navigate this new landscape and identify what solutions may be available and appropriate for them to increase safety at home.
- The interpretation of patient generated "smart home" data by clinicians requires appropriate visualizations and algorithms to facilitate clinical decision making.
- Smart home monitoring facilitates a more proactive approach whereby the focus is on prevention of adverse events rather than a reactive approach focusing on minimizing the effects of the adverse and potentially catastrophic event.

References

Aldeer M, Javanmard M, Martin R. A review of medication adherence monitoring technologies. Appl Syst Innov. 2018; https://doi.org/10.3390/asi1020014.

Berridge C. Breathing room in monitored space: the impact of passive monitoring technology on privacy in independent living. The Gerontologist. 2016;56(5):807–16.

Best JR, Liu-Ambrose T, Boudreau RM, Ayonayon HN, Satterfield S, Simonsick EM, Rosano C, et al. An evaluation of the longitudinal, bidirectional associations between gait speed and cognition in older women and men. J Gerontol Ser A: Biomed Sci Med Sci. 2016;71(12):1616–23.

Birchley G, Huxtable R, Murtagh M, Ter Meulen R, Flach P, Gooberman-Hill R. Smart homes, private homes? An empirical study of technology researchers' perceptions of ethical issues in developing smart-home health technologies. BMC Med Ethics. 2017;18(1):1–13.

Boise L, Neal MB, Kaye J. Dementia assessment in primary care: results from a study in three managed care systems. J Gerontol Ser A Biol Med Sci. 2004;59(6):M621–6.

Buchman AS, Bennett DA. Loss of motor function in preclinical Alzheimer's disease. Expert Rev Neurother. 2011;11(5):665–76.

Buracchio T, Dodge HH, Howieson D, Wasserman D, Kaye J. The trajectory of gait speed preceding mild cognitive impairment. Arch Neurol. 2010;67(8):980–6.

Burns ER, Stevens JA, Lee R. The direct costs of fatal and non-fatal falls among older adults—United States. J Saf Res. 2016;58:99–103.

Campbell AJ, Robertson MC, Gardner MM, Norton RN, Buchner DM. Falls prevention over 2 years: a randomized controlled trial in women 80 years and older. Age Ageing. 1999;28:513–8.

Carroll NV, Slattum PW, Cox FM. The cost of falls among the community-dwelling elderly. J Manag Care Pharm. 2005;11(4):307–16.

Centers for Disease Control and Prevention. 2005 Centers for Disease Control and Prevention. Web-based injury statistics query and reporting system (WISQARS). National Center for Injury Prevention and Control, Centers for Disease Control and Prevention. 2005. Available at http://www.cdc.gov/injury/wisqars/index.html

Choi Y, Lazar A, Demiris G, Thompson H. Emerging smart home technologies to facilitate engaging with aging. J Gerontol Nurs. 2019;45:41–8.

Dawadi PN, Cook DJ, Schmitter-Edgecombe M. Automated clinical assessment from smart home-based behavior data. IEEE J Biomed Health Inform. 2016;20(4):1188–94.

De Miguel K, Brunete A, Hernando M, Gambao E. Home camera-based fall detection system for the elderly. Sensors (Switzerland). 2017; https://doi.org/10.3390/s17122864.

Di Carlo A, Baldereschi M, Lamassa M, Bovis F, Inzitari M, Solfrizzi V, Inzitari D, et al. Daily function as predictor of dementia in cognitive impairment, no dementia (CIND) and mild cognitive impairment (MCI): an 8-year follow-up in the ILSA study. J Alzheimers Dis. 2016;53(2):505–15.

Dodge H, Mattek N, Austin D, Hayes T, Kaye J. In-home walking speeds and variability trajectories associated with mild cognitive impairment. Neurology. 2012;78(24):1946–52.

Florence CS, Bergen G, Atherly A, Burns E, Stevens J, Drake C. Medical costs of fatal and nonfatal falls in older adults. J Am Geriatr Soc. 2018;66(4):693–8.

Fried LP, Bandeen-Roche K, Chaves P, Johnson BA. Preclinical mobility disability predicts incident mobility disability in older women. J Gerontol Ser A: Biol Med Sci. 2000;55(1):M43–52.

Ghayvat H, Mukhopadhyay S, Gui X, Suryadevara N. WSN- and IOT-based smart homes and their extension to smart buildings. Sensors (Switzerland). 2015; https://doi.org/10.3390/s150510350.

Gonçalves J, Ansai JH, Masse FAA, Vale FAC, de Medeiros Takahashi AC, de Andrade LP. Dual-task as a predictor of falls in older people with mild cognitive impairment and mild Alzheimer's disease: a prospective cohort study. Braz J Phys Therapy. 2018.

Guralnik JM, Ferrucci L, Pieper CF, Leveille SG, Markides KS, Ostir GV, Wallace RB, et al. Lower extremity function and subsequent disability: consistency across studies, predictive models, and value of gait speed alone compared with the short physical performance battery. J Gerontol Ser A Biol Med Sci. 2000;55(4):M221–31.

Guralnik JM, Ferrucci L, Balfour JL, Volpato S, Di Iorio A. Progressive versus catastrophic loss of the ability to walk: implications for the prevention of mobility loss. J Am Geriatr Soc. 2001;49(11):1463–70.

Hayes TL, Abendroth F, Adami A, Pavel M, Zitzelberger TA, Kaye JA. Unobtrusive assessment of activity patterns associated with mild cognitive impairment. Alzheimers Dement. 2008;4(6):395–405.

Helal S, Mann W, El-Zabadani H, King J, Kaddoura Y, Jansen E. The gator tech smart house: a programmable pervasive space. Computer. 2005; https://doi.org/10.1109/MC.2005.107.

Hensel BK, Demiris G, Courtney KL. Defining obtrusiveness in home telehealth technologies: a conceptual framework. J Am Med Inform Assoc. 2006;13(4):428–31.

Holtzer R, Friedman, R, Lipton RB et al. The relationship between specific cognitive functions and falls in aging. Neuropsychology. 2007;(21):540–8 [Pubmed 17784802]; Tinetti ME, Speechley M, Ginter SF (1988) Risk factors for falls among elderly persons in the community. N Engl J Med (319): 1701–1707.

Hong A, Nam C, Kim S. What will be the possible barriers to consumers' adoption of smart home services? Telecommun Policy. 2020;44(2):101867.

Ienca M, Wangmo T, Jotterand F, Kressig RW, Elger B. Ethical design of intelligent assistive technologies for dementia: a descriptive review. Sci Eng Ethics. 2018;24(4):1035–55.

Kaye J, Maxwell SA, Mattek N, Hayes TL, Dodge H, Pavel M, Zitzelberger TA, et al. Intelligent systems for assessing aging changes. J Gerontol-Ser B Psychol Sci Soc Sci. 2011;66

Kenner AM. Securing the elderly body: dementia, surveillance, and the politics of "aging in place". Surveillance Soc J. 2008;5(3):252–69.

Lindeman DA, Kim KK, Gladstone C, Apesoa-Varano EC. Technology and caregiving: emerging interventions and directions for research. The Gerontologist. 2020;60(Suppl 1):S41–9. https://doi.org/10.1093/geront/gnz178.

McGough EL, Kelly VE, Logsdon RG, McCurry SM, Cochrane BB, Engel JM, Teri L. Associations between physical performance and executive function in older adults with mild cognitive impairment: gait speed and the timed "up & go" test. Phys Ther. 2011;91(8):1198–207.

Meiland F, Innes A, Mountain G, et al. Technologies to support community-dwelling persons with dementia: a position paper on issues regarding development, usability, effectiveness and cost-effectiveness, deployment, and ethics. JMIR Rehabilit Assist Technol. 2017;4(1):e1.

Mielke MM, Roberts RO, Savica R, Cha R, Drubach DI, Christianson T, Ivnik RJ, et al. Assessing the temporal relationship between cognition and gait: slow gait predicts cognitive decline in the Mayo Clinic Study of Aging. J Gerontol Ser A: Biomed Sci Med Sci. 2012;68(8):929–37.

Morley JE, Morris JC, Berg-Weger M, Borson S, Carpenter BD, del Campo N, Flaherty JH, et al. Brain health: the importance of recognizing cognitive impairment: an IAGG consensus conference. J Am Med Dir Assoc. 2015;16(9):731–9.

Nebeker C, Torous J, Bartlett Ellis RJ. Building a case for actionable ethics in digital health research supported by artificial intelligence. BMC Med. 2019;17:137.

Oliver D, Connelly JB, Victor CR, Shaw FE, Whitehead A, Genc Y, et al. Strategies to prevent falls and fractures in hospitals and care homes and effect of cognitive impairment: systematic review and meta-analyses. Br Med J. 2007;334(7584):82. https://doi.org/10.1136/bmj.39049.706493.55.

RAND Report. Evidence report and evidence-based recommendations: fall prevention interventions in the Medicare population. Contract # 500-98-0281; Gillespie, LD, Gillispie, WJ, Robertson, MC et al., (2004). Interventions for preventing falls in elderly people (Cochrane review). In the Cochrane library, issue 3, Chichester: Wiley; 2003.

Rantz MJ, Porter RT, Cheshier D, He Z, Alexander GL, Skubic M, Johnson RA, et al. TigerPlace, a state-academic-private project to revolutionize traditional long-term care. J Hous Elder. 2008; https://doi.org/10.1080/02763890802097045.

Rantz M, Phillips LJ, Galambos C, Lane K, Alexander GL, Despins L, Miller S, et al. Randomized trial of intelligent sensor system for early illness alerts in senior housing. J Am Med Directors Assoc (Publish Ahead of Print). 2017;

Robillard JM, Wu JM, Feng TL, Tam MT. Prioritizing benefits: a content analysis of the ethics in dementia technology policies. J Alzheimers Dis. 2019;69(4):897–904.

Salman Khan M, Yu M, Feng P, Wang L, Chambers J. An unsupervised acoustic fall detection system using source separation for sound interference suppression. Signal Process. 2015; https://doi.org/10.1016/j.sigpro.2014.08.021.

Seelye A, Leese M, Dorociak K, Bouranis N, Mattek N, Sharma N, Beattie Z, Riley T, Lee J, Cosgrove K, Fleming N, Klinger J, Ferguson J, Lamberty G, Kaye J. In-home sensor monitoring to detect mild cognitive impairment in aging military veterans: preliminary data on methods and feasibility. J Med Internet Res. 2020; https://doi.org/10.2196/16371.

Sterke CS, van Beeck EF, Looman CW, et al. An electronic walkway can predict short-term fall risk in nursing home residents with dementia. Gait Posture. 2012;36:95–101.

Thomas S, Mackintosh S, Halbert J. Does the "Otago experience programme" reduce mortality and falls in older adults? A systematic review and meta-analysis. Age Ageing. 2010;39:681–7.

Vallor S. Technology and the virtues: a philosophical guide to a future worth wanting. New York, NY: Oxford University Press; 2016.

Verghese J, Wang C, Lipton RB, Holtzer R, Xue X. Quantitative gait dysfunction and risk of cognitive decline and dementia. J Neurol Neurosurg Psychiatry. 2007;78(9):929–35.

Verghese J, Robbins M, Holtzer R, Zimmerman M, Wang C, Xue X, Lipton RB. Gait dysfunction in mild cognitive impairment syndromes. J Am Geriatr Soc. 2008;56(7):1244–51.

Verghese J, Holtzer R, Lipton RB, Wang C. Quantitative gait markers and incident fall risk in older adults. J Gerontol: Ser A. 2009;64(8):896–901.

Wangmo T, Lipps M, Kressig RW, et al. Ethical concerns with the use of intelligent assistive technology: findings from a qualitative study with professional stakeholders. BMC Med Ethics. 2019;20:98.

Whitney J, Close JC, Jackson SH, Lord SR. Understanding risk of falls in people with cognitive impairment living in residential care. J Am Med Dir Assoc. 2012;13(6):535–40.

Chapter 4
Health App by Prescription: The German Nation-Wide Model

Monika Pobiruchin and Veronika Strotbaum

Abstract In recent years, digital applications like apps or wearable devices (e.g., smart watches, fitness trackers) are discussed. They are even evaluated as promising instruments to improve healthcare and to integrate patients better into healthcare processes. Today, there are many applications for different health conditions. The provided applications are very heterogeneous in terms of manufacturers, accessibility, data privacy, and levels of quality. This makes it difficult for patients and healthcare professionals to select an adequate digital product. In fact, doctors and/or therapists were often discouraged to recommend specific apps, in addition recommendation of digital apps was not billable, either Furthermore, for manufacturers it was difficult to find a sustainable reimbursement model in the complex German healthcare system. Against this background, the "Digital Healthcare Act" (coined DVG) was passed in 2019. This law creates the legal basis for "Digital Health Applications" (coined DiGAs) to be reimbursed by the health insurance companies that cover 90% of the German population. Moreover, this law specifies certain requirements for health applications. Hence, DiGAs have to satisfy certain requirements related to technical and formal as well as medical benefits. As of July 2022, there are 32 DiGAs available. However, there is still a lot of work to be done to integrate DiGAs into the daily work of doctors and therapists.

Monika Pobiruchin and Veronika Strotbaum contributed equally.

M. Pobiruchin (✉)
GECKO Institute for Medicine, Informatics and Economics, Heilbronn University, Heilbronn, Germany
e-mail: monika.pobiruchin@hs-heilbronn.de

V. Strotbaum
ZTG Zentrum für Telematik und Telemedizin GmbH, Hagen, Germany
e-mail: veronika.strotbaum@posteo.de

© The Author(s), under exclusive license to Springer Nature Switzerland AG 2022
P.-Y. S. Hsueh et al. (eds.), *Personal Health Informatics*, Cognitive Informatics in Biomedicine and Healthcare, https://doi.org/10.1007/978-3-031-07696-1_4

After a short overview of the German Healthcare System, this article examines the main characteristics of the legal framework, the registration and the reimbursement processes of the DiGA. First experiences with DiGAs are described. Subsequently, this article provides an outlook on potential new business models for information technology companies and startups.

Keywords German healthcare system · eHealth · Digital health applications (DiGA) · Digital healthcare act (DVG) · Fast-track procedure

Learning Objectives
1. You get an overview of the German Healthcare System and the central role of the health insurance, how the process of reimbursement for "conventional" drugs and/or medical technology works, and the German eHealth strategy since 2000.
2. You know the core elements of "Digital Health Applications" (DiGAs) and the underlying legal framework.
3. You are able to assess the potential opportunities and risks associated with the German model.
4. You know conditions to be fulfilled in Germany for information technology companies and start-ups in the digital healthcare ecosystem.
5. You can derive success factors from the presented reimbursement model, and you can adapt and modify these factors to your situation/region.

Clinical Pearls
- In 2019, the legal framework for prescribing Digital Healthcare Applications (German Digitale Gesundheitsanwendungen—DiGA) was established in Germany.
- Digital Healthcare Applications must prove medical benefit or added value for care processes.
- The possibilities of Digital Healthcare Applications must be made known publicly to patients, physicians and therapists as well as health insurance employees.

Introduction

Let us think about a little 'future scenario' to start this chapter: Imagine you go to your family doctor for your annual checkup. You tell your doctor that you have back pain regularly. It is not bad, but it is a nuisance and you think it is caused by too much sitting in the office and too less physical activity in your daily life. However, you find it difficult to integrate regular exercises into your daily routine.

"No problem", your doctor tells you. "There's a new digital health app. It's connected to a wearable device and it reminds you to sit and stand up straight, do your exercises regularly, and even recommends fitness workouts based on your personal profile and needs".

"Sounds great. How much does it cost? And where can I get it?"

"Nothing, I can write you a prescription. You can download it via your preferred app store."

You are amazed: "A prescription for a digital application just like an ordinary drug?"

"Exactly."

Let us stop this scenario here. It is not so much a future scenario as one might think. Since 2020, German physicians can prescribe digital health applications. This means, health apps are now part of the services of the statutory health insurances.

In this chapter, we want to give a brief overview of the German healthcare system and its key stakeholders. We will cover the process to get new drugs—or innovative medical products in general—into the market and into the reimbursement of the health insurances which are the largest contributors in the system. Then, we will compare how this process was adapted for digital health applications. A summary of the eHealth/digitalization strategy of the German healthcare system for the last 20 years and how this culminated in the new ecosystem of digital health applications is provided in section "Electronic Health Card and Personal Health Records (2000–2020)". First experiences with the prescriptions of digital applications are described in section "First Experiences with DiGAs" and opportunities for (small) healthcare start-ups in this new environment are presented.

Overview

German Healthcare System

The basic concept of the German healthcare system dates to the nineteenth century. Germany is regarded as the first country that introduced a national system of statutory social and health insurance (SHI). This model is still called "Bismarck Model" because Otto von Bismarck instituted the SHI. In 1883, the Health Insurance for Blue-collar Workers (*Gesetz betreffend der Krankenversicherung der Arbeiter*) was passed. The aim was a mandatory universal healthcare for low-wage workers in the industrial sector that build upon an existing patchwork of SHI. The system was funded by employers and employees through health insurance companies (*Krankenkassen*) (Busse and Blümel 2014).

This basic concept is still valid today nearly 140 years after the establishment of the first health insurance system. Insured persons are members of a health insurance company and are liable to contribution. Contributions entitle them to claim benefits, e.g., medical care, drugs, etc.

The contribution to the health insurance company is a fixed universal percentage of the income. In 2021, the rate for the public insurance is 14.6%, 7.3% of which is covered by the employer (Bundesministerium für Gesundheit 2021a). On top of the universal rate, every health insurance company charges an additional rate (*Zusatzbeitrag*) (GKV Spitzenverband 2021a), on average 1.3%. That means it is a (roughly) 50:50 split between employers and employees (Sawicki and Bastian 2008). All members (and their co-insured dependents, e.g., family members, ca. 16 million people (Bundesministerium für Gesundheit 2020a)) of the health insurance company are entitled to receive the same benefits, i.e., benefits are independent of age, duration of membership, and the total amount of contributions paid. The types of benefits are defined by law (see Chap. 3 of the Social Code Book V, *Sozialgesetzbuch V*, SGB V). They comprise disease screening programs, outpatient medical care, dental care, etc.

Since 1st January 2009, every person residing in Germany is legally obligated to take out a health insurance. Today, 90% of the German population is SHI insured by 103 different health insurance companies (*Gesetzliche Krankenversicherung,* GKV) (Bundesministerium für Gesundheit 2020a; GKV Spitzenverband 2021b). Certain groups are insured by private health insurances (*Private Krankenversicherung*, PKV), e.g., civic servants, self-employed and employees above a specific income threshold.

However, for this chapter we will focus exclusively on the SHI system and how new drugs and/or medical innovations are introduced into this system. We also describe how insurants can benefit from and take advantage of these drugs as well as of medical innovations. There are two steps to consider (1) licensing, also known as market access or marketing authorization, and (2) reimbursement by the SHI.

Licensing and Marketing Authorization

Marketing authorization for new medicinal products, e.g., pharmaceuticals, contrast agents, etc., is laid down in the German Medicines Act (*Arzneimittelgesetz, AMG*). The national agency responsible for evaluation is the Federal Institute for Drugs and Medical Devices (*Bundesinstitut für Arzneimittel und Medizinprodukte, BfArM*). The criteria for licensing are based on EU-wide standards on good clinical practice and includes phase I, II (testing with healthy humans), and III (clinical trial with people affected by the disease) studies (Bundesinstitut für Arzneimittel und Medizinprodukte 2013).

These approval studies are sent to the regulatory authorities. After successful evaluation, the new drug is granted market access. This means manufacturers can sell their product in Germany. For this purpose, they set an initial price for the products by themselves. However, at this moment the new product is not yet part of the health plans of the SHI. This means physicians cannot prescribe the drug in their medical practice.

Reimbursement by the Statutory Health Insurance (SHI)

Manufacturers pursue reimbursement by the SHI because this is the main cost-bearing group in the German healthcare system. However, the price of new drugs and innovations are required to be economical (*Wirtschaftlichkeitsgebot*, see §12 SGB V). It is required that the diagnostic or therapeutic benefit and the necessity of the service must be proven. Here, the Federal Joint Committee (*Gemeinsamer Bundesausschuss, G-BA*)—the highest decision-making body of the SHI system—is responsible for the assessments (Busse et al. 2017).

The G-BA consists of 13 members: Five payer representatives, five representatives of the service providers (hospitals, physicians, etc.), and three impartial members not belonging to the aforementioned groups, one of whom is also the chairperson of the committee. Further, up to five general patient representatives and five topic-related patient representatives may attend the meetings, but are not entitled to vote.

The process for determining the price of the new drug for reimbursement in the SHI is specified in the Pharmaceuticals Market Reorganisation Act (*Arzneimittelmarktneuordnungsgesetz*, AMNOG) which came in law in 2011: Based on the Benefit Dossier (e.g., approval studies and other documents) the G-BA decides whether a new drug has an additional benefit (*Zusatznutzen*) compared to established, comparative therapies. This step in the evaluation process takes 6 months. If there is an additional benefit, the GB-A invites the manufacturer to negotiate a price with the National Association of the Statutory Health Insurance (*Spitzenverband der gesetzlichen Krankenkassen*, GKV-SV). These negotiations must take place within 6 months. If a price has been found, it becomes effective 12 months after the start of the AMNOG process. During these 12 months, the price previously set by the manufacturer is effective (Staab et al. 2018).

New Digital Services in the German Healthcare System

Electronic Health Card and Personal Health Records (2000–2020)

Attempts to introduce digital services into the German healthcare system were closely linked to the introduction of the electronic health card (*Elektronische Gesundheitskarte*, eGK). This development started in the early 2000s and originally the eGK should have been introduced on 1st January 2006. The aim was that the insured persons' data would be stored directly on the card and but that the eGK would also enable direct access to applications such as a personal, electronic health record (PHR). As early as 2005, it was determined that the German healthcare system was characterized by media disruptions, paper-based communication, avoidable duplicate examinations (Bales 2005), and fax-based communication.[1]

The necessary technical infrastructure for the eGK was named telematics infrastructure (*Telematikinfrastruktur*, TI) and developed by the gematik GmbH (shareholders of the gematik are several service providers of the German healthcare system, e.g., Federal Ministry of Health (*Bundesministerium für Gesundheit*, BMG), Federal Chamber of Physicians (*Bundesärztekammer*, BÄK), Federal Chamber of Dentists (*Bundeszahnärztekammer*, BZÄK), German Organization of Pharmacists (*Deutsche Apoth*ekerverband, DAV), German Hospital Federation (*Deutsche Krankenhausgesellschaft*, DKG), National Association of the Statutory Health Insurance (*Spitzenverband der gesetzlichen Krankenkassen*, GKV-SV), Federal Association of Statutory Health Insurance (SHI) Physicians (*Kassenärztliche Bundesvereinigung*, KBV), and the Federal Association of Statutory Health Insurance (SHI) Dentists (*Kassenzahnärztliche Bundesvereinigung*, KZBV).

The TI was designed as a virtual private network, accessible only via "connectors" (special certified card readers). Back in the early 2000s, mHealth smartphone applications or mobile access to EHRs via tablets was not envisioned. Therefore, the TI did not provide access for applications or devices that were not tied to a certified connector.

In 2005, the new eGK was announced as the key element of a new interconnected, interoperable healthcare system. Unfortunately, the eGK never met the expectations. For example, major physicians' associations rejected the eGK. The association of private health insurance companies did not participate in the roll-out of the new card. Many insured persons also feared to—partly unjustifiably—become a "transparent patient" (*Gläserner Patient*) when using the services that were tied to the eGK.

The issuance of the eGK by the SHI finally began in October 2011—with a delay of more than 6 years.

Hence, even in 2020 PHRs are not widespread and rarely used by the German population (Ploner et al. 2019). Some SHIs offered PHRs as an additional service for their members. However, PHRs were not officially introduced by the BMG until 1st January 2021. Now, access is possible without a connector and can be carried out via an app on mobile devices such as smartphones or tablets. All doctors are connected to the TI in the second half of 2021 and they will be able to transfer written notes, images, laboratory results, etc. into patient records. The use of the PHR for insurants is voluntary (Bundesministerium für Gesundheit 2020b). Patients grant accesses authorizations to their physicians, and starting in 2022, this will also be possible at the document level.

Nevertheless, the backbone of these new developments is the "old" TI. In early 2021, a technical whitepaper caused some excitement in the eHealth community and among physicians and payers: The whitepaper acknowledges that the current

---

[1] In 2020, during the COVID-19 pandemic, it must be noted that the German healthcare system would not be operable without fax and paper files. For example, the regional public health authorities (*Öffentlicher Gesundheitsdienst*, ÖGD) were still transferring lab results and address lists of infected persons via fax machine.

state of the TI reflects 10-year-old ideas, architecture, and technological background. Today, mobile applications are an essential part of daily life. Indeed, "the broad availability of apps for prevention, wellness, and fitness scenarios has resulted in an increased importance of eHealth for the healthcare industry" (Schreiweis et al. 2019). It is mandatory that the "new" TI aims to integrate innovative digital health applications alongside personal electronic health records (gematik GmbH 2020).

Digital Health Applications (Since 2020)

Following the publication of the CHARISHMA study in 2016, the BMG has commissioned several further studies to examine the current market situation with a particular focus on opportunities and remaining obstacles to a nationwide use of mHealth products (Chances and Risks of Mobile Health Apps (CHARISMHA) 2016). Several scientific institutions have also investigated the barriers with regard to mHealth products. It was shown that mHealth is mainly used in the privately funded ("second") healthcare sector. Regarding the system of the SHI ("primary" sector), mHealth products were mainly paid for in case of (pilot) projects as well as within the context of selective contractual/alternative healthcare concepts. The development of viable business models, especially for smaller information technology companies and start-ups in this sector, represents a major challenge. Access to the SHI was difficult for mHealth products. Issues such as data privacy and evidence of usefulness also contributed to this difficult situation (Leppert and Greiner 2016; Herberz et al. 2018).

In this context, the Digital Healthcare Act (*Digitale-Versorgung Gesetz,* DVG) became law in 2019. It constitutes a milestone for the further spread of mHealth applications in the German healthcare system. The main aspect of the DVG is an idea named "apps by prescription" (*App auf Rezept*). This enables doctors/physiotherapists to prescribe SHI insured patients "digital healthcare applications" *(*DiGA, *Digitale Gesundheitsanwendungen*) (§§33a and 139e SGB V). If health-related soft- and/or hardware (such as apps or wearables) is licensed as a DiGA and officially registered in the DiGA registry, it can be prescribed by doctors/psychotherapists. In this way, digital innovations can enter the SHI system more quickly. The "DiGAV—Digitale Gesundheitsanwendungen-Verordnung" (*Digital Health Applications Ordinance)* thereby instantiates the legal frame (Bundesanzeiger Verlag GmbH 2020; Bundesministerium für Gesundheit 2020c). A DiGA is supposed to fulfill the following requirements:

- Certified medicine product of the risk class I or IIa
- Focus on the use of digital technologies
- Designed for medical use
- No use for primary prevention
- Patient-focused use or shared use by doctor and patient
- Barrier-free use
- A high level of protection of data privacy and IT security
- Ensuring interoperability through the use of (international) standards

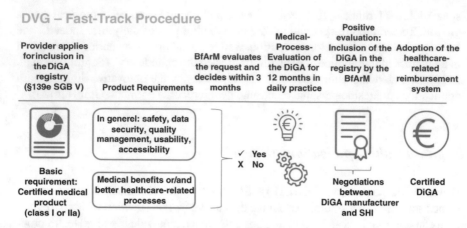

Fig. 4.1 Fast-Track Procedure of the BfArM. Own diagram (2021)

If the digital health product complies with these conditions, the manufacturer is entitled to apply for the "Fast-Track Procedure" of the BfArM (Bundesinstitut für Arzneimittel und Medizinprodukte 2022a). This procedure requires the BfArM to decide within 3 months after the application of the potential DiGA manufacturer (hence "fast" track) whether the digital product is included (temporarily or permanently) in the DiGA registry. Figure 4.1 shows the general process.

The manufacturer (given that the application already classifies as a certified medical device) applies to the BfArM and fills out a self-disclosure: It states how far the general conditions, e.g., in terms of quality management, support opportunities, data protection and data security etc., are fulfilled. Next, the manufacturer must report whether there are studies regarding the benefits of the new application. To get listed in the DiGA registry the manufacturer must supply or prove "Positive Healthcare Benefits". This can either refer to an improvement in medical use (such as positive effects regarding mortality, morbidity, or health-related quality of life) and/or to structural or process improvements (e.g., better access to supply, improvement of the health competence of the patients etc.). Provided that no studies are available yet, the DiGA will be included in the DiGA register for a limited amount of time, initially for 1 year. Within this period, the manufacturer must prove practically that his application makes improvements in one of the possible areas mentioned. The evidence of a positive supply effect must usually be carried out via a validated study design. There are no detailed requirements, however, the manufacturer must use validated instruments (e.g., the record of health-related quality of life with the SF36 or other validated questionnaires). With the entry in the DiGA registry (in accordance with § 139e SGB V) of BfArM, the positive supply effects are ensured at the beginning or after 12 months at the latest. Furthermore, the price negotiations regarding the reimbursement start in the first year between the executive committee of GKV National

Association of Statutory Health Insurance Physicians as representative of the statutory health insurance and the Executive association of Digital Healthcare (*Spitzenverband Digitale Gesundheitsversorgung,* SVDGV) as representative of the manufacturer. After 1 year, new negotiations take place between the afore-mentioned parties. The manufacturer also must provide relevant information about its product in the DiGA registry, which includes the precise indication according to ICD (International Classification of Diseases), the intended patient group, the functional conditions of the DiGA, the support potential etc. (Bundesinstitut für Arzneimittel und Medizinprodukte 2022a). Physicians are supposed to be able to find all relevant information in the DiGA registry as quickly as possible without having to search for the necessary information. In general, DiGA must always be designed for both major mobile operating systems: iOS and Android (Bundesinstitut für Arzneimittel und Medizinprodukte 2020a, b).

Following the conclusion of these formal processes, the DiGA may be prescribed to patients covered by SHI.

As Fig. 4.2 describes, the doctor's/psychotherapist's office (or hospital) selects a DiGA from the DiGA registry and prescribes the app to the insurant analogous to the regulation of medications via the "pink prescription form", i.e., the conventional format to prescribe the medication.

The insurant contacts his health insurance company with this prescription via a health insurance app or portal, in the office or by mail. The health insurance company now generates an activation code and informs the insurant via the aforementioned communication ways. The insurant can now download the DiGA from the respective app store. The manufacturer of the particular app will be informed by the health insurance company about the download of the DiGA. The manufacture clarifies the billing with the health insurance company.

DVG – DiGA Prescription by a Doctor/Therapist

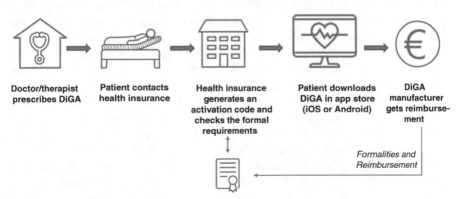

| Doctor/therapist prescribes DiGA | Patient contacts health insurance | Health insurance generates an activation code and checks the formal requirements | Patient downloads DiGA in app store (iOS or Android) | DiGA manufacturer gets reimbursement |

Formalities and Reimbursement

Fig. 4.2 Prescription process of a DiGA by a doctor/therapist. Own diagram (2021)

First Experiences with DiGAs

Acceptance and Knowledge About DiGA Among German Healthcare Professionals and Citizens

In 2020, the organizations involved in the DiGA process, especially the BMG and the GKV-SV worked intensively to clarify all technical issues and agree on common processes and standards. In fact, the DiGA manual published in April 2020 already constitutes a freely accessible document with detailed information about all aspects regarding DiGA for manufacturers, users, and suppliers. A short time later, an English version for foreign manufacturers of DiGAs was published as well.

In October 2020, the first DiGAs were included in the registry. At the same time, 21 manufactures' applications had applied for entry into the registry. Manufacturers of 75 applications had enlisted for a consultation with the BfArM (Bundesinstitut für Arzneimittel und Medizinprodukte 2020b). As of July 2022, 32 applications are listed in the DiGA registry (12 temporarily and 20 permanently). Two DiGAs have already been canceled due to different reasons. The DiGAs serve a quite broad medical field. For example, applications for, multiple sclerosis, tinnitus, mental disorders (e.g., panic disorder) or coxarthrosis etc. (Bundesinstitut für Arzneimittel und Medizinprodukte 2022b). Considering the high demands for consultations of the BfArM it can be assumed that several new applications will be accepted temporarily or permanently as DiGA this year.

Nonetheless, there is an increasing amount of critique of the current practice from various parties and several organizations are requesting changes. Especially the National Association of the Statutory Health Insurance criticize the current, relatively free pricing in the first year of the DiGA practice. In the first year, DiGA manufacturers are relatively free to define the prices per DiGA relatively freely and thus gain relatively high prices in comparison to previous profits in the private patient market. The National Association of the Statutory Health Insurance advised that the requirements for cost-effectiveness of medical benefits in SGB V must be considered. In addition, the relatively low admission criteria compared to other service areas in the healthcare system is evaluated critically from the perspective of the GKV. Another point of critique by GKV refers to the aspect of the real usage of the application, as the manufacturer receives the negotiated price after the DiGA has been cleared by the insurant—regardless of whether the application is used then. To the health insurance companies, it is not directly obvious to what extent the DiGA really plays a role in healthcare. Another issue of critique relates to the topic of data protection respectively data security. Since there is no official or governmentally acknowledged data protection seal in Germany, a self-commitment of the manufacturers is currently sufficient. An external review of data protection and data security does not (yet) exist at present (GKV-Spitzenverband 2021; Ärzteblatt online 2020).

The fact that mHealth applications are indeed a debatable aspect was already highlighted in several studies. For example, a 2019 review published in BMJ has shown that many apps both routinely pass user data to third parties—including highly sensitive data such as medication lists—and are not very transparent in their handling of user data, and that app users usually have few individual configuration options with their apps (Grundy et al. 2019).

Another aspect is the question to what extent and time duration the topic DiGA will be noticed by doctors and patients at all and especially via which channels and instruments—above all in reference to less technically savvy insurants. The same applies outside the "bubble" of GVK and manufacturer organizations (SVDGV), and how well they have taken note of the topic. One might assume that the quick implementation of the underlying processes and structures has contributed to the fact that doctors, for example, are (still) quite reluctant towards DiGAs.

In autumn 2020, a survey of 124 family doctors showed that currently 40% do not consider themselves prepared to prescribe DiGAs. Asked for the reasons, the doctors mentioned the—from their point of view—insufficient medical benefit, concerns regarding data protection, as well as the lack of binding quality criteria. However, 62% of the family doctors were convinced that health apps will have a strong or partial influence on their everyday professional life (IQVIA 2020).

Another survey among family doctors reported that respondents rated their level of information about DVG as rather poor (51%) or poor (12%). Another 12% stated that they had not yet learned anything about DVG (12%). A quarter of general practitioners currently feel rather well informed, but none consider themselves as very well informed (Radić et al. 2021).

The reluctance of physicians and therapists is certainly reflected in actual prescribing practice: Although there are no official figures on how often individual DiGAs have been prescribed to patients, there are some hints: As today (September 2021), 17,000 DiGA or less than 1000 per DiGA have been prescribed—although over 70 million people in Germany were eligible to benefit from DiGA (Ärzteblatt online 2020). Clear favorites among the available DiGAs have not yet emerged at this time (BVMed 2021).

However, the prescribing practice is influenced by the existence of reimbursement options for doctors. In this context, the SVDGV (Executive Association of Digital Healthcare) and representatives of the SHI agreed on the reimbursement options for the prescription process itself in March 2021. Doctors/Therapists will receive around two Euro for the first prescription of a permanent listed DiGA, follow-up prescriptions will not be billable. For this process, a new fee regulation position was created. Except of the DiGA "Somnio", an application that supports therapy for sleep disorders, there are no more reimbursement options for doctors, e.g., for further DiGA-related medical services. For "Somnio", doctors or therapists can receive about seven Euro for the monitoring of the patient's data (Grätzel von Grätz 2021). In can be said that doctors and therapists are relatively free in the further use of the DiGA to date as there are no medical guidelines etc. which provide information about data monitoring, follow up visits or medical consultations after the initial prescription process. This means of course that doctors and therapists currently have no financial incentives in connection with the DiGA process. In addition, there are no legal requirements or directives for transfer and/or interoperability of patient generated data between the DiGA and the medical practice management software. One possibility is the use of the national telematics infrastructure (TI); the responsible associations are currently working on that issue.

It is clear that the public relations of the cooperation partners must be improved and expanded. Therefore, the SVDGV is already planning to expand the existing information and education capacities, especially for doctors, psychotherapists and other healthcare specialists. Specific education and information for health insurance employees is to be intensified accordingly, so that they can pass on the right information to insurants and—ideally—also name contact persons for insurants and doctors as well as manufacturers. Moreover, the SVDGV reports that it is working to digitize the supply and prescription process and especially on advancing the connection of DiGA with the nationwide PHR as well as the integration with the electronic prescription (Ärzteblatt online 2021).

The German Medical Association and the Federal Association of Statutory Health Insurance (SHI) Physicians (KBV) have developed additional information material, so that doctors can better inform their patients about the possibilities and the limitations of digital health applications (Bundesärztekammer (BÄK), Kassenärztliche Bundesvereinigung (KBV) 2020).

DiGA as a New Business Model for Healthcare Start-ups and New Strategic Partnerships

The DVG not only created a market for the national health insurance companies offering DiGAs. The law also pursues the objective of stimulating digital innovations in healthcare through further measures. For example, health insurance companies may support digital medical devices, telemedical applications or other digital procedures. In addition, they are also entitled to develop or let develop, digital innovations in cooperation with third parties. In accordance with the DVG, health insurance companies may invest 2% of their financial reserves as a part of a capital commitment for a maximum of 10 years. The form and manner of this investment can be determined relatively freely by the insurance companies without the legislator having to intervene to any great extent (see §68a SGB V).

This means that health insurance companies now have the possibility, for example, to invest in promising healthcare-related start-ups and establish business incubators to specifically support founders and turn ideas into business models. The new rules of the DVG give manufacturers more planning security because it provides clear guidance to receive reimbursement for all statutory health insurances.

This new legal framework facilitates the cooperation of start-ups with well-established players in the German healthcare system. Moreover, health insurance companies can also cooperate with digital companies outside the scope of DiGAs. For example, the health insurance company IKK Südwest covers the costs of the "Nia" app, a personal assistant for better management of atopic dermatitis (ÄrzteZeitung online 2021).

As already mentioned, the German healthcare system is complex, and many stakeholders are involved. Each actor has its individual demands and conditions, be it the BMG or the DiGA manufacturers. However, the network established and the experiences gained during the planning and implementation of the DiGA process can be utilized for further digital innovation. The joint networks and the resulting "mutual trust" and debate culture represent an advantage not to be neglected the establishment of new business models. Due to precise prescription practice, health insurance companies also get the possibility to learn more about the health needs of their insurants. This provides health insurance companies the chance to co-develop digital health concepts in a more targeted way.

The "Lessons Learned" in the context of DiGA implementation certainly could mean a push in the direction of digital innovation, and not only on the part of the national healthcare insurance companies. Private health insurance companies (PKV), i.e., not SHI, are also showing their interest in developing and providing their own "DiGAs". The private health insurance companies are currently coordinating a certification procedure and are also striving for a common guideline. Similar, PKV has announced its aims to refund the DiGA certified by the BfArM. Consequently, this will result in new cooperation possibilities for start-ups in cooperation with private insurance companies (Schlingensiepen 2020).

Conclusion

The German healthcare system is (hopefully) slowly shifting towards a more innovative system that allows innovative digital applications (e.g., Web-based applications, smartphone applications) to enter the statutory healthcare system and support patients seamlessly. In 2020, laws were passed to allow digital applications to be reimbursed in the statutory health system. This is considered an essential aspect for the acceptance of digital applications in the doctors' offices. Entering the DiGA registry ensures that the applications are certified as medical device and have proved/will prove a positive effect for patients. Only those digital applications listed in the registry can be prescribed by doctors/therapists.

The process for market access and price negotiations are similar to those for "regular" drugs (AMNOG process vs. Fast-Track Procedure) with the BfArM as a central authority and a fixed period of several months that allows the manufacturers to determine the price themselves. This is one of the main points of critique from payers. In addition, physicians still do not know that DiGAs exists, what their benefits are, and how to prescribe them. Furthermore, it is quite contradictory that prescribing digital applications from the doctor or therapist is still done via the "old" pink paper-based prescription form (this is the standardized form for doctors to prescribe pharmaceuticals and devices like seeing aids or ankle-foot orthosis) as there is no widely available and well-known PHR with integrated electronic prescription functionality. With the roll-out of the PHR in 2021, it remains to be seen if this will change in the following years.

The Federal Ministry of Health wants to further advance digitalization and is focusing on nursing. With the Digital Healthcare and Nursing Modernization Act (*Digitale-Versorgung-und-Pflege-Modernisierungs-Gesetz*, DVPMG) coming into effect in 2021, Digital Care Applications (*Digital Pflegeanwendungen*, DiPA) are also to be introduced. DiPAs may include, for example, applications for fall prevention or personalized care services for dementia patients. Like the BfArM's Fast-Track procedure for DiGAs, a process evaluating DiPAs is to be established (Bundesministerium für Gesundheit 2021b).

DiGA represents a very novel and unique service area, therefore there exist no major experiences of doctors, health insurance companies and patients yet. It is still too early to evaluate the success of the "App on Prescription" approach. The major stakeholders in the German healthcare system have attempted to implement a new and quite complex area of care within a period of time that can be considered "super short" for the German system (e.g., compared to the introduction of the eGK which took more than a decade). First and foremost, the DiGA area must be understood as a learning system.

Chapter Review Questions
Questions

1. Which regulatory bodies are involved when a) a new drug, b) a new digital health application (DiGA) enters the German market and aims for reimbursement by the health insurance companies (SHI)?
2. Why is the reimbursement by the SHI so important?
3. In the early 2000s, what was considered a key element of the digitalization of the German healthcare system?
4. What are some of the main criticism of the (current) Fast-Track Procedure for DiGAs?

Answers

1. (a) For new drugs: BfArM for market access (or EMA for European market access), Federal Joint Committee decides on additional benefit based on documents ("Dossiers") from the manufacturer. (b) For a Digital Health Application (DiGA): BfArM evaluates application for DiGA registration, several stakeholders are responsible for price negotiations directly with the manufacturer.
2. Most Germans is insured in the SHI system (about 90% of the population). If a product is part of the health insurance services, it can be prescribed by doctors via an established process. Therefore, being part of the SHI system opens a large target group of potential users.
3. The electronic health card, short "eGK".
4. Manufacturers are relatively free to set the price for the first year. An external review for data protection and data security does not take place yet. The possibility of prescribing digital healthcare applications is still relatively unknown to insurants. Doctors/therapists do not consider themselves prepared to prescribe DiGAs.

Glossary

English name	German name and common abbreviation
Digital Care Application	Digitale Pflegeanwendung, DiPA
Digital Health Applications	Digitale Gesundheitsanwendungen, DiGA
Digital Health Applications Ordinance	Digitale-Gesundheitsanwendungen-Verordnung, DiGAV
Digital Healthcare Act	Digitale-Versorgung Gesetz, DVG
Digital Healthcare and Nursing Modernization Act	Digitale-Versorgung-und-Pflege-Modernisierungs-Gesetz, DVPMG
Executive Association of Digital Healthcare	Spitzenverband Digitale Gesundheitsversorgung e.V., SVDGV
Federal Association of Statutory Health Insurance (SHI) Dentists	Kassenzahnärztliche Bundesvereinigung, KZBV
Federal Association of Statutory Health Insurance (SHI) Physicians	Kassenärztliche Bundesvereinigung, KBV
Federal Chamber of Dentists	Bundeszahnärztekammer, BZÄK
Federal Chamber of Physicians	Bundesärztekammer, BÄK
Federal Institute for Drugs and Medical Devices	Bundesinstitut für Arzneimittel und Medizinprodukte, BfArM
Federal Joint Committee	Gemeinsamer Bundesausschuss, G-BA
Federal Ministry of Health	Bundesministerium für Gesundheit, BMG
German Hospital Federation	Deutsche Krankenhausgesellschaft, DKG
German Medicines Act	Arzneimittelgesetz, AMG
German Organization of Pharmacists	Deutsche Apothekerverband, DAV
Health Insurance (company)	Krankenkasse
Medical Devices Act	Medizinproduktegesetz, MPG
Medical Device Regulation (MDR)	Medizinprodukterichtlinie
National Association of the Statutory Health Insurance	Spitzenverband der gesetzlichen Krankenkassen, GKV-SV
Pharmaceuticals Market Reorganization Act	Gesetz zur Neuordnung des Arzneimittelmarktes in der gesetzlichen Krankenversicherung, in short: Arzneimittelmarkt-Neuordnungsgesetz, AMNOG
Positive Healthcare Effects, pVE	Positive Versorgungseffekte
Private Health Insurance, PHI	Private Krankenversicherung, PKV
Public Health Authorities	Öffentlicher Gesundheitsdienst, ÖGD
Social Code Book V—Statutory Health Insurance	Sozialgesetzbuch V—Gesetzliche Krankenversicherung, SGB V
Statutory Health Insurance, SHI	Gesetzliche Krankenversicherung, GKV

Acknowledgements The authors would like to thank Michaela Warzecha (ZTG) for her feedback and proof-reading of the manuscript.

References

Ärzteblatt online: Gesundheits-Apps: Sicherheitsprüfung durch BfArM unzureichend; 2020. https://www.aerzteblatt.de/nachrichten/117355/Gesundheits-Apps-Sicherheitspruefung-durch-BfArM-unzureichend. Accessed 10 Feb 2021.

Ärzteblatt online. Spitzenverband will Informationsangebot zu DiGA ausweiten; 2021. https://www.aerztezeitung.de/Wirtschaft/Spitzenverband-will-Informationsangebot-zu-DiGA-ausweiten-416480.html. Accessed 7 Feb 2021.

ÄrzteZeitung online: Auch ohne DiGA-Status: IKK Südwest fördert Neurodermitis-App; 2021. https://www.aerztezeitung.de/Wirtschaft/IKK-Suedwest-foerdert-Neurodermitis-App-416510.html. Accessed 9 Feb 2021.

Bales S. Die Einführung der elektronischen Gesundheitskarte in Deutschland [The introduction of the electronic health card in Germany]. Bundesgesundheitsbl - Gesundheitsforsch – Gesundheitsschutz. 2005;48:727–31.

Bundesanzeiger Verlag GmbH. Verordnung über das Verfahren und die Anforderungen zur Prüfung der Erstattungsfähigkeit digitaler Gesundheitsanwendungen in der gesetzlichen Krankenversicherung (Digitale Gesundheitsanwendungen-Verordnung–DiGAV) - Vom 08. April 2020. In: Bundesgesetzblatt Jahrgang 2020 Teil I Nr. 18, ausgegeben zu Bonn am 20. April 2020. Bundesanzeiger Verlag, Köln p. 768–98.

Bundesärztekammer (BÄK), Kassenärztliche Bundesvereinigung (KBV). Gesundheits-Apps im klinischen Alltag. Handreichung für Ärztinnen und Ärzte. 1st ed, Version 1; 2020. https://doi.org/10.6101/AZQ/000474

Bundesinstitut für Arzneimittel und Medizinprodukte: Organisation; 2013. https://www.bfarm.de/EN/BfArM/Organisation/_node.html. Accessed 1 Apr 2021.

Bundesinstitut für Arzneimittel und Medizinprodukte: Bundesinstitut für Arzneimittel und Medizinprodukte. Das Fast Track Verfahren für digitale Gesundheitsanwendungen (DiGA) nach § 139e SGB V: Ein Leitfaden für Hersteller, Leistungserbringer und Anwender; Version 3.1 vom 18.03.2022. 2022a https://www.bfarm.de/SharedDocs/Downloads/DE/Medizinprodukte/diga_leitfaden.pdf?__blob=publicationFile. Accessed 5 July 2022.

Bundesinstitut für Arzneimittel und Medizinprodukte: BfArM nimmt erste "Apps auf Rezept" ins Verzeichnis digitaler Gesundheitsanwendungen (DiGA) auf; 2020b. https://www.bfarm.de/SharedDocs/Pressemitteilungen/DE/2020/pm4-2020.html. Accessed 08 Feb 2021.

Bundesinstitut für Arzneimittel und Medizinprodukte: DiGA-Verzeichnis; 2022b. https://diga.bfarm.de/de/verzeichnis. Accessed 5 July 2022.

Bundesinstitut für Arzneimittel und Medizinprodukte: DiGA-Verzeichnis: Für Leistungserbringer; 2021b. https://diga.bfarm.de/de/leistungserbringer. Accessed 8 Feb 2021.

Bundesministerium für Gesundheit: Online-Ratgeber Krankenversicherung; 2020a. https://www.bundesgesundheitsministerium.de/gkv.html. Accessed 25 Mar 2021.

Bundesministerium für Gesundheit: Die elektronische Patientenakte (ePA); 2020b. https://www.bundesgesundheitsministerium.de/elektronische-patientenakte.html. Accessed 1 Apr 2021.

Bundesministerium für Gesundheit: Ärzte sollen Apps verschreiben können: Gesetz für eine bessere Versorgung durch Digitalisierung und Innovation (Digitale-Versorgung-Gesetz - DVG); 2020c. https://www.bundesgesundheitsministerium.de/digitale-versorgung-gesetz.html. Accessed 8 Feb 2021.

Bundesministerium für Gesundheit: Online-Ratgeber Krankenversicherung, Beiträge und Tarife; 2021a. https://www.bundesgesundheitsministerium.de/beitraege-und-tarife.html. Accessed 25 Mar 2021.

Bundesministerium für Gesundheit. Spahn: „Machen digitale Anwendungen jetzt auch für Pflege nutzbar: Digitale–Versorgung–und–Pflege–Modernisierungs–Gesetz (DVPMG); 2021b. https://www.bundesgesundheitsministerium.de/service/gesetze-und-verordnungen/guv-19-lp/dvpmg.html. Accessed 9 Feb 2021.

Busse R, Blümel M. Germany: health system review. Health Syst Transit. 2014;16(2):1–296.

Busse R, Blümel M, Knieps F, Bärnighausen T. Statutory health insurance in Germany: a health system shaped by 135 years of solidarity, self-governance, and competition. Lancet. 2017;390:882–97. https://doi.org/10.1016/S0140-6736(17)31280-1.

BVMed: Erste DiGA-Erfahrungen in Deutschland | Interview mit BVMed-Digitalexpertin Natalie
    Gladkov.   https://www.bvmed.de/de/versorgung/digitalhealth/digitale-medizinprodukte/
    erste-diga-erfahrungen-in-deutschland-interview-mit-bvmed-digitalexpertin-natalie-gladkov.
    Accessed 07 Sept 2021.
Chances and Risks of Mobile Health Apps (CHARISMHA) – Abridged Version, Albrecht U-V
    (Editor). 2016. http://www.digibib.tu-bs.de/?docid=00060023. Accessed 6 April 2021.
gematik GmbH. Arena für digitale Medizin. Whitepaper Telematikinfrastruktur 2.0 für ein föder-
    alistisch vernetztes Gesundheitssystem; 2020. https://www.gematik.de/fileadmin/user_upload/
    gematik/files/Presseinformationen/gematik_Whitepaper_Arena_digitale_Medizin_TI_2.0_
    Web.pdf. Accessed 25 Mar 2021.
GKV Spitzenverband: Zusatzbeiträge der Krankenkassen; 2021a. https://www.gkv-spitzenverband.
    de/krankenkassenliste.pdf. Accessed 25 Mar 2021.
GKV Spitzenverband: Die gesetzlichen Krankenkassen; 2021b. https://www.gkv-spitzenverband.
    de/krankenversicherung/kv_grundprinzipien/alle_gesetzlichen_krankenkassen/alle_gesetzli-
    chen_krankenkassen.jsp. Accessed 1 Apr 2021.
GKV-Spitzenverband: Positionspapier des GKV-Spitzenverbandes: Anforderungen und Kriterien
    an Digitale Gesundheitsanwendungen; 2021. https://www.gkv-spitzenverband.de/media/doku-
    mente/krankenversicherung_1/telematik/digitales/Positionspapier_DiGA_2021-01-07_barri-
    erefrei.pdf. Accessed 7 Feb 2021.
Grätzel von Grätz P. EBM-Ziffern für die DiGAs; 2021. https://e-health-com.de/details-news/
    ebm-ziffern-fuer-die-digas/. Accessed 24 Mar 2021.
Grundy Q, Chiu K, Held F, Continella A, Bero L, Holz R. Data sharing practices of medicines related
    apps and the mobile ecosystem: traffic, content, and network analysis. BMJ. 2019;364:l920.
    https://doi.org/10.1136/bmj.l920.
Herberz C, Steidl R, Werner P, Hagen J. Der lange Weg von der Idee bis zur Erstattung –
    ein Reisebericht [From idea to standard care—a field report]. Bundesgesundheitsbl.
    2018;61:298–303.
IQVIA Commercial GmbH & Co. OHG: Kurzbericht "Die Sicht niedergelassener Ärzte in
    Deutschland auf die COVID-19-Krise und die Bedeutung von Digital Health"; 2020. https://
    www.iqvia.com/ /media/iqvia/pdfs/germany/library/publications/iqvia-kurzbericht-rztesicht-
    auf-covid-19-und-digital-health.pdf. Accessed 8 Feb 2021.
Leppert F, Greiner W. Finanzierung und Evaluation von eHealth-Anwendungen. In: Fischer F,
    Krämer A, editors. eHealth in Deutschland: Anforderungen und Perspektiven innovativer
    Versorgungsstrukturen. Berlin: Springer Vieweg; 2016.
Ploner N, Neurath MF, Schoenthaler M, Zielke A, Prokosch HU. Concept to gain trust for a
    German personal health record system using public cloud and FHIR. J Biomed Inform.
    2019;95:103212. https://doi.org/10.1016/j.jbi.2019.103212.
Radić M, Waack M, Donner I, Brinkmann C, Stein L, Radić D. Digitale Gesundheitsanwendungen:
    Die Akzeptanz steigern. Dtsch Arztebl. 2021; 118(6):A-286/B-250.
Sawicki PT, Bastian H. German health care: a bit of Bismarck plus more science.
    BMJ. 2008;337:a1997.
Schlingensiepen I. ÄzteZeitung online. Private Versicherer wollen eigene digitale
    Gesundheitsanwendungen; 2020. https://www.aerztezeitung.de/Wirtschaft/Private-Versicherer-
    wollen-eigene-digitale-Gesundheitsanwendungen-415849.html. Accessed 9 Feb 2021.
Schreiweis B, Pobiruchin M, Strotbaum V, Suleder J, Wiesner M, Bergh B. Barriers and facilitators
    to the implementation of eHealth services: systematic literature analysis. J Med Internet Res.
    2019;21(11):e14197. https://doi.org/10.2196/14197.
Staab TR, Walter M, Mariotti Nesurini S, Charalabos-Markos D, Graf von der Schulenburg J-M,
    Amelung VE, Ruof J. Market withdrawals" of medicines in Germany after AMNOG: a com-
    parison of HTA ratings and clinical guideline recommendations. Health Econ Rev. 2018:8(23).
    https://doi.org/10.1186/s13561-018-0209-3.

Chapter 5
Patient Portal for Critical Response During Pandemic: A Case Study of COVID-19 in Taiwan

Siang Hao Lee, Yi-Ru Chiu, and Po-Lun Chang

Abstract Traditionally in Asian countries, infectious diseases are usually monitored and controlled by government health departments. Meanwhile, individuals are expected to comply to the government guidelines of disease prevention measures and seek help from medical institutions after symptom onset. Only after the medical institutions confirm the diagnosis, government agencies would then enforce quarantine and contact tracking. Unfortunately, the traditional approach was not effective in stopping the highly contagious SARS-CoV-2 virus from spreading during the COVID-19 outbreak. In response to the COVID-19 epidemic, a new model of epidemic prevention that is more efficient than the traditional approach has been developed. In this chapter, we set out to introduce the background and key design challenges of the new Smart and Connected Health (s&cHealth) model. First, we share our experience of the effective prevention measures that have been in practice in Taiwan, and summarize on the key success factors. Then, we review the design considerations of Information and Communications Technology (ICT) innovative applications that aim to enable timely response to the pandemic outbreak with personal health informatics tools. More specifically, in this chapter we present case studies to demonstrate how the new s&cHealth model works on a mobile health epidemic prevention platform launched in both China and Taiwan. Finally, the chapter ends with a discussion around the lessons learned from this case study, including the trade-off between personal privacy and the public good, the limitations of the traditional ICT approach, and the challenges of Non-ICT issues.

S. H. Lee · Y.-R. Chiu · P.-L. Chang (✉)
Institute of Biomedical Informatics, National Yang-Ming University, Taipei, Taiwan
e-mail: polun@ym.edu.tw

© The Author(s), under exclusive license to Springer Nature
Switzerland AG 2022
P.-Y. S. Hsueh et al. (eds.), *Personal Health Informatics*, Cognitive Informatics
in Biomedicine and Healthcare, https://doi.org/10.1007/978-3-031-07696-1_5

Millennium Challenges in Pandemic Prevention and Control

At the beginning of this chapter, we set out to provide some context of the Covid-19 pandemic first. This would allow us to understand the core needs that warrant effective prevention and control. In addition, we would share our experience in effective prevention and control and summarize on the success factors.

Core Needs of Effective Pandemic Prevention and Control

In order to summarize the core needs of the effective measures for pandemic prevention and control, in the following subsections we will first review the cause of the pandemic and go through the potential measures across the different stages of implementation.

Identification of Causes of Infections

First, let's review the mechanism of COVID-19 infections. Due to the highly infectious nature of the SARS-CoV-2 virus, the COVID-19 pandemic has spread rapidly, causing devastating impacts on a global scale. As such, it is essential to implement a variety of epidemic prevention monitoring and management measures, including but not limited to personal health informatics tools, in order to effectively suppress the continual outbreak.

SARS-CoV-2, similar to the SARS-CoV variant that has led to the Severe Acute Respiratory Syndrome (SARS) pandemic in 2003, is a respiratory type of virus that is highly infectious and lethal when infected. The main source of transmission of the SARS-CoV-2 virus is through the respiratory tract via splash and droplet transfer as well as via direct contact transmission (Li et al. 2020; Tingting et al. 2020).

Most of the confirmed COVID-19 cases have exhibited flu-like symptoms (Wang et al. 2020; Wu et al. 2020; Zhu et al. 2020). The Coronavirus infects host cells by identifying and binding to the host receptor ACE2 distributed in the conjunctiva (Wan et al. 2020; Zhou et al. 2020). When the respiratory tract or conjunctiva is directly or indirectly exposed to the virus, the mucosal cells will be infected (Gao et al. 2016). Since SARS-CoV-2 could replicate itself abundantly in upper respiratory epithelia, a large number of virus would be subsequently released to the lungs through the respiratory tract leading to symptoms such as fever and coughing. In addition, CT examination results would show pulmonary ground glass opacity, while respiratory failures could also happen in severe cases.

The transmission of SARS-CoV-2 occurs mainly through unprotected contact in a close proximity (within distances under two meters) with infected patients (including not only symptomatic patients, but also those who are asymptomatic). Virus transmission over a greater distance (e.g., over two meters) is uncommon but may still be possible through prolonged exposure in poorly ventilated environments, leading to the inhalation of respiratory droplets and aerosols of small particles (Burke et al. 2020; Pung et al. 2020; Chan et al. 2020; Huang et al. 2020; Tong et al. 2020; Yu et al. 2020).

Prevention of Outbreaks of Infections

Given the mechanism of COVID-19 infections and its high infection rate, the number of confirmed COVID-19 cases has been far higher than that of SARS. In the beginning phase of the disease outbreak, there are mainly two major categories of measures to prevent the outbreak: quarantine and vaccination.

On the one hand, to enforce quarantine, currently the recommended quarantine periods designated by various countries vary between 14 and 21 days (Yu et al. 2020; Lauer et al. 2020), i.e., the person who is under quarantine should stay in solitude for 14–21 days from the time of the last exposure to a confirmed case (WHO 2020a). However, quarantining for 14–21 days has been shown as insufficient in some cases. Prior studies have reported on cases wherein a significant amount of virus were detected after a long period of in-hospital negative pressure isolation; such cases could have resulted in the prolonged delays of patient discharge from hospital (Rees et al. 2020). On the other hand, vaccination is also a necessary measure to help with the prevention of infection outbreak.

However, as none of these measures are sufficient by itself, it is important that ample preventive measures continue to be adopted. In order to understand how to better advise on the timing of implementation in practice, epidemiologists and policy makers have further investigated into the epidemiological conditions of the disease (CDC, Ministry of Health and Welfare, Taiwan 2020a), including but not limited to:

1. History of travel or residing abroad or have been in contact with people from abroad who have exhibited fever or respiratory symptoms.
2. Coming into close contact with highly probable or confirmed cases exhibiting symptoms without ample protection during the process of providing care or living together, direct contact with respiratory secretions or body fluids.
3. Cluster transmissions.

These investigations have led to the setting of guideline for introducing various prevention measures in the different stages of disease outbreak. First, when cases just begin to spread rapidly in neighboring countries or regions, close surveillance must be introduced at the border. As the epidemic develops, the restriction of border access should begin as soon as necessary. Next, right after the transmission route of the disease is better understood, the government can start implementing early-stage, precautionary public health policies, such as promoting masks by the entire population, at a relatively low cost. Finally, when the number of infection cases begin to grow, government would carry out active epidemiological investigation, contract tracing and quarantine enforcement measures on those at risk of disease transmission to interrupt the known chain of transmission.

Prevention of Becoming Pandemic

In the next phase, the goal would be to stop the disease outbreak from developing into a pandemic. A dedicated disease control agency should be empowered to monitor the disease spread in the vicinity to the country in a timely manner. The sources to be monitored is not limited to official outbreak information such as the reported case information from the health department, but also social media forum discussion. The agency must establish verified sources of information to inform citizens about the early development of any major outbreaks (CDC, Ministry of Health and Welfare, Taiwan 2020b, c). The acquisition and verification of epidemic information is the highest priority among all epidemic prevention measures.

In addition, the government should establish an inter-department, cross-function response center for epidemic control. This center would help integrate all aspects of preventive measures, widely ranging from border control, risk group quarantine, disease tracking, uniform notification across medical institutions, treatment capacity inventory management, preparation for medical supplies, preparation and access control to personal preventive equipment (PPE) supplies, and communication services for epidemic prevention (CDC, Ministry of Health and Welfare, Taiwan 2020d).

The above epidemic prevention and resource management measures require the establishment of a digital management and service platform to collect accurate data for effective and timely epidemic prevention and control. To provide a closer look into what measures have been shown as effective in practice, in the following subsection we provide a briefing of the outbreak surveillance and decision-making process in Taiwan in the beginning of the current COVID-19 outbreak (CDC, Ministry of Health and Welfare, Taiwan 2020d):

In early dawn December 31, 2019, Taiwan Centers for Disease Control (CDC) learned from online sources that there had been at least 7 cases of atypical pneumonia in Wuhan, China. At 8 am, Taiwan CDC contacted the Chinese Center for Disease Control and Prevention to confirm about the latest epidemic situation. Taiwan CDC also sent an email to the International Health Regulations (IHR) focal point under the World Health Organization (WHO), informing WHO of its understanding of the disease and requesting further information. According to the standard operating procedures, Taiwan authorities have decided to initiate border control and onboard inspections for direct flights from Wuhan. On January 2, 2020, Taiwan CDC held the initial meeting to discuss "emergency response measures to pneumonia of an unknown cause originating from China", culminating in the establishment of the Epidemic Response Team. Official notices were sent to all medical institutions to request for the report of all cases with suspected symptoms and information about patients with recent travel history from Wuhan.

On January 7, 2020, Wuhan City was listed as a Level 1 (Watch) Travel Notice destination by Taiwan CDC. On January 8, Taiwan government raised the security alert level for all international and cross-strait ports of entry and exit. On January 10, Taiwan CDC formulated the "Practices and Control Measures by Primary Care Clinics in Response to Atypical Pneumonia of Unknown Cause from Wuhan, China". On January 12, Taiwan government sent two experts to Wuhan and visited the Hubei Provincial Center for Disease Control and Prevention, as well as hospitals where infected patients were being treated. On January 15, Taiwan CDC formally classified "Severe Pneumonia with Novel Pathogens" as a Category 5 Notifiable Disease to strengthen disease surveillance and prevention.

On January 23, 2020, Taiwan government announced that all airlines of Taiwan would suspend direct flights to and from Wuhan, and all Chinese nationals residing in Wuhan were prohibited from entry into Taiwan. On January 25, any Individuals with travel history in Hubei Province, China, including those with no symptoms, were subjected to health checks, which would be enforced by civil affairs personnel from their local jurisdiction for a period of 14 days after returning to Taiwan. On January 26, Taiwan government announced the entry restrictions for any Chinese citizens from entering into Taiwan, and any asymptomatic individuals with travel history in Hubei Province, China, were subjected to home quarantine. On January 30, WHO declared the novel coronavirus as "a public health emergency of international concern."

Recognition of Source Control

Once the disease outbreak has developed into a pandemic, it would incur another set of autonomous health management and medical screening measures. For example, as found in the prior cases, it is possible that the incubation period of COVID-19 cases is greater than 14 days. Hence in effect from April 5, 2020, the command center of Taiwan CDC has introduced an additional period of 7 days of autonomous health management for those whose home quarantine period expires after 14 days (CDC, Ministry of Health and Welfare, Taiwan 2020e). If anyone develops fever (≥ 38 °C), exhibits symptoms of abnormal smell or taste, diarrhea, or any other respiratory symptoms, they are advised to immediately contact the Health Bureau before proceeding to a medical institution designated by the Health Bureau for medical treatment according to the given instructions. They should also wear their face masks at all time and are prohibited from traveling by any forms of public transportation. When seeking medical treatment, they should proactively notify the doctor of the history of their recent contact, travel and residence, occupational exposures, and whether anyone around them has had similar COVID-19 related symptoms. Upon returning home, they should also wear a face mask and refrain from leaving their place of residence. They should always keep their face mask on when conversing with others and maintain a safe distance of more than 1 m from others.

In terms of the rules for additional preventive measures taken around COVID-19 testing, it is also important to ensure that the subject should stay at home and do not leave their residences until they receive the test results notification from the hospital. Should the test result be positive, the Health Bureau will arrange for treatment follow-up measures. Even if the test result returns as negative, self-health management measures are still required for a period of 7 days (CDC, Ministry of Health and Welfare, Taiwan 2020f).

Administrative, Environmental and Engineering Control

Besides the recognition of source control around the infected and suspected individuals, complementary measures are also needed at the society level to constrain the virus spread. In this subsection, we refer to the Taiwan CDC's guidelines for epidemic prevention, which describe some recommendations in three areas: Engineering Control, Administrative Control, and Safe Work Practices (U.S. Department of Labor Occupational Safety and Health Administration 2021).

Engineering Control
1. Install a high-efficiency air filter.
2. Increase the air flow rate in the work environment.
3. Install a physical barrier such as a transparent plastic anti-sneeze guard.
4. Install a pass window for customer service (such as drive-thru).
5. Set up a special negative pressure operating system such as performing procedures that produce bio-aerosol (for example, air-borne infection isolation wards and funeral sites in medical care environments).

Administrative Control
1. Encourage employees who are feeling unwell to stay at home.
2. Usage of teleconferencing functions instead of face-to-face meetings and implementing work from home procedures whenever possible minimizing face-to-face interaction between staff and customers.
3. Establish alternating shifts system to minimize contact among employees within the same organization so as to maintain safe distancing from each other in the course of their work duties.
4. Halt unnecessary travel to locations where the COVID-19 outbreak situation remains dire and checking the CDC travel advisory level regularly.
5. Develop an emergency communication plan, including a forum to address employee concerns and communication remotely via the internet (whenever feasible).
6. Provide employees with the latest education and training on COVID-19 risk factors and protective behaviors such as cough etiquette and PPE protection.
7. Provide sufficient training and education for employees who might need to use protective clothing and equipment. Training materials should be easy to understand and provided in languages at a suitable coherent level for all employees.

Safe Work Practices
1. Provide resources and a work environment that promote personal hygiene. For example, provide paper towels, non-contact trash cans, hand sanitizers containing at least 60% alcohol, disinfectants and disposable paper towels for workers to disinfect their work spaces.

2. Require regular hand washing or use of alcohol-based hand rub. Employees should wash their hands thoroughly when visibly soiled and after removing any personal protective equipment.
3. Post hand-washing signs in the restrooms.

Personal Protective Control

The complementary measures also include the following suggestions for good health habits in daily lives (CDC, Ministry of Health and Welfare, Taiwan 2020g):

- Washing one's hands frequently and donning of face masks: Use soap or alcohol-based dry wash to clean hands frequently and implement respiratory hygiene and cough etiquette.
- Avoid touching one's eyes, nose and mouth with hands: When one comes into contact with nasal secretions from sneezing or coughing, one needs to ensure thorough cleansing   with soap and water.
- Take body temperature measurements at least once a day.
- Avoid traveling and maintain social distancing: Minimize visits to public places and ensure face-mask wearing in public.
- Recuperate at home when feeling unwell: If one is experiencing symptoms of illnesses, one should recuperate at home and always wear a face mask. In the event one's face mask is stained with oral and nasal secretions, one should fold it inwards and discard it at the designated disposal area before replacing it with a new medical-grade face mask.
- Active notification of severe symptoms: If one's condition worsens or if the symptoms do not go away, one should proactively report his or her own condition to local health bureau so as to receive follow up instructions and the needed medical attention.

Effectiveness of Epidemic Prevention in Asian Cases

In Asia, many countries or regions developed mHealth applications for COVID-19 epidemic prevention earlier and actively promoted mHealth applications among the general public in the region. For example, the case study in this paper was launched in early February 2020, the China Health Code was launched in late February of 2020 (Liang 2020), the initial version of the Singapore government's TraceTogether app was released in March 2020 (Government of Singapore 2020), and the Hong Kong Health Code was officially launched in August 2020 (Wikipedia 2020).

In general, the effectiveness of the epidemic prevention in a country or region can be simply evaluated by the number of confirmations, deaths, and tests per million population (Worldometers 2020), as well as the vaccine coverage rate. The number of confirmed cases can indicate the extent of the spread of the epidemic in the local area and the efficiency of preventive measures. Using this indicator, the number of confirmed COVID-19 cases per million population as of September 9, 2021, in China, Taiwan, Hong Kong, and South Korea were 66, 673, 1603, and 5212, respectively, compared to the global average of 28,670 (WHO 2020b).

However, at the end of August 2021, the vaccination coverage rates in Hong Kong and Taiwan are only around the world average (Our World in Data 2020), which means that the major East Asian regions have not mainly used vaccination to obtain the current epidemic prevention results during the period since the global outbreak.

Critical Success Factors and Gaps of Effective Pandemic Prevention and Control

In addition to the epidemic prevention measures introduced in the previous subsections over the cycle of pandemic development, it is also important to establish the awareness about active pandemic prevention among the local population. Without sufficient public awareness of active pandemic prevention, gaps would always surface during the implementation of pandemic prevention measures. The advance deployment of pandemic prevention therefore includes at least the following four stages:

First, during the initial phase of pre-deployment, it is worthwhile noting that the preparation of public health personnel and infrastructures, as well as the notification systems, all need to be given the utmost attention prior to the occurrence of a major pandemic outbreak.

Second, during the early stages of a pandemic outbreak, the timeliness of information collection and verification on the suspected cases is of the utmost importance. After the disease mechanism is further understood, the authority in charge of the regional concern will be able to respond rapidly and come up with a decision-making process to determine whether border control or lock down measures would be needed.

Third, epidemic models should be used to generate dynamic forecasts of pandemic development, and adequate resources such as manpower and medical supplies should be prepared in advance accordingly. The key focus at this stage is to ensure active public awareness on the pandemic prevention procedures and the implementation of such procedures in their daily schedules.

Finally, in the reviewing and assessment phase after the end of the pandemic, it is important to cover all aspects of the pandemic prevention measures to identify areas that would require strengthening so as to allow for appropriate preparation of any future pandemic outbreaks.

The Overview of mHealth for Epidemic and COVID-19

The mHealth is the abbreviation for mobile health and covers the utilizing of our mobile devices to provide healthcare, medicine or public health services or support. This is achieved through wireless and remote communication to hasten the process of traditional healthcare service process by reducing costs and complexity. mHealth has been used in various healthcare applications. Many such applications have since been developed (Tirado 2011; L'Engle et al. 2014; Fortuin et al. 2016) in the field of epidemiology and this has seen continuous growth in recent years. The application of mHealth in the field of epidemiology developed between 2014 and 2020 can be divided into five main directions: (1) Public health aspects (2) Data management (3) Educational programs (4) Patient identification and diagnosis and (5) Treatment. The main diseases tracked and managed are: (1) Ebola (2) Epidemic Diseases (3) Influenza (4) Acute Respiratory Infections and (5) Tuberculosis (Aslani et al. 2020).

There are various pandemic prevention measures being utilized under the current situation of the global outbreak of the COVID-19 pandemic including: contact tracing, quarantine, personal entry and exit location controls, non-contact communication, physical and mental health monitoring and location tracking, pandemic prevention policies dissemination and the prevention of the spread of falsehoods. These epidemic prevention measures which are different from traditional healthcare service types must be carried out at reasonable social costs resulting in many countries/regions developing various types of mHealth applications to assist them in the implementation and management of pandemic prevention measures. Some of the application fields and time points of this study have been implemented in China much earlier than locally developed mHealth applications. In summarizing (Ming et al. 2020; Singh et al. 2020) the literature review as of May 2020, the application of mHealth for COVID-19 can be mainly based on (1) The unit involved in the app issuance (2) The purpose of the application and (3) The application adopted by mHealth-related technologies. There have 17 governments of the countries/regions out of the total 19 countries/regions have utilized mHealth applications to assist in pandemic prevention. Of the 29 apps utilized in total, 15 (52%) were purposely used for contact tracing, 7 (24%) for quarantine monitoring, and another 7 (24%) were used for symptoms monitoring (CDC, Ministry of Health and Welfare, Taiwan 2020h).

The mHealth platform developed in this chapter was designed from the beginning with the flexibility of application in different scenarios in different regions, so our mHealth platform has covered all the categories listed in this table in terms of the purpose of use and functionality. We try to make the most of the technology and equipment available at mHealth by considering the full usability of technology and preventive measures.

ICT Innovations for the Pandemic Prevention and Control

With the continuous development of the global COVID-19 epidemic, countries around the world are also actively engaged in the development of various Information and Communications Technology (ICT) applications to combat the pandemic on top of the main epidemic prevention measures described in the previous section. In particular, this has enabled the development of a Smart and Connected Health (s&cHealth) model in Asian countries. In this model, the applications based on personal health informatics, such as personal health records, personal health management systems, or personal health portals, have become more important as health data from personal sources contain signals more timely than those from traditional surveys in the official epidemic workflow.

Early Screening

There are three main applications of early screening: Contact Tracing, Symptoms Monitoring, and Quarantine. These are the commonly developed applications during the early stage of a pandemic outbreak. The common goal of the early screening applications is to facilitate the follow-up of systematic pandemic investigation and isolation measures through identifying the source of infection at the earliest opportunity, followed by tracking and establishing the route of infection.

The Contact Tracing application mainly uses mobile phone base station signals, Global Positioning System (GPS), and Bluetooth signals to trace and record the whereabouts of infected subjects and the conditions of those who have been in contact with them. Additionally, there are also simple questionnaires or active pop-up prompts which act as ways to establish contact history. One such example is the Contact Tracing App running on Bluetooth signal developed and openly sourced by the Singapore government.

The Symptom Monitoring application monitors and records symptoms and vital signs for individuals at risk of infection. In the event wherein suspected symptoms are detected, the individual under monitoring would be able to seek for medical attention, or undergo testing following the principles of non-contact and under appropriate protective measures.

The Quarantine application monitors the quarantine status of individuals at risk of infection. The use cases include detecting whether any at-risk individuals have left their place of quarantine, monitoring their daily physical and mental conditions during the quarantine period, and ensuring all quarantine measures to be followed until the end of the legally required quarantine period.

Given the prevalence of smartphones in Asian countries, the best practice of the above-mentioned applications is to install these applications on a smartphone that the individual carries around with them every day and to leverage the real-time data to make public health decisions.

Contact Monitoring

For those who are positively diagnosed or who are established to be at risk of infection, the s&cHealth model enables higher frequency data collection to facilitate pandemic control and personnel safety, prevent new cases of infections and provide early intervention such as medical care or any other necessary quarantine measures. Common applications for close contact monitoring include the following: location tracking, physiological measurement, and questionnaire assessment.

Location tracking: To track movement and perform contact tracing, each subject's whereabouts can be tracked through signal processing. Subjects under monitoring can also upload live photos to confirm their locations (as shown in Fig. 5.1).

Before each individual actively participates in the monitoring process, he or she must first give their informed consent. Individuals would also need to authorize the personal health application to collect their personal information such as traces and contacts and provide the health information including physiological measurements, or health status questionnaire assessment results for epidemic prevention, which can promote efficient operation and decision making of the whole epidemic prevention system.

Physiological measurement: Physiological measurement records are continuously collected through either automatic collection by wearable devices or manual recording. Among them, wearable devices have been shown in practice as a more effective solution in the sense that they can more accurately and continuously curate objective data.

Questionnaire assessment: The questionnaire scales are designed to come with one physical assessment scale and another mental assessment scale to accurately assess whether the subject's physical and mental state is affected by illness and the quarantining measures. The scales are also used to determine whether the individual under monitoring requires any health intervention during the quarantine period. The physical and mental questionnaire evaluation scales are as shown in Tables 5.1 and 5.2. In the backend, these assessment scales consisted of individuals' subjective daily records would go into the Epidemic Prevention and Health Management platform, which allows for the detection and early intervention on suspected cases.

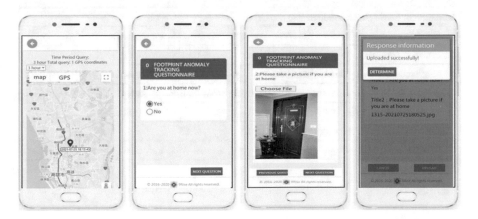

Fig. 5.1 Screenshots of the contract tracing application

Table 5.1 Simple home quarantine body status questionnaire

Total score range	Alert Color	Description
0~1	Green	Normal
2~4	Red	Suspected symptoms

Question 1: Whole Body Condition (Multiple choice)

0	Normal mental, appetite and sleep	1	Poor spirit, poor appetite

Question 2: Respiration Condition (Multiple choice)

0	No dyspnea or shortness of breath	1	Increased frequency, even breathing difficulties

Question 3: Cough Condition (Multiple choice)

0	Asymptomatic	1	Severe symptoms, mainly dry cough	1	Accompanied by sputum, wheezing

Question 4: Fever Condition (Multiple choice)

0	Asymptomatic	1	Fever within 72 hours	1	High fever more than 72 hours

Table 5.2 Simple home quarantine emotion status questionnaire

Total score range	Alert Color	Description
0~5	Green	In a good mood.
6~9	Yellow	Mild emotional distress, emotional support is recommended
10~14	Orange	Moderate emotional trauma, referral to psychiatric treatment or professional consultation is recommended
15~24	Red	Severe emotional distress, referral to psychiatric treatment or professional consultation.

Question 1: Feeling nervous (Multiple choice)

0	Absolutely not	1	Slight	2	Moderate	3	Severe	4	Very serious

Question 2: Feeling easily upset or angry (Multiple choice)

0	Absolutely not	1	Slight	2	Moderate	3	Severe	4	Very serious

Question 3: Feeling depressed(Multiple choice)

0	Absolutely not	1	Slight	2	Moderate	3	Severe	4	Very serious

Question 4: Feel inferior to others(Multiple choice)

0	Absolutely not	1	Slight	2	Moderate	3	Severe	4	Very serious

Question5: Difficulty sleeping, such as difficulty falling asleep, waking up early (Multiple choice)

0	Absolutely not	1	Slight	2	Moderate	3	Severe	4	Very serious

Question6: Have suicidal thoughts(Multiple choice)

0	Absolutely not	1	Slight	2	Moderate	3	Severe	4	Very serious

Rapid Response

Using the Early Screening and Contact Monitoring applications mentioned in the last subsection, any abnormal or alarming events of individuals under monitoring could be evaluated in real time on the epidemic prevention platform. At this time, a dedicated personnel under the governance structure would be responsible for providing a rapid response following the standard operating procedures (SOPs). The platform is also responsible to ensure the availability of front-line service personnel in order to immediately contact the individuals who are concerned about their current situations and to determine whether any intervention, such as follow-up quarantine, testing, or medical treatment, is deemed necessary under the SOPs. The platform is also responsible to support front-line service personnel when a subject under monitoring leaves his quarantine location, or when any of them becomes uncontactable. In scenarios like this, police assistance may be required for locating and route tracing.

Let's take a closer look into a home quarantine scenario to better illustrate the rapid response applications.

First, the individual under quarantine must set the home GPS location to his home quarantine address upon the first login to the Personal Health App. In conjunction with the Web API Service, the GPS signals from the smartphone would then be used to periodically collect geographic location data (Geolocation) of the quarantined individual and to gauge the relative distance from the home location to the quarantined individual's actual location. Next, if the relative distance exceeds a certain threshold, the Personal Health App would generate a warning event notification to the first responders via SMS text message and via the management Web App. Meanwhile, other units on the chain of command would also receive real-time event notifications via the management web app according to their area of responsibility and coverage.

During a pre-specified quarantine period, a "Caring Notice" questionnaire will automatically pop up on the Personal Health App. This pre-specified period can be set according to region preferences. This questionnaire will monitor the basic health status of the quarantined individuals, e.g., whether they are feeling unwell, whether they have had adequate sleep and healthy food. In the end of the questionnaire, the quarantined individuals are required to upload live photos to ensure that the operation of the Personal Health App is being done by the target quarantined individual or assisted by an approved family member. In the event wherein the questionnaire has not been responded to within a stipulated period, the platform would generate a non-responsive event notification to remind the front-line management service personnel to intervene and provide follow up instructions.

The mobile health (mHealth) platform that integrates the Personal Health App with the backend epidemic prevention management system to warrant reliable real-time location identification of individuals under home quarantine and to ensure that front-line management service personnel can respond effectively respond to any emerging needs. The user workflow of the Personal Health App on the mHealth platform is shown in Table 5.3.

Table 5.3 User workflow of geolocation monitoring and care questionnaire

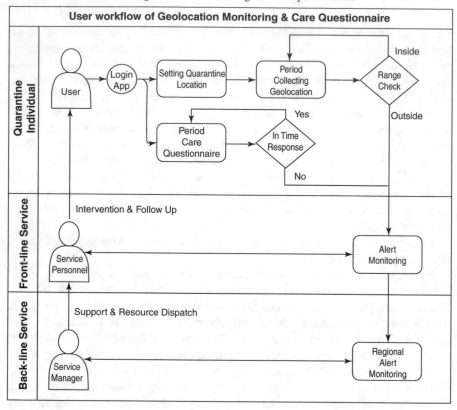

Effective Control

If the pandemic is not properly kept under control in its early stage and has spread, it is necessary to establish an organized response system for subsequent pandemic prevention procedures. The best possible solution is to utilize existing social service and law enforcement systems such as the civil administration system and the police system as a dual-system epidemic prevention and monitoring platform. In this sub-section, we would go through an example system in China to illustrate how the existing systems can contribute to pandemic prevention tasks in an organized manner and to facilitate effective implementation in pandemic prevention and control.

First and foremost, our design accounts for the local administrative region boundaries and leverages a hierarchical management structural approach to accommodate multiple administrative systems in the existing administrative region hierarchy. In the example system in China, this means that the design needs to work with at least two different administrative systems, each consisted of multiple layers. The first layer in the administrative management system is the six-layer civil administration system. The second is the system of the seven-layer police force. These two different administrative systems are both able to monitor in real-time the status of individuals under home quarantine, receive warning notifications according to its own tree structure, and provide general services and interventions with respect to their unit roles. For example, in the general case, the daily epidemic prevention measures are monitor by the service staff of the civil affairs system. However, if a home quarantine individual fails to respond to information for a long time by the regulations and an alert event is generated, and the civil affairs system staff confirms that the individual cannot be contacted, the police system will intervene to assist in locating the individual. The dual system organizational structure served by this mHealth platform is illustrated in Fig. 5.2.

Under the current design, the Personal Health App, which collects and processes personal health records, would process and provide the needed personal information related to epidemic prevention back to the hierarchical disease control system of the government organization. Personal health informatics tools can influence government disease control decisions, help epidemic control units obtain accurate data more quickly, and improve the timeliness of epidemic prevention decisions.

In terms of system design, the basic unit (leaf node) is the home quarantined individual. The system leverages an Organization Resource (c.f. HL7 FHIR Organization Resource (HL7 FHIR 2019a)), which can be flexibly applied to represent a tree-like organization structure regardless of the number of hierarchical layers.

In the real-life application of this platform, the bottommost administrative personnel (either from the grid administrator or the community police) will be responsible for front-line operations such as quarantine status monitoring, intervention after detection of abnormalities, and the provisioning of basic necessities to quarantined individuals under their jurisdiction. This platform design can ensure the essential data of quarantined individual to be effectively shared and managed while preventing unnecessary face-to-face contact between front-line personnel and quarantine individuals.

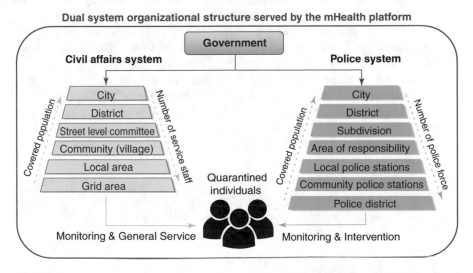

Fig. 5.2 Dual system organizational structure served by the mHealth platform in China

In the worst case scenario wherein the pandemic outbreak is still unable to be kept under effective control, it would be necessary to maintain such an organized pandemic prevention monitoring and service system until an effective vaccine has been developed and administered to a significant proportion of the population.

Take the implementation of such a system in Taiwan as another example. In response to the COVID-19 epidemic, Taiwan government has implemented a mandatory 14-days quarantine procedure since March 19, 2020, applicable to anyone entering Taiwan from other countries. In addition, the 14-days home quarantine procedure is also applied to anyone who came into contact with confirmed COVID subjects. During this home quarantine period, body temperature and health status of these subjects must be recorded, and the monitoring authorities would also take the initiative to contact the quarantined subjects on a daily basis. In the event that a quarantined individual shows any underlying symptoms during quarantine, he has to notify the health bureaus or medical institutions of their local counties or cities and seek medical treatment according to the instructions given (CDC, Ministry of Health and Welfare, Taiwan 2020h).

The overview of Taiwan's epidemic prevention strategy is depicted in the 2020 autumn and winter epidemic prevention plan, which is divided into three main axes as shown in Fig. 5.3 (CDC, Ministry of Health and Welfare, Taiwan 2020i):

1. Community Prevention:

    From December 1, 2020, masks are required in places with high risks of infection and transmission in order to effectively prevent the spread of SARS-CoV-2 in the community. Refusal to wear a mask despite being advised by local authority is subject to a fine of NT$3000 to NT$15,000 pursuant to Paragraph 1, Article 70 of the Communicable Disease Control Act (CDC, Ministry of Health and Welfare, Taiwan 2020i).

2. Border Control and Quarantine:

    As the COVID-19 pandemic rages internationally, it has been expected that the number of travelers entering Taiwan would increase significantly in the first part of 2021. To ensure that this influx of travelers would not increase risk of infection through air travel, the Central Epidemic Command Center for Severe Special Infectious Pneumonia ("CECC") in Taiwan has announced that starting from December 1, 2020, travelers arriving at any airport in Taiwan, or changing flights at an airport in Taiwan, regardless of their nationality (either Taiwanese nationals or foreign nationals) or the purpose of their visit to Taiwan (work, study, etc.), must present a COVID-19 RT-PCR test result issued within 3 days of the scheduled boarding time ("RT-PCR test report") when checking in at a foreign airport.

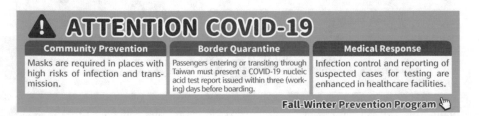

Fig. 5.3 The fall-winter prevention program of Taiwan

Travelers who do not meet the aforementioned conditions and take flights to Taiwan can enter Taiwan after submitting an Entry Quarantine Affidavit to state a specific reason for not providing a test report; such travelers are required to take a self-paid COVID-19 test at the airport and to follow the subsequent and related quarantine measures. If the reason stated by such travelers, after assessments, does not meet the requirements for related exceptions, penalties may be imposed in accordance with the Communicable Disease Control Act. Those who have COVID-19 and are suspected of having infected other persons must bear relevant criminal liability. These procedures have been drafted specifically to handle cases in which travelers have difficulty obtaining a COVID-19 RT-PCR test report in their country of departure due to emergency circumstances, and are therefore, unable to obtain a RT-PCR test report, but must enter the territory of Taiwan.

3. Medical Response

(a) Healthcare institutions are urged to fulfill their obligation of reporting confirmed and suspected cases. Local public health bureaus are instructed to strengthen the supervision of healthcare institutions under their jurisdiction, requiring them to immediately report cases that meets the criteria for "severe pneumonia with novel pathogens reporting and testing" and encouraging them to report cases that meet the criteria for "community surveillance reporting and testing."

(b) Indicators for incentive schemes, including "enhanced screening among patients with pneumonia in outpatient and emergency departments", "enhanced screening among inpatients" and "enhanced health monitoring among medical and nursing staff", are introduced to promote the reporting of suspected cases for testing through the community surveillance system.

In addition, the regulation has categorized individuals at risk of infection into four categories according to their risk levels from high to low (CDC, Ministry of Health and Welfare, Taiwan 2020h):

1. Home isolation;
2. Home quarantine;
3. Enhanced self-health management;
4. Self-health management.

Taiwan presently has a tracking management mechanism for all of the above categories. Under each category, the system captures information such as the definition and classification basis of individuals in this category, their responsible supervisory officers, the required number of days of quarantine, detailed implementation measures, and the source of local regulations. More details are shown in Table 5.4. The Personal Health App enables the curation of personal health data from individuals at varying levels of risk. The frequency, content, and detail of data collection are adjusted according to the level of regulatory compliance. In addition, on the backend, there exists a privacy control mechanism that would safeguard personal health data so that only the responsible administrative units can access the data for epidemic prevention, and the scope of access is legally bound with their pre-determined level of authority.

Table 5.4 Tracking management mechanism for persons at risk of infection

CECC measures for following up on persons at risk of infection   12.22.2020 published

Intervention	Home Isolation	Home Quarantine	Enhanced self-health management	Self-health management
Groups of persons	Persons who had contact with confirmed cases	People with travel history	Short-term business travelers from low- and medium-risk countries/regions who have applied for and been permitted entry	Reported cases who have tested negative
Responsible authorities	Local health authorities	Local civil affairs bureau or borough chief	Local health authorities	Central/Local health authorities
Enforcement	Home isolation for 14 days Active monitoring twice a day	Home quarantine for 14 days Active monitoring once or twice a day	From the end of the shortened home quarantine period to the 14th day after entry into Taiwan Active monitoring once or twice a day	Self-health management for 14 days
Notes concerning respective measures	• Health authority will issue a "Home (Self) Isolation Notice" • Health authority shall check health status of the individual twice a day	• Where the relevant authority has issued a Novel Coronavirus Health Declaration and Home Quarantine Notice, the individual is to wear a surgical mask and return home for home quarantine • The local borough chief or borough clerk shall call the individual every day during the 14-day period to ask about the individual's health status, and shall record the information obtained	• The individual is only allowed to carry out limited business activities and is prohibited from going to crowded places (such as markets, nightclubs, night markets, department stores, restaurants, tourist destinations, etc.). • The individual shall postpone all non-essential or non-urgent medical care or examinations; and make sure to inform the physician of travel history when seeking medical attention.	• Asymptomatic individuals are to avoid public places, postpone any non-urgent medical care or examination, always wear a medical mask when going out, wash hands frequently, follow respiratory hygiene and cough etiquette, and take temperature twice a day, once in the morning and once in the evening. • Individuals with fever or respiratory symptoms such as coughing or running nose are to wear a medical mask, seek medical attention immediately and not to use public transport; inform the physician of your contact history, travel history, and whether anyone else has similar symptoms; wear a surgical mask while returning home and avoid going out; and keep 1 meter away from others when talking to them.

	• During the home isolation period, the individual is to stay at home (or designated location) and not go out, and may not leave the country or use public transportation	• During the quarantine period, the individual is to stay at home (or designated location) and not go out, and may not leave the country or use public transportation	• The individual must visit leisure facilities in the quarantine hotel at staggered times to avoid contact with others; and notify quarantine hotel staff to conduct environmental disinfection after leaving those facilities.	• After being tested for COVID-19 and returning home, individuals are to stay at home and not to go out before receiving results
	• Symptomatic individuals will be sent to the hospital for medical attention	• Symptomatic individuals will be sent to designated medical facilities for tests; the relevant health authority will also begin active monitoring	• The individual must be picked up and accompanied by a designated person throughout the stay in Taiwan to ensure that protective measures are followed.	• Medical personnel are to halt work and not to come to work temporarily
	• Individuals not adhering to the CECC's prevention measures will be penalized under the Communicable Disease Control Act and be forcibly placed	• Individuals not adhering to the CECC's prevention measures will be penalized under the Communicable Disease Control Act and be forcibly placed	• A record must be kept of the individual's daily activities and the names of people he or she comes into contact with. The individual must not come into contact with anyone except the persons scheduled to meet according to the itinerary; the individual **must wear a medical mask and maintain social distance all the time.**	
	• After the home isolation period ends, the individual should conduct an additional 7-day period of self-health management	• After the home quarantine period ends, the individual should conduct an additional 7-day period of self-health management	• The individual must reply to daily text messages requesting an update on personal health status from the competent health authority.	
Legal basis	§ Article 48, Communicable Disease Control Act	§ Article 58, Communicable Disease Control Act	§ Article 58, Communicable Disease Control Act	§ Article 48, Communicable Disease Control Act; Article 58, Communicable Disease Control Act
	§ Paragraph 1, Article15, Special Act for Prevention, Relief and Revitalization Measures for Severe Pneumonia with Novel Pathogens	§ Paragraph 2, Article15, Special Act for Prevention, Relief and Revitalization Measures for Severe Pneumonia with Novel Pathogens		§ Article 67, Communicable Disease Control Act; Article 69, Communicable Disease Control Act

Central Epidemic Command Center; www.cdc.gov.tw; Communicable Disease Reporting and Consultation Hotline: ☎ 1922

Right Information to the Right People for the Right Decisions at the Right Time

To fully utilize the key innovative anti-pandemic applications listed above for pandemic prevention, the design principle of the s&cHealth model is to utilize the features of the mHealth platform and smartphones to reach each confirmed case or individuals at risk of infection. The s&cHealth model is designed to complement the administration-owned pandemic prevention policies and pandemic prevention systems. It is especially important when it comes to working with the general public to carry out tasks related to continuous monitoring, automatic warning, early screening of possible sources of infection, provisioning of warnings of abnormalities, rapid response and decision-making, and effective real-time data collection for pandemic prevention control.

For the administration, the s&cHealth model safeguards tasks related to the whole spectrum of personal health data collection through the following capabilities: (1) curate minimally necessary information required for pandemic prevention, (2) handle the compliance to the local pandemic prevention policies, (3) provide an authorization and consent mechanism for the access of personal data, (4) enable the continued collection of information documenting the occurrence and spread of the pandemic, (5) monitor in real time the steps taken by authorized personnel to determine whether further assistance or intervention is needed. This would allow the whole system to effectively perform pandemic prevention tasks, armed with the necessary information curated in the shortest time possible. The local government or health management authorities can then use the curated information to formulate follow-up pandemic prevention policies and measures and to allocate resources in response to the development of the pandemic.

For the general public, the s&cHealth model enables the Personal Health App to access reliable and transparent information sources pertaining to the development of the pandemic, understand prevention policies and the recommended preventive procedures and procedures for individuals at risk of infection, raise public awareness and promote habits of integrating pandemic prevention procedures into a daily routine. Successful pandemic prevention requires the cooperation of everyone with their regional pandemic prevention system; the s&cHealth model is designed to assist both sides in achieving the best possible outcome.

ICT Solutions

In the following subsection, we introduce how the s&cHealth model utilizes the mHealth platform developed by the authors as an example to illustrate an integrated scientific and technological epidemic prevention platform. The mHealth platform basically consists of a Personal Health App (for personal use by the general public) and a Monitor Dashboard Web App (for monitoring use by the administration).

Personal Health App

The mHealth platform service connects Personal Health App (which collects information from individuals at risk during home quarantine) with the Monitoring and Management Web Application (which is used to monitor by the administration). The right side of the Personal Health App displays the current status of the Bluetooth-based body temperature patch device in color. The orange block displays the main aspects of the quarantined individual's status summary, including (1) name, (2) temperature, (3) number of days under quarantine, (4) physical and mental state indicators and (5) location of the quarantined individual. The User Interface Exploded view is shown in Fig. 5.4, and detailed system functions are shown in Table 5.5.

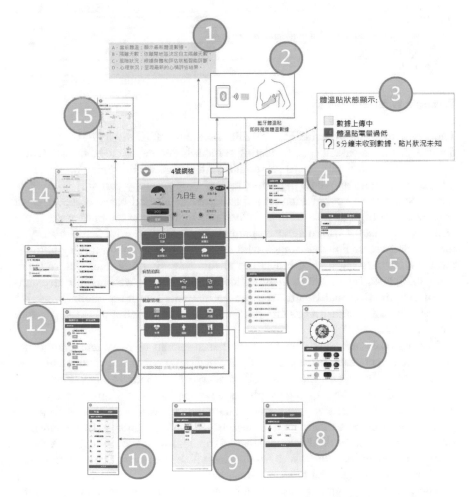

Fig. 5.4 User interface exploded view of Home Quarantine Personal Health App

Table 5.5 Personal Health App function list

Home quarantine personal health App (HTML5 cross platform App)
1. Status summary, including: (A) Current body temperature, (B) isolation days, (C) body status, (D) mental status
2. Bluetooth body temperature patch using guide
3. Bluetooth body temperature patch connection status
4. Contact history
5. Support needs message
6. Health instruction and education
7. Medication reminder (on demand)
8. Food and drink record (on demand)
9. Sport record (on demand)
10. Vital sign record
11. Physical and mental health questionnaire
12. Progress note of quarantine
13. Government declarations of epidemic prevention
14. GPS trace history
15. Home location setting

Personal Wearable Devices

There are many commercially available wearable physiological measurement devices that have passed specific testing standards and can be used to assist individuals to quantitatively record personal health status. While some products may not be as accurate as medical-grade standard devices, they can still be used to record continuously over a long period and provide a trend-based comparison of personal Vital Sign data over time. Individuals under home quarantine are those with contact history with diagnosed patients or those with prior travel history to the infected areas. For individuals who are not currently exhibiting symptoms, the most clear physiological indication at this stage is body temperature (Park et al. 2020; Hsiao et al. 2020). In the following subsection, we illustrate an example of how the Personal Health App can be integrated with a personal wearable device, in this case, a patch that comes with continuous temperature measurement.

The wearable technology enabling the measurement of body temperature has matured in recent years. In the case study, the measurement of body temperature can be continuously done via a small, rechargeable, body temperature patch (28 mm × 26 mm × 3.5 mm, 3 g weight, as shown in Fig. 5.5) without affecting the user's daily activities. Body temperature data are collected in real time from the patch, transmitted to a smartphone through Bluetooth Low Energy (BLE) transmission, synchronized by the Personal Health App, and then transmitted back to the Monitoring and Management Web Application via the platform. The automatic data collection and management process eliminates

There are many commercially available wearable errors that are often caused by manual recordings through dictation.

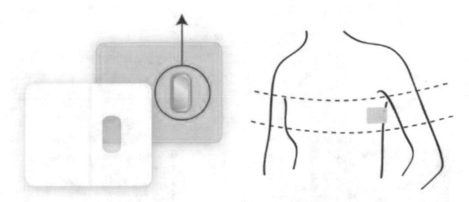

Fig. 5.5 Diagrammatic sketch of thermometer patch

The body temperature patch used on this platform is a CE certified (Conformité Européenne certified, it means the good's conformity with European health, safety, and environmental protection standards) commercially available product with a measurement accuracy threshold of within ±0.05 °C. Additionally, the patch itself is both waterproof and dustproof with coefficient standard of IP 34 (temp pal 2020). The patch is attached to the left armpit of the human body to directly measure the core temperature of the human body. The system stores an individual's body temperature data in his/her own user account. The system can also support the use of multiple user accounts.

There are many commercially available wearable on a single smartphone. Such use cases include the co-monitoring between parents and their children.

Monitoring and Management Web Application

Management personnel across all hierarchical levels in the administration log in to the same Monitor Dashboard Application, but the scope of data available to each log-in varies according to their clearance level. The main function menus of the Monitor Dashboard Web App are on the left. Figure 5.6 shows the functions from top to bottom respectively: (1) the list of monitoring personnel and their detailed status data, (2) GPS footprint tracking and query, (3) data export procedures, (4) bulletin maintenance management, (5) abnormality warning notification lists and (6) requests handled during home quarantine.

Interoperability for Big Data and Analytics

The collection of detailed data records during home quarantine are becoming an important source of reference materials for subsequent follow-up medical care, pandemic investigation and pandemic prevention research (Nair et al. 2020; Shi et al.

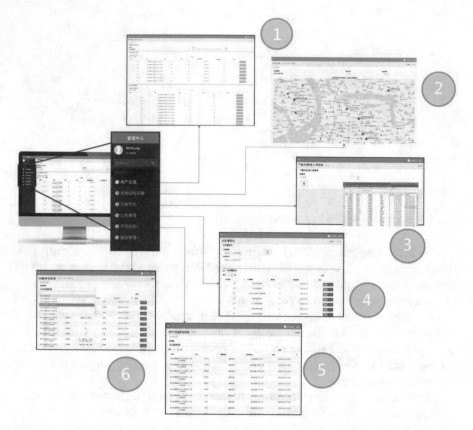

Fig. 5.6 User interface exploded view of monitoring and management web application

2020; Hedberg and Maher 2020). Therefore, the reusability of relevant home quarantine historical data collected and its interoperability managed by this platform is of ever-increasing importance. Countries around the world have proceeded with the curation of COVID-19 data sets so that administrations and medical professionals are able to jointly and effectively share consistent information in their fights against this pandemic. Example datasets collected include: The German Corona Consensus Dataset (GECCO): A standardized dataset for COVID-19 research, Logica COVID-19 (FHIR v4.0.1) Implementation Guide CI Build, and HL7 FHIR (v4.0.1) Situational Awareness for Novel Epidemic Response (SANER) IG 0.1.0 Continuous Build (Sass et al. 2020; Logica (formerly HSPC) 2020; HL7 FHIR 2019b).

To enable the interchangeability with standardized data, the s&cHealth model employs the application of Fast Healthcare Interoperability Resources (FHIR) to propose a set of APIs and Resource Collections (in the data form of JSON and XML). This design enables standardized data collection via FHIR. A unified data source can then be formed across various pandemic prevention units, health authorities, medical institutions, and relevant pandemic prevention system vendors. For the general public, the interoperable standardized data model also enables them to

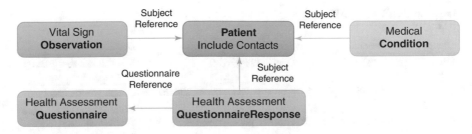

Fig. 5.7 FHIR resource combination for collecting data during quarantine

access consistent and transparent information from pandemic prevention units directly without additional investigative efforts.

To leverage the FHIR standard to increase interoperability for the personal data-attribution oriented the s&cHealth model, personal health records collected from various data sources—widely ranging from physiological measurements from wearable devices to manually input records such as individually initiated temperature measurements, physical status assessment scales and symptom recordings—can be easily with mapped back to Patient Resource. The Patient Resource ID can be used as a unique identifier to search across various data sources through the standardized FHIR API. In this way, all the information required for follow-up pandemic investigation or medical care can be integrated on the above platform. Figure 5.7 shows how a variety of information sources, including Contact History, Vital Sign Observation, Medical Condition, Health Assessment Questionnaire and Questionnaire Response, are connected back to Patient Resource.

In the scenario where the data of one specific home quarantine case is needed for further investigation, the model would allow for searching through the list of Patient Resource IDs using the standard Web API. Table 5.6 shows the different types of queries that could be enabled by FHIR Search.

s&cHealth (Smart and Connected Health): New Model to Link from the Individuals, Stakeholders, Communities, Society and the Governments

Despite the global crisis caused by the COVID-19 pandemic, it also presents an opportunity to advance a new generation of personal health informatics tools. During the process of responding to the pandemic, many countries have begun to explore solutions that would enable a larger scale, contact-free collection of objective personal physiological measurements. While the initial goal is to use the measurement data to understand the physiological changes caused by COVID-19, it can also be used to raise general public awareness and encourage healthy habits of self-care. This will allow individuals to move from seeking care only when they exhibit symptoms to managing their own health. This can help release resources to those

Table 5.6 FHIR search API for data collected by Personal Health App

HTTP Operator	FHIR Search URL sample	Description
GET	https://{FHIR_URL}/Patient/A123456789	Read patient resource by patient ID
GET	https://{FHIR_URL}/Observation?patient=A123456789	Search observation by patient ID
GET	https://{FHIR_URL}/Condition?patient=A123456789	Search condition by patient ID
GET	https://{FHIR_URL}/Condition?patient=A123456789& code=http://snomed.info/sctl386661006	Search condition by patient ID and SNOMED fever code
GET	https://{FHIR_URL}/QuestionnaireResponse?patient=A123456789	Search QuestionnaireResponse by patient ID
GET	https://{FHIR_URL}/QuestionnaireResponse?patient=A123456789&questionnaire=MentalHealthAssessment01	Search QuestionnaireResponse by patient ID and specific questionnaire ID

critically ill patients who really need health professionals' attention and would be especially helpful for the healthcare systems in regions that are already low on capacity. This would have potential impacts on changing the traditional patterns of medical care and the reimbursement policies of health insurance payers.

In the face of COVID-19 and the challenges of the new human healthcare model, we need to develop the Smart and Connected Health model and related new tools and methods across many dimensions to effectively connect data, people, and systems. Therefore, the directions of s&cHealth described in this article are summarized as follows:

1. Health Information Infrastructure: Establishing a platform for mobile health epidemic prevention to enable interoperable, distributed, and scalable digital infrastructure, as well as tools for effective sharing and use of Personal Health Record (PHR) data, networked and mobilized applications that access such data. And providing trustworthy patient identification and authentication and access control protocols, while maintaining sensitivity to the legal, cultural and ethical issues associated with making digital health data appropriately accessible by all relevant stakeholders.
2. Connecting Data: Integrate personal health information with disease control systems to support epidemic management decisions and both individual and population health. Linking data from individuals to their organizational units to healthcare institutions or regional health departments.
3. Connecting People: Develop new approaches to support individuals to effectively participate in their own health in pandemic, such as Personal Health App, accessing and daily health data collection and epidemic prevention measures that support users across gender and ethnicity. Develop multi-user roles interfaces for a variety of tasks including personnel, caregiver and epidemic prevention staff access to health data. Helping the individuals, stakeholders and communities to be in line with the government's epidemic prevention policy during the pandemic.

4. Connecting Systems: Develop protocols and interface standards to enable interoperable, temporally-synchronized, devices and systems, as well as how those systems can be utilized for continuous capture, storage and transmission of physiological, personal and organizational data. Develop and evaluate assistive technology and devices integration for personal health and decision support systems for improved epidemic prevention. Develop assessment methods and software tools that aid effectively communicate personal health information in the Government, Community, and in and around the person.

We can make use of the s&cHealth model and the mHealth platform to connect individuals, public and private organizations, and local communities with government authorities in their regions to coordinate tasks related to pandemic prevention. This would allow for effective implementation of pandemic prevention measures through a better integration of healthy habits into everyone's daily life. With the assistance of the Personal Health App, individuals can establish the habit of autonomous health management through daily activities such as establishing contact lists, physiological measurements, health status assessment scales. The data collected through the self-care process could provide information for adjusting any subsequent follow-up pandemic prevention decisions.

Smart Community Quarantine Management mHealth Platform

Beyond the goal of creating a better self-care process for pandemic prevention, the s&cHealth model and the mHealth platform can also be extended to cater for quarantine care and discharge management. Figure 5.8 shows the development of different extensions to support three key use cases: (1) developing a mobile terminal to support both discharged patient management and self-care utilized by medical professionals, (2) developing a web-based management center for hospital administrators, and (3) developing a platform to provide mobile services for patients based on their status during inpatient isolation and also after being discharged.

To handle scenarios wherein the pandemic spread continues on the escalation path, the s&cHealth model can be further catered to account for the intervention requirements of epidemic prevention. In particular, the requirements covers the following two aspects of consideration:

1. To dynamically allocate resources to balance the workload of medical staff in order to account for a large number of hospitalized and quarantine patients.
2. To accommodate the requirements for medical personnel to be quarantined and managed independently after coming in contact with patients.

In order to satisfy these requirements, our system strives to provide an electronic service intervention plan to automate the epidemic prevention workflow, starting from the in-hospital medical care of patients to the tracking and management of patients after their discharge and GPS position tracking for individuals under home

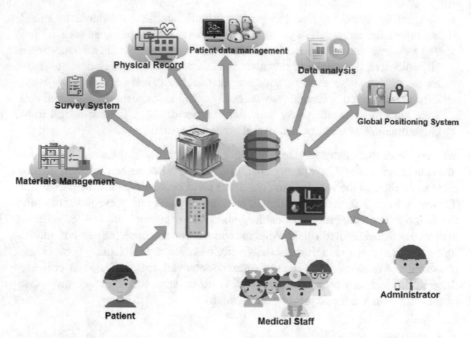

Fig. 5.8 Smart community quarantine management mHealth platform architecture diagram

quarantine. In addition, it can also be extended to include the assessment of sleep and mental health status of medical staff in order to identify workflow patterns that can help improve the efficiency and reduce the workload burden.

Figure 5.9 shows the functional system structure, which consists of two major applications: a web-based portal and a mobile application.

First, the web-based application is mainly designed to provide medical staff and institutional administrators data management functions, including (1) patient case overview, (2) GPS position tracking, (3) management of announcements and notifications, (4) inbox message history, (5) staff management, (6) patient data statistics report.

Second, the mobile application is further divided into two parts: the first part of the mobile application is tailored for hospitalized and discharged patients, while the next part is tailored for medical staff.

For in-hospital patients, the mobile application includes the following modules: (1) symptom evaluation, (2) SOS functionality, (3) a message board, and (4) health education. For discharged patients, this system provides the following modules: (1) temperature and physiological data recording, (2) GPS position tracking, (3) a question and answer (Q&A) message board, and (4) health education.

For medical staff, the mobile application includes two major modules: one for care coordination and another for off-duty self-management for medical staff. The care coordination module includes the list of patient management and another list of abnormality indicators to facilitate medical staff in their tasks of performing patient care services. The next module is designed to help off-duty medical staff to track their

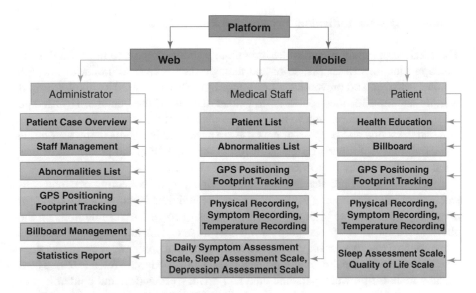

Fig. 5.9 System functional architecture diagram

own health-related information, including temperature measurements, symptoms, sleep and stress assessment questionnaires, injury records, and GPS position tracking.

Remaining Issues

Obsolescence of ICTs

Previously the development of traditional health ICT solutions was largely based on the input of medical institutions and medical personnel. For example, when individuals were feeling unwell, they would utilize a medical appointment registration system; additionally, Hospital Information System (HIS) was used to manage individual financial and management needs. These ICT solutions are developed based on a set of standard operation or management procedures. However, the traditional health ICT solutions have been put under a stress test during the COVID-19 epidemic. Many countries and regions are facing the challenges as the operational capacity of their medical system is overwhelmed. Due to the infectious nature of the SARS-CoV-2 virus, we need to maintain minimal to zero contact while providing healthcare. In response to such conditions and requirements, many healthcare solutions have been developed to incorporate new ICT technologies such as mHealth, telehealth, and wearable devices. Compared to the traditional solutions, these solutions are more personalized and focus on individual autonomy. As a result, they can enable health management applications that could better encourage the creation of healthy personal health behaviors for disease prevention and early screening. This trend is expected to continue in the post-pandemic era.

Trade-off Between Individual Privacy and Public Goods

The s&cHealth model includes the individual's active consent to use the mHealth platform functions to access, store and manage their own health data in order to conduct self-care and preventive monitoring. In the use of the mHealth platform, it is more common for individuals to download and install the Personal Health App from the mHealth platform into their mobile phones, and the scope of data collection and the scope and purpose of data use are described in details in the user terms and conditions. Informed consent is in full compliance with the principles of personal data and privacy protection (Nijhawan et al. 2013).

In a limited set of pre-specified situations, for example, collecting personal contact history and GPS tracing for home quarantine individuals, the mHealth platform is used by governments or organizations to block or force certain functions on the phones used for these special purposes. Under these circumstances, the platform is more oriented to serve for improving the effectiveness of epidemic prevention rather than protecting personal data and privacy (105. Human Rights Watch 2020). There exists a trade-off between personal data and privacy protection and epidemic prevention measures, which would be clearly stated from the beginning.

In the course of the epidemiological investigation of prior cases in Taiwan, from time to time when a suspected case does not want to reveal his or her whereabouts to help identify the possible route of infection, the situation often leads to public criticism or witch-hunting (CDC, Ministry of Health and Welfare, Taiwan 2020j), which eventually harm the implementation of any privacy protection measures during epidemiological investigation. A more ideal scenario would be to obtain informed consent from individuals at risk of infection in advance to their use of the mHealth platform. In this way, they will have their footprints collected and analyzed, and they will take the initiative to conduct their own health management assessment and fill out the report. In addition, when individuals are aware that such information will be monitored and alerted, it is also less likely for them to be engaged in unnecessary risky behaviors.

Non-ICT Challenges: Culture, ICT Literacy, Infrastructure

Besides the ICT challenges, there also exists a set of non-ICT challenges facing the successful deployment of the s&cHealth model. For one, how to strive the balance between privacy and epidemiological investigation is the key challenge to be overcome.

Take the development of a Bluetooth-based anonymous contact tracking application in Singapore for example (Government of Singapore 2020; OpenTrace 2020). While similar mobile apps have been developed in many other countries (Ministry of Science, Technology and Innovation (MOSTI), Malaysia 2020; Waltz 2020; Raskar et al. 2020), the main difference between this application and the others lies on its proactivity brought by the additional GPS component, which would further incur privacy concerns. Although the Bluetooth-based anonymous contact tracking application can operate with a higher degree of privacy protection, it can only provide passive and post hoc alerts when a contact has been confirmed in the vicinity; in addition, only then will an individual be notified of the time and place one may have been in contact with a confirmed case in the previous days. Meanwhile, the added GPS component can proactively alert individuals who should be monitored and obtain their informed consent, or routinely record the daily traces of individuals who are not at risk of infection. When an individual at risk of infection appears in public, the supervisor and the other users nearby would be notified immediately. Although users can actively turn off Bluetooth or GPS transmission from their personal phones, there might still exist privacy concerns.

This then becomes a choice at the country level. Any country would need to make decisions based on their cultures, the direction of their epidemic prevention policies, and the preferred level of proactivity in their own populations. In addition to the systematic prevention measures imposed by the government, the public also needs to take the initiative to participate in the related prevention measures in order to achieve better results in controlling this epidemic. By decentralizing the responsibility of epidemic prevention from the government to public and private organizations at all levels, the whole system could potentially become more effective. By leveraging the s&cHealth model and a mHealth platform similar to what is used in the case study reported in this chapter, the government can more proactively activate preventive measures through organizations at all levels. It can also include individuals with international communication needs and those who may be in contact with individuals at risk of infection to provide a more intact social safety net for epidemic prevention.

In addition, when a new community spread is confirmed, we should review the systemic workflow and action plans given the new ICT solutions and model, rather than simply punishing the wrongdoers. In this chapter, we would like to provide a peek into what is possible in the post-pandemic era and start exploring the potential solutions. With the demonstrated benefits brought by the co-sharing of epidemic prevention responsibilities across government, public and private organizations at all levels and the individuals in the general public, there exist endless opportunities that could enabled by the s&cHealth model and the mHealth platform.

References

105. Human Rights Watch. Mobile Location Data and Covid-19: Q&A. May 13, 2020. https://www.hrw.org/news/2020/05/13/mobile-location-data-and-covid-19-qa. Accessed 21 Apr 2021.

Aslani N, Lazem M, Mahdavi S, et al. A review of mobile health applications in epidemic and pandemic outbreaks: lessons learned for COVID-19. Iran J Clin Infect Dis. 2020;15(2):e103649. https://doi.org/10.5812/archcid.103649.

Burke RM, Balter S, Barnes E, Barry V, Bartlett K, Beer KD, et al. Enhanced contact investigations for nine early travel-related cases of SARS-CoV-2 in the United States. PLoS One. 2020;15(9):e0238342. https://doi.org/10.1371/journal.pone.0238342.

CDC, Ministry of Health and Welfare, Taiwan. Recommendations for COVID-19 case definition, specimen collection, and diagnostic tests; 2020a. https://www.cdc.gov.tw/Category/MPage/np0wef4IjYh9hvbiW2BnoQ. Accessed 21 Apr 2021.

CDC, Ministry of Health and Welfare, Taiwan. Taiwan CDC learned from online sources that there had been at least 7 cases of atypical pneumonia in Wuhan, China; 2020b. https://covid19. mohw.gov.tw/en/cp-4868-53673-206.html. Accessed 21 Apr 2021.

CDC, Ministry of Health and Welfare, Taiwan. Taiwan sent two experts to Wuhan and visited the Hubei Provincial Center for Disease Control and Prevention; 2020c. https://covid19.mohw. gov.tw/en/cp-4868-53704-206.html. Accessed 21 Apr 2021.

CDC, Ministry of Health and Welfare, Taiwan. Crucial policies for combating COVID-19; 2020d. https://covid19.mohw.gov.tw/en/sp-timeline0-206.html. Accessed 21 Apr 2021.

CDC, Ministry of Health and Welfare, Taiwan. Regulations concerning short-term business travelers' applications for shortened quarantine periods in Taiwan; 2020e. https://www.cdc.gov.tw/ En/File/Get/BeMlQQDbdUp1PK_6b0xcrQ. Accessed 21 Apr 2021.

CDC, Ministry of Health and Welfare, Taiwan. Ministry of Health and Welfare Announcement; 2020f. https://www.cdc.gov.tw/File/Get/LpahKLHrSbDVv7zfGeOeWw. Accessed 21 Apr 2021.

CDC, Ministry of Health and Welfare, Taiwan. Guidelines for prevention of SARS-CoV-2 infection; 2020g. https://www.cdc.gov.tw/En/File/Get/p6AQ9xTjwAVnArHyq-MGjQ. Accessed 21 Apr 2021.

CDC, Ministry of Health and Welfare, Taiwan. CECC measures for following up on persons at risk of infection; 2020h. https://www.cdc.gov.tw/Category/MPage/G8mN-MHF7A1t5xfRMduTQQ. Accessed 21 Apr 2021.

CDC, Ministry of Health and Welfare, Taiwan. Fall-Winter COVID-19 prevention program; 2020i. https://www.cdc.gov.tw/En/Bulletin/Detail/KIUJU0aZex70DPFUN3d66w?typeid=158. Accessed 9 Sept 2021.

CDC, Ministry of Health and Welfare, Taiwan. CECC confirms 3 more COVID-19 cases; two are colleagues of Case #760, and one arrives in Taiwan from Indonesia. December 20, 2020j. https://www.cdc.gov.tw/En/Bulletin/Detail/hQPRmEsFm8ASL0NGWr4Gxg?typeid=158. Accessed 21 Apr 2021.

Chan JF, Yuan S, Kok KH, To KK, Chu H, Yang J, et al. A familial cluster of pneumonia associated with the 2019 novel coronavirus indicating person-to-person transmission: a study of a family cluster. Lancet. 2020;395(10223):514–23. https://doi.org/10.1016/ s0140-6736(20)30154-9.

Fortuin J, Salie F, Abdullahi LH, et al. The impact of mHealth interventions on health systems: a systematic review protocol. Syst Rev. 2016;5:200. https://doi.org/10.1186/s13643-016-0387-1.

Gao H, Yao H, Yang S, Li L. From SARS to MERS: evidence and speculation. Front Med. 2016;10:377–82. https://doi.org/10.1007/s11684-016-0466-7.

Government of Singapore. TraceTogether, safer together March 20, 2020. https://wwwtracetogeth-ergovsg/. Accessed 9 Sept 2021.

Hedberg K, Maher J. The CDC field epidemiology manual: collecting data. Official website of CDC US; 2020. https://wwwcdcgov/eis/field-epi-manual/chapters/collecting-datahtml. Accessed 21 Apr 2021.

HL7 FHIR. FHIR organization resource. FHIR Specification (v401: R4); 2019a. https://www.hl7. org/fhir/organization.html. Accessed 21 Apr 2021.

HL7 FHIR. Situational awareness for novel epidemic response implementation guide 0.1.0 - STU Ballot. FHIR Specification (v4.0.1: R4); 2019b. http://build.fhir.org/ig/HL7/fhir-saner/. Accessed 21 Apr 2021.

Hsiao S-H, Chen T-C, Chien H-C, Yang C-J, Chenb Y-H. Measurement of body temperature to prevent pandemic COVID-19 in hospitals in Taiwan: repeated measurement is necessary. J Hosp Infect. 2020;

Huang R, Xia J, Chen Y, Shan C, Wu C. A family cluster of SARS-CoV-2 infection involving 11 patients in Nanjing. China. Lancet Infect Dis. 2020;20(5):534–5. https://doi.org/10.1016/ s1473-3099(20)30147-x.

L'Engle K, Raney L, D'Adamo M. mHealth resources to strengthen health programs. Glob Health Sci Pract. 2014;2(1):130–1. https://doi.org/10.9745/GHSP-D-14-00013.

Lauer SA, Grantz KH, Bi Q, Jones FK, Zheng Q, Meredith HR, et al. The incubation period of coronavirus disease 2019 (COVID-19) from publicly reported confirmed cases: estimation and application. Ann Int Med. 2020;2020(172):577–82.

Li H, Wang Y, Ji M, et al. Transmission routes analysis of SARS-CoV-2: a systematic review and case report. Front Cell Dev Biol. 2020;8:618. https://doi.org/10.3389/fcell.2020.00618.

Liang F. COVID-19 and health code: how digital platforms tackle the pandemic in China. Social Media + Society; 2020. https://doi.org/10.1177/2056305120947657

Logica (formerly HSPC). Logica COVID-19 FHIR Profile Library IG 0.11.0 - CI Build; 2020. https://covid-19-ig.logicahealth.org/index.html. Accessed 21 Apr 2021.

Ming LC, Untong N, Aliudin NA, Osili N, Kifli N, Tan CS, Goh KW, Ng PW, Al-Worafi YM, Lee KS, Goh HP. Mobile health apps on COVID-19 launched in the early days of the pandemic: content analysis and review. JMIR Mhealth Uhealth. 2020;8(9):e19796. https://doi.org/10.2196/19796.

Ministry of Science, Technology and Innovation (MOSTI), Malaysia. MyTrace, a Preventive Counter Measure and Contact Tracing Application for COVID-19 May 3, 2020. https://www-mostigovmy/web/en/mytrace/. Accessed 21 Apr 2021.

Nair SP, Moa A, Macintyre R. Investigation of early epidemiological signals of COVID-19 in India using outbreak surveillance data. Global Biosecurity. 2020;1(4):10.31646/gbio.72.

Nijhawan LP, Janodia MD, Muddukrishna BS, et al. Informed consent: issues and challenges. J Adv Pharm Technol Res. 2013;4(3):134–40.

OpenTrace. OpenTrace Github repositories. April 9, 2020. https://githubcom/opentrace-community. Accessed 21 Apr 2021.

Our World in Data. Coronavirus (COVID-19) vaccinations; 2020. https://ourworldindata.org/covid-vaccinations. Accessed 9 Sept 2021.

Park S, Brassey J, Heneghan C, Mahtani K. Managing fever in adults with possible or confirmed COVID-19 in primary care. Centre for Evidence Based Medicine. 2020;

Pung R, Chiew CJ, Young BE, Chin S, Chen MI, Clapham HE, et al. Investigation of three clusters of COVID-19 in Singapore: implications for surveillance and response measures. Lancet. 2020;395(10229):1039–46. https://doi.org/10.1016/s0140-6736(20)30528-6.

Raskar R, Schunemann I, Barbar R, Vilcans K, Gray J, Vepakomma P, et al. Apps gone rogue: maintaining personal privacy in an epidemic. arXiv. 2020:A.

Rees EM, Nightingale ES, Jafari Y, et al. COVID-19 length of hospital stay: a systematic review and data synthesis. BMC Med. 2020;18:270. https://doi.org/10.1186/s12916-020-01726-3.

Sass J, Bartschke A, Lehne M, et al. The German Corona consensus dataset (GECCO): a standardized dataset for COVID-19 research in university medicine and beyond. BMC Med Inform Decis Mak. 2020;20:341. https://doi.org/10.1186/s12911-020-01374-w.

Shi L, Li Q, Li K, et al. Quarantine at home may not enough!-from the epidemiological data in Shaanxi Province of China. BMC Res Notes. 2020;13:506. https://doi.org/10.1186/s13104-020-05342-5.

Singh J, Couch D, Yap K. Mobile health apps that help with COVID-19 management: scoping review. JMIR Nursing. 2020;3(1):e20596. https://doi.org/10.2196/20596.

temp pal. temp pal Temp Pal skin temperature epidermal patch; 2020. https://www.iweecare.com/tw/product. Accessed 21 Apr 2021.

Tingting H, Liu Y, Zhao M, et al. A comparison of COVID-19. SARS and MERS, PeerJ. 2020;8:e9725. https://doi.org/10.7717/peerj.9725.

Tirado M. Role of mobile health in the care of culturally and linguistically diverse US populations. Perspect Health Inf Manage. 2011;8(Winter):1e.

Tong ZD, Tang A, Li KF, Li P, Wang HL, Yi JP, et al. Potential presymptomatic transmission of SARS-CoV-2, Zhejiang Province, China, 2020. Emerg Infect Dis. 2020;26(5):1052–4. https://doi.org/10.3201/eid2605.200198.

U.S. Department of Labor Occupational Safety and Health Administration. Guidance on preparing workplaces for COVID-19. https://www.osha.gov/sites/default/files/publications/OSHA3990.pdf. Accessed 21 Apr 2021.

Waltz E. Halting COVID-19: the benefits and risks of digital contact tracing. IEEE Spectrum 2020 Mar 25. https://spectrumieeeorg/the-human-os/biomedical/ethics/halting-covid19-benefits-risks-digital-contact-tracing. Accessed 21 Apr 2021.

Wan Y, Shang J, Graham R, Baric RS, Li F. Receptor recognition by novel coronavirus from Wuhan: an analysis based on decade-long structural studies of SARS. J Virol. 2020;94:e00127–0. https://doi.org/10.1128/JVI.00127-20.

Wang D, Hu B, Hu C, Zhu F, Liu X, Zhang J, et al. Clinical characteristics of 138 hospitalized patients with 2019 novel coronavirus-infected pneumonia in Wuhan, China. JAMA. 2020;323:1061–9. https://doi.org/10.1001/jama.2020.1585.

WHO. Transmission of SARS-CoV-2: implications for infection prevention precautions; 2020a. https://www.who.int/news-room/commentaries/detail/transmission-of-sars-cov-2-implications-for-infection-prevention-precautions. Accessed 21 Apr 2021.

WHO. WHO Coronavirus Disease (COVID-19) Dashboard; 2020b. https://covid19.who.int/. Accessed 9 Sept 2021.

Wikipedia. Hong Kong health code; 2020. September 9, 2021. https://enwikipediaorg/wiki/Hong_Kong_Health_Code. Accessed 9 Sept 2021.

Worldometers. COVID-19 coronavirus pandemic; 2020. https://www.worldometers.info/coronavirus/. Accessed 9 Sept 2021.

Wu F, Zhao S, Yu B, Chen YM, Wang W, Song ZG, et al. A new coronavirus associated with human respiratory disease in China. Nature. 2020;579:265–9. https://doi.org/10.1038/s41586-020-2008-3.

Yu P, Zhu J, Zhang Z, Han Y. A familial cluster of infection associated with the 2019 novel coronavirus indicating possible person-to-person transmission during the incubation period. JInfect Dis. 2020;221(11):1757–61. https://doi.org/10.1093/infdis/jiaa077.

Zhou P, Yang XL, Wang XG, Hu B, Zhang L, Zhang W, et al. A pneumonia outbreak associated with a new coronavirus of probable bat origin. Nature. 2020;579:270–3. https://doi.org/10.1038/s41586-020-2012-7.

Zhu N, Zhang D, Wang W, Li X, Yang B, Song J, et al. A novel coronavirus from patients with pneumonia in China, 2019. N Engl J Med. 2020;382:727–33. https://doi.org/10.1056/NEJMoa2001017.

Chapter 6
The Integration of Patient-Generated Health Data to Clinical Care

Sarah Collins Rossetti and Victoria Tiase

Abstract Patients are increasingly capturing and tracking their own health data, known as Patient-generated health data (PGHD), through mobile or remote patient monitoring (RPM) devices. The rise of mobile health applications (mHealth apps) combined with the twenty-first Century Cures Act and related regulations, are making the sharing and transferring of PGHD data increasingly accessible across clinical settings. PGHD have been used successfully to help in self-management of chronic disease and remote patient monitoring, and when incorporated into clinical care have the potential to benefit the experiences of both patients and clinicians, as well as improve care outcomes. However, barriers to adoption still exist, including lack of trust, incentives for use, and efficient workflows. Moreover, low adoption in specific patient populations may risk increasing health inequities. Several key organizations and frameworks have been created to guide mHealth app developers and support patients in selecting mHealth apps to use. The integration of PGHD into clinical care can advance patient engagement, self-management, and shared decision making, though requires further optimization. Advancement in trust of data, incentives for use, and efficient workflows will allow for greater integration of PGHD into the clinical care setting and support a shift from episodic care to increased continuity of information exchange and tracking of data, which may benefit both patients and clinicians.

Keywords Patient generated health data · Patient portals · Personal health information · Personal health records · eHealth · mHealth

S. C. Rossetti (✉)
Department of Biomedical Informatics, Columbia University, New York, NY, USA
e-mail: sac2125@cumc.columbia.edu

V. Tiase
Department of Biomedical Informatics, University of Utah, Salt Lake City, USA
e-mail: vtiase@nyp.org

© The Author(s), under exclusive license to Springer Nature
Switzerland AG 2022
P.-Y. S. Hsueh et al. (eds.), *Personal Health Informatics*, Cognitive Informatics
in Biomedicine and Healthcare, https://doi.org/10.1007/978-3-031-07696-1_6

Learning Objectives for the Chapter
1. Articulate the barriers to adoption of PGHD
2. Identify exemplars and facilitators to adoption of PGHD
3. Articulate how twenty-first Century Cures Act may advance integration of PGHD into clinical care
4. Identify key organizations and frameworks to guide mHealth app developers

Introduction

In the digital world, the use of technology is commonplace, data generation is rampant, and social behaviors are changing. The ubiquity of devices and availability of data have implications for new solutions and provide opportunities for transformation, especially in healthcare. Healthcare providers and patients alike rely on mobile devices and have data at their fingertips. With the rise of mobile health applications (mHealth apps), digital healthcare consumers not only collect data but use their data to make everyday decisions and solve real-world problems, and most importantly, expect the same of healthcare providers and the healthcare system. The abundance of health data created, collected, and gathered by patients or their caregivers—known as patient-generated health data (PGHD)—when incorporated into clinical care, have the potential to shape the future of healthcare (Office of the National Coordinator for Health IT [ONC] 2021).

In the clinical setting, PGHD can help complete the sometimes-incomplete picture of the patient. They can be a source of important components of the patient history that may be unattainable or incomplete. In addition to a comprehensive view of the patient, PGHD have been shown to prevent readmissions, improve outcomes, and support tailored care that is more personalized (Genes et al. 2018). However, clinicians are already suffering from documentation burden—and another data source must be carefully introduced into clinical workflows. As patients continue to get more access to their health data and have a greater desire to share with all clinicians, it is critical to overcome the current integration challenges and seek to balance the inclusion of this potentially beneficial data source into clinical workflows.

This chapter describes the challenges, facilitators, and opportunities for integrating PGHD into clinical care. We begin with a description of the current types of PGHD, the issues associated with the transfer of PGHD on the part of the patient, and the difficulties clinicians face while using PGHD within the context of clinical care. Through use cases demonstrating the impact of PGHD integration, we will highlight best practices and propose several areas for future research and exploration.

Capture and Sharing of PGHD

PGHD can be tracked and shared using multiple approaches and are primarily captured and shared through patient portals, personal health records, and patient-facing mHealth apps that connect to EHRs.

A patient portal, according to HealthIT.gov, is a secure online website that gives patients access to personal health information and provides 24 h access from anywhere with an Internet connection (Healthit.gov 2017). Patient portals typically are affiliated with a particular healthcare organization, or 'tethered', and connect to personal health information from that organization's EHR. In doing so, patient may be able to access information such as recent appointments, discharge summaries, medications, immunizations, allergies and laboratory results (Healthit.gov 2017). Some patient portals also provide the ability to securely message your clinician, request prescription refills, schedule non-urgent appointments, and make payments. If configured to do so, PGHD can be readily captured by patients and shared with clinicians through patient portals in between episodes of care, increasing the opportunities for communication and engagement.

Alternatively, personal health records (PHRs) also store and can share personal health information, but are typically not connected to a healthcare organization (i.e., 'untethered'). According to HealthIT.gov, a PHR is an electronic application that allows patients to maintain and manage their own health information in a private, secure, and confidential environment (HealthIT.gov 2016). A PHR can also be used to maintain and manage health information of others by authorized individuals (HealthIT.gov 2016).

The number of available patient-facing mHealth apps are rapidly increasing. Many apps have been developed for use within the healthcare domain. Chronic disease self-management, for example, is a common goal for many types of patient facing apps. Tracking wearable data (e.g., Fitbit) is also a common feature. Given the early stages of patient use, objective appraisal of apps is important to ensure the vendor/developer follows recommended guidelines for mHealth app design and development, such as maintaining privacy (Xcertia 2019).

Transfer of PGHD

PGHD may be manually entered into a portal, PHR or mHealth app; however, large amounts of PGHD are typically collected through sensors, medically approved devices, and biometrics outside of the clinical care setting, while the patient is at home or goes about their daily activities. Adler-Milstein and Nong (2019) identified three categories of PGHD: health history, surveys or questionnaires, and biometric and patient activity (Adler-Milstein and Nong 2019). See Table 6.1 for PGHD types and associated examples and values. Health history data may include allergies, medications, past surgeries or even family history. Survey data encompass patient

Table 6.1 PGHD Types

Type	Example	Value
Health history	Allergy	Latex
Surveys or questionnaires	Asthma control test (ACT)	16, partially controlled
Biometric or patient activity	Blood glucose level	132 mg/dl

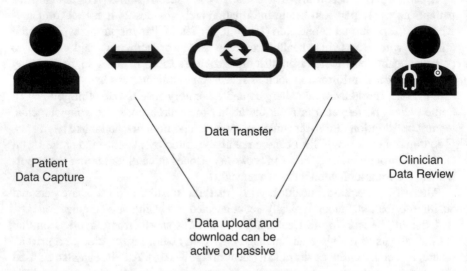

Patient
Data Capture

Data Transfer

Clinician
Data Review

* Data upload and
download can be
active or passive

Fig. 6.1 Data transfer between patient data capture and clinician data review

responses to validated tools such as patient reported outcomes, patient reported experience measures or other health questionnaires that assess for depression (PHQ-9) or asthma control (ACT). Generally collected through US Federal Drug Administration (FDA) technologies approved for a specific use, biometric data consist of blood pressure, heart rate or blood glucose values. Exercise or food log data are also considered a part of this third category of PGHD.

One key aspect of PGHD collection is the method by which the patient uploads their data to the app or platform of their choosing. This may be accomplished by active or passive transfer of the data (see Fig. 6.1). Active transfer indicates that the patient has to do something to 'actively' get their data to the device (Shapiro et al. 2012). On the other hand, passive transfer means that the data are automatically transferred to the device without any effort on the behalf of the patient (Shapiro et al. 2012). The methods for collection often align with the types of data collected. While health history and survey PGHD are actively transferred, biometric data are commonly collected through passive methods.

Individuals may wish to not only track and trend their data for self-management purposes, but also share with their healthcare providers. The PGHD transmission may be purposes of review, surveillance or simply incorporation into either an in person or virtual visit. Depending on the capabilities of the technology and the type of platform used, there may be additional work needed to transfer PGHD to the provider, or generally the EHR. This process can also be described as active or passive. In supporting the movement of PGHD on the part of the patient, both the device being used to capture the data and method of transfer to the EHR must be considered.

Challenges Incorporating PGHD into Clinical Care

Although PGHD have the potential to improve patient outcomes, little progress has been made to incorporate PGHD into direct patient care due to multiple barriers and challenges (Demiris et al. 2019; Tiase et al. 2021). Some are technical in nature and closely related to historical sociotechnical and broad interoperability issues with electronic health data. Many of the challenges concern the passive and active aspects of transfer and which user is responsible for the success of the integration. Other challenges are unique to particular aspects of PGHD such as the role of the user, the role of the provider and qualities of the data themselves in relation to their use within the context of clinical care.

Although over 3000 health related apps exist in smartphone app stores, there has been little guidance on how apps should be developed and there is scant evidence on their ability to improve care. Due to rapid development and small-scale implementations, details on user testing and validity studies are ongoing. Additional details on effectiveness, usefulness, benefits, and safety can be difficult to find. Also, privacy and security are concerns for patients when it is unclear as to what methods an app or device uses to protect PGHD and how data are protected during transfers.

Aspects of design, usability, and functionality of apps and devices can be daunting for patients or caregivers, especially when there are limited opportunities for onboarding and education. Without proper assessment of preferences and onboarding support, both technical literacy as well as health literacy can limit use and potentially incur patient harm if the data app or device is used inappropriately. This is especially important with vulnerable populations, including the elderly, those with non-medical social needs, and the disabled. In studies of portal use, vulnerable populations are reported to use portals less often, leading to intervention-generated inequity—a situation in which well-intentioned interventions may worsen existing health inequities (Grossman et al. 2019). Outreach efforts to patients, including access to technology and connectivity, may encourage adoption of PGHD transfer and specific outreach activities could be targeted at vulnerable populations as an effort to reduce health inequities. It is also plausible that active and continued buy-in from patients to upload their PGHD for integration with the EHR is contingent on patients receiving consistent feedback from clinicians (Ancker et al. 2019).

In addition to challenges to patient engagement, there are a number of barriers from a provider perspective. The quality and reliability of PGHD sources may vary. Without clear documentation and transparency into the design aspects of the app and studies evaluating its impact on patient outcomes, provider trust of PGHD and associated apps is a major barrier. Evidence to demonstrate the validity and reliability of the data collected is needed, as well as studies to examine efficiencies in care and reduced costs. Given the lack of trust, financial concerns related to liability and insurance may also inhibit the use of PGHD in clinical care. Healthcare providers must understand the requirements and associated policies that stipulate when they must view PGHD and what happens if they are unable to act upon the PGHD provided by the patient. Also, there are very few incentives in place for the review of PGHD outside of routine clinical care. New payment models to support review processes have the potential to increase the utilization of PGHD.

After addressing trust and incentives for use of PGHD, effective workflow integration is key to ongoing provider engagement. It will be difficult to bring meaningful value to patient care without clear expectations on how PGHD is used within existing and new clinical workflows. Studies have found that presentation of PGHD within the EHR is important to consider (Tiase et al. 2021; Lewinski et al. 2019). Extra steps to login to a separate system or platform to access PGHD may discourage use. Depending on the use case, the level of summarization and contextualization of PGHD must facilitate ease of interpretation in real time. As adoption increases, methods to introduce the information generated from PGHD into clinical decision-making algorithms may be beneficial.

The healthcare community is in a position to provide guidance to mHealth app developers and to encourage transparency to support users that wish to collect, share and use PGHD. Both patient and provider concerns must be addressed. Moreover, many of these concerns can be mitigated through the engagement of users in participatory design and coproduction methods for PGHD that support optimal care outcomes.

Facilitators for Incorporating PGHD into Clinical Care

Patient participation in their care has increased over the last decade with a desire for individuals to access their own health data. In addition, efforts to increase patient engagement through the use of patient facing applications as a means to facilitate self-care management are expanding. Along with the introduction of new care models requiring the integration of PGHD, the regulatory landscape is changing in a way that promotes technical integration and supports data sharing activities. As the patient demand for the sharing and integration of PGHD increases, we expect the following frameworks and initiatives to facilitate greater use of PGHD.

In recent years, hospitals and healthcare providers across the United States have expanded services to include remote patient monitoring (RPM) programs. Through RPM, FDA approved devices are used to collect PGHD from individuals outside of a care facility. Data are then transmitted to clinicians that may be a part of care management services to monitor patients remotely, trend data, and act on the information to adjust treatment plans as needed. As part of RPM programs, patients are provided support, education, and feedback. Given its potential to reduce readmissions and hospitalizations and allow older populations to live at home longer, Medicare provides reimbursement for remote physiologic monitoring to offset costs connected to onboarding, patient education and devices.

Consumer health and fitness app spending continues to increase year over year—indicating a desire to track and use these data on the part of the consumers; however, the clinical evidence related to use of mobile health apps must keep pace to ensure increased integration and use by healthcare organizations and clinicians. Efforts such as the new HIMSS Health App Guidelines Work Group will evolve the Xcertia guidelines and create a comprehensive framework to guide healthcare organizations, clinicians, consumers and developers on what is needed to ensure apps are safe, effective and evidenced-based (HIMSS 2020). In 2019, Germany signed the Digital Healthcare Act into law which includes a register of healthcare apps that have met requirements related to safety, quality, data protection and data security (Gesley 2020). In the U.S., the Food and Drug Administration (FDA) issued a guidance document entitled, "Policy for Device Software Functions and Mobile Medical Applications", to describe the oversight of mobile health apps that are connected to health devices (United States Food and Drug Administration [FDA] 2019). Moreover, in late 2020, the FDA established the Digital Health Center of Excellence to serve as centralized resource for expertise and knowledge to accelerate the development of safe and effective digital health technology (United States Food and Drug Administration [FDA] 2020). The healthcare professional community is also driving scientific progress along with clinician engagement by forming organizations such as the Digital Medicine Society (DiMe) and NODE.Health (Network of Digital Evidence in Health). Although many of these efforts and organizations are in their infancy, the recognition of the need to organize around PGHD is promising.

From a data sharing perspective, a spectrum of initiatives is in place to move this work forward. See Table 6.2 for an example list of Organizations and Resources with a focus on PGHD. To support patients in obtaining and sharing their own health data with less friction, the CARIN Alliance developed a trust framework and Code of Conduct which serve as a set of principles for how healthcare organizations can support consumers and their authorized caregivers to easily get, use, and share their digital health information. In 2020, the CARIN Alliance launched the My Health Application website as a transparent way to help consumers select a consumer-facing health application that has attested to the Code of Conduct and is affiliated with other trusted sources (CARIN Alliance 2021).

In addition, recent federal guidance, The twenty-first Century Cures Act, includes provisions for interoperability to combat information blocking, defined as practices

Table 6.2 Organizations and resources with a focus on PGHD

Organization	Website
CARIN Alliance	https://www.carinalliance.com/
DiMe	https://www.dimesociety.org/
NODE health	https://nodehealth.org/
SMART on FHIR	https://docs.smarthealthit.org/

that discourage the access, exchange, or use of electronic health data so that patients can request and obtain their data with less friction (Office of the National Coordinator for Health IT [ONC] 2021). Patient-facing mHealth apps are rapidly increasing and application programming interface (API) technology allows third party apps to exchange data to and from the EHR, with the patient's permission. Two accompanying initiatives focus on the promotion of patient-initiated data sharing. A regulation from the Centers for Medicare and Medicaid Services requires that healthcare facilities support open APIs, allowing for real-time data exchange between patients and clinicians. The ONC proposed another rule that encourages communication between patients and care providers in a standard, secure way without special effort on the part of the user (Office of the National Coordinator for Health IT [ONC] 2021). These rules also lay the groundwork for EHRs to "speak" with third-party applications using a common language via SMART on FHIR—or Substitutable Medical Apps, Reusable Technologies that leverage Fast Healthcare Interoperability Resources—a specification for internet-based exchange that is considered best practice for health data. Advances in this space can potentially simplify both technical and clinical workflow integration (Mandel et al. 2016).

Although there is demonstrative progress with some of the technical and clinical workflow hurdles, there are some areas that are in need of greater attention. In particular a deeper and more comprehensive of understanding of patient needs is necessary to reduce exacerbation of inequities and identify effective approaches to connect with patients that would benefit from connection with clinicians in-between visits, such as those with at home monitoring needs or those who are unable to travel due to rural settings or other types of geographical or physical restrictions. Incentives for providers to use the data are also essential, including making the data easier to consume, summarize, and integrate into decision support activities.

Evidence of Impact

The capture of PGHD offers unique and novel benefits stemming from the opportunity to re-engineer health information flow that is not dependent on healthcare encounters. Patients may enter data at regular intervals or in response to symptomatology for immediate review by clinicians in-between visits. Further, these new patient information workflows allow for a longitudinal trending of patient data in-between visits and ultimately a deeper understanding of patient symptomatology. In doing this, information loss is minimized and patient continuity is maximized. The minimization of information loss and maximization of patient continuity may directly benefit care quality and safety. More complete EHR data will likely benefit secondary uses of data, such as for research and evidence-generation. Finally, the connection in the home can benefit both: (1) patients that already receive homecare services, and (2) patients that do not qualify for home services but have chronic conditions that benefit from trending of trackable device data and symptomatology.

In 2019, Tiase and colleagues conducted a rigorous scoping review to explore and summarize current evidence related to the integration of PGHD into electronic health records. The scoping review resulted in 19 studies that met inclusion criteria suggesting that PGHD integration into EHRs appears to be at an early stage (Tiase et al. 2021). Themes emerged concerning resource requirements, data delivery to the EHR, and preferences for review. This review underscored the need for best practices and better reporting of technical requirements to integrate PGHD into EHRs to leverage the potential value of PGHD.

Exemplars of PGHD Integration and Using in the Clinical Care Setting

Successful PGHD integration have been implemented for chronic disease management, self-management and patient engagement, and telehealth/remote patient monitoring. Ancker et al. (2019) described the characteristics of patients and providers that engaged in data uploads for chronic disease management of diabetes (Ancker et al. 2019). PGHD uploads were associated with improved blood glucose control and body mass index, but it was noted that overall blood glucose monitoring via PGHD uploads still suffered from slow adoption and that patients that uploaded their data had more visits and portal log-ins than patients that did not upload data (Ancker et al. 2019). Uploading of blood glucose data by patients for integration into the EHR has also been shown to be a feasible part of a diabetes telemedicine intervention to assist in diabetes self-management (Lewinski et al. 2019). Importantly, a user-friendly presentation format and automatic transfer of data from the patient's monitoring device into the EHR are essential considerations for use, adoption, and data interpretation by patients (Lewinski et al. 2019). Kumar et al. demonstrated in a pilot study the capability to integrate continuous glucose monitor data from pediatric patients/parents smartphones between scheduled clinic visits (Kumar et al. 2016). This study emphasized the feasibility of using existing technology that is widely available to consumers (e.g., commonly owned mobile devices, Apple Healthkit) as a means to increase wide-scale replication, as well as efficient workflows and intuitive visualizations within the EHR for clinicians.

Pevnick et al., investigated efficient and safe protocols for cardiologists' select review of heart rate monitor data, which is high volume data per patient (Pevnick et al. 2020). Their protocol included the development of a dashboard highlighting concerning values and logic that would trigger a cardiologist review. This work points to the importance of a governance framework and associated clinical protocol when integrating high volume PGHD into EHRs that have important clinical and safety implications requiring urgent review (Pevnick et al. 2020). Finally, while patient reported outcomes (PROs) have been widely used and are a best practice in cancer care, more recently PGHD has been used to actively support smoking cessation for patients with cancer by increasing screening and treatment referral (May et al. 2020).

Future Work and Opportunities

The ubiquitous capture and use of PGHD within healthcare delivery will require strong and widespread endorsement within patient communities by clinicians. PGHD can align with and promote the Quadruple Aim of decreasing cost, improving outcomes, improving the patient experience and increasing provider engagement (Bodenheimer and Sinsky 2014). It is possible that movement away from episodic care to increased continuity of information exchange and tracking of data from patients' daily lives as preventative interventions may facilitate achievement of the Quadruple aim (Bodenheimer and Sinsky 2014). The greater patient-provider communication and engagement that arises from increased capture and use of PGHD could also contribute to improved patient experience and clinician engagement. Some aspects of documentation burden—a key driver of clinician burnout—may be alleviated when patients directly capture more of their data themselves. However, reduced clinician documentation burden is dependent on efficient integration of PGHD into existing clinician workflows. Finally, the alignment of PGHD with the increased use of telehealth visits may expand patient access and increase continuity of care. Each of these areas are ripe for further investigation, exploration and innovation, as described in more detail below.

Efficient and Usable Clinical Workflow Integration

Data interpretation can be challenging and moreover, clinicians are already suffering from documentation burden. Adding another data source such as PGHD must be carefully introduced into clinical workflows. An exploration of information and visualization needs related to PGHD for varied and complex clinical conditions should be explored in the context of the clinical setting. Clinicians are already burdened with information overload during the use of EHRs and will require tools that surface and simplify data in context, including PGHD, using visualizations and other decision support tools. While there exist some solutions already that can minimize the burden of clinicians sifting through voluminous PGHD, such as clinical decision support alerts, intervening on and minimizing information overload will require novel approaches to the design and integration of PGHD within the clinical record. The use of cognitive task analyses should be employed to understand the utility of PGHD in complex decision making and how best to include PGHD in decision support algorithms to provide actionable insights. To understand needs related to visualization and discovery within the EHR, investigations of interactive displays with PGHD alongside EHR data, viewed within the EHR should be conducted to explore its impact on decision making and patient outcomes.

Telehealth and PGHD

The acceleration of telehealth virtual visits during the COVID-19 pandemic accentuated the need to provide PGHD, generally in the form of RPM data, to the provider at the point of the virtual visit. Since these PGHD may be generated from multiple devices, research is needed to investigate the optimal way to present PGHD, including the type of user interface and the appropriate level of synthesis and analysis (Abdolkhani et al. 2019). Further, as clinical care and decision-making is increasingly moved into virtual spaces, it will be important to identify best practices related to the role of shared decision making.

Conclusion

With an abundance of PGHD, we now have a wealth of data with the potential to predict and prevent disease—at a time where 60% of Americans suffer from a chronic condition (Irving 2017). PGHD have been used successfully to help in self-management of chronic disease and remote patient monitoring. However, these applications still suffer from overall low adoption and without careful consideration of the implications of engaged versus non-engaged patient populations may risk increasing health inequities. The twenty-first Century Cures act, related regulations, and consumer expectations promise to accelerate the use of patient-facing technologies, and with it the integration of PGHD as key ingredients to the disruption—and advancement—of health and healthcare.

Clinical Pearls
- Patient-generated health data are collected from patients outside of the clinical visit and may be categorized as health history, survey and questionnaire responses, or biometric data.
- Incorporation of PGHD into clinical workflows must consider the effort on the part of the patient to collect and transfer the data as well as the effort on the part of the clinician to introduce PGHD into their workflow. At each point, the transfer can be described as active or passive. This is critical to assess for implementation purposes.
- Several barriers to the integration of PGHD within clinical care exist, including trust, incentives for use, and efficient workflows, that must be addressed in order for the use of PGHD within the clinical setting to become standard and valuable information that help to improve care outcomes.
- The implementation of PGHD into care workflows is an important step to advance patient engagement, self-management, and shared decision making.

Chapter Review Questions
Review Questions

Q1. Which of the following is a primary benefit of PGHD integration into the clinical care setting?

a. Decreased need for post-discharge follow-up visits.
b. Increased longitudinal trending of patient data in-between visits.
c. Higher reimbursement for combined visits.
d. Additional data and workflows available to clinicians.

Q2. As a mobile health app developer, what are the factors that should be considered in the design of an app?

a. Safe, effective, and evidenced-based.
b. Trust, workflows, and incentives.
c. Active and passive transfer.
d. Patient engagement, self-management, and shared decision making.

Answers.

Q1:

Answer choice B. Rationale: New patient information workflows allow for a longitudinal trending of patient data in-between visits and ultimately a deeper understanding of patient symptomatology.

Q2:

Answer choice A. Rationale: The HIMSS Health App Guidelines Work Group is creating a framework to guide mHealth app developers on what is needed to ensure apps are safe, effective and evidenced-based.

References

Abdolkhani R, Gray K, Borda A, DeSouza R. Patient-generated health data management and quality challenges in remote patient monitoring. JAMIA Open. 2019;2:471–8.

Adler-Milstein J, Nong P. Early experiences with patient generated health data: health system and patient perspectives. J Am Med Informatics Assoc. 2019;26:952–9.

Ancker JS, Mauer E, Kalish RB, Vest JR, Gossey JT. Early adopters of patient-generated health data upload in an electronic patient portal. Appl Clin Inform. 2019;10:254–60.

Bodenheimer T, Sinsky C. From triple to quadruple aim: Care of the Patient Requires Care of the provider. Ann Fam Med. 2014;12:573–6.

CARIN Alliance. Trust framework and code of conduct; 2021.

Demiris G, Iribarren SJ, Sward K, Lee S, Yang R. Patient generated health data use in clinical practice: a systematic review. Nurs Outlook. 2019;67:311–30.

Genes N, Violante S, Cetrangol C, Rogers L, Schadt EE, Chan Y-FY. From smartphone to EHR: a case report on integrating patient-generated health data. Npj Digit Med. 2018;1:23.

Gesley J. Germany: new law allows health apps by prescription 2020.

Grossman LV, Masterson Creber RM, Benda NC, Wright D, Vawdrey DK, Ancker JS. Interventions to increase patient portal use in vulnerable populations: a systematic review. J Am Med Informatics Assoc. 2019;26:855–70.

HealthIT.gov. What is a personal health record? 2016.

Healthit.gov. What is a patient portal? 2017.

HIMSS. HIMSS continues improving health app effectiveness and safety; 2020.

Irving D. Chronic conditions in America: Price and prevalence. RAND Rev. 2017;

Kumar RB, Goren ND, Stark DE, Wall DP, Longhurst CA. Automated integration of continuous glucose monitor data in the electronic health record using consumer technology. J Am Med Inform Assoc. 2016;23:532–7.

Lewinski AA, Drake C, Shaw RJ, Jackson GL, Bosworth HB, Oakes M, et al. Bridging the integration gap between patient-generated blood glucose data and electronic health records. J Am Med Inform Assoc. 2019;26:667–72.

Mandel JC, Kreda DA, Mandl KD, Kohane IS, Ramoni RB. SMART on FHIR: a standards-based, interoperable apps platform for electronic health record. J Am Med Informatics Assoc JAMIA. 2016;23:899–908.

May JR, Klass E, Davis K, Pearman T, Rittmeyer S, Kircher S, et al. Leveraging patient reported outcomes measurement via the electronic health record to connect patients with cancer to smoking cessation treatment. Int J Environ Res Public Health. 2020;17

Office of the National Coordinator for Health IT [ONC]. ONC's Cures Act Final Rule; 2021.

Pevnick JM, Elad Y, Masson LM, Riggs RV, Duncan RG. Patient-initiated data: our experience with enabling patients to initiate incorporation of heart rate data into the electronic health record. Appl Clin Inform. 2020;11:671–9.

Shapiro M, Johnston D, Wald J, Mon D. Patient-generated health data; 2012.

Tiase VL, Hull W, McFarland MM, Sward KA, Del Fiol G, Staes C, et al. Patient-generated health data and electronic health record integration: a scoping review. JAMIA Open. 2021;3:619–27.

United States Food and Drug Administration [FDA]. Policy for Device Software Functions and Mobile Medical Applications; 2019.

United States Food and Drug Administration [FDA]. FDA Launches the Digital Health Center of Excellence; 2020.

Xcertia. Xcertia mHealth App Guidelines; 2019.

Part II
Methods for Translating Biomedical Research and Real World Evidence into Patient-Centric Precision Health Application

Chapter 7
Role of Digital Healthcare Approaches in the Analysis of Personalized (N-of-1) Trials

Thevaa Chandereng, Ziwei Liao, Stefani D'Angelo, Mark Butler, Karina W. Davidson, and Ying Kuen Cheung

Abstract The advancement in digital healthcare approaches, including health applications (apps) and wearable devices have allowed health system scientists to rapidly develop and implement innovative trial designs (e.g., Personalized, or N-of-1 trials). In this type of trial, the effect of one treatment is compared with one or more other treatments or a placebo condition, and the differences are calculated within-person. Thus, these designs are essentially multiple cross-over trials conducted on single persons. The ultimate goal of a Personalized trial is to determine the best tailored treatment for the participant using an objective data-driven criterion. Unlike traditional trial designs, the outcomes of the trial are continuously or repeatedly assessed throughout the study period. The ability to collect data instantly using health apps and wearable devices have eased the implementation of Personalized trials. In this chapter, we will elaborate on the role of health apps and other digital healthcare approaches in the design and analysis of an exemplar series of chronic lower back pain study (CLBP), personalized trials. We will discuss the collection of trial data (ecological momentary assessment (EMA) three-times daily of participant-reported pain, stress, and fatigue) using text messages and additionally weekly electronically delivered survey questionnaires. We will share the details of the analysis of the CLPB series of personalized trials using generalized least squares (GLS) regression. We will also elaborate on the computing platform (an R shiny app that is patient friendly) built to analyze the trial data. We will emphasize

T. Chandereng (✉) · Z. Liao · Y. K. Cheung
Department of Biostatistics, Columbia University, New York, NY, USA
e-mail: tc3123@cumc.columbia.edu; zl2417@cumc.columbia.edu; yc632@cumc.columbia.edu

S. D'Angelo · M. Butler · K. W. Davidson
Institute of Health System Science, Feinstein Institutes for Medical Research, & Donald and Barbara Zucker School of Medicine at Hofstra/Northwell, Northwell Health, Manhasset, NY, USA
e-mail: SDAngelo1@northwell.edu; markbutler@northwell.edu; kdavidson2@northwell.edu

© The Author(s), under exclusive license to Springer Nature
Switzerland AG 2022
P.-Y. S. Hsueh et al. (eds.), *Personal Health Informatics*, Cognitive Informatics in Biomedicine and Healthcare, https://doi.org/10.1007/978-3-031-07696-1_7

the importance of personalized trials by displaying the heterogeneity of the treatment effect in the study participants.

Keywords Personalized trials · Health apps · Computing platforms · N-of-1 trials · Pooled analysis · Time-series analysis

Learning Objectives for the Chapter
The objective of this chapter is to provide insight of using health apps to implement N-of-1 trials. By reading this chapter, the reader will learn to perform the following:

1. Learn how to use health apps to analyze Personalized trials
2. Learn how a series of Personalized (N-of-1) trials were conducted CLBP study
3. Learn how to analyze time-series data for Personalized trials
4. Compute and interpret patient-by-patient analysis for the CLBP study

Introduction

R shiny app is an interactive web app built from the R language. Shiny is an open source R package that provides an elegant and powerful web framework for building web applications using R without requiring HTML, CSS, or JavaScript knowledge. In recent years, researchers have begun to utilize R shiny for graphical representation and analysis of patient data for a variety of conditions and treatments (Chandereng et al. 2020; Yanhong Zhou et al. 2021; Yi Zhou et al. 2020). The utility of web applications for the analysis and presentation of participant data is twofold: (1) Descriptive statistics and treatment effects can be accessed for individual patients at any time and (2) No knowledge of statistical methods is required to generate the results. In addition, R shiny is a package freely available in the open-source R language and requires zero software costs or licensing fees for research use. As a result, a web-based shiny app for presenting patient data is both cost-effective and scalable.

In this chapter, we discuss the role of health apps in the analysis of a chronic lower back pain study. First, we compare personalized trials with traditional randomized controlled trials (RCT). Second, a brief overview of the prevalence of chronic low back pain (CLBP) is provided. Next, we discuss the study design of the CLBP personalized trial and recruitment of the participants. Fourth, we discuss how the EMA (fatigue, pain, and stress) and weekly survey data were collected using text messages. We discuss our use of generalized least squares (GLS) to analyze the EMA data. We will also demonstrate how an R shiny app is used to analyze the EMA data. Our analysis indicates that the treatment effect of both yoga and massage differ among participants. We observe the pooled analysis fails to capture the treatment effect of both yoga and massage due to heterogeneity in treatment effect among participants.

Personalized Trials

Clinicians usually apply evidence drawn from a large group of patients in a traditional RCT. In a traditional RCT, the patients are randomly allocated to two or more treatment groups and the treatment groups are compared with respect to the measured outcome. However, a single treatment/intervention is not always universally better than the others (Gabler et al. 2011; Zucker, Ruthazer, and Schmid 2010; Mahon et al. 1996). Heterogeneity in both treatment efficacy and side effects often lead clinicians to make an educated guess without a proper data-driven approach (Davidson et al. 2018). Single patient, multiple cross-over design (Personalized or N-of-1) is an alternative approach to tailor the most optimal therapy. Personalized trials consider an individual participant as the sole unit of observation in a study investigating the efficacy or side-effect of different treatments/interventions. In a personalized trial, the effect of one treatment is compared with one or more treatments, and the differences are calculated within-person (Davidson et al. 2021).

Table 7.1 summarizes a number of characteristics well suited for conducting personalized trials. Clinical problems with substantial uncertainty about the optimal intervention are suitable for personalized trials. Chronic conditions are ideal for personalized trials because the treatment target must be measurable over time and must exhibit some variation (Shaffer et al. 2018). It is important to ensure the effects of an intervention are reversible once withdrawn and the washout period is short and estimable (Duan, Kravitz, and Schmid 2013; Kravitz et al. 2014).

Background on CLBP

More than 25% of the U.S. adult population are affected by lower back pain (LBP) lasting a whole day in the past 3 months (Deyo et al. 2006). Chronic lower back pain (CLBP) is defined as lower back pain lasting 12 weeks or more, exceeding the usual time frame for tissue healing. CLBP is the fifth most common cause for physician visits and 80% of all healthcare costs (Khan et al. 2014). It is estimated that seven million adults in the U.S. have limitations in daily activities due to CLBP (Chou

Table 7.1 Considerations for conducting personalized trial

Features	Suitable for personalized	Not suitable for personalized
Heterogeneity of treatment	Treatment effects vary across patients	Homogeneity of treatment effects
Nature of disease	Slowly progressing, chronic, or stable	Rapid or acute
Assessment of outcomes	Outcomes can be assessed multiple times	Outcomes are measured at a single point
Effect onset and carryover	Significant individual differences in intervention response, minimal washout period across time	Small individual differences in intervention response, long washout period across time

2010). There is a high cost affiliated with CLBP due to limitations in daily activities and frequent physician visits.

The clinical guidelines on the pain management of CLBP in the U.S. have suggested changes to the use of pharmacotherapy when treating CLBP (Qaseem et al. 2017). Medications, primarily opioid therapy, should only be prescribed at the lowest dose for the shortest amount of time. Research has concluded that opioids are beneficial for pain relief and should only be prescribed where the benefits outweigh the risks (Saragiotto et al. 2016). The Centers for Disease Control and Prevention (CDC) have recommended the use of a non-opioid treatment and the need for additional research on managing chronic pain due to the danger of addiction and accidental overdose of opioid treatment (Dowell et al. 2016).

Both yoga and massage are non-opioid treatments that have been shown to be useful to treat CLBP patients. Both interventions were associated with reduced levels of pain compared to a placebo group with CLBP. Yoga treatments for CLBP were also associated with improvements in quality of life. However, the treatment effects of both yoga and massage for CLBP are not homogeneous for all patients. Some participants with CLBP benefit more from these interventions than others and vice versa. To study the individual treatment effect from these interventions, a personalized trial design is ideal. By utilizing digital healthcare approaches, including mobile devices, texting, and other digital communication strategies, both the design and analysis of a personalized trial were conducted to study the effectiveness of yoga, massage, and usual care from November 20, 2019 to January 31, 2021. The trial is registered with clinicaltrials.gov ("Personalized Trial for Chronic Lower Back Pain" n.d.).

Study Design

In this section, we discuss the design of the CLBP personalized trials, and then how participants were recruited for the study, including inclusion and exclusion criteria. The study is a series of 60 randomized personalized trials examining the effects of Swedish massage and yoga versus usual care on CLBP from November 20, 2019 to January 31, 2021. Yoga poses were selected based on those previously used by (Sherman et al. 2005) in a study assessing the effect on chronic lower back pain. Participants received a series of treatments of yoga and massage through a commercial wellness service called Zeel®. Zeel® allows people to book in-home massages with licensed massage therapists. For this study, Zeel® also allowed participants to book in-home one-on-one yoga sessions with a certified yoga instructor.

Once a participant was recruited to the study, the participant underwent a baseline assessment period for the first 2 weeks (as shown in Fig. 7.1). Participants were discouraged from receiving yoga and/or massage treatments during this period. The participants were asked to rate the EMA of their pain, fatigue, and stress at three random times daily during their waking hours, wear a fitbit device 24 h a day, and answer a number of surveys sent electronically each week. The details of the data collection are included below. Participant adherence to the protocol was assessed during the first 14 days of the baseline assessment period. Participants who did not achieve a minimum of 80% adherence to protocol requirements (including EMA, device wear, and survey response) were not permitted to continue to the intervention portion of the study. Participants maintaining 80% adherence or more were randomized to one of two different treatment sequences. The order of the treatment sequences is illustrated in Fig. 7.1. Participants were randomized 1:1 to the treatment sequences (i.e. 30 participants each treatment sequence).

As shown in Fig. 7.1, the treatment sequences were designed to deliver two intervention arms (massage and yoga) and a usual care arm (no intervention) in a multiple-crossover design of six treatment blocks. Each treatment block lasted a total of 2 weeks. During intervention treatment blocks, participants were asked to

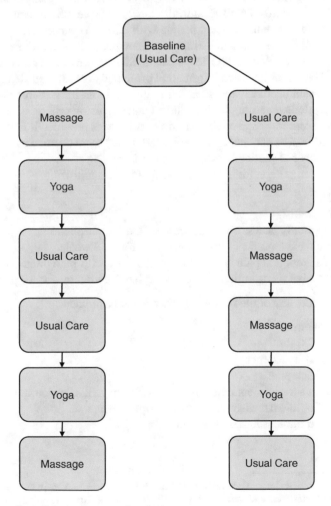

Fig. 7.1 Flowchart of the treatment assignments

use Zeel® to book two 1-h sessions of in-home Swedish massage (massage treatment blocks) or two 1-h sessions of in-home yoga (yoga treatment blocks) each week, at least 48-h apart. No treatment was provided to participants during usual care treatment blocks; instead, participants were asked to use techniques they normally would have used to manage their CLBP. Participants were discouraged from receiving additional massage or yoga sessions outside of the eight massage sessions and eight yoga sessions delivered throughout the study.

Recruitment and Study Population

The potential candidates for the study were primarily recruited using emails sent out to all employees at Northwell Health, the largest private health care employer in New York State. The email invited people with CLBP to participate in a personalized trial. Other recruitment strategies included referrals from Northwell Occupational Health Services (OHS), social media advertising, flyers distributed to Northwell Health facilities, and information presented at Northwell Health Wellness events. Interested candidates were asked to complete an initial screening measure covering questions regarding both inclusion and exclusion criteria of the trial. The electronic consent form and additional information was provided if the candidate is deemed eligible. The candidates were notified if they were deemed ineligible or the sufficient number of participants had been recruited.

The inclusion criteria for a participant included the following:

- Age ≥ 18
- Fluent in English
- Able to regularly access an email account and a smartphone
- Experiencing symptoms of lower back pain for ≥12 weeks
- Have a self-reported pain intensity>8 on the[1] PROMIS pain intensity scale
- Able to receive therapeutics (2× per week; between 8 a.m. and 10 p.m.)

Persons who met any of the following criteria were excluded:

- Pregnant women
- Weight ≥ 500 lbs.
- History of spinal surgery
- Complex back pain
- History of a serious mental health condition or psychiatric disorder
- History of opioid use disorder or current opioid users
- History of treatment for any substance abuse

---

[1] The PROMIS pain scales version 1.0 are used to measure intensity of pain symptoms (Revicki et al. 2009) and interference (Amtmann et al. 2010) (Wang et al. 2017) with daily life due to pain symptoms over the past 24 hours.

- Current physical activity restrictions or previously advised that yoga or massage is unsafe for their condition
- Planned travel outside of the United States within treatment period
- Planned surgery/procedures within 6 months of recruitment

Although the original goal of the study was to randomize 60 participants to receive the protocol, all study activities were halted in March 2020 as a result of the COVID-19 crisis in New York. The analysis below describes the data of 26 study participants that were able to complete their intervention treatment blocks before the study was ended for infection-control purposes.

Data Collection (EMA Pain, Fatigue, and Stress)

The ecological momentary assessment (EMA) of pain, fatigue, and stress data were collected via text messages. These assessments were collected three times daily and the timing is randomized throughout the day. An interval of at least 30 minutes was added between two texts. The text messages asked participants to rate their pain, fatigue, and stress in the current moment on a scale of 0–10. Table 7.2 summarizes the EMA stress ratings. The ratings were interpreted in the same manner for both EMA pain and fatigue. These assessment tools have been used extensively before the spurt of information age and have been used with smartphones in recent studies (Smyth et al. 2009; Shiffman et al. 2008; Cheung et al. 2017; Wang et al. 2017).

Analyzing EMA Data

Unlike traditional RCT designs, the treatment arms are not independent in Personalized trials. Statistical analyses that account for correlation structure (time-series analyses) are essential to analyze Personalized RCTs (Shaffer et al. 2018). We analyzed the ecological momentary assessment (EMA) of pain, fatigue, and stress data using GLS regression. The GLS estimator of a linear regression is a generalization of the ordinary least square (OLS) estimator. When the OLS estimator violates

Table 7.2 EMA stress rating scales

Rating	Stress level
0	No stress
1–3	Mild stress
4–6	Moderate stress
7–10	Severe stress

one of the assumptions of the Gauss-Markov theorem,[2] namely that of equal variances, the GLS estimator is used.

In a standard linear model,

$$Y = X\beta + \varepsilon,$$

where Y is the $n \times 1$ response vector, X is an $n \times p$ model matrix, β is a $p \times 1$ vector of estimated regression coefficients, and ε is an $n \times 1$ vector of errors. The ordinary-least squares (OLS) estimator of β assuming that $\varepsilon \sim N(0, \sigma^2 I_n)$ (i.e. the errors are uncorrelated),

$$\beta_{OLS} = \left(X^T X\right)^{-1} X^T Y,$$

with the covariance matrix

$$Var\left(\beta_{OLS}\right) = \sigma^2 \left(X^T X\right)^{-1}.$$

However, in time-series data, the errors from the regression model are unlikely to be independent. Generalized least-squares (GLS) regression extends OLS estimation of the standard linear model by providing for possibly unequal error variances and for correlations between different errors. In these cases, the intervals (time) are usually equally spaced. Let V = Var($\varepsilon \mid X$), where V is an $n \times n$ symmetric positive definite matrix.

In a GLS regression, the covariance matrix has the following structure:

$$V = Var\left(\varepsilon\right) = \begin{bmatrix} \sigma_1^2 & \rho_{1,2}\sigma_1\sigma_2 & \cdots & \rho_{1,n}\sigma_1\sigma_n \\ \rho_{2,1}\sigma_1\sigma_2 & \sigma_2^2 & \cdots & \rho_{2,n}\sigma_2\sigma_n \\ \vdots & \vdots & \ddots & \vdots \\ \rho_{n,1}\sigma_n\sigma_1 & \rho_{n,2}\sigma_n\sigma_2 & \cdots & \sigma_n^2 \end{bmatrix}$$

There is an invertible matrix, such that $V = WW^T$. If we multiply the regression equation by W^{-1}, we get

$$W^{-1}Y = W^{-1}X\beta + W^{-1}\varepsilon.$$

Replacing $Y^* = W^{-1}Y$, $X^* = W^{-1}X$, $\varepsilon^* = W^{-1}\varepsilon$, we get

$$Y^* = X^*\beta + \varepsilon^*.$$

---

[2] The Gauss Markov theorem states that if the errors OLS estimator are uncorrelated, have equal variances, and expected value (mean) of 0, the errors do not need to be normal, nor do they need to be independently identically distributed.

Thus,

$$\beta_{GLS} = \left(X^{*T} X^* \right)^{-1} X^{*T} Y^*$$

$$= \left(X^T V^{-1} X \right)^{-1} X^T V^{-1} Y^*.$$

We can fit several time-series models with GLS. Autoregressive model with order 1 (AR(1)) is one of the most frequently used models. In an AR(1) model, the regression errors are assumed to be stationary. In other words, the errors are assumed to have the same expectation and the same variance:

$$\sigma^2 = \sigma_1^2 = \cdots = \sigma_n^2$$

In addition, the model postulates that correlations diminish as observations are farther apart in a specific form:

$$\rho_{a,a+k} = \rho_{a+k,a} = \rho^k, \quad -1 \le \rho \le 1, \quad a,k > 0.$$

If both the values of ρ and σ^2 are known in an AR(1) model, the GLS estimator of β can be easily obtained. However, these parameters are generally unknown.

R Shiny App for the CLBP Trial and Trial Results

We developed a user-friendly R shiny app for analyzing the EMA data from the CLBP trial using GLS (video attached). The R shiny app code is available at https://github.com/ROADMAP-Columbia/patient-report. A sample data is included in the Data folder. The Shiny app performs GLS if the data is provided and the outcomes, (multiple columns) and treatment columns are selected for patient-by-patient basis as shown in Fig. 7.2. The R shiny app can serve as a tool to analyze the data for trial coordinators.

Table 7.3 shows the R shiny app output for the treatment effect of all three variables measured using EMA (i.e. pain, fatigue, and stress) for a single patient. The baseline treatment for comparison is usual care (no yoga or massage). Based on Table 7.3, there is no difference for all mean EMA averaged between usual care and yoga for this particular patient. There is a significant difference for both EMA pain and fatigue between yoga and massage (p-value <0.05). The patient reported lower scores for both EMA pain and stress during massage treatments compared to usual care. However, the mean EMA fatigue scores reported by the patient were the same for both massage and usual care.

This example illustrates how easily the R shiny app can be used to generate analyses and descriptive statistics for the effectiveness of three outcomes of the two treatments utilized in this particular trial. By displaying results in this manner,

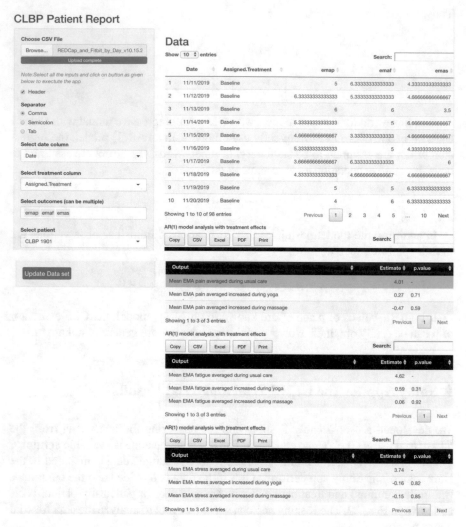

Fig. 7.2 An R shiny app developed to perform GLS to estimate the treatment effect for individual patients

research team members can easily identify the most effective treatments for each particular participant simply by clicking on the participant's ID number within the R shiny app. Without the flexibility of this R shiny app, study staff would need to consult with a statistician or attempt to run analyses themselves to generate these results. This would lead to both wasted time and increased potential for research errors.

In addition, the app runs based on the linked participant data set. This allows the analysis results to be continuously updated as participant data is added, easily generating interim and final results for each participant through the course of the study.

Table 7.3 Treatment effect obtained from all three EMAs (pain, fatigue, and stress) for a single patient

Output	Estimate	p value
Mean EMA pain averaged during usual care	3.49	–
Mean EMA pain averaged increased during yoga	−0.22	0.57
Mean EMA pain averaged increased during massage	−1.05	0.01
Mean EMA fatigue averaged during usual care	4.25	–
Mean EMA fatigue averaged increased during yoga	−0.24	0.52
Mean EMA fatigue averaged increased during massage	−0.71	0.07
Mean EMA stress averaged during usual care	3.61	–
Mean EMA stress averaged increased during yoga	−0.46	0.11
Mean EMA stress averaged increased during massage	−1.25	0.00

Further, the analyses utilized in this R shiny app can be easily modified to fit various N-of-1 designs to account for variations in number of treatment blocks, duration of treatment, and other design elements essential to N-of-1 trials.

The EMA data (pain, fatigue, and stress) are obtained three times daily. We summarize the data collected 3 times daily by taking the daily mean for each EMA. The treatment effect (point estimate) is obtained from daily mean EMAs using GLS regression with AR(1) model. We used the R package *nlme* for all analyses (Pinheiro et al. 2017).

Table 7.4 displays the treatment effect obtained from all three daily mean EMAs using GLS for all 26 patients. More than 50% (14 of the 26) of the participants had no difference in all three EMAs for both yoga and massage compared to usual care. Table 7.5 summarizes the outcomes of Table 7.4. Table 7.5 shows the number of participants with no, positive, and negative effects that are statistically significant for all three daily mean EMAs comparing both yoga and massage to usual care. None of the participants had lower daily mean EMA stress when they received yoga treatment compared to usual care and only one participant had a higher daily mean EMA stress when he/she/they received yoga treatment compared to usual care. However, as noted above, this study was conducted during the beginning of the COVID-19 pandemic in New York city, and stress levels reported by many in the area were very high. Tables 7.4 and 7.5 clearly show the heterogeneity in treatment effect for both yoga and massage compared to usual care in CLBP patients.

Conclusion

In this chapter, we presented the CLBP study, a Personalized RCT. We discuss the role of health apps in the design and analysis of a Personalized trial. We presented how health apps are used for the daily data collection of the participants' outcomes (three different EMAs). Besides data collection, we also illustrate how an R shiny app is used to analyze the outcomes of the trial participants by the trial coordinator.

Table 7.4 Treatment effect obtained from all three daily mean EMAs (pain, fatigue, and stress) for all 26 patients. For each EMA, we reported the mean EMA value during usual care in the first column and the difference between yoga and usual care and the difference between massage and usual care in the second and third columns respectively. If the difference is significant (p-value < 0.05), we used * to denote it after the magnitude of the difference

Patient ID	Daily average EMA pain			Daily average EMA fatigue			Daily average EMA stress		
	Mean during usual care	Difference between yoga and usual care	Difference between massage and usual care	Mean during usual care	Difference between yoga and usual care	Difference between massage and usual care	8Mean during usual care	Difference between yoga and usual care	Difference between massage and usual care
1901	4.01	0.27	−0.47	4.62	0.59	0.06	3.74	−0.16	−0.15
1902	3.49	−0.22	−1.05*	4.25	−0.24	−0.71	3.61	−0.46	−1.25*
1904	1.36	−0.05	0.65	3.73	−0.51	−0.17	1	0.62	1.22*
1905	2.48	−0.56*	−0.54*	2.68	−0.41*	−0.4	1.48	0.04	−0.07
1911	1.49	0.02	−0.21	2.83	0.07	0.16	1.24	0.06	−0.04
1920	3.77	0.52	−0.22	3.05	0.13	0.02	2.55	−0.13	0.79
1923	0.73	0.68	0.7	1.62	0.1	−0.01	1.18	−0.14	−0.56
1925	2.31	−0.05	0.07	2.76	−0.2	0.05	4.31	−0.58	−0.23
1928	4.5	−0.27	−0.16	4.56	−0.09	−0.3	4.47	−0.12	−0.17
1930	3.95	−0.05	0.22	4.04	−0.4	−0.37	3.81	−0.25	0.16
1931	1.62	0.56	0.24	3.08	−0.65*	−1.1*	2.68	−0.35	−1.03*
1934	2.71	0.42	0.86	4.68	0.65	1.44*	3.7	0.5	0.61
1935	2.21	−0.21	−0.48	5.78	0.11	0.07	5.1	0.11	0.04
1941	3.67	−0.14	−0.22	0.22	0.12	−0.44*	0	0.01	0
1949	2.35	−0.56	−1.08	2.09	0.01	0.52	2.02	−0.45	−0.71
1956	3.2	0.87	0.48*	2.17	0.49	0.17	3.88	−0.07	−0.64*
1959	2.01	−0.02	0.13	4.86	−1.97*	−1.25	3.03	−0.69	−0.31
1960	4.71	1.32*	2.57*	5.18	1.39*	2.31*	5.25	1.09*	2.27*

1961	5.45	−0.84	−0.82	5.C5	0.2	−0.12	5.21	−0.37	−0.74*
1975	6.66	−0.03	−0.36	6.14	−0.5	−0.79	6.07	−0.58	−0.44
1979	3.31	−0.69*	0.04	3.66	−0.06	0.37	3.56	0.11	0.35
1980	3.2	−0.05	0.16	1.98	0.02	−0.44	0.99	0	0.01
1984	2.45	0.02	−0.58	2.88	0.12	0.55	2.27	−0.32	−0.03
1986	3.86	−0.69	0.59	3.5	−0.29	1.25*	1.79	−0.11	0.34
1990	4.21	−0.18	−0.23	4.52	−0.12	−0.16	2.23	0.08	−0.48
1994	3.66	0.17	−0.45	6.48	0.39	0.43	4.3	0.96	−0.39

Table 7.5 Number of participants with no, positive, and negative significant effects for all three daily average EMAs comparing both yoga and massage to usual care

		Positive effect (lower EMA)	Negative effect (lower EMA)	No effect
Daily average EMA pain	Yoga vs Usual Care	2	1	23
	Massage vs Usual Care	2	2	22
Daily average EMA fatigue	Yoga vs Usual Care	3	1	22
	Massage vs Usual Care	2	3	21
Daily average EMA stress	Yoga vs Usual Care	0	1	25
	Massage vs Usual Care	4	2	20

The R shiny app can be used to securely transfer trial results to the participants. The ability to collect data instantly using health apps and wearable devices have eased the implementation of Personalized trials. In the near future, we are planning to streamline the process using a single mobile app that sends a push notification for data collection and provide the trial results instantly once the trial is completed. We also plan to build a simplified version of the shiny app that app helps trial participants understand their data and the effect of each treatment. The ultimate goal is to provide a tool to patients for the insight of their data and select the best treatment using a data-driven approach.

Review Questions
1. List two differences between Personalized RCTs and traditional RCTs.
2. Why is generalized least square (GLS) regression is preferred over ordinary least square for time-series data?

Answers
1. (a) In Personalized RCTs, the effectiveness of a treatment is compared on an individual by individual basis. However, in traditional RCTs the effectiveness of a treatment is computed using net benefit from a large population.

    (b) In Personalized RCTs, a patient is the entire trial compared to traditional RCTs, where a large population of subjects are required.
2. Time-series data are usually correlated and not independent. Generalized least-squares (GLS) regression extends ordinary least-squares (OLS) estimation of the standard linear model by providing for possibly unequal error variances and for correlations between different errors.

References

Amtmann D, Cook KF, Jensen MP, Chen W-H, Choi S, Revicki D, Cella D, et al. Development of a PROMIS Item Bank to measure pain interference. Pain. 2010;150(1):173–82.

Chandereng T, Wei X, Chappell R. Imbalanced randomization in clinical trials. Stat Med. 2020;39(16):2185–96.

Cheung YK, Hsueh P-YS, Qian M, Yoon S, Meli L, Diaz KM, Schwartz JE, Kronish IM, Davidson KW. Are nomothetic or ideographic approaches superior in predicting daily exercise behaviors? Methods Inf Med. 2017;56(6):452–60.

Chou R. Pharmacological Management of low Back Pain. Drugs. 2010;70(4):387–402.

Davidson KW, Cheung YK, McGinn T, Claire Wang T. Expanding the Role of N-of-1 Trials in the Precision Medicine Era: Action Priorities and Practical Considerations. NAM Perspectives. 2018. https://doi.org/10.31478/201812d.

Davidson KW, Silverstein M, Cheung K, Paluch RA, Epstein LH. Experimental designs to optimize treatments for individuals: personalized N-of-1 trials. JAMA Pediatr. 2021. February; https://doi.org/10.1001/jamapediatrics.2020.5801.

Deyo RA, Mirza SK, Martin BI. Back pain prevalence and visit rates: estimates from U.S. National Surveys, 2002. Spine. 2006;31(23):2724–7.

Dowell D, Haegerich TM, Chou R. CDC guideline for prescribing opioids for chronic pain—United States, 2016. JAMA. 2016;315(15):1624–45.

Duan N, Kravitz RL, Schmid CH. Single-Patient (n-of-1) Trials: A Pragmatic Clinical Decision Methodology for Patient-Centered Comparative Effectiveness Research. J Clin Epidemiol. 2013, 66(8 Suppl):S21–28.

Gabler NB, Duan N, Vohra S, Kravitz RL. N-of-1 Trials in the Medical Literature: A Systematic Review: A Systematic Review. Medical Care. 2011;49(8):761–68.

Khan I, Hargunani R, Saifuddin A. The lumbar high-intensity zone: 20 years on. Clin Radiol. 2014;69(6):551–8.

Kravitz R, Duan N, Eslick I, Gabler NB, Kaplan HC. Design and Implementation of N-of-1 Trials: A User's Guide. Agency for Healthcare. 2014. https://scholar.google.ca/scholar?cluster=14387607499423024105&hl=en&as_sdt=0,5&sciodt=0,5.

Mahon J, Laupacis A, Donner A, Wood T. "Randomised Study of N of 1 Trials versus Standard Practice." BMJ. 1996; 312(7038):1069–74.

Personalized Trial for Chronic Lower Back Pain. n.d. Accessed March 31, 2021. https://clinicaltrials.gov/ct2/show/NCT04203888.

Pinheiro J, Bates D, DebRoy S, Sarkar D, Heisterkamp S, Van Willigen B, and Maintainer R. "Package 'nlme.'" *Linear and nonlinear mixed effects models, Version* 2017 3 (1). http://cran.rapporter.net/web/packages/nlme/nlme.pdf

Qaseem A, Wilt TJ, McLean RM, Forciea MA, Clinical Guidelines Committee of the American College of Physicians. Noninvasive treatments for acute, subacute, and chronic low back pain: a clinical practice guideline from the American College of Physicians. Ann Intern Med. 2017;166(7):514–30.

Revicki DA, Chen W-H, Harnam N, Cook KF, Amtmann D, Callahan LF, Jensen MP, Keefe FJ. Development and psychometric analysis of the PROMIS pain behavior Item Bank. Pain. 2009;146(1–2):158–69.

Saragiotto BT, Machado GC, Ferreira ML, Pinheiro MB, Shaheed CA, Maher CG. Paracetamol for low back pain. Cochrane Database Syst Rev. 2016;6(June):CD012230.

Shaffer JA, Kronish IM, Falzon L, Cheung YK, Davidson KW. N-of-1 Randomized Intervention Trials in Health Psychology: A Systematic Review and Methodology Critique. Annals of Behavioral Medicine: A Publication of the Society of Behavioral Medicine. 2018;52(9):731–42.

Sherman KJ, Cherkin DC, Erro J, Miglioretti DL, Deyo RA. Comparing Yoga, Exercise, and a Self-Care Book for Chronic Low Back Pain: A Randomized, Controlled Trial. Annals of Internal Medicine. 2005;143(12):849–56.

Shiffman S, Stone AA, Hufford MR. Ecological momentary assessment. Annu Rev Clin Psychol. 2008;4:1–32.

Smyth JM, Wonderlich SA, Sliwinski MJ, Crosby RD, Engel SG, Mitchell JE, Calogero RM. Ecological momentary assessment of affect, stress, and binge-purge Behaviors: day of week and time of day effects in the natural environment. Int J Eat Disord. 2009;42(5):429–36.

Wang R, Chen F, Chen Z, Li T, Harari G, Tignor S, Zhou X, Ben-Zeev D, Campbell AT. StudentLife: using smartphones to assess mental health and academic performance of college students. In: Rehg JM, Murphy SA, Kumar S, editors. Mobile health: sensors, analytic methods, and applications. Cham: Springer International Publishing; 2017. p. 7–33.

Zhou Y, Lin R, Ying-Wei Kuo J, Lee J, Yuan Y. BOIN suite: a software platform to design and implement novel early-phase clinical trials. JCO Clinical Cancer Informatics. 2021;5(January):91–101.

Zhou Y, Leung S-W, Mizutani S, Takagi T, Tian Y-S. MEPHAS: an interactive graphical user Interface for medical and pharmaceutical statistical analysis with R and shiny. BMC Bioinformatics. 2020;21(1):183.

Zucker DR, Ruthaze R, Schmid CH. Individual (N-of-1) trials can be combined to give population comparative treatment effect estimates: methodologic considerations. J Clin Epidemiol. 2010;63(12):1312–23.

Chapter 8
Early Detection of Cognitive Decline Via Mobile and Home Sensors

Holly Jimison, Maciej Kos, and Misha Pavel

Abstract Cognition is a significant determinant of our intellectual capacity and quality of life. Our cognition enables our perception, recognition, memory, attentional control, reasoning, and decision-making and is therefore involved in most of our behaviors. In this chapter we will discuss the large spectrum of cognitive functions ranging from high-level executive functions to their implication in the "simplest" repetitive, nearly automatic movements of one's finger. The only behaviors that are not completely tied to cognition are purely reflexive and certain habitual behaviors. Because of the importance of cognition, the assessment and understanding of cognitive functionality have been the foci of many research initiatives and projects ranging from basic science to applied assessment. A recent report from the U.S. Center for Disease Control (Taylor et al. Morb Mortal Wkly Rep 67:753, 2018) included results showing that the prevalence of subjective cognitive decline in the U.S. was 11.1%, or 1 in 9 adults. It was slightly higher for adults 65 years and older (11.7%) and somewhat lower for adults 45–64 years of age. Clearly, cognitive impairment with its resulting impacts on health and welfare is widespread and important to address.

Keywords Cognitive monitoring · Cognitive decline · Health coaching · Aging · Neurological conditions

Learning Objectives: 4–6 Short Learning Objectives
- Describe the clinical aspects of cognitive health and disorders and their traditional clinical assessment.

H. Jimison (✉) · M. Kos · M. Pavel
Khoury College of Computer Sciences, Northeastern University, Boston, MA, USA

Bouvé College of Health Sciences, Boston, MA, USA
e-mail: h.jimison@northeastern.edu

© The Author(s), under exclusive license to Springer Nature Switzerland AG 2022
P.-Y. S. Hsueh et al. (eds.), *Personal Health Informatics*, Cognitive Informatics in Biomedicine and Healthcare, https://doi.org/10.1007/978-3-031-07696-1_8

- Explain current and future cognitive assessment techniques and intervention approaches.
- Compare the wide array of data acquisition techniques, including sensors available for monitoring health and cognitive states.
- Articulate computational modeling approaches for inferring patient cognitive function from observed data collected using mobile and home sensors.
- Describe how computer games and interactions with technology can be used to cognitive function.
- Summarize the opportunities and challenges associated with monitoring cognitive health and associated sensing technologies.

Introduction

Cognition is one of the most important functions underlying individuals' ability to perform most of tasks, thereby enabling independence and quality of life (QoL). Qualitative results indicate that older adults, rate cognitive function above most of their other capabilities (H Jimison et al. 2010). This should not be surprising as noted by philosophers some 500 years ago, cogito, ergo sum, (Plato, Rene Descartes, *Meditations on First Philosophy*) that our cognition defines our existence and identity. In fact, our cognition enables our perception, recognition, memory, attentional control, reasoning, decision-making and is therefore involved in most of our behaviors. Later in this chapter, we will discuss the large spectrum of cognitive functions ranging from high-level executive functions to their implication in the "simplest" repetitive, nearly automatic movements of one's finger. The only behaviors that are not completely tied to cognition are purely reflexive and certain habitual behaviors.

Cognition is a significant determinant of our intellectual capacity and quality of life. Because of its importance, the assessment and understanding of cognitive functionality have been the foci of many research initiatives and projects ranging from basic science to applied assessment. A recent report from the U.S. Center for Disease Control (Taylor et al. 2018) included results showing that the prevalence of subjective cognitive decline in the U.S. was 11.1%, or 1 in 9 adults. It was slightly higher for adults 65 years and older (11.7%) and somewhat lower for adults 45–64 years of age. Clearly, cognitive impairment with its resulting impacts on health and welfare is widespread and important to address.

Since the birth of experimental psychology in the realm of basic science, researchers have studied cognitive functions in well-controlled laboratory studies with participants trained to perform well-designed, sophisticated experimental paradigms. These experimental efforts accumulated vast amounts of knowledge and understanding but, with notable exceptions, these results were frequently did not generalized to real-life situations. For a variety of mostly practical reasons, many of the rigorous theoretical frameworks and laboratory-based experimental assessment techniques and paradigms were rarely adopted in clinical settings (e.g., signal detection theory).

In the healthcare domain, there are several motivators for clinicians to be interested in the assessment of cognitive functions. From a practical point of view, understanding the everyday functioning of individuals is useful to gain insights into difficulties that affect the quality of life frequently due to deficits in cognitive functionality. This knowledge is especially important as the demographic in most countries comprises dramatically increasing proportions of older adults (National Institute on Aging 2022; Possin et al. 2018; United Nations Department of Economic and Social Affairs Population Division 2019; US Census Bureau 2021). Everyday functioning encompassing daily functional activities such as hygiene, dressing (i.e., activities of daily living, ADL) as well as cooking, managing finances, driving (instrumental activities of daily living, IADL) all require certain levels of cognitive functioning. Informal assessments of the ability to perform ADLs and IADLs are often taken as indicators of cognitive and or physical decline. Unfortunately, these assessments, frequently based on self-reports and informant responses to questionnaires, provide only subjective measures that are corrupted by biases and distortions. To get more accurate assessments, clinicians often resort to neuropsychological tests that have been normed on large pools of participants. Although these instruments have been validated, their sensitivity and specificity are limited by the variability across populations in cultural background, socio-economic status, native language, education, and prior experiences with assessment tests (De Santi et al. 2008). Since cognitive functions represent a significant component of human neurological processes, it is possible to asses changes by monitoring brain changes with imaging techniques such as MRI, but these techniques are also plagued by the variability among individuals and their functional cognitive performance (Dinse 2006; Driscoll et al. 2009).

Another issue associated with most of the cognitive measures is the sparsity of the assessments relative to the within and across subject variability. As it turns out, most of the variables associated with cognitive function have significant dynamics (variability over time)(Gamaldo et al. 2012) that motivated researchers and clinicians to consider collect and use intensive longitudinal data (ILD). A simultaneous realization of the need to assess ad model individuals leads to designs that enable the acquisition of individuals' data over long periods of time (Hekler et al. 2019; Misha Pavel et al. 2016; M. Pavel et al. 2015).

While collecting ILD for individuals has been very challenging, recent advances in sensor technology, computation, data science, and artificial intelligence (AI) opened the opportunity to mitigate many of the shortcomings within the area of Digital Health. In the remainder of this chapter, we discuss several important topics underlying approaches to cognitive assessments, focusing on self-motivating computer games. We will briefly review the most relevant cognitive processes and their relationship to observable behaviors that enable assessment. We then address the fundamental concepts of measurements and their application to cognitive functionality. We will discover that most measurements require assumptions that are best described and specified in terms of computational measurement models. We will then extend the notion of models and modeling to the domain of cognitive monitoring. Equipped with the notions of measurement and computational modeling, we will describe ways that we can use streams of data from unobtrusive sensors and associated algorithms to.

Cognitive Processes and Related Behaviors

As noted above, cognitive competency comprises a multitude of mental processes that include memory and the ability to learn new things, judgment and decision-making, attention, problem-solving, linguistic functions, and even many perceptual processes necessary to recognize objects and relationships (Center for Disease Control and Prevention 2016). These processes are necessary to enable fluid intelligence (solving novel problems) as well as crystalized intelligence (knowledge) (Cattell 1963). As noted above, cognitive competence is necessary for independence and high QoL at any age. Yet cognitive functionality is affected by many conditions ranging from chronic decline due to aging and non-communicative disease to adverse events such as traumatic brain injury, strokes or even complete anesthesia.

During most of the twentieth century, laboratory experiments and many clinical tests were developed to assess specific cognitive processes. Many of these tests are based on the assumption that using carefully designed paradigms enable clinicians to isolate and assess specific cognitive processes without regard to other, concurrent processes. Although this may be true by training the participants in the experiments, this independence assumption can be challenged in several ways. First, in almost every task assessing cognitive processes, the participants must perform in addition to the target cognitive task perceptual and motor task that appear to interfere. A classic example is the speed-accuracy tradeoff that can be interpreted as a competition for resources such as time. Another example is based on the observations that many of the results of these assessment procedures did not generalize to real-life situations (Katz et al. 2018) Although there are several possible explanations, one possible reason for the failure to generalize is that in real life, most people need to perform multiple functions simultaneously. We frequently talk while walking, have to recall from memory while paying attention to the traffic, etc. The results of several recent dual tasks experiments suggest that performance on one task can frequently interfere with another concurrent task (Beauchet et al. 2005). These considerations led researchers to consider the conditions that govern the relationship between performance on multiple tasks (Sperling and Dosher 1986). We will briefly address these notions in the section discussing attention.

Memory

Human memory employing neurological processes that encode, store and retrieve information is not a single homogeneous process. Many experimental results suggest that there are distinct types of memory that differ in the processes that underlie creating and accessing memories (Cowan 2008; Kadlec 2015). A simplified diagram of the relationships among different types of memories is shown in Fig. 8.1. The memory types differ in the processes generating the memory traces, including independent variables such as time (short, long term, or prospective), information

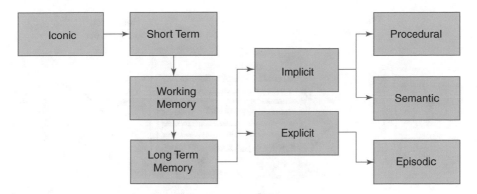

Fig. 8.1 Graphical representation of various memory types after (Kadlec 2015)

types (objects, symbols, linguistic elements, procedures, etc.), sensory inputs (colors, sounds, etc.). For the purpose of this discussion, an important aspect of the relationships among different types of memories is that aging significantly affects the short-term and working memories and thereby impairing the transition of information to long-term memory.

Current memory assessments are typically focused on working memory and the transfer of information to long-term memory. For example, a typical test trial consists of presenting a list of words to participants and asking them to recall them immediately or after another interposed task. Although this process addresses working memory and the transfer to long term memory, it is somewhat artificial in that the participant has no interest in the meaning of the words.

Attention

Attention represents the ability of human perceptual and cognitive systems to process multiple sources of information (divided attention) or to concentrate on a particular task while ignoring most of other stimuli and events (focused attention). Although attention has been the subject of many research efforts over the last couple of centuries (James 1890), a modern interpretation of attentional control is typically described in terms of allocation of processing resources, for different views see (Anderson 2005; Sperling 1984). The illustration in Fig. 8.2 is an oversimplified view of different attentional processes controlling individual task performance by assigning perceptual, cognitive, and resources to each task. Multimodal inputs impinging on an individual are represented on the left side of Fig. 8.2. The first attentional "filter" may reduce the amount of processing allocated to different sensory inputs. For example, while driving in heavy traffic, one may ignore any auditory inputs. The next filter, represented by a set of parallel channels, designates processes in the cognitive domain; for example, one may perceive visual stimuli but not recognize their symbolic meaning. There is a certain limited capacity for each

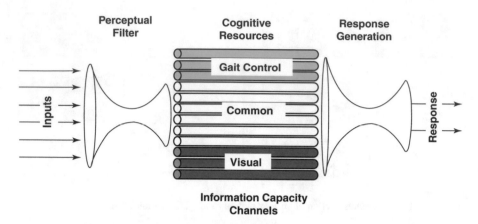

Fig. 8.2 Capacity-limited performance of dual tasks represented in terms of information channels. The top blue channels are dedicated to walking, the bottom red are memory, and the remaining channels can be allocated by the attentional processes

process that cannot be allocated to other modalities, but the common channels are available to be shared among tasks.

Finally, one may determine the appropriate response, but another task (like driving) may require sensory-motor control. The allocation of processing resources is assumed to be controlled by the relative utility of each task (Sperling and Dosher 1986). Important, high utility tasks are allocated more resources than low utility tasks. This dependence of performance on the relative task utility is particularly important in dual-task experiments. In a well-designed experiment, the experimenter would provide guidance to the participats' internalization of each task utility.

Consider an experiment with two concurrent tasks, for example, walking fast and perhaps on a challenging terrain while performing cognitive task such as navigation (recognition of landmarks in a complex environment. If they pay full attention to the cognitive task, they will do well recognizing landmarks, but they will slow down their gait. As the experimenter increases the participants' utility to the walking task, they will speed up but are more likely to miss their landmak targets. As the relative utility is shifted between the tasks, the performance follows the Performance Operating Characteristics shown in Fig. 8.3.(Navon and Gopher 1979; Sperling and Dosher 1986) The performance of each task is plotted on the corresponding coordinate—Task 1 is indicated on the abscissa and Task 2 on the ordinate; a point represents the operating point selected by the participant to reflect a given set of relative utilities of the two tasks. The reader may notice that if the operating point is near the points R_1 or R_2 the cocncurrent task will only have a small effect. The key take-home message is that degree of observed interaction can only be well described by tracing out the entire curve.

Although these empirical curves are useful, it is important to consider its theoretical implications so that the qualitative results of "observed interference between tasks" can be used to estimate the individuals' processing abilities associated with each task.

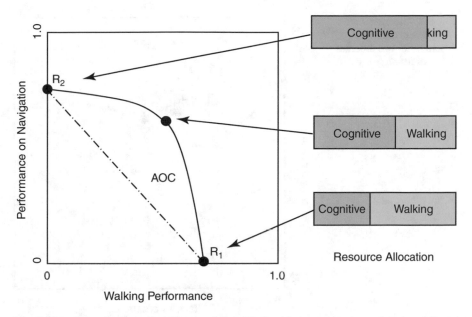

Fig. 8.3 Performance Operating Characteristics (POC) with three operating points that differ in terms of resources allocated to different tasks

Using the channel model, the performance tradeoff described by a POC can be represented by varying the allocation of channels between the two tasks. To illustrate the approach, let us assume that each of the M channels is a symmetric binary channel characterized by the probability q of correct transmission of a binary symbol (designated by "1") across the channel. Such a channel has information-theoretic channel capacity C given by the channel entropy $H(q)$ (Cover and Thomas 2012), $C = 1 - H(q)$ where entropy is computed as $H(q) = -q \log(q) - (1-q) \log(1-q)$. Intuitively, channel capacity can be interpreted as the efficiency of a channel to transmit or process information. Suppose we assume that N of the M channels (where $N < M$) are allocated to Task 1 (e.g., walking); then $M-N$ could be used to support the secondary task. Let us assume an ideal "performer" produces a response by maximizing the posterior probability of the correct response over all channels associated with a given task. In our example, if there are k outputs "1" in the N channels allocated to Task 1, the observer should respond "1" if.

$$\pi q^k (1-q)^{N-k} > (1-\pi) q^{N-k} (1-q)^k \tag{1}$$

where π is the prior probability of response ("1"). The results over a number of trials will enable us to estimate the POC curve shown in Fig. 8.4 Given the decision rule in Eq. (1), we can compute the threshold θ for k that satisfy the inequality for input symbol "1" as $k > \theta = [M - a(\pi)/a(p)]/2$. where $a(p) = \log[p/(1-p)]$ is the logit function, and $p > 0.5$. The probability that the observer responds correctly on Task 1 is given by the binomial distribution $P(\theta) = 1 - Binomial(\theta, M, p)$. In practice,

Fig. 8.4 *Empirical POC with fitted* continuous functions for two different levels of functionality

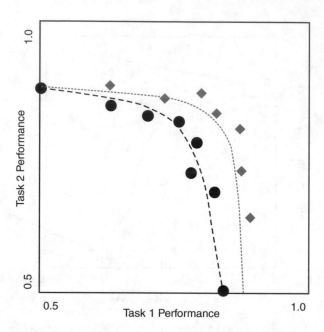

with a large number of channels, we can simplify the calculation by approximating the binomial distribution by a Gaussian distribution.

The performance of a person on Task 2 is then given by the same equation with the number of remaining channels not used by Task 1, i.e., N-M. A particular POC curve is then specified by the two parameters N and p as M takes on values between 1 and N. This simplest version of the resource allocation model captures the tradeoff by two parameters, M and p, but the data may require a more complex representation to capture various aspects of the data such as asymmetries between tasks. One way to capture asymmetries is to use different channel capacities for different tasks.

The important lessons from these analysis are similar as those from the signal detection and include:

1. The need to measure performance on both tasks rather than only one so that it is possible to assess the relative allocation of attention
2. Perform the task at multiple assignments of utility, i.e., the relative importance of each task.

Measurement & Computational Modeling

Measurement is generally defined as the process of converting aspects of physical, neurological or behavioral "objects" to numerical quantities. To estimate an individual's BMI we must assess the their mass and height. Measuring height is the subject of extensive measurement (Charles and Pasupathi 2003; Krantz et al. 1971) by directly comparing objects with known length to the height of a standing individual. To measure their mass, however, is not that simple and is based on several mathematical models of physical phenomena. First, we convert mass to force using Newton's law relating acceleration (gravity) to force. But measurement of force requires other physical laws that govern conversion between forces and more directly measurable quantities (using a balance or Hooke's law). In this simple example we illustrated how measurement of unobservable or difficult to observe phenomena can be implemented by using known relationships that transform the unobservable quantities to observable and measurable.

Physical measurements can be frequently relized because we know the underlying modeling components, such as Newton's laws. This is frequently not the case in psychology and even physiology. In medicine, for example, clinician would like to assess the state of the patient's heart and the state of their cardiovascular system, but she may only be able to measure the blood pressure. In this situation we need to empirically estimate the transformations between the blood pressure and the blockage of the vessels.

An example relevant to continuous monitoring is the assessment of impact of a persons weight on their health status. Noticing that a higher heavier individuals had lower life expectancy, insurance companies in the first half of 20th century used the ratio $Q = M/H$ to assess predict the life expectancy where M is mass in kilograms and H is the height in meters. The ratio Q was taken as the measure of people's fitness. Subsequently this measure found to underestimate life exptancy of taller people and new formulas were derived taking into account the three-dimensional nature of human body by modifying the expression for $q = M/H^3$ which overestimated the health status. After more empirical investigation, realizing that fat does not accumulate uniformly over the body, the exponent was reduced to the current definition of BMI, i.e. $BMI = M/H^2$ (Nuttall 2015; Romero-Corral et al. 2008) approximately reflecting the distribution of fat over a human body.

BMI has been used as a measure of health status or at least the proportion of fat. Although the validity of this measurement model is still scrutinized (Nuttall 2015), it is an example of a measurement model that is continuously improving as we gather more data combined with knowledge of physics physiology and the relationship of adipose to health.

The main point of this brief discussion is that any quantification or measurement requires a model that relates the properties to be measured to the outputs of the measuring instrument. This is particularly important in psychology, where many of the measured phenomena are represented by latent variables, and the only way to assess them (other than physiological measurements) are behavioral responses. Examples of the quantitative outputs include responses to questionnaires and Likert scales as well as performance on behavioral tasks such as walking, typing or drawing. Based on our brief description of the performance operating curve, computational models of measurement should include contextual variables such as the subjective utility allocated to a given task. For instance, if an individual is focusing on their health state, they may not allocate as much attention to the memory task they face in a clinic. Inferring these contextual aspects of the measurement process is essential during the interpretation of the results and may account for a significant proportion of the variability.

Computer-Based Assessment of Cognitive Function

The approach to the traditional assessment of cognitive functions has been fragmented so that decions on the type of assessment are difficult and frequently suboptimal. A 2011 survey of 25 European countries found over 200 neuropsychological instruments used in those countries to assess dementia in clinical practice (Maruta et al. 2011). The choice of the assessment instruments typically depends on contextual factors such as the effort required to administer the tests, the cost, and on the clinician's experiences and training. Another important shortcoming of the typical paper-and-pencil test is the lack of adaptability to individuals' levels of performance resulting in significant ceiling and floor effects (Hessl et al. 2016). One of the frequently used test is the mini-mental state examination (MMSE) which is very simple and fast but insensitive (Brainin et al. 2015), culturally biased, and cannot be administered repeatedly without significant practice results. Moreover MMSE does not leverage most of the insights and advances in psychological science underlying assessment of cognitive and executive functions.

During the last several decades, clinicians and researchers recognized many of the limitations of even the best traditional pen-and-paper tests including lack of standardization of test administration, inability to accurately measure response latencies, lack of adaptability to individuals, and difficulties in detecting trends over time. The detection of variability and trends is hampered by the fact that repeated applications of the same paper-and-pencil test introduces biases and distortions trough practice effects. These shortcomings are particularly important for measurement targeting older adults since the dynamics of cognitive changes and the variability are important aspects of the assessment.

The advances in computer technology provided the opportunity to develop many computerized tests, but only a small portion of these tests are based on rigorous theoretical frameworks. See (Wild et al. 2008) for an early review of computer-based testing (CBT). Most of the CBTs are designed to reproduce as closely as possible the paper-and-pencil versions without taking advantage of the computer capability. A subset of these tests, however, do take advantage of the flexibility of the computing environment and are able to make two important modifications: (1) randomize aspects of the task so the same type of tests can be used repeatedly and (2) adapt the difficulty of the test to the capabilities of the individual participants. In this way, they are able to assess a wider ranges of the functionality without censoring due to the ceiling and floor effects. Perhaps the best known set of tests is the validated NIH Toolbox Cognitive Battery (NIH-TBC) (Hessl et al. 2016). These tests improve the uniformity of the test administration and scoring although there are still many unresolved issues (Maruta et al. 2011) .

Although these tests represent significant improvement vis a vis the paper and pencil tests, they fail to provide motivations for the participants to use them frequently enough to assess the variability of the cognitive abilities. As we noted earlier, variability over time is likely to be more important in early detection than the average performance. To rectify this problem, it is useful to turn to computer games that require cognitive abilities and executive function since hey provide the much needed internal motivation.

Assessment Using Computer Games

Computer games can alleviate many of the issues raised in the previous sections. Games are generally designed to be motivating for the participants to play frequently so that the game makers have a large volume. The motivation is also useful for the clinicians and researchers to collect large amounts of densely sampled longitudinal data. The difficulty of each game can be adapted to track the instantaneous skills of individuals, maintaining their successful performance while collecting useful data. Games are frequently considered to be promising training instruments to maintain and enhance the abilities of aging people (National Academies of Sciences, Engineering, and Medicine, 2017) but they often fail to make measurable generalizable differences. We therefore focus on using games for assessment.

Although this adaptive tracking of users' performance is useful in encouraging improvements as the difficulty increases, the game's actual score is likely not to reflect the level of the associated cognitive functionality. Therefore, for assessment purposes, it is necessary to develop computational models of each game that include the changing game difficulty to quantify the players' ability.

Metrics of Cognition

As examples of using user interactions with computer games to assess cognitive function, we describe our experiences in designing and evaluating computer games for older adults for this purpose. In the early design process we first conducted focus groups and surveys to discover which computer games were most popular and enjoyable for older adults, given that it would be critical to have users play the games repeatedly over time. Then from this information we chose the metrics associated with each game based on computational models of basic cognitive processes associated with the neuropsychological tests. This process resulted in the selection and reworking of nine popular cognitive computer games. Table 8.1 describes the cognitive performance variables we measure with our nine adaptive computer games. The first column defines the variables and the second column describes the measurement method.

Table 8.1 Methods for measuring cognitive variables. Adapted from Jimison et al. (2008). Home-based cognitive monitoring using embedded measures of verbal fluency in a computer word game. Conf Proc IEEE Eng Med Biol Soc, 2008, 3312–3315. ©2008 IEEE.

Component definition	Measurable aspects and test
Visual perception – Converts physical signal to internal representations	Psychophysics of visual detection, discrimination and categorization
Visual scan – Extracting information from the display	Situational awareness
Visual search – finding a specific target	Target detection
Mental rotation – ability to reason about two or three dimensional objects in different orientations	Performance on same/different tasks for rotated images of 2D and 3D objects
Working memory – ability to store and retrieve information to accomplish a short-term task	Probability of correct answers to questions pertaining to stimuli or situations within seconds and minutes
Long-term memory – access to sustained items in memory	Probability of correctly retrieving item from previous knowledge
Selective attention – ability to ignore irrelevant inputs, Features, goals and responses	Decline in performance due to introduction of a distracting stimuli or dual tasks
Divided attention – ability to simultaneously process information from multiple sources	Performance on dual tasks as a function of the utilities and probabilities of the tasks
Vigilance – ability to maintain best possible performance over time	Change in performance as measured by sensitivity and bias over long period of time with rare stimuli
Phonemic fluency – ability to recall words under phonemic constraints (letters, length, etc)	Performance measured by the number of words generated
Semantic fluency – ability to recall words under semantic constraints (categories)	Performance measured by the number of words generated
Executive function – supervisory control, ability to allocate resources, deploy strategies, allocate priorities to processes	Performance following change in task contexts or objectives, planning performance
Motor speed – ability to generate and control movements quickly and accurately	Speed, accuracy, and repeatability of movements

Game Development

Our project on cognitive monitoring with in-home computer games consisted of three phases: (1) a needs assessment, (2) game infrastructure and the development of embedded cognitive metrics, and (3) evaluation. For the needs assessment we used focus groups and surveys to define older adult preferences for computer game applications and potential barriers to computer use (H. B. Jimison et al. 2007) to determine a set of 15 possible game activities. We then performed a cognitive task analysis on each of the games to characterize its appropriateness for providing information on one of the cognitive dimensions from standard cognitive tests. Our resulting set of nine interactive cognitive computer games measure most aspects of the standard neuropsychological tests, while still being engaging enough to play on a routine basis so that we could take frequent measures and detect within-user trends.

Measure of Verbal Fluency

Two of our computer games have fairly direct measures of verbal fluency (ability to generate a class of words within time constraints). Figure 8.5 shows a word jumble game, where the user is challenged to create as many words a possible from a scrambled set of seven letters. The simple measure of rate of word generation in this game most directly corresponds to standard measures of verbal fluency. However, we also measure the word complexity of the generated words. Our complexity measure is related to the entropy and orthographic complexity of the words generated by the user, and defined as $h(w) = - [\log p(w) + \log q(w)]$, where p corresponds to the word frequency and q to the frequency of the bigrams within the word in the English language (greater rare word usage corresponding to higher cognitive function). As with all of our games the embedded cognitive metrics, in this case a verbal fluency metric) are different from the game score used to motivate play.

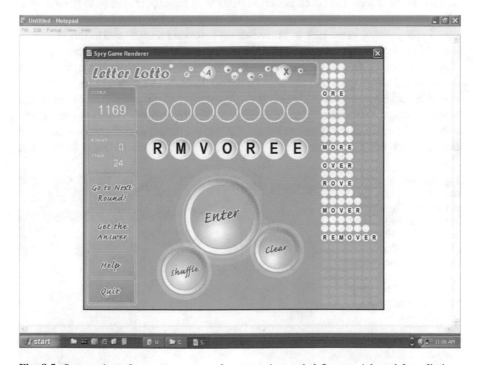

Fig. 8.5 Screen shot of a computer game for measuring verbal fluency. Adapted from Jimison et al. (2008). Home-based cognitive monitoring using embedded measures of verbal fluency in a computer word game. Conf Proc IEEE Eng Med Biol Soc, 2008, 3312–3315. ©2008 IEEE

Measure of Executive Function

Most of the computer games we have created require multiple cognitive processes and yield multiple measures of cognitive performance, reflecting the nature of everyday tasks. As an example of a game that is closely related to one of the neuropsychological tests, and at the same time measures a combination of multiple processes, is our adaptation of the standard Trail Making Test into a game (shown in Fig. 8.6). The Trail Making Test requires subjects to connect a sequence of numbered circles as quickly as possible, and then connect a sequence of alternating numbers and letters (e.g., 1, A, 2, B, 3, C…). This process of set switching (from numbers to letters) requires memory, visual search, motor speed, divided attention, and mental flexibility. Standard test scores only reflect overall timing and number of errors for this test—a two dimensional representation of the complex processes. In our game environment, we are able to measure each move and model the performance dependent on the complexity of the search. In addition, we can measure the incremental effects of changing the complexity of the task. For example, measuring an individual subject's speed in following a single highlighted target with the mouse device provides a baseline measure of motor speed. Following the sequence of numbers requires a combination of working memory and visual search. However, adding distracters to the task allows us to measure the effect of visual search without changing the memory requirement. The time difference in progressing to the task of set switching between numbers and letters is indicative of the relative cognitive difficulty of tracking two simultaneous sequences.

Our model of executive function using the user interactions with this game decomposes a move into a sequence of three statistically independent stages: (1) the *recall & update* stage during which the subject calls to mind the next target in the search string; (2) the *search* stage during which the subject searches among the unselected targets game board to locate the current target; and (3) the *motor* stage during which the subject moves the mouse or pen to the located target to select it.

Fig. 8.6 Screen shot of a cognitive computer game based on the Trail Making Test of executive function. Adapted from Hagler et al. (2014). Assessing executive function using a computer game: Computational modeling of cognitive processes. IEEE Journal of Biomedical and Health Informatics, 18(4), 1442–1452. ©2014 IEEE

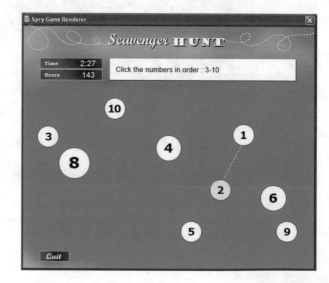

The statistical independence is based on the idea that each stage is affected by different aspects of the task and that the effect is limited to that stage. We expect that the duration of the recall & update stage would vary with the type of the search string (i.e., it should take a different amount of time to recall the next target when the search string is purely alphabetic or numeric as opposed to an alphanumeric search string). The duration of the search stage should depend on the number of additional distractors and unselected targets on the board, with the time spent in search decreasing on average as the subject moves to the end of the round (Hagler et al. 2014) Finally, the length of the motor stage should depend only on the distance on the board from the previously selected target to the new target—assuming that the target size is constant.

Figure 8.9 shows the results of our validation of this model of executive function. Thirty older adults (25 female and 5 male, average age 80 ± 6.0 years, average level of education 15 ± 2.7 years, MMSE = 28 ± 1.1, ADL = 0.071 ± 0.30) participated in a 1 year study in which a set of computer games that included Savenger Hunt was placed into their homes. The results shown in Fig. 8.7 indicate very strong correspondence

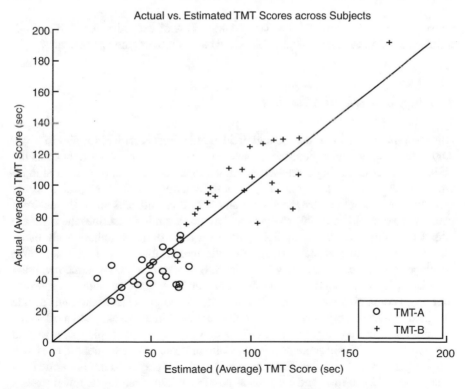

Fig. 8.7 Actual versus estimated TMT scores across subjects. Each of the 23 subjects has two values shown, one for TMT-A and one for TMT-B, each representing the average of the three administrations of TMT. The model fit has $R^2 = 0.82$ and $p < 0.0001$. A line with slope one passing through the origin is shown for reference. Adapted from Hagler et al. (2014). Assessing executive function using a computer game: Computational modeling of cognitive processes. IEEE Journal of Biomedical and Health Informatics, 18(4), 1442–1452. ©2014 IEEE

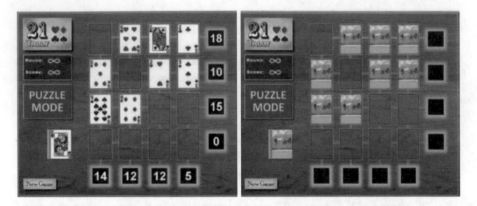

Fig. 8.8 Two screenshots from "21 Tally" used to measure divided attention. Left: stimulus, displayed for a certain duration based on the participant's previous correct or incorrect responses. Right: awaiting response, in which the participant could see card placement but nothing else. Adapted from McKanna et al. (2009). Divided attention in computer game play: analysis utilizing unobtrusive health monitoring. Conf Proc IEEE Eng Med Biol Soc, 2009, 6247–6250. ©2009 IEEE

between scores on a conventional Trail Making Test of executive function and our estimates on how each individual would score based on their game performance.

Measure of Divided Attention

Attention (including both focused and divided attention) is critical for almost every cognitive action we take. Focused, or selective, attention can be thought of as the ability to focus on a single relevant stimulus, or a single stream of such stimuli, while excluding other (less relevant) stimuli. Without this skill, cognition would quickly be overwhelmed by the simple amount of stimuli present in the environment, and we would be unable to function. Divided attention describes the ability to attend to multiple tasks, or multiple parts of a task, either simultaneously or by switching back and forth fast enough that the measurable effect is the same. We developed a game called 21 Tally (see Fig. 8.8), which is a puzzle game involving blackjack played in two dimensions simultaneously. A player is shown a four-by-four board containing a certain number of cards and empty spaces, and must decide in which of these empty spaces to place the next card in the deck, shown off to the bottom-left of the board (as in Fig. 8.6). When this next card is played, rows and columns totaling 21 will score positively, while those summing to more than 21 will score negatively (bust). Thus, for each new board, the player attempts to obtain as many totals of 21 in rows and columns as possible while receiving as few over-21 s (busts) as possible. New boards are shown for a certain period of time (the "stimulus period"), as in the left side of Fig. 8.6, after which they are flipped face-down (as in the right side) to await player response (McKanna et al. 2009). During the game testing we used algorithm-generated boards that were designed to emphasize divided

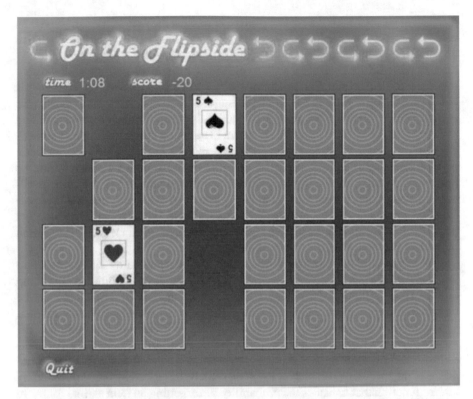

Fig. 8.9 Screen shot on a computer game used to assess working memory. Adapted from Jimison et al. (2007). A neural informatics approach to cognitive assessment and monitoring. Proceedings of the third International IEEE EMBS Conference on Neural Engineering, 696–699. ©2007 IEEE

attention; specifically, each one had equal numbers of cards and empty spaces (eight each), contained no aces (to avoid confusion between scores of 1 and 11), had only one best answer, and required decisions in one or both directions. The stimulus period was varied utilizing a staircase algorithm to determine the point at which participants could answer 50% of the boards correctly. Comparing the performance of participants across age groups on the 21 Tally game and the standard Useful Field-of-View test of divided attention, varying the difficulty of each individual task independently, we found a large correlation (Pearson's $r = 0.89$) between the magnitude of the interaction between the two tasks as difficulty increased in each.

Measure of Working Memory

Although many of the cognitive computer games and standard tests involve short-term and working memory we rely on one game in particular to provide us with a more direct measure of working memory. For this game, we adapted the standard card game of Concentration, as shown in Fig. 8.9. Users must remember the location of various cards they select (turn over to view the face of the card) and then match pairs. Game difficulty is adapted based on number of cards and the cognitive difficulty of the matches. These range from simple shape and color matches to cognitively more difficult matches, such as matching a digital clock time with the analogue picture equivalent. The model of the cognitive performance on this game is based on a "leaky" memory buffer. The average "life expectancy" of the items in the memory buffer derived from a survival function is used to characterize the working memory size. The derivation of this measure is based on the concept of a hypothetical memory buffer for an ideal player. For example, a card that has been seen at a given location would enter the buffer and remain there until its match would be uncovered. When the matching cards are removed from the board, the corresponding cards are dropped from the buffer. Using this approach to the analysis, it is possible to determine the maximum and average buffer sizes required for perfect performance. We then normalize the observed average memory buffer size for an individual player to obtain a metric of memory.

The actual working memory performance is characterized by a leaky buffer in which each item's state can be described by modeling the probability of forgetting at each stage. Although the actual values of the transition probabilities must be determined empirically for each individual, the probability that a card seen t moves ago remains in memory can be well approximated by a Weilbull distribution of the form $P(t) = \Pr\{\text{Recal}; t\} = \exp((-t/v)^k)$, where v and k are parameters. An interesting aspect of this formulation is analogous to survival analysis in that the dependence of the forgetting parameters $1 - pt$ on t can be described by the corresponding hazard function that indicates the probability of forgetting an item at time (or move number) t given that it has been in memory until time t. For example, if all the probabilities pt were identical, the forgetting curve would be exponential, and the hazard function would be constant. Prior to an attempt to use this model to characterize individual players, it is necessary to consider responses that are due to guessing rather than remembering. For example, if there are three cards left on the board, the correct card can be chosen by chance with probability 1/3. To correct for this type of chance effect, we need incorporate a model for guessing $Q(t,n) = g_n + (1 - g_n)P(t)\,P(t)$ where n represents the state of the board and g_n is the chance of being correct by chance. In practice, the estimation of $Q(t,n)$ may require a more sophisticated analysis, as the player may remember some of the cards, and the probability of randomly choosing the correct card may be $P\,n\,guess\,n\,(\,)>1$.

In order to demonstrate the model-based approach described above, we asked 30 older adults (25 female and 5 male, age 80 ± 6.0 years) to participate in longitudinal study by playing computer games using their home computers (Jimison et al. 2004; Jimison et al. 2007). Following informed consent and a series of neuropsychological tests, the enrolled participants were encouraged to play as many games as they could over a period of 1 year. The neuropsychological tests were repeated at the end of 6 months and then again at the end of the year. We restricted our data analysis to those participants who played at least a minimum number of rounds throughout the monitoring period. This reduced the cohort to 19 individuals.

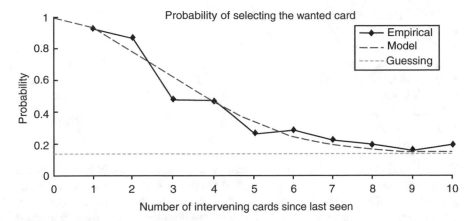

Fig. 8.10 Probability of selecting the wanted card for a single subject. An empirical estimate of the probabilities (black), the probabilities according to the model with guessing included (red), and the estimated contribution of guessing the correct card (green) are indicated. Adapted from Jimison et al. (2007). A neural informatics approach to cognitive assessment and monitoring. Proceedings of the third International IEEE EMBS Conference on Neural Engineering, 696–699. ©2007 IEEE

As an example, Fig. 8.10 shows the probability of a particular participant recalling a card after the number of intervening events (card flips) shown on the abscissa and the corresponding Weibull fit. The buffer size derived from the parametric representation of the Weibull fit for this participant is 3.0 cards, and the individual's hazard function is approximately constant, suggesting that an exponential model would also account for the data. By monitoring and tracking changes in this estimated working memory buffer length for an individual over time we are able to detect within-subject trends that may be useful in providing earlier detection and intervention.

Summary Model of Cognitive Assessments

We conducted a study with 30 elderly computer users in their homes over a period of 1 year to collect cognitive game metrics and compare the results to standard neuropsychological tests. The mean age of these subjects was 81.3 ± 6.6 years. They had an average level of 14.6 ± 2.7 years of education, and most were female (79%). We assessed their cognitive status using a standard neuropsychological test battery at baseline, 3 months, 6 months and 1 year. At all points in time we found that none of the participants had mild cognitive impairment, as determined by a self-report version of the Clinical Dementia Rating. Similarly, all Mini Mental Status Exams (MMSE) continued to be within normal range (all were 27–30). The depression scores, as measured by the CESD-10 depression scale all fell within the normal range (all scores were ≤ 5). We used the following tests to measure specific dimensions of cognitive performance to use as a standard for testing our cognitive metrics:

- Verbal Fluency (letter and semantic)
- Word-List Acquisition
- Word list Recognition
- Trail-Making Test
- Symbol Digit Modalities Test
- Digit Span
- Block Design
- Boston Naming Test
- Picture Completion Test

Overall, subjects continued to play the computer games frequently throughout the study. We used a factor-analytic approach to decompose the set of cognitive skills, see Fig. 8.11. There were clear patterns, however, where most subjects would only play a subset of the games regularly. Early on we discovered that it was important to intervene with messages to encourage the use of all of the games, in order to have complete cognitive assessments. In fact, we have since developed a coaching platform for delivering the games as part of a cognitive health coaching intervention with weekly contact with all participants. The resulting monitoring data from users' game performance and the neuropsychological test scores at four points in time allowed us to develop a model for developing metrics within each game and for developing a model of the correspondence between each participant's performance

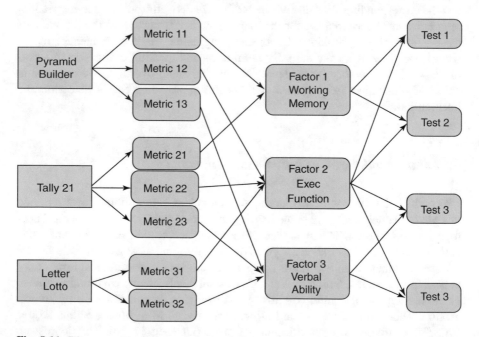

Fig. 8.11 Diagram representing a factor analytic approach to relating computer game performance to the standard neuropsychological tests. Jimison HB (2010). ©2007 IEEE

on the cognitive computer games and the participant's performance on our standard battery of neuropsychological tests.

Differential Privacy and Federated Learning

The availability of data acquisition approaches in recent years stimulated concerns about data security and privacy violations resulting in the emergence of new research and technological developments focused on data privacy. Differential Privacy and Federated Learning are two approaches that enable using individual-level data in training and deploying machine learning algorithms while maintaining individual privacy.

Let us consider the following example. We are interested in testing whether ceteris paribus decreased cognitive abilities predict increased use of ride-hailing services among patients with mild cognitive impairment (MCI). We think this hypothesis may be true because patients with reduced cognitive ability would have difficulty performing daily tasks on time. Therefore, to avoid being late, the patients would use Uber or Lift to get to work and medical appointments more often.

To develop a predictive model and test the hypothesis, the app could send all recorded data to a server, where it would be stored with patients' names replaced by subject IDs, as is typical in many research projects. However, from a privacy point of view, this approach has a significant flaw. If the data ever become public, combining it with a third-party dataset can be used to identify patients. (Importantly, research data can become public not only due to security breaches but also by simply publishing it as is required by an increased number of academic journals.) In their paper, Narayanan and Shmatikov showed that they were able to uniquely identify 99% of subscriber records in a "de-identified" dataset published intentionally by Netflix, simply by joining these data with public Internet Movie Database (IMDb) ratings. In our example, any person with access to Uber or Lift's user data could easily identify patients by combining our dataset with users' ride history. Federated Learning and Differential Privacy were developed to address this and similar issues.

A dataset is considered Differentially Private if removing any individual from it does not meaningfully change the patterns existing in the data. For this characteristic to hold true, no individual in the data can be substantially different from others. If this is the case, then the risk of patient reidentification is substantially reduced. While the development of algorithms to ensure Differential Privacy is an active area of highly technical research, the general idea behind them is relatively intuitive. Broadly speaking, to reduce individuals' distinguishability from others, we can add noise to each patient's data, using the Laplace mechanism or response randomization, in such a manner that (a) the noise across all patients either cancels out or makes an insignificant impact on the estimated predictive model and (b) the noise cannot be removed using existing filtering methods. When applicable, patients' privacy can be further protected by using algorithms to identify and discard specific identifying data, e.g., age, or replacing raw values with broader categories, e.g., age range.

Federated Learning shifts the location of where a predictive model is trained on user data. Instead of training it on all patient data in a central location, e.g., our study server, separate instances of the model are trained on patients' smartphones such that each instance is trained on data of a single individual. It is only the parameters of the trained model that are sent back to the server, where they are averaged with parameters of other individuals' models. Patients' data never leaves their devices and can be deleted after model training, thus practically eliminating the risk of ever becoming public. Additional methods are being developed to improve this approach's effectiveness further.

Conclusions and Future Work

We have described several principles and metrics for measuring cognitive function in real time in a home environment, as well as mechanisms to ensure the privacy and security of cognitive monitoring data. Although the examples from our work show promising opportunities, there remains much to be done in several key areas. First, our ability to develop effective computational models characterizing behaviors in the wild is in its early stages. Advances are required in the development of new computational frameworks to capture the complexities, uncertainties, and most importantly, dynamics inherent in the behavioral informatics approach (Hekler et al. 2016). Closely related is the need to capture and characterize contextual information and its effect on the monitoring results. In addition to the rapid advances in monitoring behaviors, similar advances in monitoring physiological metrics are beginning to open the possibility of inferring instantaneous affective states of individuals and assessing their effects on cognitive functions. The ability to infer instantaneous cognitive and affective states in the wild also opens the possibility for interventions that would amplify an individual's cognitive abilities. Steps along this line of research include work on augmented cognition. Similar advances are expected in precision education and training with a combination of behavioral and physiological interventions, such as transcranial current stimulation.

References

Anderson JR. Cognitive psychology and its implications. Macmillan; 2005.

Beauchet O, Dubost V, Gonthier R, Kressig RW. Dual-task-related gait changes in transitionally frail older adults: the type of the walking-associated cognitive task matters. Gerontology. 2005;51(1):48–52. Retrieved from http://www.ncbi.nlm.nih.gov/entrez/query.fcgi?cmd=Retrieve&db=PubMed&dopt=Citation&list_uids=15591756

Brainin M, Tuomilehto J, Heiss WD, Bornstein NM, Bath PM, Teuschl Y, et al. Post-stroke cognitive decline: an update and perspectives for clinical research. Eur J Neurol. 2015;22(2):229–e216.

Cattell RB. Theory of fluid and crystallized intelligence: a critical experiment. J Educ Psychol. 1963;54:1–22.

Center for Disease Control and Prevention. Healthy aging. Retrieved from 2016., https://www.cdc.gov/aging/pdf/perceptions_of_cog_hlth_factsheet.pdf

Charles ST, Pasupathi M. Age-related patterns of variability in self-descriptions: implications for everyday affective experience. Psychol Aging. 2003;18(3):524–36. https://doi.org/10.1037/0882-7974.18.3.524.

Cover TM, Thomas JA. Elements of information theory. John Wiley & Sons; 2012.

Cowan N. What are the differences between long-term, short-term, and working memory? Prog Brain Res. 2008;169:323–38.

De Santi S, Pirraglia E, Barr W, Babb J, Williams S, Rogers K, et al. Robust and conventional neuropsychological norms: diagnosis and prediction of age-related cognitive decline. Neuropsychology. 2008;22(4):469.

Dinse HR. Cortical reorganization in the aging brain. Prog Brain Res. 2006;157:57–387.

Driscoll I, Davatzikos C, An Y, Wu X, Shen D, Kraut M, Resnick S. Longitudinal pattern of regional brain volume change differentiates normal aging from MCI. Neurology. 2009;72(22):1906–13.

Gamaldo AA, An Y, Allaire JC, Kitner-Triolo MH, Zonderman AB. Variability in performance: identifying early signs of future cognitive impairment. Neuropsychology. 2012;26(4):534.

Hagler S, Jimison HB, Pavel M. Assessing executive function using a computer game: computational modeling of cognitive processes. IEEE J Biomed Health Inform. 2014;18(4):1442–52. https://doi.org/10.1109/JBHI.2014.2299793.

Hekler EB, Michie S, Pavel M, Rivera DE, Collins LM, Jimison HB, et al. Advancing Models and Theories for Digital Behavior Change Interventions. Am J Prev Med. 2016;51(5):825–32.

Hekler EB, Klasnja P, Chevance G, Golaszewski NM, Lewis D, Sim I. Why we need a small data paradigm. BMC Med. 2019;17(1):1–9.

Hessl D, Sansone SM, Berry-Kravis E, Riley K, Widaman KF, Abbeduto L, et al. The NIH toolbox cognitive battery for intellectual disabilities: three preliminary studies and future directions. J Neurodev Disord. 2016;8(1):1–18.

James W. Habit. H. Holt; 1890.

Jimison H, Pavel M, Hatt W, Chan M, Larimer N, & Yu C. Delivering a multi-faceted cognitive health intervention to the home. In: Gerontechnology 2010.

Jimison HB, McKanna J, Ambert K, Hagler S, Hatt WJ, & Pavel M. Models of Cognitive Performance Based on Home Monitoring Data, Proceedings of the 32nd Annual International IEEE EMBS Conference, 2010, pp. 5234–7.

Jimison H, Pavel M, Le T. Home-based cognitive monitoring using embedded measures of verbal fluency in a computer word game. Conf Proc IEEE Eng Med Biol Soc. 2008;2008:3312–5. https://doi.org/10.1109/IEMBS.2008.4649913.

Jimison HB, Pavel M, McKanna J, & Pavel J. Unobtrusive monitoring of computer interactions to detect cognitive status in elders. IEEE Trans Inf Technol Biomed. 2004;8(3):248–52.

Jimison HB, Pavel M, Wild K, Bissell P, McKanna J, Blaker D, & Williams D. A neural informatics approach to cognitive assessment and monitoring. Proceedings of the 3rd International IEEE EMBS Conference on Neural Engineering. 2007;696–699. https://doi.org/10.1109/CNE.2007.369768.

Kadlec, R. (2015). DyBaNeM: Bayesian Model of episodic memory.

Katz B, Shah P, Meyer DE. How to play 20 questions with nature and lose: reflections on 100 years of brain-training research. Proc Natl Acad Sci. 2018;115(40):9897–904.

Krantz, D., Luce, D., Suppes, P., & Tversky, A. (1971). Foundations of measurement, Vol. I: Additive and polynomial representations.

Maruta C, Guerreiro M, De Mendonça A, Hort J, Scheltens P. The use of neuropsychological tests across Europe: the need for a consensus in the use of assessment tools for dementia. Eur J Neurol. 2011;18(2):279–85.

McKanna JA, Jimison H, Pavel M. Divided attention in computer game play: analysis utilizing unobtrusive health monitoring. Conf Proc IEEE Eng Med Biol Soc. 2009;2009:6247–50. https://doi.org/10.1109/IEMBS.2009.5334662.

National Academies of Sciences, Engineering, & Medicine. (2017). Preventing cognitive decline and dementia: a way forward.

Navon D, Gopher D. On the economy of the human-processing system. Psychol Rev. 1979;86(3):214.

National Institute on Aging, Cognitive Health and Older Adults. https://www.nia.nih.gov/health/cognitive-health-and-older-adults, last viewed Jun 28, 2022.

Nuttall FQ. Body mass index: obesity, BMI, and health: a critical review. Nutr Today. 2015;50(3):117.

Pavel, M., Jimison, H., & Spring, B. (2016). *Behavioral informatics: Dynamical models for measuring and assessing behaviors for precision interventions.* Paper presented at the Engineering in Medicine and Biology Society (EMBC), 2016 IEEE.

Pavel M, Jimison HB, Korhonen I, Gordon CM, Saranummi N. Behavioral informatics and computational modeling in support of proactive health management and care. IEEE Trans Biomed Eng. 2015;62(12):2763–75. https://doi.org/10.1109/TBME.2015.2484286.

Possin KL, Moskowitz T, Erlhoff SJ, Rogers KM, Johnson ET, Steele NZ, et al. The brain health assessment for detecting and diagnosing neurocognitive disorders. J Am Geriatr Soc. 2018;66(1):150–6.

Romero-Corral, A., Somers, V. K., Sierra-Johnson, J., Thomas, R. J., Collazo-Clavell, M., Korinek, J., . . . Lopez-Jimenez, F. (2008). Accuracy of body mass index in diagnosing obesity in the adult general population. Int J Obes, 32(6), 959–966.

Sperling G. A unified theory of attention and signal detection. In: Parasuraman R, Davies DR, editors. Varieties of attention. New York, N. Y: Academic; 1984. p. 103–81.

Sperling G, Dosher BA. Strategy and optimization in human information processing. In: Boff K, Kaufman L, Thomas J, editors. Handbook of perception and performance. New York, NY: Wiley; 1986.

Taylor CA, Bouldin ED, McGuire LC. Subjective cognitive decline among adults aged≥ 45 years—United States, 2015–2016. Morb Mortal Wkly Rep. 2018;67(27):753.

United Nations Department of Economic and Social Affairs Population Division. World Population Ageing 2019: Highlights (ST/ESA/SER.A/430) 2019.

US Census Bureau. (2021, October 8, 2021). Older population and aging. Retrieved from https://www.census.gov/topics/population/older-aging.html

Wild K, Howieson D, Webbe F, Seelye A, Kaye J. The status of computerized cognitive testing in aging: a systematic review. Alzheimers Dement. 2008;4(6):428–37.

Chapter 9
The Role of Patient-Generated Data in Personalized Oncology Care and Research: Opportunities and Challenges for Real-World Implementation

Luis Fernandez-Luque, Francisco J. Núñez-Benjumea, Sergio Cervera-Torres, José Luis López-Guerra, Zhongxing Liao, José A. Pagán, and Francisco Zambrana

Learning Objectives
- To provide an overview of current practices on data collection for routine cancer care.
- To identify the exogenous determinants of health-related quality of life (HRQoL) in cancer survivorship.
- To understand how data science can be leveraged to accelerate real-world evidence (RWE) discovery.

L. Fernandez-Luque (✉) · F. J. Núñez-Benjumea
Adhera Health, Inc., Palo Alto, CA, USA
e-mail: luis@adherahealth.com

S. Cervera-Torres
Open University of Catalonia (UOC), Barcelona, Spain

J. L. López-Guerra
Radiation Oncology, University Hospital Virgen del Rocio, Seville, Spain

Z. Liao
The University of Texas MD Anderson Cancer Center, Houston, TX, USA

Radiation Oncology Department, The University of Texas MD Anderson Cancer Center, Houston, TX, USA

J. A. Pagán
New York University, New York, NY, USA

F. Zambrana
Department of Medical Oncology, Hospital Universitario Infanta Sofía, Madrid, Spain

© The Author(s), under exclusive license to Springer Nature Switzerland AG 2022
P.-Y. S. Hsueh et al. (eds.), *Personal Health Informatics*, Cognitive Informatics in Biomedicine and Healthcare, https://doi.org/10.1007/978-3-031-07696-1_9

- To describe the concepts of learning healthcare system and value-based care.
- To identify current regulatory issues for a real-world implementation of using patient-generated data in personalized care and ongoing actions to overcome them.

Introduction

People living with cancer and its associated treatments can experience important physical, psychological, and social burdens. Furthermore, these burdens compromise health-related quality of life (HRQoL) not only of individuals living with cancer but also their caregivers. Objective quantitative assessment of these health-related domains is sparse in oncology due to key factors such as the lack of patient-generated data and limitations in traditional assessment methods (e.g., questionnaires). In this chapter, we provide an overview of the current practices and trends in real-world data (RWD) collection from longitudinal patient observations in routine cancer care. In addition, data science methods that can be applied to gain insights from the data will be reviewed so that it can be leveraged to provide real-world evidence (RWE) that can further inform the development and update of clinical practice guidelines (CPGs) in the oncology domain.

We discuss the growing interest in gathering patient-generated longitudinal information about context-specific cognitive and behavioral patient experiences. This includes biometric, psychometric, and other patient-reported outcome measurements (PROMs) and patient-reported experience measurements (PREMs) relevant across the patient journey, and how consumer-grade health and wellness devices and wearables are fueling this trend. At this point, it should be brought into the discussion how the management and analysis of these large, heterogeneous datasets, and its derived implications, is lately being addressed by an emerging field of research under the umbrella term of exposome informatics (Martin Sanchez et al. 2014a).

The initial shift from fee-for-service to value-based care schemas in oncological healthcare delivery is also promoting the use of PROMs and PREMs to better measure the real impact that clinical interventions have on patients' HRQoL, beyond the traditional clinical outcomes of such interventions. This shift also promotes the continuous improvement of quality-of-care delivery and, when combined with the latest trends and applications in health technology and informatics, it opens the door to the implementation of learning healthcare systems.

Finally, we close the chapter with a discussion about the types of questions posed by policymakers and regulatory bodies for the real-world deployment and implementation of strategies to foster a patient-generated data grounding for care delivery. These challenges arise mainly from the Food and Drug Administration (FDA) in the United States and the Medical Device Regulation (MDR) recently approved by the European Commission.

Current Practices and Trends about RWD collection in Routine Cancer Care

Overview of CPG in Cancer Care

A Clinical Practice Guideline (CPG) is a set of recommendations on how to diagnose and treat a medical condition, summarizing the most updated medical knowledge and supporting them with the scientific evidence behind those recommendations. They are meant to ensure that patients receive the appropriate care at every stage of the disease journey, and therefore they are written for doctors and healthcare providers. They serve as a framework for clinical decisions and supporting best practices, but they are not legally binding and must be adapted to the limitations and strengths of each setting and country.

Recently, CPGs coming from internationally recognized organizations have also included recommendations concerning follow-up care, psychosocial support and rehabilitation for cancer patients, as well as guidelines for patients and their caregivers, aiming to assist them in other practical and emotional issues related to living with cancer and treatments. Furthermore, cancer patients, their caregivers and patient advocacy groups are now more than ever working to ensure that patients receive appropriate care that not only focus on traditional survival outcomes, but also on a broader concept of the cancer experience. It is within this more holistic and multidimensional view of cancer care that the quality of life (QoL), PROMs and PREMs have emerged as important endpoints that matter to people with cancer.

Some authors have shown that lung cancer patients have a lower risk of mortality when they have a higher QoL prior to radiation therapy (Nieto-Guerrero Gomez et al. 2020). Quality of life scores towards the beginning of treatment and resulting changes in those scores may anticipate the survival term independently of the treatment. Unfortunately, besides the traditional and indispensable documentation of medical history and the continuity of care that provides clinicians with the signs and symptoms through the disease course, there is not a unique, established method for assessing the QoL of cancer patients in routine care, nor have the PROMs and PREMs been formally included in patient's records. Interestingly, modern clinical trial designs seeking the approval of new drugs currently include extensive assessments of the patient's QoL and functionality as important outcome variables, with multiple questionnaires that aim to score many aspects of the patient experience. The report of these QoL measurements in trials covers only the intervention period and are usually taken during the clinical encounters and, therefore, they leave just a snapshot or short-lived information of how the patient's QoL really is.

The Electronic Health Record (EHR) is the standard repository of any patient data used in most developed countries and has shown to improve quality of healthcare in multiple ways (Campanella et al. 2016) and to be feasible for evaluating the quality of cancer care (Caldarella et al. 2012). EHR systems can also integrate all kinds of patient-generated data that can be utilized in many ways, retrospectively or prospectively, for the benefit of the patient care and research. Of special interest is the ability that this integration provides for the remote monitoring of QoL, symptoms and the toxicities derived from the treatment of cancer. In summary, EHRs are currently the most important sources for obtaining RWE of the effects of any medical intervention (Garrison Jr et al. 2007), and a powerful tool to augment and speed up the identification of patient needs but often lack dat from patients lifestyle and behaviors due lack of integration with mobile applications and wearables.

What constitutes the minimum clinical data to be obtained from the clinical encounter or directly from the patients is an important field of study. In an effort to advance cancer data sharing and improve the quality and coordination of patient care, the American Society of Clinical Oncology (ASCO) has partnered with other organizations to develop the mCODE (Minimal Common Oncology Data Elements) for establishing a core set of structured data elements for oncology EHRs (Anon. n.d.-a). This initiative will contribute to analyze not only patients and populations, but also cancer practices to improve treatments and the full patient experience. Equipped with this knowledge, an immense opportunity for clinical interventions (physical, psychological, social) opens up, tailoring interventions to outcomes that actually matter the most to people with cancer.

Current Practices on RWD Collection across the Patient Journey

National health systems usually provide guidelines for collecting datasets useful to support the management of the oncological patient across the patient journey based on recommendations released by scientific and professional organizations such as ASCO and the National Cancer Comprehensive Network (NCCN), among others.

As an example, in the UK, Public Health England (PHE) encourages oncology specialists to follow the recommendations derived from the Cancer Outcomes and Services Dataset (COSD), which is the national standard for reporting cancer in the NHS in England since January 2013. The COSD specifies the items to be submitted electronically by service providers to the National Cancer Registration and Analysis Service (NCRAS) on a monthly basis. This registry, which is revised and updated yearly, addresses the collection of data related to cancer incidence, mortality, survival, prevalence, routes to diagnosis, stage at diagnosis, treatment (radiotherapy, chemotherapy, etc.), and timings of the oncology care delivery process to support service provision and commissioning in the NHS, clinical audits, and public health and epidemiological research (Anon. n.d.-b).

Some PROMs are increasingly being implemented into the routine care of patients with cancer, as the scientific evidence backs its positive impact on health outcomes. A study conducted by Kelleher et al. (Kelleher et al. 2016) aimed to examine how the PROMs of self-efficacy for pain and other symptoms assessed at the point of service were associated with pain, symptom severity and distress, and physical and psychosocial functioning in a cohort of breast and gastrointestinal cancer patients. Their results suggested that self-efficacy for pain and symptom management may be a beneficial addition to clinic-based PROM assessment batteries for patients with cancer and other chronic diseases.

Regarding clinical research in oncology, data collection instruments usually include questionnaire surveys and patient self-reported data, use of proxy/informant information, hospital and ambulatory medical records, and analysis of biologic materials (Saczynski et al. 2013). Nevertheless, an approach addressing the systematic collection of longitudinal patient-generated data in oncology routine care has not been implemented yet in a real-world setting.

Use of Other Tools for Longitudinal Patient Data Collection

Besides the current practices on RWD collection across the patient journey discussed in the previous section, other data sources should be considered to fulfil the HRQoL assessment needs of patients and caregivers regarding perceived quality of care, symptom management and other outcomes relevant for the subject of care.

The use of PROMs and PREMs are deemed as a suitable tool to put the patient at the center of the care process.

Definitions
- **PROMs**: Psychometric tools (e.g., questionnaires) that measure patients' views of e.g. health status, perceived level of impairment, disability, or health-related quality of life. PROMs are a means of measuring clinical effectiveness and safety. PROMs can be classified as either generic or disease specific.
- **PREMs**: PREMs are psychometric tools that measure patients' views of their experience whilst receiving care. They are an indicator of the quality of patient care, although do not measure it directly. PREMs look at the impact of the process of the care on the patient's experience e.g. communication and timeliness of assistance. PREMs can be classified as either relational (identify patients' experience of their relationships during treatment, e.g. did they feel listened to) or functional (examine more practical issues, such as the facilities available). PREMs measure whether patients have experienced certain care processes rather than their satisfaction with the care received (which may be subject to bias).

The key aspect of these tools is that they enable to self-report the perceived status on different HRQoL domains. It should be noted that the standardization of the psychometric development process is quite recent and mainly led by specific initiatives such as the COnsensus-based Standards for the selection of health Measurement Instruments (COSMIN) initiative (Mokkink et al. 2018) (https://www.cosmin.nl/), the International Consortium for Health Outcomes Measurement (ICHOM) (http://www.ichom.org/), or the work published by the International Society for Pharmacoeconomics and Outcomes Research (ISPOR) (Rothman et al. 2009; Coons

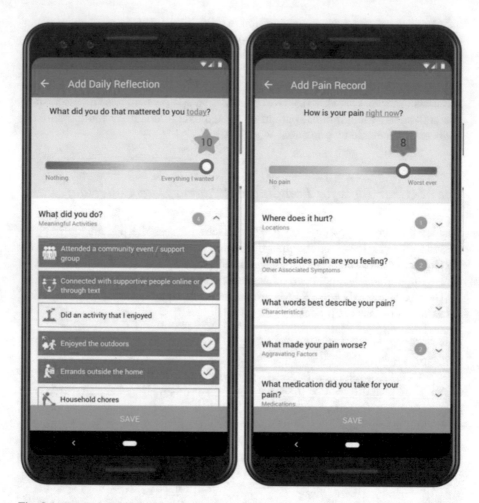

Fig. 9.1 Screenshots of the Manage My Pain app to collect patient-reported outcomes (Bhatia et al. 2021)

et al. 2009). As such, it is paramount that PROMs and PREMs that are considered for use in clinical practice and/or research are selected based on a thorough evaluation of their psychometric properties to ensure that valid and reliable person-reported data are captured. These can be captured using mobile devices as shown in the Fig. 9.1.

And, what can be measured with PROMs and PREMs in the oncology field? A recent systematic search conducted in the frame of the LifeChamps H2020 European project (https://lifechamps.eu/) identified up to 51 unique target outcomes and up to 12 unique target experiences that could be measured with the questionnaires already available in the literature, which can be grouped under the following categories:

PROMs	PREMs
Body image/sexual functioning	Care process coordination/continuity
Cognitive decline	Patient-clinician communication
Emotional/psychological responses (fear of recurrence, depression, anxiety, etc.)	Patient centeredness/empowerment in care services
Frailty	Preferences of goals of care
Functional status/dependency	Quality of care/satisfaction with care
HRQoL/Well-being	
Nutritional status/cachexia	
Healthcare needs	
Physical activity/ability/mobility	
Social isolation	
Symptom burden/distress (multisymptom burden, fatigue, pain, sleep appetite, etc.)	

Overall, 79 PROMs and 11 PREMs were recommended for use in the oncology field based on the psychometric validity of the questionnaires used to measure them. Nevertheless, ultimate selection of any of these PROMs and PREMs for use in research and/or clinical practice must take into account the unique requirements of the outcomes, end-points and frequency of measurement as well as the unique characteristics and abilities of the patient population (e.g. respondent burden, cognitive capacity).

User-centered psychometric information provided by PROMs/PREMs can be complemented with biometric information regarding patient's lifestyle behavior in a way that it can yield a comprehensive overview of patients' health status at every step of their journey. Even though the use of activity trackers and biometric sensors has not become the gold standard in the routine care yet, there is a growing trend in their use as a means to collect valuable information about the behavioral evolution of the user throughout the patient journey for clinical research purposes.

A quick search through ClinicalTrials.gov (a database of privately and publicly funded clinical studies conducted around the world) made in April 2021 for the keywords "wearable sensor" yielded 99 completed studies and 165 active clinical studies addressing mainly neurological and mental disorders. Nevertheless, up to 52 oncology-related conditions such as infection, pain, fatigue, and inflammation, among others, are currently under investigation in 11 clinical trials, according to the ClinicalTrials.gov registry. The successful completion of these trials will support the growing evidence on the utility and cost-efficacy that the introduction of this technology may bring into the routine care for the healthcare providers and payers, which will eventually be leveraged by the scientific associations such as the ASCO and NCCN to be included in their catalogue of good clinical practices for the management of oncological patients, which would ultimately trigger its implementation in the routine care delivery for this population.

Biometric variables (and the parameters related to them) relevant for the oncology scenario that can be measured with off-the-shelf wearable sensors are:

- Mental health (depression, anxiety, fear of recurrence): heart rate (HR), HR variability, activity tracking, sleep monitoring
- Infection: HR, HR variability, body temperature
- Sleep quality: sleep monitoring
- Cardiac events: HR, HR variability, oxygen saturation (SpO2), ECG, activity tracking
- Physical activity: HR, HR variability, sleep monitoring, activity tracking
- Oxygen consumption: SpO2, HR variability, sleep monitoring
- Vital signs: SpO2, HR, ECG

It is expected that, as technology evolves and the biggest technology providers turn their focus into the health and wellness business (Google, Apple and Amazon are already in competition for collecting health and wellness related information from their users), the number of different biometric variables will increase, thus enabling its further application to broader health concepts and covering a wider range of health determinants.

An open issue remains the accuracy of the measurements provided by regular wellness wearable devices and activity trackers, which hampers their adoption in the routine clinical care. Some vendors have already made the decision to step into the medical device regulatory process for clearing its fitness for clinical purposes. This issue will be further discussed in the latest section of this chapter.

Precision Oncology Care beyond Genes: The Role of Exposome Informatics in a Holistic Healthcare Delivery Model

Introduction to Exposome Informatics

The role of the environment in health has been conceptualized as the exposome, that includes a wide range of factors such as behaviors and social influences among others (see Fig. 9.2). It is also well known that environmental exposures, such as poor sleep habits, influence physio pathological processes and which have been measured using biomarkers. In oncology, a clear example is cancer-related fatigue which is a quite common symptom in most types of cancer and there are many variables from the exposome, such as sleep or nutritional habits, which can be affecting the pathological process of the development of that important symptom (Bower 2014).

The increased availability of sensors and the use of mobile PROMs allow to monitor a wide range of parameters that eventually can be used to provide new insights into the oncological process. The combination of these more continuous,

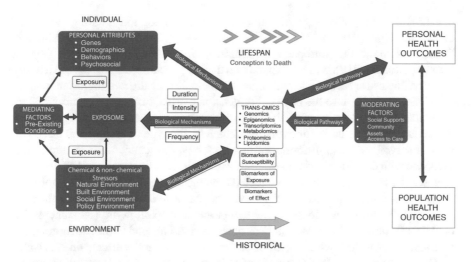

Fig. 9.2 Applying an exposome approach to cardio-vascular disease onset, progression, and outcomes (Juarez et al. 2020)

comprehensive and personalized data sources require new approaches for the analysis of such data and how to apply them into the clinical practice (Martin Sanchez et al. 2014b).

Determinants of HRQoL of Cancer Survivors

This section highlights current approaches to health-related quality of life (HRQoL) in cancer survivorship. Advances in early detection and treatment have contributed in great measure to increase the rates of cancer survivorship. From a broad point of view, survivorship starts at the moment of diagnosis and extends to the rest of one's lifespan (National Cancer Institute 2019), yet it could also be understood as the stage where no evidence of active cancer is detected following curative-intent treatment (Marzorati et al. 2017). Special cases of cancer survivors are children, who can experience chronic conditions and premature aging after treatment (Ness et al. 2015) and older adults, whose care usually requires geriatric expertise. It is important to note, however, that the care of cancer survivors has not reached an adequate integration in the cancer care continuum yet. For example, communication between oncologists and primary care providers needs to be substantially improved (Shapiro 2018).

Furthermore, according to the World Health Organization, health is "a state of complete physical, mental, and social-wellbeing and not merely the absence of disease or infirmity" (WHO, 1948). This is leading to increasingly consider HRQoL in cancer survivorship from a bio-psycho-social perspective, namely, accounting for physical, mental, and social dimensions of health (Lehman et al. 2017; Van Leeuwen et al. 2018). In the following paragraphs, core recommendations guiding the care of cancer survivors in line with the ASCO (Shapiro et al. 2016) and Survivorship and Rehabilitation of the European Commission Joint Action on Cancer Control (Lagergren et al. 2019), will be mapped into the bio-psycho-social model of HRQoL.

Surveillance for recurrence and side effects monitoring are two important recommendations tapping into the physical dimension of HRQoL in cancer survivorship. Surveillance facilitates the early detection of new primary cancers (e.g., age-related) and recurrences in cancer survivors. Nonetheless, the type of testing and effectiveness of surveillance can differ depending on the type of cancer. For example, surveillance with computerized tomography scans enhances the likelihood of detecting metastasis associated with lung cancer (Dingemans et al. 2021) but has not been recommended in early breast cancer survivors who have completed primary therapy with curative intent and do not show symptoms in the follow-up (Khatcheressian et al. 2013; Runowicz et al. 2016). Fear of recurrence can lead to pursue more intensive and costly testing with limited or unclear evidence on the effects on survival.

On the other hand, improvement of side or late effects such as fatigue, pain, sexual dysfunction, insomnia or depression and anxiety among others, has been linked to HRQoL too (American Society of Clinical Oncology n.d.). In this regard, being able to adopt and maintain healthy lifestyles is a pivotal recommendation. As mentioned before, innovative digital technologies are rising as a scalable and cost-effective approach to objectively monitor symptoms and coach personalized health-related goals (Aaronson et al. 2014). For example, wearables such as smartwatches are increasingly used in oncology settings to monitor sleep patterns and physical activity (Gresham et al. 2018a). Mobile health solutions (mHealth) are also being developed to promote, for example, smoking cessation, which is a key risk factor of lung cancer (Carrasco-Hernandez et al. 2020) or self-care management and support of mental wellbeing for cancer survivors (Nápoles et al. 2019). That introduces a second dimension of HRQoL deeply intertwined with the physical domain, namely, the psychological functioning.

As already noticed, motivational aspects (e.g., decisions to implement health behaviors or follow-up indicated surveillance/screening) and emotional aspects (e.g., fear of cancer recurrence or symptoms of anxiety and depression) cannot be disentangled from the physical experience of living with and surviving to cancer and therefore are critical in HRQoL. In general, distress is used as an umbrella term to assess the unpleasant psychological experience characterizing those aspects. Indeed, the NCCN has labelled emotional distress as the "sixth vital sign" after pulse, respiration, blood pressure, temperature, and pain (Holland and Bultz 2007). However, it is only in recent years when the connection between physical and psychological functioning associated with cancer, in general, and with cancer survivorship, in particular, is being taken in more serious consideration (Aaronson et al. 2014). Current recommendations include distress management guidelines (Smith et al. 2018; Goedendorp et al. 2009) or non-pharmacological interventions for pain and fatigue management (Audell and Rosner 2012). Most of these guidelines adopt principles of well-known psychological interventions such as the Cognitive-Behavior Therapy approach (CBT (Gabriel et al. 2020)), although variants based on

Mindfulness are also promising (Goedendorp et al. 2009; Gonzalez-Hernandez et al. 2018).

Nonetheless, as for the definition of health by the WHO, HRQoL in terms of mental health should not be uniquely defined by the absence of mental illness or distress. According to the WHO, mental health is "a state of well-being in which the individual realizes his or her own abilities, can cope with the normal stresses of life, can work productively and fruitfully, and is able to make a contribution to his or her community" (World Health Organization 2014). Such definition is in line with some challenges in cancer survivorship, which may differ from those during cancer treatment. For example, coping with financial, family role and job-related issues and worries, could be more salient after treatment. In line with this reasoning, the European Organization for Research and Treatment of Cancer (EORTC) investigates HRQoL assessment tools specifically developed to account in addition to physical symptoms, this type of stressors and adaptive psychological functioning in terms of psychological strengths and post-traumatic growth (Van Leeuwen et al. 2018).

In the face of the foregoing, it can be inferred that psychological (and physical) aspects co-exist with individual social circumstances. Here, the role of caregivers in social support during and after cancer treatment requires especial attention. Hence, caregiving has been shown associated with some symptoms like those of individuals living with cancer (e.g., fatigue, insomnia, or distress (Girgis et al. 2013)). That makes necessary to include caregivers in psychological and educational programs for HRQoL enhancement (Gabriel et al. 2020). Transitions to life after treatment, job re-engagement and reducing social inequity are also topics capturing increasing attention to properly target HRQoL (Handberg et al. 2019).

Revisiting the Roles of the Oncology Team to Deliver a Holistic Care

Clinical management of cancer patients is a complex issue that needs to be tackled from several angles. The ASCO, through its patient information portal Cancer.Net (Anon n.d.), recently published a statement referring to the desirable roles that an oncology team should include in order to deliver a holistic care. Besides specialized oncologists (either by treatment, i.e. medical, radiation, surgical; or by etiology, i.e. gynecologic, pediatric or hematologist) and nurses, the oncology team should also include the following roles: nurse practitioners, physician assistants, patient navigators, palliative care doctors and nurses, social workers, genetic counselors, pathologists, clinical pharmacists, dietitian nutritionists, diagnostic radiologists, rehabilitation therapists, spiritual support advisors and, importantly, mental health professionals .

Among these roles, we can find both medical-, lifestyle- and mental health-related professionals that act in coordination to provide care and support to the patient. Besides the traditional roles that mainly deal with the purely clinical aspects of the disease management, it is remarkable the presence of patient navigators (also called patient educators) who guide patients from diagnosis through survivorship, social workers to provide patients and caregivers access to support groups and help them cope with the challenges posed by the cancer, dietitians to help patients cope with treatment and cancer side effects, and mental health professionals to provide counseling and promote coping strategies for common mental distress symptoms such as anxiety, depressive mood and fear of recurrence.

Although these recommendations are intended to guide the composition of the oncology team in a routine care scenario, few healthcare providers implement all these roles described before. In low- and middle-income countries (LMICs), it can be due to a lack of resources to afford the costs of specialized staff such as cancer patient navigators, psycho-oncologists or nutritionists specialized in cancer, but also the lack of trained professionals able to play these roles and the poor awareness on the benefits that such roles may bring to the patient's health outcomes poses a significant challenge to the adoption of a more holistic care approach. Where available, non-for-profit cancer patient organizations take over some of the duties mentioned before, mostly related to provide patients and relatives with support across their journey not only about how to better cope with all the side effects of cancer, but also helping them to find counsel, financial, and mental health support, among other services.

Nonetheless, ASCO statement underscores the relevance and impact that these not-so-traditional roles may have in the patient support towards achieving an optimal quality of life throughout the patient journey. However, when compared to the patient-related information that clinical roles can leverage to effectively manage the oncological patient (lab tests, CT scans, clinical outcomes, etc.), it is evident the huge gap in the routine practice that these roles experience when it comes to effectively monitoring the patient status in their respective domains.

Building a Learning Healthcare System in Oncology Care upon a Value-Based Care Schema

Introducing the Learning Health System Concept

In the last decade there have been great advances in both pharmacology and technology (Zheng et al. 2016; Fitzgerald et al. 2016) to fight cancer and to improve the results in terms of survival, side effects and quality of life. The increased understanding of cancer biology, with special emphasis on the tumor microenvironment and adaptive immune response, has contributed to the development of numerous target drugs that have been reaching clinical practice through clinical trials.

The term Learning Health System (LHS) emerged in 2007 as a definition of a conceptual strategy to guide the transformation that a health system should pursue to improve its efficiency based on how the organization generates and applies the available scientific knowledge, knowledge that is generated and updated at a pace that is difficult for current health systems to chase (Etheredge 2007). The LHS model is based on the mutual influence between research and clinical practice, and on how to manage and integrate the advances made in both areas in the organization in such a way that they translate into improvements in efficiency and quality of care. In a healthcare model based on an LHS, the knowledge generated through the experience acquired during daily clinical practice should be taken into account when making decisions in the healthcare setting, in addition to the CPGs (Fig. 9.3).

For the implementation of this strategy, EHR systems and patient-generated data play a fundamental role as a means to guide professionals in the use of clinical guidelines and in the application of care protocols, as well as serving as a meeting point between researchers and clinical leaders (Greene et al. 2012). The reuse of this is crucial for the generation of new evidence that should be considered when

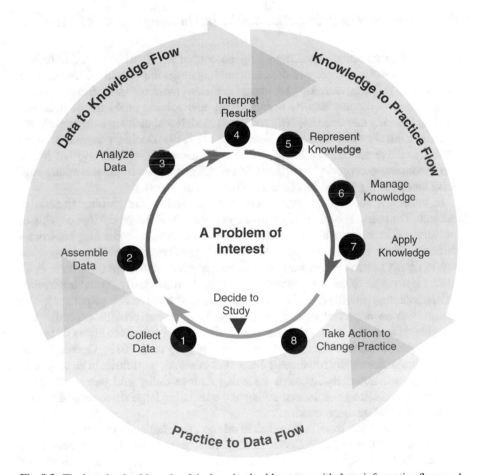

Fig. 9.3 The learning health cycle of the learning health system with three information flows and eight steps (Flynn et al. 2018)

making care and therapeutic decisions. Its main advantage is the availability of a large amount of information about the disease, treatment, and health outcomes of a large number of patients, thus eliminating sample size bias in the generation of evidence, as commonly occurs in clinical trials. By being able to generate significant cohorts of patients with specific particularities, it is possible to make proposals for personalized treatments with better health outcomes and cost-effectiveness (Lambin et al. 2013). Given that the information contained in EHR systems and patient-generated data repositories is often fragmented in different databases, commonly referred to as information silos due to their lack of capacity to integrate with other EHR systems, an integrative strategy based on technical and semantic interoperability standards is necessary to enrich and increase the quality and availability of the information.

Patient-Generated data Actionability in Oncology Routine Care

Clinical practice requires handling a large amount of information related to patient care. The escalating quantity of data and, consequently, the way in which that data can relate to patients, is making healthcare decisions more complex. Smart systems are intended to support experts in identifying and solving problems of decision-making. Systems that combine both statistical models and data are being developed to assist clinical decision-makers (Moreira et al. 2019). Decision support systems (DSSs; assistive technology for clinicians, who have limited time and are facing ever-increasing complexity) are hailed as a possible solution to the increasing cognitive burden being placed on clinicians (Walsh et al. 2019).

In oncology, specifically, consumer wearable devices are gaining traction in research. The market continues to evolve and expand, with some devices capable of measuring skin temperature and blood oxygen saturation or collecting electrocardiograms. Many of these wearable devices have been tested providing an opportunity to obtain patient health measures to an unprecedented degree (Alberts et al. 2020; Gupta et al. 2018; Gresham et al. 2018b). Commercially available physical activity monitors provide clinicians an opportunity to obtain oncology patient health measures to an unprecedented degree. These devices can provide objective and quantifiable measures of physical activity, which are not subject to errors or bias of self-reporting or shorter duration of formal testing (Beg et al. 2017). Oncology programs can systematically implement these tools into their workflows in an adaptable and iterative manner. But, besides assessing their usability and perceived utility there exists a challenge of understanding and translating large amounts of data collected to support decision making.

Data visualization has the potential to address the challenge of integrating and using large amounts of data collected to support the personalized care of individuals with cancer (Backonja et al. 2018). Data visualizations are representations of data through the application of visual encodings (e.g., position and color) (Bertin 1983; Few 2009). Visualization can leverage a user's cognitive strengths such as pattern recognition, and it helps them overcome their cognitive limitations including calculating and remembering strings of numbers. Appropriate, well thought out visualizations can ultimately support understanding, task completion, and decision making (Padilla et al. 2018).

Leveraging Data science for Boosting RWE Discovery

Data science methods can leverage large datasets of longitudinal patient data to provide empirically-based support to healthcare professionals in their decision-making process. Predictive models can be built upon these large datasets to anticipate potential clinical outcomes for a given patient according to the knowledge embedded in the retrospective experiences registered in the database. These methods, commonly referred to as clinical decision support systems (CDSS), are typically designed to integrate a medical knowledge base, a patient database and an inference engine to generate case-specific suggestions and facilitate the achievement of diagnoses. These types of systems pose technological challenges of great complexity and diversity, establishing new computational requirements and paradigms for the representation, use and acquisition of the biomedical knowledge necessary for their implementation (Mitchell et al. 2011).

In this sense, predictive models based on data science techniques are becoming a key tool for both biomedical research and clinical practice (Bellazzi and Zupan 2008). These techniques will play a fundamental role in the future for the discovery, extraction, generation, and application of new biomedical knowledge. To achieve this goal and related to the role that longitudinal patient-generated data will play in this strategy, significant advances must be made in the following areas: (a) Integration of different data sources, (b) Normalization, sampling, and pre-processing, (c) Pattern analysis and discovery, (d) Interactive visualization and decision support, and (e) Information security, privacy, and protection (Holzinger et al. 2014).

The techniques used to generate predictive models can be classified into different categories according to the underlying algorithms and the intended applications of each one of them. Some of these categories are artificial neural networks, dynamic prediction algorithms and evidence-based predictive systems, among others (Liao et al. 2012). For these techniques to be useful, they must be applied to a repository of data that includes all the relevant information to the research, in the case of oncology, detailed information about the patient's pathology, treatments administered, side effects derived from the treatment (toxicity), and evolution of the disease (survival). In the field of radiation oncology, the use of data mining techniques for automatic feature extraction has been shown to improve the quality of the information collected (Pontes et al. 2021a), as well as to reduce the time spent on manual collection of this information (Roelofs et al. 2013). At the international level, several initiatives have been developed aiming at establishing multicenter repositories accessible to the research community with the objective of increasing the sample size of quality information sets and thus improving the accuracy and reliability of new therapeutic models, as well as facilitating the generation and discovery of new knowledge (Roelofs et al. 2014). The use of these techniques in the field of cancer treatments based on chemical agents (chemotherapy, immunotherapy, targeted therapy) and/or radiation parameters (Pontes et al. 2021b) has also proved useful for the discovery and design of new pharmacological multidisciplinary approaches (Ilardi et al. 2014).

On the other hand, to achieve an optimal level of automation when generating new therapeutic models and decision support rules, it is essential to incorporate self-learning techniques so that the system can adapt its recommendations based on the retrospective analysis of health outcomes obtained in the past to the incorporation of new cases and, therefore, new information about the health outcomes of new systemic and radiotherapy treatments administered to patients. It is these self-learning techniques that should provide a LHS with the flexibility and agility necessary to continuously adapt to the new evidence available, whether it comes from updates in the available CPGs and scientific evidence or from the experience derived from the healthcare routine.

The Shift from Fee-for-Service to Value-Based Care Schema

Population health management (PHM) focuses on the delivery and coordination of patient-centered health care services to optimize the patient care experience, improve health, and manage health care costs (NACHC (National Association of Community Health Centers) 2016). As health care delivery systems move from fee-for-service (paying for the volume of services delivered) to value-based care (paying for health and quality outcomes attained), interest in PHM strategies is increasing rapidly. PHM relies on the use of patient registries that include clinical data as well as the utilization of health insurance claims data to effectively manage health care utilization. Risk stratification is used to identify patients and groups of patients with different health care needs, assess how health care coordination teams should be structured, and build partnerships with different entities (e.g., hospitals, clinics, specialists, community organizations providing social services) to better coordinate care (NACHC (National Association of Community Health Centers) 2016).

Health care systems and payers have at their disposal increasingly sophisticated ways of analyzing and visualizing clinical data but what most of them do not have is access to patient-generated data. The lack of patient-generated data is a major challenge to manage any patient with complex chronic health conditions; having access to patient-generated data is particularly important in oncology care given the physical, psychological, and social distress associated with cancer treatment. Although clinical, genomic, and financial data are critical for PHM given the inherent complexities of cancer care coordination (Goede 2019), patient-generated data collected over time can be useful not only to assess when patients are at risk of events such as emergency department visits and hospitalizations but also to identify different points for interventions and referrals.

Patient-generated data and sophisticated predictive analytics are more likely to be used in health systems and organizations that are moving toward value-based contracting. Under a fee-for-service payment system, these types of investments cannot be easily allocated to the delivery of a specific service; rather, they are investments that benefit everyone that is being managed at a given time and, as such, systems to use patient-generated data are more likely to be adopted and thrive whenever the data and analytic tools are used to gain actionable insights for a given population in a value-added way.

Payers are critical to increase the adoption of PHM strategies in general, but they are even more important to increase the use of PHM for cancer patients. The main reason for this is that payers are moving to value-based care reimbursement, and they have experience integrating complex data from different sources (Goede 2019). Every organization in the health care delivery space shares data with payers if they want to get reimbursed for any services provided. As such, the role of payers as partial data integrators together with the fact that they interact directly with every organization involved in providing care and support for cancer patients means that they also have a responsibility to be part of the solution to fully understand the patient experience and better manage oncology care.

Some payers have developed value-based oncology programs that seem promising (COA (Community Oncology Alliance) 2020). Humana developed the Oncology Model of Care (OMOC) for their Medicare Advantage and commercial members. The OMOC program provides a monthly care coordination fee to practices, and it is designed to improve the patient experience by using care coordination strategies (patient navigation) and providing analytics to support oncology providers (Kent 2019). Cigna designed the Collaborative Care Oncology Focus Program to help providers improve health care quality of patients in cancer treatment. The Cigna program includes a shared savings value-based reimbursement component and a care coordination fee for providers. UnitedHealthcare has an Episodes of Care model that focuses on the delivery of evidence-based care, quality improvement, and shared savings based on decreases in cancer care costs (COA (Community Oncology Alliance) 2020).

Perhaps the most comprehensive value-based oncology program in existence is the Oncology Care Model (OCM) from the Center for Medicare & Medicaid Innovation. OCM centers on controlling health care costs by improving care coordination and access to care for chemotherapy patients. As of 2020, a total of 138 practices and 10 commercial payers are participating in the OCM (Center for Medicare and Medicaid Innovation (CMMI) 2021).

The OCM is based on an episode-based payment model to incentivize better health care quality and coordination for Medicare fee-for-service beneficiaries on cytotoxic chemotherapy, biologic therapy, immunotherapy, or hormonal therapy for cancer. Each episode last 6 months. Practices can receive a Monthly Enhanced Oncology Services (MEOS) payment per episode for each beneficiary (US$160) and a performance-based payment for a chemotherapy episode of care. The MEOS payment is designed to cover patient management and care coordination during the episode of care whereas the performance-based payment is designed to improve health care quality and lower costs during the episode of care.

A recent evaluation of the OCM model showed that, for high-risk episodes, the OCM led to reductions in payment increases related to hospitalizations, post-acute care, physician services, and outpatient drug treatment, compared to comparison episodes of care (Abt (Abt Associates) 2021). However, for low-risk episodes, payments increased more for OCM episodes than for comparison episodes. The evaluation also found no changes in the use of chemotherapy drug treatments or radiation therapy between the OCM and comparison episodes. When it comes to patient-centered care, the evaluation found that OCM patients rate their care experience highly both at the start of the model and through time; and there were no differences between the OCM model and the comparison group. There was also a slight decrease in hospitalizations in the last month of life for OCM patients who died compared to patients in the comparison group (1.1 percentage point relative reduction in hospitalizations) (Abt (Abt Associates) 2021).

The collection of longitudinal patient-generated data through devices, surveys, and wearables is a key missing piece in the PHM data puzzle. Although the OCM evaluation found no impact of the model on patient-reported composite measures of the patient health care experience, the evaluation study found that shared decision making, enabling patient self-management, and symptom management were rated relatively low (Abt (Abt Associates) 2021). OCM patients were asked if they were bothered by cancer symptoms or cancer treatment (i.e., pain, energy level, emotional problems, nausea, breathing, coughing, constipation, and neuropathy); the evaluation found that the OCM did not have an effect on these patient-reported symptoms (Abt (Abt Associates) 2021).

Longitudinal patient-generated data collection efforts have the potential to address data gaps by generating more precise patient information—either continuously or in shorter time intervals than what is possible through traditional patient surveys. Patient-generated data could also lead to improvements in cancer symptoms and treatment with the use of data science and the development of new tools such as digital health coaching systems (Konstantinidis et al. 2021). The shift from fee-for-service to value-based care is a trend that may be providing the right financial and clinical care incentives to collect, integrate, and analyze longitudinal patient-generated data to develop new digital tools to best support PHM in cancer care.

Challenges for Real-World Deployments of Longitudinal Patient-Generated Data Collection Digital Tools

Regulatory Challenges

Regulatory aspects concerning the deployment of technologies that may enable the systematic collection of longitudinal patient-generated data in a routine care environment may limit their adoption by the healthcare providers. Health authorities are continuously exploring and advancing a regulatory framework for the validation and clearance of the emerging technologies to ensure their safety and accuracy to be used in a clinical environment. However, novel technologies with potential indications for this context are being released at a faster pace, which makes difficult for regulators' policies to evolve as quick as the market demands. These technologies are usually referred to as medical devices, which is an umbrella term for technological devices that are used during the healthcare delivery process (including both implantable and non-implantable devices), software processing clinical information to support the patient management (SaMD) and platforms which deliver services intended to be used by the healthcare professionals (PaMD).

At global level, the International Medical Device Regulators Forum (IMDRF) oversees the release of regulatory guidance that can be further applied at national and regional level by the related health authorities. It also encourages local regulators to apply a classification of the medical devices based on the risk that its use could imply for human safety (IMDRF 2014). In USA, the Center for Devices and Radiological Health (CDRH) is the entity within the FDA that deals with the clearance of proposed technologies to be classified as medical devices considering their intended use, indications to use, and the potential risk that it may pose for the human being. In the EU, this work is carried out by the Notified Bodies, which are private organizations accredited by the relevant national health authorities.

Therefore, the first challenge that medical devices manufacturing companies face when trying to bring to the global market their technology to enable longitudinal patient-generated data collection is the fragmentation of the regulatory framework itself despite the efforts of initiatives such as the IMDRF, given that every country has their own accreditation and clearance process in place, thus burdening a deployment of the technology at global scale.

Another challenge is related to the fast pace that SaMD technologies evolve to be adapted to respond to glitches, adverse events, and other safety concerns quickly. Traditional regulatory frameworks usually perform their assessments based on specific products, and when it comes to software products, it may happen that whenever the assessment is completed, which may take several months, the software product needs to be updated, thus with the potential need to go through the assessment process again.

To tackle this issue, the FDA is running the Pre-Cert Pilot Program (Digital Health Software Precertification (Pre-Cert) Program 2019) to inform the development of a future regulatory model that will provide more streamlined and efficient regulatory oversight of SaMD developed by manufacturers who have demonstrated a robust culture of quality and organizational excellence. In this sense, the FDA is working to establish a regulatory framework that is equally responsive when issues arise to help ensure consumers continue to have access to safe and effective products.

Technological Challenges

This section addresses the set of the most salient technological challenges when it comes to the real-world deployment of longitudinal patient-generated data collection tools in routine care, as highlighted in a systematic review by Baig et al. (Baig et al. 2017) In order to produce reliable and accurate data, sensors usually require to be placed on a specific part of the body (Martin et al. 2000). Body movements and gestures can interfere with the data acquisition process, thus, hampering sensor reliability. This is a common challenge for sensors that rely on the contact with the skin to acquire the information such as ECG and EEG sensors. Furthermore, these sensors usually must deal with other sources of external noise related to electromagnetic interferences. Several signal processing strategies can be applied to overcome this issue, mainly based on adaptive signal filtering (Malghan and Hota 2020), and can be performed on hardware and/or software platforms.

In wireless devices, connectivity is another challenging area that patient-generated data collection sensors must face to accomplish their objectives. Connectivity issues can happen due to low signal strength between the sensor and the receiver, low battery life because of an intensive use of network interfaces, and/or low transmission speed, which can lead to a poor user experience due to data loss, intermittent connectivity and higher waiting periods than expected. Furthermore, connectivity-related issues should also be thoroughly tested in real-world settings as the working conditions may change over time and are hardly replicable on a laboratory setting (Rault et al. 2017). It seems that 5G-enabled technologies might enter in this landscape as a rule-changer and could potentially help to overcome most (if not all) of these connectivity challenges, becoming the cornerstone for future smart healthcare technologies (Ahad et al. 2020), but this is to be evidenced under real-world working conditions yet.

In the artificial intelligence and machine learning era, the collection of large cohorts of longitudinal patient-generated data becomes a fundamental step to train predictive models and classification algorithms at the core of clinical decision support systems. The main challenge for these technologies to roll-out in the routine care is their transparency, accuracy and reliability, which takes us to the data quality issue. In order to produce such models and algorithms with a reasonable performance level to be used in the clinical practice, patient-generated data needs to be cleaned, structured, labelled, and pre-processed to meet the requirements posed by the different algorithms. Due to its high degree of complexity and specialization needed for the final purpose of the clinical decision support system, these tasks are usually performed following an ad-hoc approach that hinders its scalability to different areas. In order to overcome this challenge, initiatives like the OMOP Common Data Model (Observational Health Data Sciences and Informatics 2021) supported by the Observational Health Data Science and Informatics, strive to provide data standardization tools and vocabularies to harmonize concepts so they can be further processed and made actionable disregarding the data source.

One of the main hypotheses that could explain why some people do not respond as expected to digital therapeutic interventions delivered by mHealth solutions puts the focus on the engagement level. Since this digital health approach needs the active participation and implication of patients to function correctly, it is essential to find parameters to measure the engagement and adherence to these interventions. Engagement can be conceptualized in terms of both "experience and behavior and sits within a complex system involving the application, the context of use, the mechanisms of action of the application and the target behavior"(Perski et al. 2017). Qualitatively, it has been conceptualized as the amount, duration, breadth, and depth of intervention usage (Pham et al. 2019). Nonetheless, these parameters only consider the user-app interaction. Other authors, in contrast, propose two categories to measure engagement in digital behavior change interventions (DBCI): health behavior engagement or Big E, and DBCI engagement or Little E (Cole-Lewis et al. 2019). Since Little E can be analyzed and generalized easily, most studies only focus on the user-app interaction. Nevertheless, it is essential to keep in mind that the main purpose of these studies of engagement in mHealth apps transcends the commercial and economic interests, since the objective is to improve the health condition of different people by changing their lifestyle or intervening in their disease management. To this end, the incorporation of the Big E bridges the gap between app use and adherence or effectiveness.

Conclusions

Despite of the potential benefits in terms of HRQoL that people living with cancer (and their caregivers) may achieve from healthcare providers adopting systematic longitudinal patient-reported data collection in oncology care, this is not a common practice in the routine oncology care field. Given the importance of appropriately selecting patients best suited for certain definitive treatments, incorporating PROMs that better report the overall well-being and symptoms important to the patient into the clinical decision-making process may better identify patients that may benefit from a specific treatment approach. There is a growing body of evidence about the efficacy of using not only PROMs and PREMs, but also biometric measurements, to have a closer view into the actual patient status and to provide a more personalized care management. Leveraging on this evidence will hopefully support the translation of these findings into the real-world settings.

Care of cancer survivors generates another challenge that requires to be properly addressed. Besides late (after treatment) physical symptoms (e.g., pain and fatigue), cancer survivors can also face specific psychosocial stressors related to family role and job re-engagement. Behavioral and lifestyle aspects impacting on patients' HRQoL can be better analyzed and understood making use of tools that enable the collection of variables and health determinants not only from a strictly clinical point of view, but also from the patient exposure to external factors. In this setting, digital health (eHealth), and particularly mobile health solutions start playing a pivotal role as scalable and cost-effective intervention systems.

Advances in supporting patients to enjoy a better experience through their patient journey have been recently attained, stressing on the importance of accounting for a multidisciplinary care team to facilitate their transition throughout their care pathway. This support broadens from strictly clinical care towards a more holistic care approach, also addressing psychosocial, financial, and spiritual support for both patients and caregivers.

Healthcare systems need to undertake a trade-off between the quality of care delivered and the cost-effectiveness of their interventions. In the big data and AI era, technology is ready to provide insights beyond the traditional quality of care indicators by making use of other valuable sources of information that can help in shaping personalized patients' performance across their patient journey. Additionally, the analysis of longitudinal patient-generated data can provide support to healthcare providers in anticipating potential worsening of patients' conditions, thus enabling the adoption of preventive strategies which have proven to be more cost-effective when compared to the traditional reactive approach. Furthermore, the LHS paradigm would trigger a virtuous cycle where the clinical outcomes can be used to generate new knowledge on top of CPGs and scientific evidence that, in turn, can be used to improve the clinical outcomes in the next iteration in a seamless, continuous way. It is in this context where the shift from fee-for-service to value-based care models makes sense to promote a better quality of care delivered, as this model is driven by longitudinal patient-generated data on top of clinical, genomic, and financial data.

Real-world deployments of digital tools to enable the systematic collection of longitudinal patient-generated data also brings regulatory challenges that need to be taken under consideration. The most remarkable ones are related to the fragmentation of the regulatory framework that hinders the application of scalable strategies at global level for technological vendors, and the lack of regulatory agility to keep the pace of the ever-evolving technology.

Chapter Review Questions
- Can you identify current practices on data collection for routine cancer care?
- Besides the variables derived from clinical and genomic fields, which other determinants of HRQoL should be considered in cancer care?
- How are the concepts of learning healthcare system and value-based care aligned?
- What is the role of longitudinal patient-generated data in cancer care?

References

Aaronson NK, Mattioli V, Minton O, Weis J, Johansen C, Dalton SO, et al. Beyond treatment–psychosocial and behavioural issues in cancer survivorship research and practice. Eur J Cancer Suppl. 2014;12(1):54–64.

Abt (Abt Associates). Evaluation of the oncology care mode: performance periods 1-5. January 2021. Rockville, MD. https://innovation.cms.gov/data-and-reports/2021/ocm-evaluation-pp1-5

Ahad A, Tahir M, Sheikh MA, Ahmed KI, Mughees A, Numani A. Technologies trend towards 5G network for smart health-care using IoT: a review. Sensors. 2020;20(14):4047. https://doi.org/10.3390/s20144047.

Alberts NM, Leisenring WM, Flynn JS, Whitton J, Gibson TM, Jibb L, et al. Wearable respiratory monitoring and feedback for chronic pain in adult survivors of childhood cancer: a feasibility randomized controlled trial from the childhood cancer survivor study. JCO Clini Cancer Informatics. 2020;4:1014–26.

American Society of Clinical Oncology. Survivorship care clinical tools and resources. http://www.asco.org/practice-research/survivorship-care-clinical-toolsand-resources.

Anon.   https://www.cancer.net/navigating-cancer-care/cancer-basics/cancer-care-team/oncology-team, n.d.

Anon. https://mcodeinitiative.org/, n.d.-a

Anon. https://www.cancerdata.nhs.uk/, n.d.-b

Audell L, Rosner HL. The alternatives for chronic pain management in cancer survivors. J Support Oncol. 2012;10(3):96.

Backonja U, Haynes SC, Kim KK. Data visualizations to support health practitioners' provision of personalized care for patients with cancer and multiple chronic conditions: user-centered design study. JMIR Hum Factors. 2018;5(4):e11826.

Baig MM, GholamHosseini H, Moqeem AA, et al. A systematic review of wearable patient monitoring systems—current challenges and opportunities for clinical adoption. J Med Syst. 2017;41:115. https://doi.org/10.1007/s10916-017-0760-1.

Beg MS, Gupta A, Stewart T, Rethorst CD. Promise of wearable physical activity monitors in oncology practice. J Oncol Pract. 2017;13(2):82–9.

Bellazzi R, Zupan B. Predictive data mining in clinical medicine: current issues and guidelines. Int J Med Inform. 2008;77(2):81–97., ISSN 1386-5056. https://doi.org/10.1016/j.ijmedinf.2006.11.006.

Bertin J. Semiology of graphics; diagrams networks maps (No. 04; QA90, B7.), 1983.

Bhatia A, Kara J, Janmohamed T, Prabhu A, Lebovic G, Katz J, Clarke H. User engagement and clinical impact of the manage my pain app in patients with chronic pain: a real-world, multisite trial JMIR. Mhealth Uhealth. 2021;9(3):e26528. URL: https://mhealth.jmir.org/2021/3/e26528. https://doi.org/10.2196/26528.

Bower JE. Cancer-related fatigue—mechanisms, risk factors, and treatments. Nat Rev Clin Oncol. 2014;11(10):597–609. https://doi.org/10.1038/nrclinonc.2014.127.

Caldarella A, Amunni G, Angiolini C, Crocetti E, Di Costanzo F, Di Leo A, Giusti F, Pegna AL, Mantellini P, Luzzatto L, Paci E. Feasibility of evaluating quality cancer care using registry data and electronic health records: a population-based study. Int J Qual Health Care. 2012;24:411–8.

Campanella P, Lovato E, Marone C, Fallacara L, Mancuso A, Ricciardi W, Specchia ML. The impact of electronic health records on healthcare quality: a systematic review and meta-analysis. Eur J Pub Health. 2016;26:60–4.

Carrasco-Hernandez L, Jódar-Sánchez F, Núñez-Benjumea F, Conde JM, González MM, Civit-Balcells A, et al. A mobile health solution complementing psychopharmacology-supported smoking cessation: randomized controlled trial. JMIR Mhealth Uhealth. 2020;8(4):e17530.

Center for Medicare & Medicaid Innovation (CMMI). Oncology Care Model (OCM). April 2021. https://innovation.cms.gov/innovation-models/oncology-care

COA (Community Oncology Alliance). 2020 Community Oncology Alliance Payment Reform Model Brief. October 1, 2020. https://communityoncology.org/wp-content/uploads/2020/10/COA-2020_Payment_Reform_Brief-FINAL.pdf

Cole-Lewis H, Ezeanochie N, Turgiss J. Understanding health behavior technology engagement: pathway to measuring digital behavior change interventions. JMIR Form Res. 2019;3(4):e14052. https://doi.org/10.2196/14052.

Coons SJ, Gwaltney CJ, Hays RD, et al. Recommendations on evidence needed to support measurement equivalence between electronic and paper-based patient-reported outcome (PRO) measures: ISPOR ePRO good research practices task force report. Value Health. Epub ahead of print. 2009; https://doi.org/10.1111/j.1524-4733.2008.00470.x.

Digital Health Software Precertification (Pre-Cert) Program 2019. https://www.fda.gov/medical-devices/digital-health-center-excellence/digital-health-software-precertification-pre-cert-program. Accessed April 2021.

Dingemans AM, Früh M, Ardizzoni A, Besse B, Faivre-Finn C, Hendriks LE, et al. Small-cell lung cancer: ESMO Clinical Practice Guidelines for diagnosis, treatment and follow-up. Ann Oncol. 2021;32:839.

Etheredge LM. A rapid-learning health system. Health Aff (Millwood). 2007;26:w107-18.

Few S. *Now you see it: simple visualization techniques for quantitative analysis* (No. Sirsi) i9780970601988) 2009.

Fitzgerald R, Owen R, Hargrave C, Pryor D, Barry T, Lehman M, Bernard A, Mai T, Seshadri V, Fielding A. A comparison of three different VMAT techniques for the delivery of lung stereotactic ablative radiation therapy. J Med Radiat Sci. 2016;63(1):23-3.

Flynn A, Friedman C, Boisvert P, Landis-Lewis Z, Lagoze C. The knowledge object reference ontology (KORO): a formalism to support management and sharing of computable biomedical knowledge for learning health systems. Learning Health Systems. 2018;2 https://doi.org/10.1002/lrh2.10054.

Gabriel I, Creedy D, Coyne E. A systematic review of psychosocial interventions to improve quality of life of people with cancer and their family caregivers. Nurs Open. 2020;7(5):1299–312.

Garrison LP Jr, Neumann PJ, Erickson P, Marshall D, Mullins CD. Using real-world data for coverage and payment decisions: the ISPOR real-world data task force report. Value Health. 2007;10:326–35.

Girgis A, Lambert S, Johnson C, Waller A, Currow D. Physical, psychosocial, relationship, and economic burden of caring for people with cancer: a review. J Oncol Pract. 2013;9:197–202.

Goede P. Achieving the "Holy Grail" of population health management in cancer care. MedCity News. 2019; https://medcitynews.com/2019/03/achieving-the-holy-grail-of-population-health-management-in-cancer-care/?rf=1

Goedendorp MM, Gielissen MF, Verhagen CA, Bleijenberg G. Psychosocial interventions for reducing fatigue during cancer treatment in adults. Cochrane Database Syst Rev. 2009;1:CD006953.

Gonzalez-Hernandez E, Romero R, Campos D, Burychka D, Diego-Pedro R, Baños R, et al. Cognitively-based compassion training (CBCT®) in breast cancer survivors: a randomized clinical trial study. Integr Cancer Ther. 2018;17(3):684–96.

Greene SM, Reid RJ, Larson EB. Implementing the learning health system: from concept to action. Ann Intern Med. 2012;157(3):207–10.

Gresham G, Hendifar AE, Spiegel B, Neeman E, Tuli R, Rimel BJ, et al. Wearable activity monitors to assess performance status and predict clinical outcomes in advanced cancer patients. NPJ Digit Medicine. 2018b;1(1):1–8.

Gresham G, Schrack J, Gresham LM, Shinde AM, Hendifar AE, Tuli R, et al. Wearable activity monitors in oncology trials: current use of an emerging technology. Contemp Clin Trials. 2018a;64:13–21.

Gupta A, Stewart T, Bhulani N, Dong Y, Rahimi Z, Crane K, et al. Feasibility of wearable physical activity monitors in patients with cancer. JCO Clin Cancer Inf. 2018;2:1–10.

Handberg C, Svendsen ML, Maribo T. A cross-sectional study evaluating potential differences in the need for cancer survivorship Care in Relation to patients' socioeconomic status. J Clin Med Res. 2019;11(7):515.

Holland JC, Bultz BD. The NCCN guideline for distress management: a case for making distress the sixth vital sign. J Natl Compr Cancer Netw. 2007;5(1):3–7.

Holzinger A, Dehmer M, Jurisica I. Knowledge discovery and interactive data Mining in Bioinformatics—State-of-the-Art, future challenges and research directions. BMC Bioinformatics. 2014;15(6):I1. https://doi.org/10.1186/1471-2105-15-S6-I1.

Ilardi EA, Vitaku E, Njardarson JT. Data-mining for sulfur and fluorine: an evaluation of pharmaceuticals to reveal opportunities for drug design and discovery. J Med Chem. 2014;57:2832–42. https://doi.org/10.1021/jm401375q.

IMDRF   2014.   http://www.imdrf.org/docs/imdrf/final/technical/imdrf-tech-140918-samd-framework-risk-categorization-141013.pdf. Accessed April 2021.

Juarez PD, Hood DB, Min-Ae S, Aramandla R. Use of an exposome approach to understand the effects of exposures from the natural, built, and social environments on cardio-vascular disease onset, progression, and outcomes. Front Public Health. 2020;8:379. https://doi.org/10.3389/fpubh.2020.00379.

Kelleher SA, Somers TJ, Locklear T, Crosswell AD, Abernethy AP. Using patient reported outcomes in oncology clinical practice. Scand J Pain. 2016;13:6–11. https://doi.org/10.1016/j.sjpain.2016.05.035. Epub 2016 Jun 16. PMID: 27818717; PMCID: PMC5094273

Kent J. Humana launches value-based care oncology program for MA members. Health Payer Intelligence. 2019; https://healthpayerintelligence.com/news/humana-launches-value-based-care-oncology-program-for-ma-members

Khatcheressian JL, Hurley P, Bantug E, et al. American Society of Clinical Oncology: breast cancer follow-up and management after primary treatment: American Society of Clinical Oncology clinical practice guideline update. J Clin Oncol. 2013;31:961–5.

Konstantinidis EI, Vellidou E, Fernandez-Luque L, Bamidis PD. Editorial: coaching systems for Health and Well-being. Front Digit Health. 2021;3:18. https://doi.org/10.3389/fdgth.2021.658023.

Lagergren P, Schandl A, Aaronson NK, Adami HO, de Lorenzo F, Denis L, et al. Cancer survivorship: an integral part of Europe's research agenda. Mol Oncol. 2019;13(3):624–35.

Lambin P, Roelofs E, Reymen B, et al. Rapid learning health care in oncology'–an approach towards decision support systems enabling customised radiotherapy. Radiother Oncol. 2013;109(1):159–64.

Lehman BJ, David DM, Gruber JA. Rethinking the biopsychosocial model of health: understanding health as a dynamic system. Soc Personal Psychol Compass. 2017;11(8):e12328.

Liao S-H, Chu P-H, Hsiao P-Y. Data mining techniques and applications—a decade review from 2000 to 2011. Expert Syst Appl. 2012;39(12):11303–11., ISSN 0957-4174. https://doi.org/10.1016/j.eswa.2012.02.063.

Malghan PG, Hota MK. A review on ECG filtering techniques for rhythm analysis. Res Biomed Eng. 2020;36:171–86. https://doi.org/10.1007/s42600-020-00057-9.

Martin Sanchez F, Gray K, Bellazzi R, Lopez-Campos G. Exposome informatics: considerations for the design of future biomedical research information systems. J Am Med Inform Assoc. 2014a;21(3):386–90.

Martin Sanchez F, Gray K, Bellazzi R, Lopez-Campos G. Exposome informatics: considerations for the design of future biomedical research information systems. J Am Med Inform Assoc. 2014b;21(3):386–90. https://doi.org/10.1136/amiajnl-2013-001772. Epub 2013 Nov 1. PMID: 24186958; PMCID: PMC3994854

Martin T, Jovanov E, and Raskovic D. Issues in wearable computing for medical monitoring applications: a case study of a wearable ECG monitoring device. In: Wearable Computers, The Fourth International Symposium on. IEEE, 2000.

Marzorati C, Riva S, Pravettoni G. Who is a cancer survivor? A systematicreview of published definitions. J Cancer Educ. 2017;32:228–37.

Mitchell JA, Gerdin U, Lindberg DAB, et al. 50 years of informatics research on decision support: What's next. Methods Inf Med. 2011;50(6):525–35.

Mokkink L, Prinsen C, Patrick D, et al. COSMIN methodology for systematic reviews of patient-reported outcome measures (PROMs): user manual. Amsterdam Public Health Research Institute. 2018:1–78.

Moreira MW, Rodrigues JJ, Korotaev V, Al-Muhtadi J, Kumar N. A comprehensive review on smart decision support systems for health care. IEEE Syst J. 2019;13(3):3536–45.

NACHC (National Association of Community Health Centers). Population health management. 2016. Bethesda, MD. http://www.nachc.org/wp-content/uploads/2015/12/NACHC_pophealth_factsheet_FINAL.pdf

Nápoles AM, Santoyo-Olsson J, Chacón L, Stewart AL, Dixit N, Ortiz C. Feasibility of a mobile phone app and telephone coaching survivorship care planning program among Spanish-speaking breast cancer survivors. JMIR Cancer. 2019;5(2):e13543.

National Cancer Institute. Office of Cancer Survivorship. 2019 (http://cancercontrol.cancer.gov/ocs/).

Ness KK, Armstrong GT, Kundu M, et al. Frailty in childhood cancer survivors. Cancer. 2015;121:1540–7.

Nieto-Guerrero Gomez JM, Silva Vega GP, Cacicedo J, Delgado León BD, Herrero Rivera D, Praena Fernández JM, et al. Impact of pre-radiation therapy quality of life in lung cancer survival: a prospective, intention-to-treat, multicenter study. Clin Transl Oncol. 2020;22(9):1635–44.

Observational Health Data Sciences and Informatics. The book of OHDSI; 2021. https://ohdsi.github.io/TheBookOfOhdsi/

Padilla LM, Creem-Regehr SH, Hegarty M, Stefanucci JK. Decision making with visualizations: a cognitive framework across disciplines. Cogn Res Princ Implic. 2018;3:29. https://doi.org/10.1186/s41235-018-0120-9.

Perski O, Blandford A, West R, Michie S. Conceptualising engagement with digital behaviour change interventions: a systematic review using principles from critical interpretive synthesis. Transl Behav Med. 2017;7(2):254–67. https://doi.org/10.1007/s13142-016-0453-1.

Pham Q, Graham G, Carrion C, Morita PP, Seto E, Stinson JN, Cafazzo JA. A library of analytic indicators to evaluate effective engagement with consumer mHealth apps for chronic conditions: scoping review. JMIR Mhealth Uhealth. 2019;7(1):e11941. https://doi.org/10.2196/11941.

Pontes B, Núñez F, Rubio C, Moreno A, Nepomuceno I, Moreno J, et al. A data mining based clinical decision support system for survival in lung cancer. Rep Pract Oncol Radiother. 2021a;26:839.

Pontes B, Núñez F, Rubio C, Moreno A, Nepomuceno I, Moreno J, Cacicedo J, Praena-Fernandez JM, Rodriguez GAE, Parra C, León BDD, del Campo ER, Couñago F, Riquelme J, Guerra JLL. A data mining based clinical decision support system for survival in lung cancer. Rep Pract Oncol Radiother. 2021b; e-ISSN 2083–4640. ISSN 1507–1367

Rault T, et al. A survey of energy-efficient context recognition systems using wearable sensors for healthcare applications. Pervasive Mob Comput. 2017;37:23–44.

Roelofs E, Dekker A, Meldolesi E, van Stiphout RGPM, Valentini V, Lambin P. International data-sharing for radiotherapy research: an open-source based infrastructure for multicentric clinical data mining. Radiother Oncol. 2014;110(2):370–4., ISSN 0167-8140. https://doi.org/10.1016/j.radonc.2013.11.00.

Roelofs E, Persoon L, Nijsten S, Wiessler W, Dekker A, Lambin P. Benefits of a cli-nical data warehouse with data mining tools to collect data for a radiotherapy trial. Radiother Oncol. 2013;108(1):174–9., ISSN 0167-8140. https://doi.org/10.1016/j.radonc.2012.09.019.

Rothman M, Burke L, Erickson P, et al. Use of existing patient-reported outcome (PRO) instruments and their modification: the ISPOR good research practices for evaluating and documenting content validity for the use of existing instruments and their modification PRO task force report. Value Health. 2009;12:1075–83.

Runowicz CD, Leach CR, Henry NL, et al. American Cancer Society/American Society of Clinical Oncology breast cancer survivorship care guideline. J Clin Oncol. 2016;34:611–35.

Saczynski JS, McManus DD, Goldberg RJ. Commonly used data-collection approaches in clinical research. Am J Med. 2013;126(11):946–50. https://doi.org/10.1016/j.amjmed.2013.04.016.

Shapiro CL. Cancer survivorship. N Engl J Med. 2018;379(25):2438–50.

Shapiro CL, Jacobsen PB, Henderson T, et al. ReCAP: ASCO core curriculum for cancer survivorship education. J Oncol Pract. 2016;12(2):145. e108-e117

Smith SK, Loscalzo M, Mayer C, Rosenstein DL. Best practices in oncology distress management: beyond the screen. Am Soc Clin Oncol Educ Book. 2018;38:813–21.

Van Leeuwen M, Husson O, Alberti P, Arraras JI, Chinot OL, Costantini A, et al. Understanding the quality of life (QOL) issues in survivors of cancer: towards the development of an EORTC QOL cancer survivorship questionnaire. Health Qual Life Outcomes. 2018;16(1):1–15.

Walsh S, de Jong EE, van Timmeren JE, Ibrahim A, Compter I, Peerlings J, et al. Decision support systems in oncology. JCO Clin Cancer Informatics. 2019;3:1–9.

World Health Organization. "Mental health: strengthening our response". World Health Organization. August 2014. Retrieved 4 May 2014.

Zheng H, Wang M, Wu J, Wang ZM, Nan HJ, Sun H. Inhibition of mTOR enhances radiosensitivity of lung cancer cells and protects normal lung cells against radiation. Biochem Cell Biol. 2016; [in press]

Chapter 10
Semantic Technologies for Clinically Relevant Personal Health Applications

Ching-Hua Chen, Daniel Gruen, Jonathan Harris, James Hendler, Deborah L. McGuinness, Marco Monti, Nidhi Rastogi, Oshani Seneviratne, and Mohammed J. Zaki

Abstract Despite recent advances in digital health solutions and machine learning, personal health applications that aim to modify health behaviors are still limited in their ability to offer more personalized decision support. Moreover, while many personal health applications cater to general health and well-being, there remains a significant opportunity to increase the clinical relevance of the insights being generated. This chapter describes the motivation for, and illustrative applications of, semantic technologies for enabling clinically relevant personal health applications. We present two use cases that demonstrate how semantic web technologies, in combination with machine learning and data mining methods, can be used to provide personalized insights to support behaviors that are consistent with nutritional guidelines for people with diabetes.

Keywords Semantic web · Knowledge graphs · Artificial intelligence · Personal health · Health behavior · Diabetes self-management · Consumer health · Decision support systems

C.-H. Chen (✉)
Center for Computational Health, IBM Research, Yorktown Heights, NY, USA
e-mail: chinghua@us.ibm.com

D. Gruen · J. Harris · J. Hendler · D. L. McGuinness · N. Rastogi · O. Seneviratne · M. J. Zaki
Rensselaer Polytechnic Institute, Troy, NY, USA
e-mail: gruend2@rpi.edu; harrij15@rpi.edu; hendler@cs.rpi.edu; dlm@cs.rpi.edu; nidhi.rastogi@rit.edu; senevo@rpi.edu; zaki@cs.rpi.edu

M. Monti
Cognitive AI and Analytics, IBM Global Business Services, Circonvallazione Idroscalo, Segrate, Milan, Italy
e-mail: marco.monti@it.ibm.com

© The Author(s), under exclusive license to Springer Nature
Switzerland AG 2022
P.-Y. S. Hsueh et al. (eds.), *Personal Health Informatics*, Cognitive Informatics
in Biomedicine and Healthcare, https://doi.org/10.1007/978-3-031-07696-1_10

Decision Support for Health Behavior Change

Health outcomes are known to be driven by a combination of medical, genetic and lifestyle factors. In the United States, a disproportionate emphasis is placed on medical treatment, as compared to lifestyle modifications (Bipartisan Policy Center 2012). Where the former is primarily delivered in reaction to poor health status, the latter is often used as a form of disease prevention and/or health maintenance. As such, efforts to implement lifestyle modifications often rest on the shoulders of patients (or more generally, health consumers) with sufficient means, skills and motivation. The process of behavior change is well-studied. Yet, sustained behavior change remains challenging to intervene effectively on (Bouton 2014). While behavior change is recognized by experts as being a complex process involving dynamic and stochastic factors that span the psychological, social and physical domains, popular misconceptions are that changing one's behavior requires no more than 'common sense' or a good marketing campaign, and that most people will rationally process relevant knowledge and information (Kelly and Barker 2016). Arguably, interventions that are adaptive and sensitive to an individual's psychological, social and environmental context, are in a better position to address behavior change than those that are static, or adopt a 'one-size-fits-all' approach.

With the rapid adoption of mobile phones and wearable sensing technologies, most people now have access to mobile applications that can provide real-time sensing and feedback to their users. This trend has led to the development and study of several 'context-aware' digital technologies for tackling health behavior change (Thomas Craig et al. 2020). Common approaches of incorporating contextual awareness into digital behavior change interventions include the use of statistical and machine learning models to generate feedback based on user generated data (e.g., step counts and other forms of physical activity, food logs, sleep logs), as well as the use of rule-based dialog systems, or chat bots, that provide deterministic responses to user textual inputs that conform to anticipated patterns. However, most mobile health applications, while popular among patients, have not seen significant levels of acceptance from clinicians (Gordon et al. 2020). This lack of clinical acceptance is partly explained by factors pertaining to regulations, payment systems, and clinical workflows. It may also be explained by the limited incorporation of evidence-based, clinical guidelines into the function and design of mobile health applications.

Semantic technologies are well-suited for representing clinical knowledge that has been curated by medical and health experts. When semantic technologies that can represent and reason over clinical knowledge are used together with machine learning methods that learn from and adapt to the 'big data' that is continuously generated by activities of daily living, there is the potential to improve the clinical relevance of personal health applications. With a few notable exceptions (Michie et al. 2017; Dragoni et al. 2020; Chen et al. 2021) there has been limited work exploring the use of semantic technologies for health behavior change. This chapter aims to introduce readers to semantic technologies and the potential benefits that they present for enhancing the personalization, interpretability and clinical utility of personal health applications.

The objective of this chapter is to provide an introduction to semantic technologies to health informatics researchers and practitioners, and to demonstrate their application in combination with other artificial intelligence methods (e.g., data mining and machine learning) via exemplary use cases pertaining to people with diabetes. These use cases were selected to highlight how clinical and health knowledge can be combined with "big data" sources of personal behaviors and personal context, to provide insights that are relevant to both health consumers and the clinicians who serve them. The remainder of this chapter is organized as follows: In Sect. "Semantic Technologies and the Personal Health Knowledge Graph", we provide an introductory overview of semantic technologies, highlighting key concepts related to knowledge graphs and defining Personal Health Knowledge Graph (PHKG). In Sect. "Combining Learning and Logic for Personal Health Applications", we explain how methods that combine machine learning and semantic technologies are able to exploit the best of machine learning and knowledge graphs, allowing computers to simultaneously tap into deep data and deep knowledge. To ground our discussion in a personal health application, Section "Nutrition Self-Management for People with Type 2 Diabetes" describes the experiences of people with type 2 diabetes who are engaging in self-management behaviors, and includes two examples of how semantic technologies have been used in conjunction with machine learning and data mining to generate personalized and context-aware meal recommendations. We close our chapter with a discussion of the many opportunities we see for using semantic technologies in the pursuit of improving personal health applications for health consumers.

Semantic Technologies and the Personal Health Knowledge Graph

Semantic technologies are used to enable computers to process data in ways that leverage the meaning of terms, such as through the use of logical reasoning. At the heart of these technologies is the *knowledge graph* (KG), which has been defined as "as a graph of data intended to accumulate and convey knowledge of the real world, whose nodes represent entities of interest and whose edges represent relations between these entities." (Hogan et al. 2022) DBpedia, YAGO and Wikidata are examples of public knowledge graphs generated from content available in Wikipedia, a crowd-sourced encyclopedia available on the Internet (Ringler and Paulheim 2017; Abián et al. 2018; Pillai et al. 2019). Knowledge graphs inherit from classic artificial intelligence such formalisms as semantic networks and description logics (Baader et al. 2007). The advantages of using knowledge graphs to represent knowledge are that they are amenable to the linking of knowledge across multiple sources and domains (through identifying overlapping semantic concepts across ontologies). To be regarded as high-quality, knowledge represented in knowledge graphs should be consistent, and feature a certain degree of completeness, accuracy and timeliness (i.e., degree to which knowledge is kept up-to-date) along with containing provenance content (where the knowledge came from). *Semantic reasoners* are capable of inferring new knowledge from the data contained in knowledge graphs. These reasoners may be based on logic (e.g., first-order logic, predicate logic, non-monotonic logic), fuzzy logic, or machine learning. The use of machine learning methods for reasoning over KGs has been of rising interest in the artificial intelligence community, due to the rapid and parallel growth in availability of very large, electronic data sets and access to computing power. Section "Combining Learning and Logic for Personal Health Applications" of this chapter discusses the advantages of combining machine learning and semantic technologies, and our subsequent use cases in Sect. "Nutrition Self-Management for People with Type 2 Diabetes" demonstrate a combined use of both types of approaches for personal health applications. For a recent survey on methods for reasoning over knowledge graphs, the reader is referred to Chen et al. (Chen et al. 2020).

Semantic technologies are often at the core of interactive decision-support systems that have to deal with complex knowledge. They are useful for addressing key challenges in knowledge management such as finding, summarizing or answering questions pertaining to information contained in electronic medical records, legal documents and scientific literature. Typical functions performed using semantic technologies include: entity summarization, faceted search, and question answering. Entity summarization involves generating a concise description of what is known about an entity, such that it satisfies users' information needs (Liu et al. 2021; Cheng et al. 2020). Faceted search is a method of finding information that allows users to progressively navigate towards more relevant results using filters that are meaningful within the search domain (e.g., searching for recipes based on filters for nutritional content, cuisine, preparation time, etc.) (Arenas et al. 2016). Question and answering over knowledge bases allows users to seek answers (from the knowledge graph) to questions posed in natural language (Arenas et al. 2016; Moschitti et al. 2017). Before the invention of the World Wide Web (WWW), semantic technologies were used within large organizations with significant institutional knowledge bases, and wherein knowledge representation could be centralized (Pan et al. 2017). With the invention of the WWW, the potential for semantic technologies to enable intelligent agents that could 'traverse' globally linked knowledge became an exciting and real proposition (Berners-Lee et al. 2001; Hendler 2003). Applications using the KG should be able to provide a set of knowledge services, which should be feature high reliability (e.g., fast response time, and high fault tolerance) and high usability (e.g., good learnability).

When constructing knowledge graphs, the usual assumption is that the entities and the relationships between entities are shaped by domain experts, who define an *ontology*. The ontology defines the vocabulary that is used to describe the various concepts, relations and axioms that need to be represented in the knowledge graph.

The knowledge graph then uses the terms from that ontology when representing assertions regarding individuals, instances within the domain of interest. The ontology may be partially or entirely contained within the knowledge graph itself. The process of ontology engineering (Kendall and McGuinness 2019) lies in capturing necessary and sufficient conditions for including terms, and connections between terms, in the ontology. Complementary to such a 'top-down' approach is a 'bottom-up' approach, wherein new knowledge is generated (through descriptive statistics and/or logical inference) from specific instances of the data. Using this approach, new categories and related concepts can be derived, resulting in the creation of new knowledge. Since the construction of large knowledge graphs can be time consuming, various efforts exist to increase the degree of automation of knowledge graph construction. For example, the Semantic Data Dictionary (SDD) approach is able to facilitate automatic creation of knowledge graphs by semantically annotating tabular data with concepts from existing ontologies (Rashid et al. 2020). Furthermore, the automated knowledge base construction community has been employing natural language processing techniques to develop knowledge graphs (Suchanek et al. 2013a), and these efforts have given rise to the Automated Knowledge Base Construction workshop series (Suchanek et al. 2013b), that has now become a full-fledged conference (https://www.akbc.ws), which supplements parallel efforts by the larger semantic web community.

The World Wide Web Consortium (W3C) has established standards for implementing semantic technologies. The Resource Description Framework (RDF) is the basic mechanism through which basic statements can be made. The RDF data model is based upon the idea of making statements about resources in expressions of the form *subject–predicate–object*, known as an RDF *triple*. The *subject* denotes the resource, and the *predicate* denotes traits or aspects of the resource and expresses a relationship between the subject and the *object*. For example, one way to represent the statement "The lasagna contains meat" in RDF is as the triple: a subject denoting "the lasagna", a predicate denoting "contains", and an object denoting "meat". RDF triples can be serialized using several alternative syntaxes, including *N-Triples*, *Turtle*, *RDF/XML*, and *JSON-LD*. Examples of how the triple for "the lasagna"-"contains"-"meat" using the alternative RDF data formats are shown below.

Using *N-Triples* syntax:

```
<http://example.com/exampleOntology#Lasagna>
<http://example.com/exampleOntology#contains>
<http://example.com/exampleOntology#Meat> .
```

Using *Turtle* syntax:

```
@prefix ex: <http://example.com/exampleOntology#> .
ex:Lasagna ex:contains ex:Meat .
```

Using *RDF/XML* syntax:

```
<?xml version="1.0" encoding="utf-8" ?>
  <rdf:RDF xmlns:rdf="http://www.w3.org/1999/02/22-rdf-syntax-
      ns#" xmlns:ns0="http://example.com/exampleOntology#">

<rdf:Description rdf:about="http://example.com/
    exampleOntology#Lasagna">
<ns0:contains rdf:resource="http://example.com/
    exampleOntology#Meat"/>
</rdf:Description>
</rdf:RDF>
```

Using the *JSON-LD* syntax:

```
[
  { "@id":"http://example.com/exampleOntology#Lasagna",
    "http://example.com/exampleOntology#contains":[
            {"@id":"http://example.com/exampleOntology#Meat"}
    ]
  },
  {"@id":"http://example.com/exampleOntology#Meat"}
]
```

While RDF is a way of representing knowledge graphs, languages such as the RDF Schema (RDFS) language and the Web Ontology Language (OWL) can be used to define ontologies. While OWL is more expressive than RDFS, it is also more complex to use. Both OWL and RDFS are recommended standards by the W3C. For more on semantic modeling in RDFS and OWL, readers are referred to an introductory text by Allenmang and Hendler (Allemang et al. 2020) and Ontology Engineering text by Kendall and McGuinness (Kendall and McGuinness, 2019).

The predominant query language for RDF graphs is SPARQL, (pronounced *spahr- kuhl*, and it is the recursive acronym for SPARQL Protocol And Query Language) is an SQL-like query language for RDF that has been standardized by the W3C. The following is an example of a SPARQL query to show all foods contained within a menu named `italian_menu`, using a fictional ontology called `exampleOntology`:

```
PREFIX ex: <http://example.com/exampleOntology#>
SELECT ?food ?menu
WHERE {
    ?x ex:foodname ?food ; ex:isContainedin ?y .
    ?y ex:menuname ?menu ; ex:isInMenu ex:italian_menu .
}
```

While most popular knowledge graphs capture entities that are of global relevance (i.e., of interest to the general population), knowledge graphs that capture data that is relevant only to a particular individual (i.e., a *personal knowledge graph*), can also be useful. Given the large amount of data that is now being tracked and recorded from personal activities, and increased consumer demand for more personalized services, in particular for health and wellness, reasoning over a personal knowledge graph presents an opportunity for generating insights highly relevant to the person whose data is represented in the knowledge graph. Moreover, if data in a personal knowledge graph is linked to data in general knowledge graphs, a reasoner could generate insights that relate a personal experience to those in the general population. Balog and Kenter (Balog and Kenter 2019) present the concept of the personal knowledge graph and how it differs from general knowledge graphs. They note an increased, but fragmented amount of research relating to personal knowledge graphs, and propose a research agenda for personal knowledge graphs. Meanwhile, Gyrard et al. (Gyrard et al. 2018) specifically consider the concept of a personal knowledge graph for health, which integrates and represents all health information specific to an individual, including their medical history and health behaviors, as well as relevant socio-environmental factors that the individual may be exposed to. They also identify several research challenges for advancing the state-of-the-art in personal knowledge graphs for health, including how to model and integrate general health and personal health knowledge, and how to analyze data from the Internet-of-Things (IoT) to produce meaningful contextual information for supporting health behavior change. For additional perspectives on personal knowledge graphs for health, the reader is referred to (Rastogi and Zaki 2020) and (Shirai et al. 2021). In this chapter, we consider a *Personal Health Knowledge Graph* (PHKG) to be a knowledge graph representation of a person's health and wellness data. This data may come from various sources (e.g., physical activity trackers, digital food logs, personal health records). In Sect. "Populating a Personal Health Knowledge Graph with Personalized Assessments of Dietary Needs and Preferences" we will describe how a PHKG can be automatically constructed from a user's temporal food log data, and how the PHKG can be used (along with general health knowledge) to derive a user's dietary needs and preferences. Then, in Sect. "Personalizing Dietary Recommendations" we describe how to identify recipes that satisfy these needs and preferences.

Combining Learning and Logic for Personal Health Applications

In the context of personal health, the combination of knowledge graphs and machine learning opens up new possibilities for designing effective digital health assistant applications (Thomas Craig et al. 2020). The use of conversational agents in digital health applications is a popular design choice because it supports natural language queries from the user. These natural language queries need to be converted into SPARQL queries if one wants to answer the query by retrieving information from a knowledge graph. While SPARQL is well-suited to retrieve factual information stored in the knowledge graph, and also to infer answers via reasoning, it is not well-suited for answering ranking based queries (i.e., multiple answers that are sorted in order of relevance) that arise in recommendation settings. Indeed, in personal health applications, users may seek recommendations and/or facts to support decisions about what health behaviors to engage in. In recommendation settings, the answer to the user's query should ideally be personalized to take into account a user's intent, context and constraints. As it turns out, such personalized responses can be provided via machine learning based methods, such as knowledge base question answering (KBQA).

Learning-based methods have the advantages of discovering and leveraging implicit semantics, and can scale to large datasets. However, learning is data-intensive, can produce trivial or known insights and insights are often difficult to explain. Knowledge-based methods have the advantages of being able to explicitly represent and use knowledge without requiring "big data", and this knowledge is easier to transfer between projects. On the other hand, capturing knowledge is labor intensive and logical inference can be computationally intensive. The best of both approaches can be captured via a hybrid approach that injects semantics within machine learning methods, and on flip side, leverages machine learning to scale up semantic approaches. In this section we will highlight the interaction between logic and learning for answering personalized user queries.

Since knowledge graphs store high quality information in a structured format, they are well-suited for answering factual queries by leveraging the underlying semantics. For example, a query like "What are some physical exercises I can try?" can be converted into the following SPARQL query.

```
SELECT DISTINCT ?exerciseName
WHERE {
    ?exercise <http://purl.org/dc/terms/subject> <http://dbpedia.
org/resource/Category:Physical_exercise>;
    <http://www.w3.org/2000/01/rdf-schema#label> ?exerciseLabel .
BIND (STR(?exerciseLabel) AS ?exerciseName)
}
```

Interpreted as a factual retrieval question, this query would return a list of physical exercises, which can then be displayed to the user. However, it is clear that returning a long list of exercises is probably not what the user intends as the response. Rather, the user's context and preferences should be taken into account while answering such a query. For example, taking into consideration the fact that the user might be at the gym, or taking into account their health goals (e.g., lose weight) and their exercise preferences and also their physical ability, and so on. Going even further, this query can be interpreted as asking for recommendation of physical exercises, e.g., "what are some physical exercises I can try that are good for

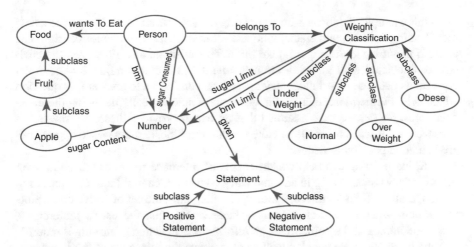

Fig. 10.1 Example of the inference rules and ontology for answering the query "Can I eat a Gala apple?"

me?" Instead of simple retrieval this may require the system to compare alternatives, and then suggest the most beneficial activities at that given place, time, and context, potentially along with an explanation of the suggestion.

As another example, consider the query "Can I eat a Gala apple?" To answer this question well, the system should recognize that there could be an implicit context at play. Namely, the user may be concerned about weight management, or other relevant underlying health conditions. To answer this query we need to rely on a reasoning engine over the personal knowledge graph, as illustrated in Fig. 10.1.

The logic for the inference required to answer this query is captured by the inference rules below.

```
Rule 0:
Subclass Transitivity
Rule 1:
(Person and
(person:bmi > WeightClassification:bmiLimit))
=>
Person belongsTo
[owl:equivalentClass WeightClassification] .

Rule 2:
(Person and
(WeightClassification and (Person:wantsToEat Food) and
(Person:sugarConsumed + Food:sugarContent > WeightClassification:s
ugarLimit))))
=>
Person given NegativeStatement .
```

In this example, the focus is on comparing the sugar limit for the person based on their health condition and status, who are returning that they cannot eat the Gala apple if they exceed the sugar intake limit. This example also illustrates the challenges associated with inferring the user intent and health conditions. Additional constraints besides sugar intake may have to be considered to answer this question adequately. Furthermore, there is the question of automatically deducing the inference rules. So far, we have assumed that an expert provides these. However, this approach is not scalable, and is a challenge that machine learning-based approaches are in a good position to address.

Machine learning can help construct sets of inference rules for reasoning over the KG. They can also help in automatically converting natural language queries to SPARQL queries. Furthermore, learning can help infer the set of active constraints to consider when answering a query—these would span the user's preferences, health guidelines, and all other relevant information. In general, learning is required to hone in on the user intent, as well as to evaluate the relevance of the input constraints and responses. On the other hand, machine learning methods can benefit tremendously from the structured knowledge in the knowledge graphs by leveraging the underlying semantics of the concepts and relationships. For example, knowledge graph embedding methods (Bordes et al. 2011) can be employed to learn concept and relationship embeddings, or representations, that can be used in a deep learning framework to answer user queries.

The combination of semantics and machine learning is even more important when dealing with queries that involve providing recommendations. For example, a user may ask "What is a good breakfast for me?" To answer this type of query, the machine learning framework would have to leverage the interlinked knowledge graphs such as their personal health knowledge graph, a medical guidelines knowledge graph, and a food knowledge graph.

If all of the constraints (e.g., food preferences, allergies, ingredient availability, etc.) are treated as mandatory constraints, the answer is likely to be a null set. While SPARQL provides the OPTIONAL clause to allow for optional constraints, the resulting answer set is not trivial to rank based on relevance to the query (Feyznia et al. 2014). Such queries can be answered by KBQA based methods such as BAMNET (Chen et al. 2019), which is an end-to-end bidirectional attention memory network for complex question answering over a knowledge graph. Readers are referred to Fu et al. (Fu et al. 2020) for an in-depth review of KBQA methods. In more recent work, we have developed a novel system for personalized food recommendation, called *pFoodReq* (Chen et al. 2021) that uses constrained question answering over a food knowledge graph to help users search for relevant recipes. We describe *pFoodReq* in detail in Sect. "Personalizing Dietary Recommendations".

Nutrition Self-Management for People with Type 2 Diabetes

Diabetes is a chronic health condition that affects approximately 10.5% of the United States population (National Diabetes Statistics Report 2020). People with diabetes are typically advised to engage in several self-management behaviors in order to improve their health outcomes. People newly diagnosed with diabetes or pre-diabetes, and advised to modify their diet face numerous challenges. In addition to understanding which specific dietary guidelines apply to them, they must also understand how these guidelines translate into specific actions and food choices they can make. Then they must actually implement these changes. Successful behavior change requires understanding and knowledge of the guidelines and nutritional content of different foods and their impact. It requires introspection on their current dietary behavior to understand what changes need to be made and the relative importance of making those changes. Beyond understanding what to do, changing one's diet is notoriously difficult. It can require changing long-term habits, eschewing foods one enjoys, and avoiding foods that are prominent in social gatherings or play an important role in their cultural cuisine. As such, the challenges are both informational—understanding (and remembering) what changes to make and specifically how to implement them, and motivational—providing messages, options, and specific suggestions to encourage making good choices and making doing so as appealing and non-disruptive as possible.

Our current efforts aim to address these challenges by surfacing the health guidelines relevant to a specific user, explaining why those guidelines apply to them, and suggesting foods the user could eat. We also aim to help the user understand their current dietary behavior to see where they are successfully adhering to the guidelines and what changes would be most beneficial to make.

We describe two use cases in the following subsections. In the first use case described in Sect. "Populating a Personal Health Knowledge Graph with Personalized Assessments of Dietary Needs and Preferences", we review a user's food log (i.e., a daily diary of meals consumed) through the lens of a set of relevant dietary guidelines, and generate semantic expressions in the OWL language to represent the gaps between their actual and expected food consumption patterns. In this use case, we combine semantic technologies with data mining methods. In the second use case described in Sect. "Personalizing Dietary Recommendations", suggests specific foods that will fit a user's dietary guidelines and food preferences. In this use case we combine semantic technologies with machine learning. An essential knowledge resource common to both use cases is the Food Knowledge Graph (FoodKG). The FoodKG was constructed by Haussmann et al. (Haussmann et al. 2019) and integrates recipe data from the Recipe1M+ data set (Marín et al. 2021) with ingredient nutritional information from the United States Department of Agriculture's National Nutrient Database for Standard Reference (Haytowitz et al. 2019). The FoodKG uses the FoodOn ontology (Dooley et al. 2018). Resources and instructions for constructing the FoodKG are provided at `https://foodkg.github.io/foodkg.html`.

Populating a Personal Health Knowledge Graph with Personalized Assessments of Dietary Needs and Preferences

In this section, we demonstrate how semantic technologies can be combined with data mining techniques to generate semantic expressions of a user's dietary needs and preferences. In this example, the user's dietary needs are assessed by comparing the user's recent eating patterns with relevant health guidelines set by the American Diabetes Association (ADA) (American Diabetes Association 2021). Any gaps between the user's behaviors and the guidelines are considered to represent the user's current dietary needs. The user's dietary preferences can also be discovered from their reported eating patterns. These dietary needs and preferences can be captured in the user's personal health knowledge graph (PHKG) and queried by downstream applications. Unlike most efforts for automatic KG population, which extract entities and relationships from unstructured text using natural language processing methods, we discover relevant patterns from time-series data in our use case. To support this use case, we created the Personal Health Ontology (PHO) based on a set of interviews conducted with 21 people who declared themselves to be within five years of being diagnosed with type 2 diabetes. Using a semi-structured interview style, we asked participants to describe their eating patterns and probed specifically about the contextual, health and lifestyle factors that influenced their eating behaviors. The PHO differs from existing efforts such as (Puustjarvi and Puustjarvi 2011), which have put a focus on interoperability of various e-health tools through a shared vocabulary. In contrast, our focus was on capturing the personal behavioral preferences. The essential steps involved in populating a PHKG with the user's dietary needs and preferences are four-fold: (i) relevant eating patterns need to be discovered from temporal food log data (ii) eating patterns need to be mapped to a personal health ontology (iii) eating patterns need to be assessed against medical nutrition therapy guidelines (iv) semantic 'directives' for health needs need to be inferred. These steps are depicted in Fig. 10.2.

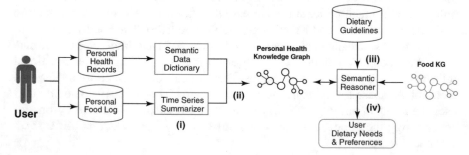

Fig. 10.2 Illustration of how personal health data from the user is transformed by the Time Series Summarizer (Harris et al. 2021) and Semantic Data Dictionary (Rashid et al. 2020) into RDF triples that populate a PHKG. A semantic reasoner is used to generate expressions of the users dietary needs and preferences based on the PHKG and clinical dietary guidelines

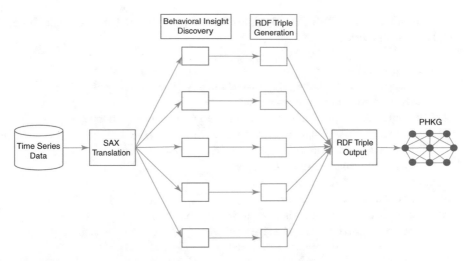

Fig. 10.3 Workflow to discover behavioral insights within a user's food log data and generate RDF triples to populate the PHKG

To implement the use case depicted in Fig. 10.2, we customized an existing Time-Series Summarization (TSS) framework (Harris et al. 2021) to generate RDF triples representing a user's temporal personal health data (e.g., digital food diaries, personal wearables logs). The TSS applies advanced data mining approaches to discover patterns within time-series data. In order to identify 'interesting' patterns, the TSS framework relies on a dimensionality reduction algorithm called Symbolic Aggregate Approximation (SAX) (Lin et al. 2007) to translate the raw time-series data into a string of alphabetical letters (e.g., 'abbbacdac'). Each of these letters can represent different time granularities (e.g., 'a' can represent a day or a week in the data). Data mining algorithms, such as the frequent item-set mining tool called SPADE (Zaki 2001) and the categorical clustering algorithm called *Squeezer* (He et al. 2002), are used to search the data for patterns once the data is translated into categorical data. Once a pattern is retrieved, it is represented as a template-based natural language summary, or 'protoform'. An example protoform is "On *<quantifier><sub-time window (plural)>* in the past *<time window (singular)>*, your *<attribute>* was *<summarizer>*." Within this protoform, there are five defined placeholders that are each filled with words/phrases chosen from a predefined vocabulary. An example of how this example protoform could be filled is "On *most of the days* in the past *week*, your *calorie intake* was *high*." This framework uses extended versions of rule-based linguistic summarization algorithms that use fuzzy logic to select the correct words/phrases for a protoform (Zadeh 2002; Zadeh 1983; Zadeh 1975; Kacprzyk et al. 2002). TSS was customized to produce RDF triples that would conform with the PHO. The TSS workflow is shown in Fig. 10.3.

An example set of TSS PHKG triples with respect to the user's carbohydrate intake is as follows[1]:

```
:Alice  a prov:Person;
        sio:has-attribute  :AliceInsulinMedicationDosage,
        :AliceCarbIntakePattern  .
:AliceInsulinMedicationDosage a pho:FixedMedicationDosage.
:AliceCarbIntakePattern a pho:ConsistentPattern;
        sio:has-attribute        chebi:carbohydrate,
        :AliceCarbIntakePatternSumm,
:AliceCarbIntakePatternCV,
:AliceCarbIntakeTimeWindow.
:AliceCarbIntakePatternSumm a pho:Summarizer;
        sio:has-value "considerably" .
:AliceCarbIntakePatternCV a stato:CoefficientofVariation;
        sio:has-value "0.99" .
:AliceCarbIntakeTimeWindow a pho:TimeWindow;
        sio:has-value sio:week  .
```

Once the RDF triples from the user's daily personal logs have been generated, we implemented a semantic reasoner to evaluate the generated graph against guidelines that determine whether the user has complied with the applicable medical and dietary guidelines. To that end, we modeled several ADA guidelines related to diet and activity into a computable form using OWL. As an example, consider the following ADA guideline recommendation (American Diabetes Association 2021), which we will refer to as 'Dietary-Guideline-01':

> For individuals whose daily insulin dosing is fixed, a consistent pattern of carbohydrate intake with respect to time and amount may be recommended to improve glycemic control and reduce the risk of hypoglycemia.

The guideline contains a *rule* portion that indicates the necessary and sufficient conditions, and a *directive* that indicates what action to take if the rule was evaluated to be true. A semantic reasoner can ingest such ADA guidelines implemented as *rules* and the PHKG triples output from the TSS to recommend a course of action in the form of a *directive*,

---

[1] The full form of the prefixes used in the code listings are as follows:

- **chebi** http://purl.obolibrary.org/obo/chebi#
- **owl** http://www.w3.org/2002/07/owl#
- **pho** http://idea.rpi.edu/heals/pho#
- **prov** http://www.w3.org/ns/prov#
- **rdf** http://www.w3.org/1999/02/22-rdf-syntax-ns#
- **rdfs** http://www.w3.org/2000/01/rdf-schema#
- **sio** http://semanticscience.org/resource/
- **stato** http://purl.obolibrary.org/obo/stato.owl#

The *rule* (i.e., Dietary-Guideline-01) is represented in OWL as follows. First, this rule applies an OWL property restriction on any instances of the `pho:FixedMedicationDosage` on its *has-attribute* property (i.e., our patient should be taking a fixed medication dose for this rule to take effect). Then we check to see if the patient has been following a `pho:ConsistentPattern` of `chebi:carbohydrate` consumption, which is again implemented as an OWL property restriction.

```
pho:Dietary-Guideline-01 rdf:type owl:Class ;
   owl:equivalentClass
     [ owl:intersectionOf (
        [ rdf:type owl:Restriction ;
            owl:onProperty sio:has-attribute ;
            owl:someValuesFrom pho: FixedMedicationDosage ]
        [ rdf:type owl:Restriction ;
            owl:onProperty sio:has-attribute ;
            owl:someValuesFrom [
              owl:intersectionOf (
                 pho:ConsistentPattern
                    [ rdf:type owl:Restriction ;
                      owl:onProperty sio:has-attribute ;
                      owl:someValuesFrom chebi:carbohydrate ] ) ;
                    rdf:type owl:Class]
              ] ) ;
          rdf:type owl:Class] ;
   rdfs:subClassOf pho:DietaryGuideline ;
   rdfs:label "For a diabetic individual, if their daily insulin
dosing is fixed, and there is a consistent pattern of carbohydrate
intake with respect to time and amount, that pattern should be main-
tained." .
```

Note that concepts such as `pho:FixedMedicationDosage`, `pho:ConsistentPattern`, and `chebi:carbohydrate` that are mentioned in the rule are defined in the corresponding ontologies, i.e. Personal Health Ontology (PHO) and Chemical Entities of Biological Interest (ChEBI). For example, the consistent pattern is defined as follows, which indicates that a `pho:ConsistentPattern` should consist of some `pho:TimeWindow` (i.e., week, day, month, etc.) and a `pho:Summarizer` (slightly, considerably, etc.):

```
pho:ConsistentPattern rdf:type owl:Class ;
    owl:equivalentClass [
    owl:intersectionOf (
        [ rdf:type owl:Restriction ;
            owl:onProperty sio:has-attribute ;
            owl:someValuesFrom pho:TimeWindow ]
        [ rdf:type owl:Restriction ;
            owl:onProperty sio:has-attribute ;
            owl:someValuesFrom pho:Summarizer ] ) ;
    rdf:type owl:Class] ;
    rdfs:subClassOf pho:TemporalPattern .
```

The *directive* is represented in OWL in the following manner. This is a custom declaration to suit our specific application, which simply states that if a certain PHKG instance is conforming to the above *rule*, that instance would be classified under Dietary-Guideline-01 and has an associated pho:hasDirective Representation that provides the python programmatic representation for the *constraints* (i.e., the lower and upper limits of the carbohydrate intake along with the daily total limit) that would be plugged into KBQA as an input.

```
pho:ConsistentCarbIntakeDirective rdf:type owl:Class ;
    owl:equivalentClass [ rdf:type owl:Restriction ;
        owl:onProperty sio:has-attribute ;
        owl:someValuesFrom pho:LowCarb] ,
        [ rdf:type owl:Restriction ;
        owl:onProperty sio:is-associated-with ;
        owl:allValuesFrom pho:Dietary-Guideline-01] ;
        rdfs:subClassOf pho:Directive ;
        pho:hasDirectiveRepresentation
        """{'carbohydrate' :
        { 'unit': 'g', 'meal' : { 'type': 'range', 'lower' : '30',
        'upper': '45' }, 'daily total' : '150'}}""" ;
        rdf:label "Baseline carbohydrate level should be 30g - 45g
per carbs per meal and for the whole day 150g max.".
```

Using the available set of OWL formalizations for ADA guidelines and the PHKG, a semantic reasoner can be used to infer whether our user, i.e., *Alice*, has been adhering to behaviors consistent with the guidelines. A corresponding set of rules can be created to capture any cases of guideline violations. Then the semantic representations allow us first to identify the eventual deviation and then to provide evidence-based recommendations based on their lifestyle and diabetes condition.

Ongoing and future work is focused on expanding the set of addressable queries and integrating personal health records with the PHO. Therefore, our ongoing work includes: (1) expanding the PHO to further accommodate concepts important for comparing behaviors to ADA guidelines, (2) applying the semantic data dictionary (Rashid et al. 2020) approach to the conversion of personal health records into RDF triples that are consistent with the PHO, and (3) linking the PHKG to other semantic resources such as the Healthy LifeStyle (HeLiS) ontology (Dragoni et al. 2018).

Personalizing Dietary Recommendations

In this section, we present the personalized food recommender *pFoodReq* (Chen et al. 2021), a recommender system for answering questions that seek relevant food recommendations (e.g., "What is a Chinese dish with beef that does not include ginger?"). *pFoodReq* frames the recommender problem as that of performing knowledge base question and answering (KBQA). While recommender systems (De Croon et al. 2021) need not use semantic technologies, KBQA methods do, by definition, require a knowledge graph. Specifically, KBQA systems assume that a subset of the nodes in the knowledge graph contains answers to a general class of questions, and that the relationships between graph entities are useful for identifying good answers. Typically, questions are posed in natural language and the function of the KBQA system is to efficiently and effectively identify relevant and correct answers to the question, from the knowledge graph. Here, we will describe the specific approach used by *pFoodReq* to retrieve recipes from the FoodKG. Figure 10.4 shows the core elements of the *pFoodReq* system. At the heart of the system is a KBQA component that retrieves recipes from the FoodKG. In Fig. 10.4, the "User Dietary Needs & Preferences" could be extracted from users'

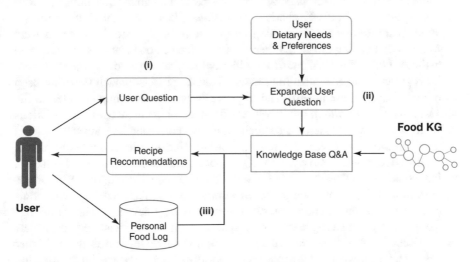

Fig. 10.4 Illustration of how a user's question is combined with a directive regarding the user's general dietary needs and preferences to produce an expanded question that is provided to a KBQA model, resulting in a set of recipes retrieved from the Food Knowledge Graph

PHKG by a semantic reasoner, as presented in Sect. "Populating a Personal Health Knowledge Graph with Personalized Assessments of Dietary Needs and Preferences".

The KBQA model in *pFoodReq* has been trained to retrieve recipes from the FoodKG as answers to questions that are expressed as a combination of 'positive' (i.e., attributes to be included) and 'negative' (attributes to be excluded) constraints. Attributes that can be accommodated include recipe ingredients (e.g., mushrooms, peanuts), nutritional content (e.g., carbohydrates, fat), and cuisine/ diet/dish type (e.g., Korean, vegan, dessert). Examples of these questions are: *What are jellies recipes that contain orange? What turkish or dinner-party recipes can I cook without milk? Can you recommend low protein russian recipes which have onions?* Although the user's question (refer to (i) in Fig. 10.4) represents the user's immediate preferences, people with diabetes also have long-term health needs. For example, according to the ADA guidelines (American Diabetes Association 2021), diabetics may need to control their caloric intake, target high fiber foods, or avoid carbohydrates with high protein content. Since any recipes recommended by *pFoodReq* would be expected to accommodate these needs, *pFoodReq* may expand the user's question (refer to (ii) in Fig. 10.4) to include constraints related to these needs, even though the user does not include them in their question. For example, the user's question *"What turkish or dinner- party recipes can I cook without milk?"* would be expanded by *pFoodReq* to become *"What turkish or dinner-party recipes can I cook without milk and includes carbohydrates within the desired range of 5 g to 30 g?"* In general, if a user typically avoids certain foods, these foods can also be appended to the user's question as a negative constraint.

Rather than semantically parsing the user's natural language questions and converting them into SPARQL queries, *pFoodReq* adopts an information retrieval approach that relies on a large training set of 'ground-truth' questions and answers to train a deep learning model that learns how to locate good answers to a question from the *FoodKG*. However, questions with positive and negative constraints are not easily represented in deep learning models. Hence, a new approach for using deep learning to handle these positive and negative constraints was implemented in the KBQA model in *pFoodReq*. Intuitively, the deep learning model learns associations between words in the question sentence and the corresponding answer (recipe) entity, or entities, and its nearby (recipe and non-recipe) entities and relationships in the knowledge graph. Unlike a SPARQL query (without an OPTIONAL clause), which would treat all answers satisfying the query as equally relevant, *pFoodReq*'s deep learning KBQA approach produces a continuous, scalar score for each candidate answer, allowing them to be ranked in priority of 'relevance.' These rankings are generated by comparing learned representations of the candidate recipe answers (Li and Zaki 2020) with recipes in the user's historical food log and assigning higher scores to recipe answers that are more semantically similar to recipes in the food log (refer to (iii) in Fig. 10.4). The full details of the deep learning model used for KBQA in *pFoodReq* are provided in an earlier methodological paper by Chen, Wu and Zaki (Chen et al. 2019).

Summary

In this chapter, we have described how semantic technologies and machine learning can be used to bring both logic and learning to personal health applications. We have shared two use cases related to supporting dietary behaviors for people with diabetes. In our first use case, we showed how semantic technologies and data mining were used to extract, represent and reason over applicable dietary health guidelines and past user behaviors, resulting in a personal health knowledge graph that contains knowledge about a user's health preferences and needs. In our second use case, the user's health preferences and needs provide context to a user's question, allowing the recommendations to the user to consider the user's immediate and ongoing interests. There remains a significant opportunity to enhance and expand upon the ideas presented in this chapter. For example, the scope of the PHO is still limited, as are the number of ADA guidelines represented in OWL and the types of RDF triples that the TSS generates. Several dimensions of the user context could also be incorporated, such as geographical location, social context and financial constraints. Additionally, KBQA remains an active area of research from both a methodological and an application-oriented perspective.

A major advantage of using semantic models (particularly in comparison to machine learning models) is that they are inherently interpretable, and therefore amenable to providing explanations for their results. Readers are referred to works by Dragoni et al. (Dragoni et al. 2020; Dragoni et al. 2018), which present state-of-the-art applications of semantics for explainable, personalized health insights. Further, extending the work described in this chapter, we are modeling an ontology for food and diet recommendation explanations, called the Food Explanation Ontology (FEO) (Padhiar et al. 2021). FEO can be used to generate various types of explanations, such as contextual, contrastive, and counterfactual. Many of these facets can supplement the clinically relevant personal health applications in promoting effective behavior change through suitable explanations. Ideally, a personal health application would be able to provide explanations for any suggestions and recommendations, to improve their overall understanding of their health condition, the health guidelines, and their behaviors.

To keep the scope of this chapter amenable to readers new to semantic technologies, we have limited our discussion to the most salient and essential ideas and trends. There is a vast body of literature on semantic technologies, such as various reasoning techniques (higher order (Eiter et al. 2006), probabilistic (Giugno and Lukasiewicz 2002), causal (Gudivada et al. 2008)), OWL2 profiles (Motik et al. 2009), and linking data using protocols such as Linked Data Platform (Mihindukulasooriya et al. 2013), all of which are quite useful when considering the next generation personal health applications powered by semantics. The software and ontologies described in this chapter are available at `https://github.com/semantics-for-personal-health/semantics-for-personal-health.github.io`. This work was conducted as part of the

Health Empowerment by Analytics, Learning and Semantics (HEALS) project (HEALS 2017). The primary goal of the HEALS (Health Empowerment by Analytics, Learning, and Semantics) project is to apply advanced cognitive computing capabilities to help people understand and improve their own health conditions.

Acknowledgements This work is supported by IBM Research AI through the AI Horizons Network.

References

Abián D, Guerra F, Martínez-Romanos J, Trillo-Lado R. Wikidata and DBpedia: a comparative study. In: Szymański J, Velegrakis Y, editors. Semantic keyword-based search on structured data sources. Cham: Springer International Publishing; 2018. p. 142–54.

Allemang D, Hendler J, Gandon F. Semantic web for the working ontologist: effective modeling for linked data, RDFS, and OWL. 3rd ed. New York, NY: Association for Computing Machinery; 2020.

American Diabetes Association Standards of Medical Care in Diabetes—2021; 2021. https://doi.org/10.2337/dc21-S005.

Arenas M, Cuenca Grau B, Kharlamov E, Marciuška Š, Zheleznyakov D. Faceted search over RDF-based knowledge graphs. Journal of Web Semantics. 2016;37–38:55–74. https://www.sciencedirect.com/science/article/pii/S1570826815001432.

Baader F, Calvanese D, McGuinness D, Nardi D, Patel-Schneider P. The description logic handbook: theory, implementation and applications. 2nd ed. Cambridge University Press; 2007.

Balog K, Kenter T. Personal knowledge graphs: a research agenda. In: Proceedings of the ACM SIGIR International Conference on the Theory of Information Retrieval (ICTIR); 2019.

Berners-Lee T, Hendler J, Lassila O. The semantic web. Sci Am. 2001;284(5):34–43. http://www.jstor.org/stable/26059207.

Bipartisan Policy Center. What makes us healthy vs. what we spend on being healthy [Internet]; 2012 [cited April 15, 2021]. https://www.bipartisanpolicy.org/ report/ what-makes-us-healthy-vs-what-we-spend-on-being-healthy/.

Bordes A, Weston J, Collobert R, Bengio Y. Learning structured embeddings of knowledge bases. In: Proceedings of the Twenty-Fifth AAAI Conference on Artificial Intelligence. AAAI'11. AAAI Press; 2011. p. 301–306.

Bouton ME. Why behavior change is difficult to sustain. Prev Med. 2014;68:29–36.

Chen X, Jia S, Xiang Y. A review: knowledge reasoning over knowledge graph. Expert Syst Appl. 2020;141:112948. https://www.sciencedirect.com/science/article/pii/S0957417419306669

Chen Y, Subburathinam A, Chen CH, Zaki MJ. Personalized food recommendation as constrained question answering over a large-scale food knowledge graph. In: Proceedings of the 14th ACM International Conference on Web Search and Data Mining. WSDM '21. New York, NY, USA: Association for Computing Machinery; 2021. p. 544–552. https://doi.org/10.1145/3437963.3441816.

Chen Y, Wu L, Zaki MJ. Bidirectional attentive memory networks for question answering over knowledge bases. In: Annual Conference of the North American Chapter of the Association for Computational Linguistics; 2019.

Cheng G, Gunaratna K, Kharlamov E. Entity summarization in knowledge graphs: algorithms, evaluation, and applications. In: Companion Proceedings of the Web Conference 2020. WWW '20. New York, NY, USA: Association for Computing Machinery; 2020. p. 301–302: https://doi.org/10.1145/3366424.3383108.

De Croon R, Van Houdt L, Htun NN, Štiglic G, Vanden Abeele V, Verbert K. Health Recommender systems: systematic review. J Med Internet Res. 2021;23(6):e18035. https://www.jmir.org/2021/6/e18035

Dooley D, Griffiths E, Gosal G, Buttigieg P, Hoehndorf R, Lange M, et al. FoodOn: a harmonized food ontology to increase global food traceability, quality control and data integration. NPJ Sci Food. 2018;2:23.

Dragoni M and Bailoni T et al. Helis: An ontology for supporting healthy lifestyles. In: ISWC. Springer; 2018. p. 53–69.

Dragoni M, Donadello I, Eccher C. Explainable AI meets persuasiveness: translating reasoning results into behavioral change advice. Artif Intell Med. 2020;105:101840. https://www.sciencedirect.com/science/article/pii/S0933365719310140.

Eiter T, Ianni G, Schindlauer R, Tompits H. Effective integration of declarative rules with external evaluations for semantic-web reasoning. In: European Semantic Web Conference. Springer; 2006. p. 273–287.

Feyznia A, Kahani M, Zarrinkalam F. COLINA: A Method for Ranking SPARQL Query Results through Content and Link Analysis. In: Proceedings of the 2014 International Conference on Posters & Demonstrations Track – Volume 1272. ISWC-PD'14. Aachen, DEU: CEUR-WS. org; 2014. p. 273–276.

Fu B, Qiu Y, Tang C, Li Y, Yu H, Sun J. A survey on complex question answering over knowledge base: Recent advances and challenges. arXiv preprint arXiv:2007.13069. 2020 Jul 26.

Giugno R, Lukasiewicz T. P-SHOQ (D): a probabilistic extension of SHOQ (D) for probabilistic ontologies in the semantic web. In: JELIA. vol. 2. Springer; 2002. p. 86–97.

Gordon WJ, Landman A, Zhang H, Bates DW. Beyond validation: getting health apps into clinical practice. npj Dig Med. 2020;3:14.

Gudivada RC, Qu XA, Chen J, Jegga AG, Neumann EK, Aronow BJ. Identifying disease- causal genes using semantic web-based representation of integrated genomic and phenomic knowledge. J Biomed Inform. 2008;41(5):717–29.

Gyrard A, Gaur M, Thirunarayan K, Sheth AP, Shekarpour S. Personalized Health Knowledge Graph. In: CKGSemStats@ISWC; 2018.

Harris JJ, Chen CH, Zaki MJ. A framework for generating explanations from temporal personal health data. ACM Trans. Comput. Healthcare. 2021;02(21):1–43.

Haussmann S, Chen Y, Seneviratne O, Rastogi N, Codella J, Chen CH, et al. FoodKG enabled Q&A application. In: ISWC Satellites; 2019. p. 273–276.

Haytowitz DB, Ahuja JKC, Wu X, Somanchi M, Nickle M, Nguyen QA, et al. USDA National Nutrient Database for Standard Reference, Legacy Release [Data File]; 2019. [Cited 02 Apr 2021]. Nutrient Data Laboratory, Beltsville Human Nutrition Research Center, ARS, USDA. https://data.nal.usda.gov/dataset/usda-national-nutrient-database-standard-reference-legacy-release.

He Z, Xu X, Deng S. Squeezer: an efficient algorithm for clustering categorical data. J Comput Sci Technol. 2002;09(17):611–24.

HEALS: Health empowerment by analytics, learning, and semantics [Internet]; 2017 [updated April 2021; cited April 15, 2021]. https://idea.rpi.edu/research/projects/heals.

Hendler J. Science and the semantic web. Science. 2003;299(5606):520–1. https://science.sciencemag.org/content/299/5606/520.

Hogan A, Blomqvist E, Cochez M, d'Amato C, de Melo G, Gutierrez C, et al. Knowledge graphs. ACM Comput. Surv. 54(4), Article 71 (May 2022), 37 pages. https://doi.org/10.1145/3447772.

Kacprzyk J, Yager RR, Zadrozny S. In: Abramowicz W, Zurada J, editors. Fuzzy Linguistic summaries of databases for an efficient business data analysis and decision support. Boston, MA: Springer US; 2002. p. 129–52. https://doi.org/10.1007/0-306-46991-X_6.

Kelly MP, Barker M. Why is changing health-related behaviour so difficult? Public Health. 2016;136:109–16. https://www.sciencedirect.com/science/article/pii/S0033350616300178.

Kendall E, McGuinness D. Ontology engineering. In: Synthesis Lectures on The Semantic Web: Theory Technology. vol. 9; 2019. p. i–102.

Li D, Zaki MJ. RECIPTOR: an effective pretrained model for recipe representation learning. In: Proceedings of the 26th ACM SIGKDD International Conference on Knowledge Discovery & Data Mining. KDD '20. New York, NY, USA: Association for Computing Machinery; 2020. p. 1719–1727. https://doi.org/10.1145/3394486.3403223.

Lin J, Keogh JE, Wei L, Lonardi S. Experiencing SAX: a novel symbolic representation of time series. Data Min Knowl Disc. 2007;08(15):107–44.

Liu Q, Cheng G, Gunaratna K, Qu Y. Entity summarization: state of the art and future challenges. Journal of Web Semantics. vol. 69; May 2021.

Marín J, Biswas A, Ofli F, Hynes N, Salvador A, Aytar Y, et al. Recipe1M+: a dataset for learning cross-modal embeddings for cooking recipes and food images. IEEE Trans Pattern Anal Mach Intell. 2021;43(1):187–203.

Michie S, Thomas J, Johnston M, Aonghusa P, Shawe-Taylor J, Kelly M, et al. The human behaviour-change project: harnessing the power of artificial intelligence and machine learning for evidence synthesis and interpretation. Implement Sci. 2017;12(1):121.

Mihindukulasooriya N, Garcia-Castro R, Gutiérrez ME. Linked Data Platform as a novel approach for Enterprise Application Integration. In: COLD; 2013.

Moschitti A, Tymoshenko K, Alexopoulos P, Walker A, Nicosia M, Vetere G, et al. In: Pan JZ, Vetere G, Gomez-Perez JM, Wu H, editors. Question answering and knowledge graphs. Cham: Springer International Publishing; 2017. p. 181–212. https://doi.org/10.1007/978-3-319-45654-6_7.

Motik B, Grau BC, Horrocks I, Wu Z, Fokoue A, Lutz C, et al. OWL 2 web ontology language profiles. W3C Recommendation. 2009;27:61.

National Diabetes Statistics Report. Atlanta, GA; 2020.

Padhiar I, Seneviratne O, Chari S, Gruen D, McGuinness DL. Semantic modeling for food recommendation explanations; 2021. https://arxiv.org/abs/2105.01269.

Pan JZ, Vetere G, Gomez-Perez JM, Wu H, editors. Exploiting linked data and knowledge graphs in large organisations. Springer International Publishing; 2017.

Pillai SG, Soon LK, Haw SC. Comparing DBpedia, Wikidata, and YAGO for web information retrieval. In: Piuri V, Balas VE, Borah S, Syed Ahmad SS, editors. Intelligent and interactive computing. Singapore: Springer Singapore; 2019. p. 525–35.

Puustjarvi J, Puustjarvi L. Personal health ontology: towards the interoperation of e-health tools. Int J Electron Healthc. 2011;6(1):62–75.

Rashid SM, McCusker JP, Pinheiro P, Bax MP, Santos HO, Stingone JA, et al. The semantic data dictionary–an approach for describing and annotating data. Data Intelligence. 2020;2(4):443–86.

Rastogi N, Zaki MJ. Personal health knowledge graphs for patients. arXiv:2004.00071; 2020. https://doi.org/10.48550/arxiv.2004.00071.

Ringler D, Paulheim H. One knowledge graph to rule them all? Analyzing the differences between DBpedia, YAGO, Wikidata & co. In: Kern-Isberner G, Fürnkranz J, Thimm M, editors. KI 2017: advances in artificial intelligence. Cham: Springer International Publishing; 2017. p. 366–72.

Shirai S, Seneviratne O, McGuinness DL. Applying personal knowledge graphs to health. arXiv:2104.07587; 2021. https://doi.org/10.48550/arxiv.2104.07587.

Suchanek F, Fan J, Hoffmann R, Riedel S, Talukdar PP. Advances in automated knowledge base construction. SIGMOD Records journal, March. 2013a.

Suchanek FM, Riedel S, Singh S, Talukdar PP. AKBC 2013: third workshop on automated knowledge base construction. In: Proceedings of the 22nd ACM international conference on Information & Knowledge Management; 2013b. p. 2539–2540.

Thomas Craig KJ, Morgan LC, Chen CH, Michie S, Fusco N, Snowdon JL, et al. Systematic review of context-aware digital behavior change interventions to improve health. Transl Behav Med. 2020:10. https://doi.org/10.1093/tbm/ibaa099.

Zadeh LA. The concept of a linguistic variable and its application to approximate reasoning–I. Inf Sci. 1975;8(3):199–249.

Zadeh LA. A computational approach to fuzzy quantifiers in natural languages. Comput Math Appl. 1983;9(1):149–84.

Zadeh LA. A prototype-centered approach to adding deduction capability to search engines-the concept of protoform. In: IEEE Symposium on Intelligent Systems; 2002.

Zaki MJ. SPADE: an efficient algorithm for mining frequent sequences. Mach Learn. 2001;42(1):31–60.

Chapter 11
Privacy Predictive Models for Homecare Patient Sensing

Luyi Sun, Bian Yang, Egil Utheim, and Hao Luo

Abstract The pace of population aging has promoted the development of homecare monitoring systems and assisted living technologies. On the one hand, these technologies are supposed to help patients and the elderly at home to get help in any medical emergencies. On the other hand, such monitoring systems have raised the concern about patients' privacy. Though privacy-enhancing technologies for homecare sensing have been developed to protect patients' privacy, there have been few researches on patients' privacy attitudes towards different homecare sensing technologies, which may impact the practical performance of these sensing systems. Since individuals have different privacy attitudes towards the sensing systems and their needs in health monitoring, it would be interesting for the healthcare service providers and technology vendors to know about patients' privacy attitudes and how to model them into actionable privacy settings. In this chapter, we discuss the research state of the arts in this area and describe a preliminary study on this topic conducted recently. The chapter includes the following parts: first, an overview of homecare sensing and assisted living technologies; second, patients' privacy attitudes towards healthcare monitoring and video surveillance systems; third, legal and ethical considerations of using camera for patient monitoring; and finally, our findings from the preliminary study consists of focus group discussions and questionnaire used to collect people's privacy attitudes, and test results of applying different methods to predict patients' privacy preferences.

L. Sun (✉) · B. Yang
Department of Information Security and Communication Technology, NTNU i Gjøvik, Gjøvik, Norway
e-mail: luyi.sun@ntnu.no; bian.yang@ntnu.no

E. Utheim
VP Home and Healthcare, Halodi Robotics AS, Moss, Norway
e-mail: egil.utheim@sykehuset-innlandet.no

H. Luo
Zhejiang University, Yuquan Campus, Hangzhou, China
e-mail: luohao@zju.edu.cn

Keywords Privacy attitudes · Assisted living technologies · Machine learning · Privacy predictive model · Homecare sensing · Homecare monitoring system

Learning Objectives
1. Knowledge of the state of the arts in privacy-preserving health monitoring technologies
2. Knowledge of needs and concerns towards health monitoring technologies and the associated legal and ethical context
3. Skills in organizing focus group discussions and questionnaires to collect the privacy preference and the knowledge of preliminary analysis results from the collected data
4. Skills of using qualitative methods for characterizing personal privacy preferences and using quantitative methods for predicting personal privacy decisions
5. Skills of creating the personal privacy models and summarizing the limit of current work

Introduction

The deployment of intelligent sensing services today brings people great convenience. For instance, the broad deployment of video surveillance in recent years causes lots of benefits. In supermarkets, banks, airports, or any other public places, it helps detect events and suspicious behaviors, therefore enhancing security and safety (Socha and Kogut 2020). For patients at home or nursing homes, installing cameras helps people, especially health staff, to determine whether the care given to them is appropriate (Socha and Kogut 2020). For example, if accidents happen, the video surveillance system can detect and report it, and health care providers will be able to take measures in time. In the commercial sector, service providers can adopt intelligent sensing services to help them gather and analyze the user data, and then reach target consumers based on the analysis results (Adelman et al. 2014).

Nevertheless, in the meantime, these intelligent sensing services make preserving one's privacy increasingly tricky because people may have different attitudes towards these intelligent sensing services regarding how they could collect and use the collected data. Though the European General Data Protection Regulation (GDPR) endows data subjects with the right to be informed about the collection and use of their personal data (Anon. 2015), i.e., the data subject has the right to grant or deny permissions for a service provider to access his/her personal data, data subjects have very few technical tools to encode their needs in privacy and to define how their personal data is used by the service provider. If a patient lacks the awareness and knowledge of exercising his/her privacy rights, it will increase the service provider's difficulty to preserve their privacy appropriately (Art. 13 GDPR and Art. 14 GDPR n.d.; Anon. n.d.-a). Even if patients are aware of their privacy needs, they often have no other choices but to give a Yes-or-No-to-All consent in order to use a service

(Annenberg School for Communication 2015). The previous studies have reflected this phenomenon. According to a survey conducted in the U.S., most people give consents to sharing their personal data in exchange for free services (Annenberg School for Communication 2015). As a matter of fact, the study has revealed that more people believe they have already lost control of their personal information even though they are not willing to. Human behavior is another factor that can impact one's privacy decision-making because people have the tendency to choose the default option and maintain the status quo (Annenberg School for Communication 2015). Another study from the Norwegian Data Protection Authority also found how the questions about consent are asked can affect whether one says yes or no to give a consent (Anon. 2019). In addition to that, the two surveys carried out in the study have also shown that demographic characteristics, such as age, gender, and education, may influence one's tendency to give a consent to share his/her personal data.

There are other challenges with regard to giving a consent. Medical decision-making is one of the complicated challenges. Though researchers are facilitating the implementation of shared decision-making (SDM), an SDM scheme does not provide solutions when patients are incapable of making decisions (Anon. n.d.-b). Pursuant to Article 9 (Art. 7 GDPR n.d.) in the GDPR, "when the hospital is monitoring a patient who is physically or legally incapable of giving his consent, in order to protect the vital interests of the patients, the data controller has to justify the necessity of processing special categories of data." Although according to Recital 46 (Vollmer 2020), vital interests only cover the essential interest of a data subject's life, parents and legal guardians, as well as health care providers (HCPs), rather than the patients themselves, have significant roles in medical decision-making under certain circumstances. Based on the fact that different people have their own tendency to give a consent, and some decisions must be made case by case (Coughlin 2018), it could be useful to develop personal privacy models so that consents could be given based on one's personal privacy model as a possible reference for guardians. A privacy model is developed from learning one's privacy preferences previously indicated or captured from life events. When a patient is receiving a healthcare service, his or her own privacy preferences will be recorded by the system. As time goes by, when the patient loses the cognitive ability to make rational decisions, this privacy model may be referred to for inferring a decision respecting the patient's "willingness" learned from previous incidents. Another daily-life use case of such a personal privacy model is to use it as a privacy setting template that can be learned and configured automatically on the IoT endpoints or services without the need of administrating the configuration one by one manually.

With the challenges we have mentioned above, we attempt to construct a privacy model based on individual's preferences and serve as a reference when one is giving consents to the deployment of patient sensing systems.

The rest of the chapter is organized as follows: In Sect. "Related Works", we provide an overview of the state of the arts of homecare sensing and assisted living technologies, people's privacy attitudes towards them, as well as their legal and ethical context. In Sect. "Description of the Questionnaire Design and Predictor Selection", we describe the design of our questionnaire, model selection, and result analysis. And in Sect. "Challenges, Opportunities, and Future Scope", we discuss and understand the problems in the created models and suggest potential approaches to testing the questionnaire in a larger group of people in the future.

Related Works

In this section, we will first introduce and provide an overview of the homecare monitoring systems and assisted living technologies. Next, we'll discuss people's privacy attitudes and concerns about ambient assisted living technologies. Finally, the legal and ethical considerations, as well as the problem of privacy paradox, will be discussed.

The State of the Arts: Homecare Monitoring System and Assisted Living Technologies

Homecare monitoring systems today allow the elderly to stay independent and healthier and therefore age in place (Caine 2009). In the meantime, not only older adults but also patients with chronic diseases can benefit from the homecare monitoring systems. From a financial perspective, it will cost less for a person to stay at his or her home rather than stay in an assisted living facility (Caine 2009). From another perspective, it eases the burden of the healthcare service providers and healthcare organizations as well as assisted living facilities because it helps save medical resources.

With the benefits we have listed above, a large number of medical devices for homecare monitoring have been designed to meet the requirements of different groups of people. These healthcare devices and services for home care can be categorized into three groups (Magjarevic 2007): First, stationary medical devices which are used to measure physiological parameters like blood pressure, electrocardiogram (ECG), and photoplethysmography (PPG) regularly. Second, embedded devices are used to raise alarms in case of a medical emergency or safety accident. Third, wearable sensors and sensor networks are used to monitor physiological parameters continuously (Magjarevic 2007). Apart from the technologies that can achieve the prevention of diseases, researchers are making efforts to substitute traditional sensors with smart textiles in health monitoring as well (Lymberis and Paradiso 2008).

Applying the medical devices and the homecare technologies and implementing them into a system is another area. Many implemented systems and architectures are designed for ambient assisted living (AAL). The GiraffPlus system (Palumbo et al. 2014), which is funded by EU FP7,[1] for example, is a complete system that

---

[1] http://www.giraffplus.eu/

collects daily behavioral and physiological data from distributed sensors. Currently, smart homes are the commonly used assisted living technology that serves as a facilitating factor for independent living of older adults (Thorstensen 2018). Some smart home projects in the EU through the use of AAL technologies include iDorm (Pounds-Cornish and Holmes 2002), PROSAFE (Chan et al. 2005) and CareLab (Nick and Becker 2007).

Apart from smart homes and healthcare devices like mobile and wearable sensors, assistive robots are developed to help the elderly to overcome their physical limitations by helping them with their daily activities (Rashidi and Mihailidis 2013). These assistive robots have different functions based on their types (Rashidi and Mihailidis 2013; Lawton 1990): robots assisting with activities of daily living (ADL) can help with tasks such as feeding, grooming, bathing, and dressing, etc. Robots assisting with instrumental activities of daily living (IADL) can help with activities such as housekeeping (iRobot® n.d.), meal preparation, medication management, laundry, shopping, telephone use, etc. Robots assisting with enhanced activities of daily living (EADL) can help with tasks such as hobbies, social communication, and new learning (Smarr et al. 2011).

In Norway, there are various assisted living technology projects currently. To illustrate, the Assisted Living Project (ALP) led by Oslo and Akershus University College aims at the use of welfare technology among the elderly with mild cognitive difficulties and develop smart technological solutions for them. It has shown that cognitive impairment is one of the factors which impedes people from staying at home independently for a longer time. The researcher intends to overcome this problem by applying machine learning and developing self-learning systems for those who suffer mild cognitive impairment. (Assisted Living-prosjektet n.d.)

Privacy Attitudes and Concerns in Homecare Monitoring Systems

It is significant to preserve privacy and confidentiality when designing the assisted living technologies. All communications should be encrypted and secure to avoid invasive threats (Rashidi and Mihailidis 2013). However, not only the privacy of the system and data processing procedures should be taken into consideration, but also people's privacy concerns and their willingness to disclose their information in a monitoring environment.

Currently, a series of privacy research for homecare monitoring systems are focusing on ensuring users' awareness and control of when and to whom their information is transmitted. According to a scenario provided by Kelly E. Caine (Caine 2009), for an old adult who wants to live in his or her own home, a visual sensing system will enable someone to check up on him and provide help when needed. In this way, his/her privacy is not only affected by the technology but also possibly traded with his/her well-being. Another survey carried out by the Oregon Center for Aging and Technology (ORCATECH) invited older adult participants to the

Intelligent Systems for Assessment of Aging Changes study (ISAAC) regarding their privacy attitudes about unobtrusive home monitoring (Boise et al. 2013). From the previous focus group and interviews (Andersson et al. 2002) and surveys (Malone et al. 2005) the researchers found that older adults have seen the value of the monitoring systems, expressed their willingness to adopt in-home monitoring technologies, and had relatively few concerns about privacy or security. But most of the studies have not considered how participation over time may affect people's privacy attitudes and response to the technologies (Boise et al. 2013). Therefore, the researchers in the ISAAC study tested participants at two surveys, the baseline survey which happened at the beginning and year one survey which happened after 1 year, to examine the change of attitudes and concerns over time and to measure their willingness to share health data with the healthcare service provider or family members.

Legal and Ethical Consideration Regarding Homecare Sensing

A paper regarding privacy and future consent in smart homes (Thorstensen 2018) found out several ethic issues which should be considered for future consent giving. First, the General Data Protection Regulation (GDPR) has stated in Article 14 that the controller shall provide the data subject with "meaningful information about the logic involved, as well as the significance and the envisaged consequences of such processing for the data subject" (Art. 14 GDPR n.d.). Second, it has also been stated in Article 5 that personal data shall follow the data minimization principle, and it shall be "adequate, relevant and limited to what is necessary in relation to the purposes for which they are processed" (Art. 5 GDPR n.d.). Third, Article 22 has stipulated that "the data subject shall have the right not to be subject to a decision based solely on automated processing, including profiling, which produces legal effects concerning him or her or similarly significantly affects him or her", but it shall not apply when the automated decision-making "is based on the data subject's explicit consent" (Art. 22 GDPR n.d.).The second issue might cause conflicts for data controllers because providing appropriate care services may need more data collected, which seems to be against the data minimization principle, while the first and third cases clarify the importance of making the data subject informed and have a thorough understanding of the automated decision-making and the background so that they can give informed consents.

The Privacy Paradox

Even though individuals' privacy attitudes and preferences are collected, there is a phenomenon known as the privacy paradox (Barth and de Jong 2017). The term privacy paradox was raised by Norberg in 2007 (Norberg et al. 2007). It was raised because research has revealed that there are discrepancies between user privacy attitudes and user privacy behavior. Norberg's study confirmed the hypothesis that individuals would disclose more personal information than their stated intentions indicated, and decision-making takes place on an irrational level rather than a rational level to a great extent (Barth and de Jong 2017). Considering this phenomenon, we aim to set up several user groups in our research. One is "text-based" and participants' privacy attitudes are collected online or via papers. While another one will be "situated" and participants will be invited to a real-world environment to provide their privacy preferences. We plan to compare the results from these groups and validate if privacy paradox exists. In the next sections, we are going to describe the experiment of the first group. The situated group will be presented in our future work.

Description of the Questionnaire Design and Predictor Selection

Based on the background and the state-of-the-art work we mentioned, our research intends to develop personal privacy models based on one's personal privacy attitudes, analyze the patients' privacy preferences towards homecare patient sensing, and investigate the legal and ethical background of homecare patient sensing. In this vein, we conducted a series of studies to collect and analyze people's opinions and privacy attitudes.

To prepare for a large-scale study in the future, we recruited 20 participants as a preliminary study for our research project this round. These participants are divided into five groups. (1) four employees/students from the department of information security and communication technology in NTNU (2) four employees/students from the department of public health and nursing or department of health science in NTNU (3) four health management staff from health organizations (4) four people over sixties from their private homes in Norway (5) four people over sixties from their private homes in Indonesia.

The first four groups of participants are recruited from Norway. Since patients or the elderly who stay at home are the targeted people who are most in need of homecare monitoring, their privacy preferences are of great value to us. Thus, we planned to invite two groups of people over sixties to take part in the research. Because of the limited time and COVID-19 in Norway, it's hard for us to recruit enough old people in Norway. Therefore, the participants of the last group are recruited from Indonesia.

Second, we conducted five focus group discussions, each of which consists of four participants from the same group and one moderator, who is not a member of the group but will inspire the participants and guide the discussion. Then we collected people's privacy attitudes regarding their privacy towards home sensing through the online questionnaire. The focus group discussions are conducted before the questionnaire because the questions in the focus group discussion will raise participants' privacy awareness and help them have a better overview of the project when answering the questionnaire. Finally, we analyze the collected data and select some algorithms to derive a privacy predictive model.

Focus Group Discussion

Focus groups are usually conducted by a moderator, and it is easier to have a homogeneous group as people with the similar background may find it easier to talk with each other (Adams and Cox 2008). A focus group discussion before distributing the questionnaire can help participants have a better understanding of the research project and give more practical answers to the questionnaire. In common cases, the number of participants who take part in the discussion should not be larger than eight and smaller than three (Adams and Cox 2008). The first focus group discussion is conducted offline. Nevertheless, due to the COVID-19 situation, the other four focus group discussion in this research are conducted virtually. The participants in Group 4 and Group 5 don't have to work, and it's easy to get them together for a discussion. But it's difficult for us to get all the participants in Group 2 and Group 3 together at the same time online. Therefore, the participants in these two groups are divided into two subgroups practically, and a subgroup consisting of two people is invited into the discussion online. The moderator conveys the answers of the first subgroup to the second subgroup and contacts the first subgroup if new ideas are raised up by the second subgroup.

A consent form and an information letter are distributed to the participants. And everyone is informed of the background of the research in the information letter. The following questions are asked in each session:

Q1: List a few activities (e.g., getting dressed, taking a shower) monitored by the monitoring system (e.g., camera, microphone, etc.) that may concern your privacy at home.

Q2: Rank the following factors in terms of importance for you, related to the monitoring system – (1) my health status; (2) my privacy and dignity; (3) medical emergencies; (4) disturbance to my family member and other caregivers; (5) how much I should pay for the system.

Q3: List the indoor places that you think are private, semi-private, public at home.

A summarization of the findings is described below.

When asked about the activities at home, the participants in Group 1 state that taking a shower, having sex with partners, playing with children may concern their privacy. Then the moderator asks about their attitudes towards talking with someone else in the house. One participant doesn't think that speaking with a girlfriend or someone else is private because if he calls someone else for help, it can help him a lot if the system can monitor him. If he were the elderly, he would not consider dialing a phone number is private because he thinks most of the phone numbers are not private. Another participant says that watching a laptop and using a bank account can be private for him, and the monitoring system can even identify some sensitive information by the audio. But the participants agree that even sensitive information can be protected, and privacy-enhancing technologies can be used from technologists' perspective. The participants in Group 2 and Group 3 agree that showering, dressing, sleeping are the most private activities at home. Different from the participant in Group 1 who thinks that talking with others doesn't affect his privacy, a participant in Group 2 thinks talking with others is sensitive, and he even doesn't want anything to be published when he is talking on the phone. Another participant in Group 2 claims that she thinks every room in her house is private, and she doesn't want any activities to be monitored. She takes the example of her daughter and says even if she wants to monitor her daughter to ensure her safety, she has to respect her privacy and dignity. So she has to accept the possibility of risks and prefers not to monitor her. Apart from the activities above, the participants in Group 5 add that praying unless it's a congregational prayer can concern their privacy as well.

When asked to rank the factors from the most to the least important to them, many participants in the first three groups take medical emergency and privacy as the most important factors. And they claim that the importance could change over time based on their health status. The participants who think all the activities are private hold the view that privacy and dignity are the most important. But a participant in Group 2 says she will always set medical emergencies prior to privacy and dignity because she has a medical background, and she can bypass privacy and dignity when emergencies happen. The unique answer is from a participant from Group 3 who is the manager of the healthcare organization. He says since he is a doctor, he will say medical emergency is the most important, but if he were the patient, he would take it as the least important related to the monitoring system because we already have other solutions for medical emergencies. And another one in Group 3 thinks privacy and dignity are not so important because caregivers should have access to the monitoring system and they can check the recordings, and she would trust the caregivers. However, old people from Group 4 and Group 5 have reached the agreement that their health status is the most important factor though they have different cultural background and the discussions are conducted separately. A couple in Group 4 claim that once they need help, everything will be public even if they are at home. There will no longer be private activities and private rooms in the house. The bathroom and bedroom, which should be private in most younger people's view, are not important to them because they need caregivers to assist them in case accidents happen or even help them during showers. The most important thing for them is that their laptop should be kept private and should not be monitored at all so that no one will take their credentials. It coincides with our findings from the previous groups that financial activities should be protected.

When asked about the participants' interpretation of private, semi-private, and public places in a house, we got the two most common responses. Some of them regard bedrooms and bathrooms are the most private places in a house. When asked about the rest parts of the rooms, most of them have shown their hesitation because it's hard to distinguish the privacy level, and they provide various answers; However, some insist that all places in a house are private. The latter participants have already given their answer in the first question that they don't want any activities to be monitored at all in their houses.

Questionnaire Design and Data Collection

In the questionnaire, we asked the participants about nine scenarios to gather their privacy preferences for daily activities that they may encounter at home. These scenarios differed from each other and are the combination of the following three contextual parameters: place, activity, and incident.

The criteria categorization of the contextual parameters in the scenarios shown in Table 11.1 are:

Place Distinguishing the level of privacy that certain spaces demand in a house is an important though difficult part. There is no sufficient evidence defining the private levels in a house by now. Though according to the interview and focus groups conducted by the researchers (Abbott-Chapman and Robertson 2009), adolescents have shown the preferences of redefining the boundaries of private spaces like homes, especially their own bedrooms, and places in the natural environment, we lack the standard or regulation of the boundary in a house. Besides, digital spaces and the existence of social media make things more complex (Lincoln 2015). A doctoral thesis regarding video mediated communication (VMC) stated that rather than the traditional concept where the boundaries between public space and private space are precise, video conferences could link private and public at home

Table 11.1 Scenario parameters

Place (A1)	(1) Private level 1	Bedroom
		Bathroom
	(2) Private level 2	Living room
Activity (A2)	(1) Most sensitive activities	Getting dressed
		Taking a shower
	(2) Sensitive activities	Processing personal finance
	(3) Normal activities	Sitting by the bed
		Making the bed
		Washing hands
		Talking with friends
		Putting things in place
Incident (A3)	(1) Medical emergency	Have a heart attack
		Hurt in a slip/stumble-and-fall accident
		Suffer a syncope
	(2) Chronic disease symptom	Facial weakness detected
		Barely noticeable tremor detected
	(3) Other incidents	Get a heavy cough
		Suffer a sharp injury

(Junestrand 2004). Spaces in a home where you can be seen and heard by a VMC session should become public, while places where you can not be seen nor be heard, should become private in the new and specific sense.

As has been mentioned in the focus group discussion section, the answers we get from the participants concerning the private level in a house are different. To get the subdivision results, we adopt the interpretation of the former group of people who hold the view that bedrooms and bathrooms are the most private places in a house. Because of the lack of standard division of the places in a house and unified interpretations by now, we label the places into "private level 1" and "private level 2" rather than "private", "semi-private", and "public" places.

Activity We put forward three activity levels varying from most sensitive activities to normal activities based on their privacy level. In our research, the most sensitive activities include getting dressed, taking a shower; the sensitive activities include processing personal finance, while all the other activities are categorized into normal activities.

Incident The incidents that people might need healthcare help are consist of a medical emergency (have a heart attack, suffer a syncope), chronic disease symptoms (facial weakness detected which might be a symptom of facial nerve paralysis (Altuntas et al. 1998), barely noticeable tremor detected which might be a symptom of Parkinson's disease (Mayo Clinic n.d.), and other incidents.

After providing the participants with scenarios, five questions are asked in each scenario: who are the persons they want to inform when the incident happens, how they would like the incident to be recorded, how they would like the monitoring system to report the incident, the data type they would like to include when reporting, and what data (if coded in different privacy levels) they want to report.

Data Analysis and Algorithm Selection

Scikit-learn, a software machine learning library used for the Python programming language and suitable for medium-scale supervised and unsupervised problems, is adopted in the data analysis (Pedregosa et al. 2011). As the training data in our research is relatively smaller and concerns multi-class classification problems, traditional machine learning algorithms used for classification problems like support vector machine (SVM) (Anon. n.d.-c), logistic regression (Anon. n.d.-d), and Naïve Bayes (Anon. n.d.-e) are selected. These algorithms are also widely used in privacy decision support systems. We utilized the *place* (A1), *activity* (A2), and *incident* (A3) contextual factors as input features to predict how participants' preferences under different scenarios. We learn machine learning models to predict parameters *person* (Q1), *how to be recorded* (Q2), *how to report* (Q3), *data type included when reporting* (Q4), and *what to report* (Q5). We adopt "one-vs-the-rest" multi-class strategy when using SVM and logistic regression, while we select multinomial naïve Bayes classifier, which is suitable for classification with discrete features in our experiment (Anon. n.d.-e).

To illustrate, the participants can select multiple options when answering Q1, Q3, and Q4. Therefore, despite the order shown in Table 11.2, we rearrange the label based on the privacy level of each combination when analyzing the results in Table 11.3. The combinations of multi-choices in the first question are ordered from the least private to the most private. When a participant informs the caregivers and family members at the same time, he/she might get healthcare help in time at the cost of disclosing more information to others. If he/she prefers not to inform anyone else, we assume the system will protect his privacy, but he/she cannot get medical aid in time.

We set the label according to the rearranged order. For example, when the user is taking a shower in the bathroom and suffers a syncope by accident, he prefers to inform his care service provider for help. He would like the activity to be

Table 11.2 Privacy preference parameters

Person (Q1)	(1) Care service provider
	(2) A person I am familiar with
	(3) Myself
How to be recorded (Q2)	(1) Continuously recording
	(2) Automatically recording when the incident is detected (event-triggered)
	(3) Manually recording (human-triggered) – Voice command
	(4) Manually recording (human-triggered) – Press the button
	(5) No recording at all (not able to send recording data when informing people, but a text message or a call still works)
How to report (Q3)	(1) I'd like the person I want to inform to remotely monitor me 24 h 7 days whenever they like
	(2) The system should report the event automatically after recording the incident
	(3) Manually report (human-triggered)—Voice command
	(4) Manually report (human-triggered)—Press the button
Data type included when reporting (Q4)	(1) Video
	(2) Image
	(3) Audio
	(4) I would like the technologist to decide it for me
	(5) None of the above (text-only)
What to report (Q5)	(1) Raw recording data
	(2) Privacy-enhanced recording data
	(3) Text message describing the event
	(4) Text message calling for human aids immediately but no description of the event

Table 11.3 Privacy level

Person (Q1)	1. (1)(2)(3), (1)(2)
	2. (1), (1)(3)
	3. (2)(3), (2)
	4. (3)
How to be recorded (Q2)	1. (1)
	2. (2)
	3. (3), (4)
	4. (5)
How to report (Q3)	1. (1)(2)(3)
	2. (1)(2)
	3. (1)(3)
	4. (2)(3)
	5. (1)
	6. (2)
	7. (3)
Data type included when reporting (Q4)	1. (4), (1)(4), (2)(4), (3)(4), (1)(2)(4), (1)(3)(4), (2)(3)(4), (1)(2)(3)(4)
	2. (1)(2)(3), (1)(3)
	3. (2)(3)
	4. (1), (3), (1)(2)
	5. (2)
	6. (5)
What to report (Q5)	1. (1)
	2. (2)
	3. (3)
	4. (4)

continuously monitored but only automatically trigger the recording and store the data when the incident happens. He would like the system to report the event automatically after recording the incident. Only privacy-enhanced recording data with a video attached will be reported to his care service provider. The labels in this case would be: Q1 = 1, Q2 = 2, Q3 = 6, Q4 = 4, Q5 = 2.

Results

We adopt boxplots to show the distribution of the privacy preferences for all the participants P1–20 (see Figs. 11.1, 11.2, 11.3, 11.4 and 11.5). The minimum, first quartile, median, third quartile, and maximum are shown in the figures. The orange line and green triangle represent the median and mean value of the corresponding participant's preferences.

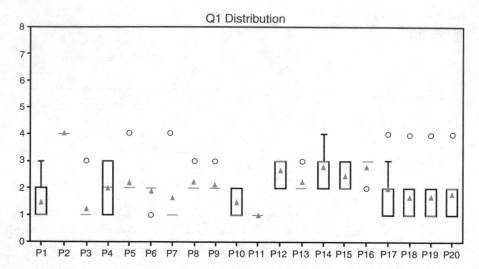

Fig. 11.1 Preference distribution of Q1

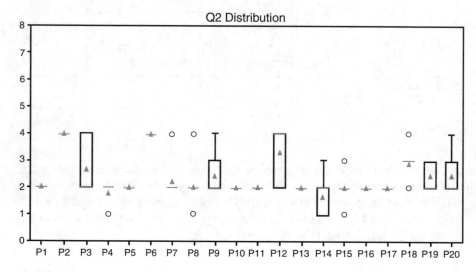

Fig. 11.2 Preference distribution of Q2

Data Analysis and Algorithm Selection

Instead of ten-fold cross-validation, we used five-fold cross-validation accuracy to estimate the accuracy of the models because of the limited dataset we collect from the participants. Among the three algorithms we select, linear kernel SVM performs the best. Therefore, we present its results instead of the other two in this

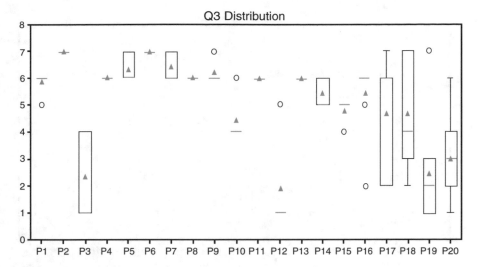

Fig. 11.3 Preference distribution of Q3

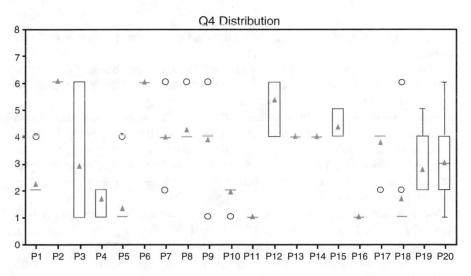

Fig. 11.4 Preference distribution of Q4

essay. Table 11.4 reports the weighted average accuracy of it. In the table, "P" represents a participant, and "G" represents the group which the participant belongs to.

We apply the direct observation method to figure out the reasons for the low accuracy results we get from Table 11.4 and notice that the "SVM-based" predictor works better when predicting the decisions of those who tend to select the same options in different scenarios. To validate the observation, we calculate the

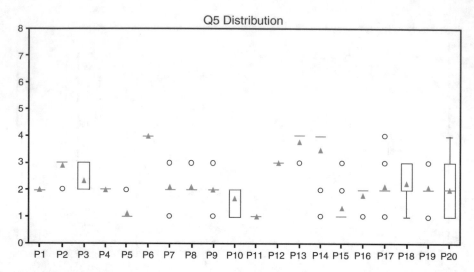

Fig. 11.5 Preference distribution of Q5

maximum frequency of each person when answering the same question in different scenarios and get the results in Table 11.5.

After comparing the results in Table 11.4 and Table 11.5, we come to the conclusion that the more similar preferences the users are provided in these scenarios, the better predictive results the model will perform.

In addition to the predictors mentioned above, we utilize the vector quantization (VQ) method (Hammer et al. 2014) based on the assumption that privacy decisions could be the same as the ones made by the same person earlier under the same or the most similar contextual parameter condition. We search the label in the training set by calculating the closest Euclidean distance between the training set and test set and get the results in Table 11.6.

More intuitively, we plot the line charts of the accuracy of each question in Figs. 11.6, 11.7, 11.8, 11.9 and 11.10. The results reflect a positive correlation between the "maximum-frequency-based" predictor and the "SVM-based" predictor. In general, these predictors have better performances compared to the "vector-quantization-based" predictor.

The mean squared error (MSE) (Anon. n.d.-e) is introduced to measure the quality of the predictors as well. The closer the MSE is to zero, the better quality the predictors are. In Figs. 11.11, 11.12, 11.13, 11.14 and 11.15, we plot the mean squared error of the predictors for each question. Other than that, we calculate the median value of the dynamic range of each participant's preferences as a benchmark. It is obvious that the MSE of the three predictors are much smaller than that of the median value of the dynamic range most of the time.

Table 11.4 Weighted average accuracy of "SVM-based" predictor

Person	Q1	Q2	Q3	Q4	Q5
P1-G1	66.7%	100.0%	88.9%	88.9%	100.0%
P2-G1	100.0%	100.0%	100.0%	100.0%	100.0%
P3-G1	88.9%	66.7%	11.1%	11.1%	66.7%
P4-G1	33.3%	77.8%	100.0%	66.7%	100.0%
P5-G2	88.9%	100.0%	66.7%	88.9%	88.9%
P6-G2	88.9%	100.0%	100.0%	100.0%	100.0%
P7-G2	77.8%	88.9%	11.1%	77.8%	66.7%
P8-G2	77.8%	66.7%	100.0%	88.9%	88.9%
P9-G3	88.9%	66.7%	77.8%	77.8%	77.8%
P10-G3	22.2%	100.0%	77.8%	88.9%	66.7%
P11-G3	100.0%	100.0%	100.0%	100.0%	100.0%
P12-G3	66.7%	66.7%	77.8%	66.7%	100.0%
P13-G4	77.8%	100.0%	100.0%	100.0%	77.8%
P14-G4	55.6%	0.0%	11.1%	100.0%	77.8%
P15-G4	11.1%	77.8%	77.8%	66.7%	77.8%
P16-G4	77.8%	100.0%	77.8%	100.0%	77.8%
P17-G5	22.2%	100.0%	0.0%	88.9%	55.6%
P18-G5	22.2%	66.7%	44.4%	77.8%	33.3%
P19-G5	44.4%	11.1%	33.3%	66.7%	66.7%
P20-G5	11.1%	66.7%	22.2%	11.1%	44.4%

Table 11.5 Weighted average accuracy of "maximum-frequency-based" predictor

Person	Q1	Q2	Q3	Q4	Q5
P1-G1	66.7%	100.0%	88.9%	88.9%	100.0%
P2-G1	100.0%	100.0%	100.0%	100.0%	100.0%
P3-G1	44.4%	66.7%	11.1%	55.6%	66.7%
P4-G1	0.0%	77.8%	100.0%	66.7%	100.0%
P5-G2	88.9%	100.0%	66.7%	88.9%	88.9%
P6-G2	88.9%	100.0%	100.0%	100.0%	100.0%
P7-G2	77.8%	88.9%	11.1%	77.8%	66.7%
P8-G2	77.8%	66.7%	100.0%	88.9%	88.9%
P9-G3	88.9%	66.7%	77.8%	77.8%	77.8%
P10-G3	22.2%	100.0%	77.8%	88.9%	66.7%
P11-G3	100.0%	100.0%	100.0%	100.0%	100.0%
P12-G3	66.7%	66.7%	77.8%	66.7%	100.0%
P13-G4	77.8%	100.0%	100.0%	100.0%	77.8%
P14-G4	55.6%	0.0%	11.1%	100.0%	77.8%
P15-G4	11.1%	77.8%	77.8%	66.7%	77.8%
P16-G4	77.8%	100.0%	77.8%	100.0%	77.8%
P17-G5	11.1%	100.0%	0.0%	88.9%	55.6%
P18-G5	55.6%	66.7%	22.2%	77.8%	55.6%
P19-G5	55.6%	11.1%	22.2%	66.7%	66.7%
P20-G5	22.2%	66.7%	33.3%	0.0%	44.4%

Table 11.6 Weighted average accuracy of "vector-quantization-based" predictor

Person	Q1	Q2	Q3	Q4	Q5
P1-G1	88.9%	100.0%	44.4%	77.8%	100.0%
P2-G1	100.0%	100.0%	100.0%	100.0%	100.0%
P3-G1	77.8%	77.8%	44.4%	33.3%	77.8%
P4-G1	55.6%	66.7%	100.0%	77.8%	100.0%
P5-G2	66.7%	100.0%	55.6%	44.4%	77.8%
P6-G2	77.8%	100.0%	100.0%	100.0%	100.0%
P7-G2	44.4%	77.8%	11.1%	55.6%	44.4%
P8-G2	55.6%	22.2%	100.0%	77.8%	77.8%
P9-G3	66.7%	77.8%	55.6%	55.6%	44.4%
P10-G3	44.4%	100.0%	33.3%	77.8%	22.2%
P11-G3	100.0%	100.0%	100.0%	100.0%	100.0%
P12-G3	33.3%	33.3%	44.4%	33.3%	100.0%
P13-G4	88.9%	100.0%	100.0%	100.0%	66.7%
P14-G4	33.3%	33.3%	66.7%	100.0%	55.6%
P15-G4	0.0%	55.6%	88.9%	77.8%	66.7%
P16-G4	55.6%	100.0%	66.7%	100.0%	55.6%
P17-G5	11.1%	100.0%	22.2%	77.8%	44.4%
P18-G5	44.4%	33.3%	0.0%	66.7%	44.4%
P19-G5	22.2%	55.6%	33.3%	22.2%	77.8%
P20-G5	66.7%	55.6%	22.2%	0.0%	11.1%

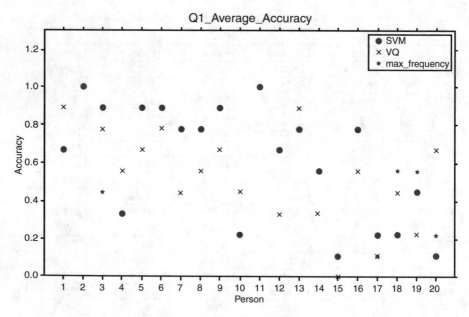

Fig. 11.6 Average accuracy of Q1

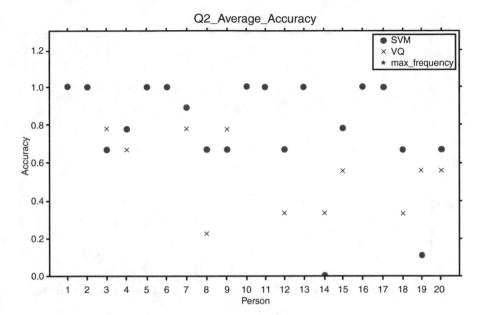

Fig. 11.7 Average accuracy of Q2

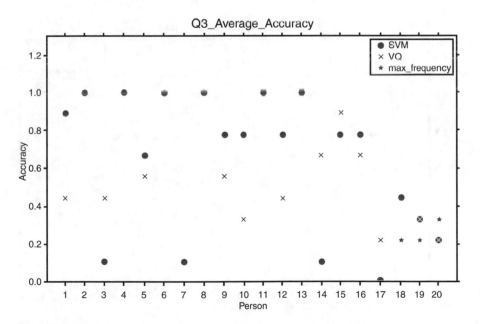

Fig. 11.8 Average accuracy of Q3

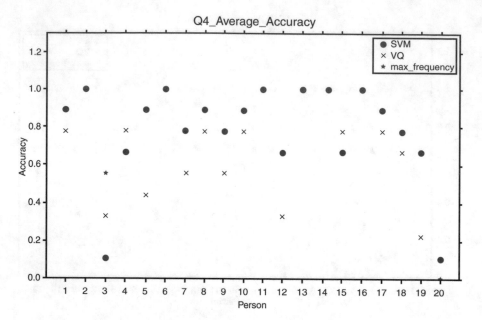

Fig. 11.9 Average accuracy of Q4

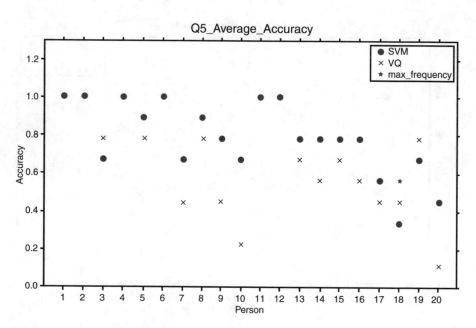

Fig. 11.10 Average accuracy of Q5

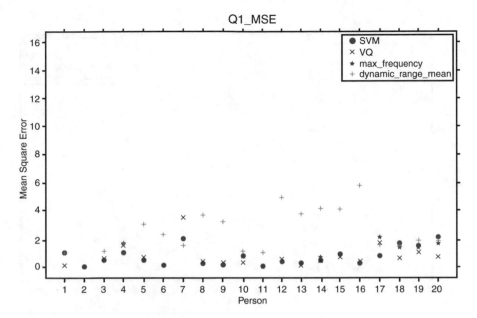

Fig. 11.11 Mean squared error of Q1

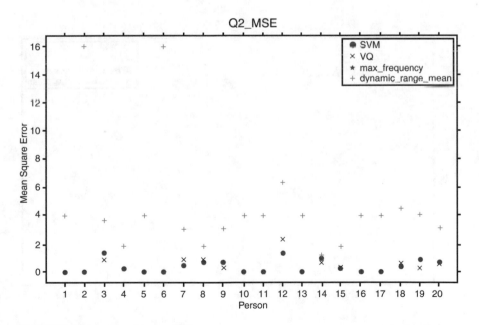

Fig. 11.12 Mean squared error of Q2

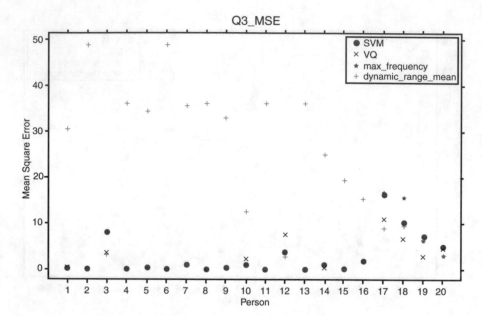

Fig. 11.13 Mean squared error of Q3

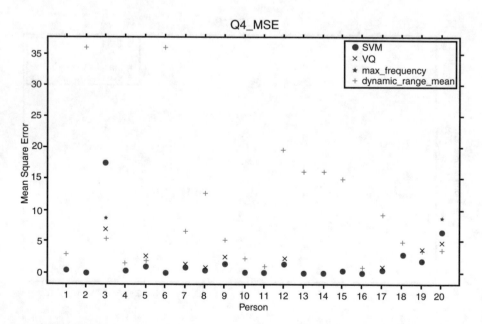

Fig. 11.14 Mean squared error of Q4

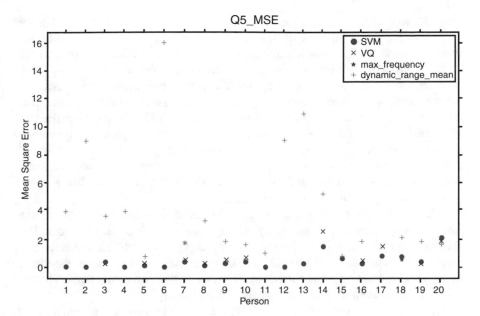

Fig. 11.15 Mean squared error of Q5

Challenges, Opportunities, and Future Scope

To summarize, we introduced three predictors when analyzing the results: "SVM-based" predictor, "maximum-frequency-based" predictor, and "vector-quantization-based" predictor. The "SVM-based" predictor and "maximum-frequency-based" predictor perform well and can help predict an individual's decision-making to some extent. The "maximum-frequency-based" predictor showing good performance indicates that most participants have a relatively stable personal model in privacy preferences in spite of the varied scenario private levels. However, it relies on the assumption that participants have stable preferences in different scenarios. For those participants who have given different answers in different scenarios, the predictor has shown worse performance, and it might not perform well in newly designed scenarios.

We further investigate participants who have fewer stable preferences. Other than those participants who tend to provide similar answers under every scenario, the rest of participants like P3, P14, P15, P17, P19, and P20 tend to report different data types based on privacy level because the privacy levels differ from each other in most of the scenarios, they consider disclosing privacy information case by case. We contact them again and ask for their opinions. In general, they will not want to share more information than the minimum of what is strictly necessary for the care providers to assess their situation properly and understand the degree of severity, while they will not hold back information that is necessary to understand the incident. Furthermore, they want the highest level of autonomy, so they want to assess and take care of the situations as much as possible themselves before asking for help. Last but not least, some of them consider the scenarios are totally different even if we have labeled some scenarios to the same privacy level in our experiments.

In conclusion, with the data we have collected by now, it's difficult to judge whether the "machine-learning-based" predictors can have a good performance on a larger scale of the dataset. Even though it has a good performance on participants who have stable preferences, there might be a probability that the questionnaire was not sufficiently well designed and cannot incentivize the participants to differentiate the scenarios. Ideally, we expect the "machine-learning-based" predictors would perform better and get more accurate results with the increase of the dataset. More scenarios will be designed, and the questionnaire will be distributed to a larger group of participants in the future to validate it.

Also, as we have mentioned above, participants' demographic information, like age, religion, education, or nationality, might influence their privacy attitudes. The focus group discussion results have also shown that participants with different cultural backgrounds have different privacy considerations. For example, they have come up with different private activities. Thus, we will utilize demographic characteristics when developing privacy models in the next step.

Apart from that, because of the privacy paradox phenomenon we have stated above, we plan to test the questionnaire in a situated-based environment to ensure that participants' behavior of disclosing information and reporting data is closer to reality.

Clinical Pearls
- We noticed that participants who held the view that all activities should not be monitored at home in the first question thought privacy and dignity were the most important to them.
- The focus group discussion results have shown that participants with different backgrounds have different privacy considerations.
- The privacy predictive models have been developed and can help with medical decision-making in health monitoring to some extent, but they may need further investigation.

Review Questions
1. What is actually a personal privacy model? Are there any definitions, literature references, or some examples?
2. As privacy paradox is an important impact in the experiment, how is the phenomenon validated and discussed in the chapter?

Answers
1. It was stated in the introduction part that a privacy model is developed from learning one's privacy preferences previously indicated or captured from life events.
2. As a matter of fact, the privacy paradox hasn't been validated yet in the research. However, we plan to invite several groups to validate the phenomenon. The

group we have invited in the chapter is mainly questionnaire-based and all participants are asked to answer the questionnaire. However, in the next step, there will be scenario-based groups so that participants will be able to give privacy preferences in an environment where they feel the incidents happen in their own room. By comparing the results from different groups, we will be able to validate the privacy paradox phenomenon.

References

Abbott-Chapman J, Robertson M. Adolescents' favourite places: redefining the boundaries between private and public space. Space Cult. 2009;12:419–34.

Adams A, Cox A (2008) Questionnaires, in-depth interviews and focus groups. Res. Methods Hum.-Comput. Interact.

Adelman RD, Tmanova LL, Delgado D, Dion S, Lachs MS. Caregiver burden: a clinical review. JAMA J Am Med Assoc. 2014;311:1052–60.

Altuntas A, Unal A, Aslan A, Ozcan M, Kurkcuoglu S, Nalca Y. Facial nerve paralysis in chronic suppurative otitis media: Ankara Numune hospital experience. Auris Nasus Larynx. 1998;25:169–72.

Andersson N-B, Hanson E, Magnusson L, Nolan M. Views of family carers and older people of information technology. Br J Nurs Mark Allen Publ. 2002;11:827–31.

Annenberg School for Communication. "The tradeoff fallacy: how marketers are misrepresenting American consumers and opening them up to exploitation." Annenberg School for Communication, 2015. I Annenberg School for Communication. https://www.asc.upenn.edu/news-events/publications/tradeoff-fallacy-how-marketers-are-misrepresenting-american-consumers-and.

Anon. (2015) THE GREAT DATA RACE - How commercial utilisation of personal data challenges privacy [Internet]. Norwegian Data Protection Authority (Datatilsynet). https://www.datatilsynet.no/globalassets/global/english/engelskkommersialisering-endelig.pdf.

Anon. (2019) Nordmenn og deling av persondata.

Art. 13 GDPR, Art. 14 GDPR (n.d.) - Right to be informed. Gen. Data Prot. Regul. GDPR.

Anon. (n.d.-a) storbyuniversitetet O- Jürgen Kasper. https://www.oslomet.no/om/ansatt/jurgenka.

Anon. (n.d.-b) 1.4. Support Vector Machines—scikit-learn 0.24.2 documentation. https://scikit-learn.org/stable/modules/svm.html.

Anon. (n.d.-c) sklearn.linear_model.LogisticRegression—scikit-learn 0.24.2 documentation. https://scikit-learn.org/stable/modules/generated/sklearn.linear_model.LogisticRegression.html.

Anon. (n.d.-d) 1.9. Naive Bayes—scikit-learn 0.24.2 documentation. https://scikit-learn.org/stable/modules/naive_bayes.html.

Anon. (n.d.-e) sklearn.metrics.mean_squared_error—scikit-learn 0.24.2 documentation. https://scikit-learn.org/stable/modules/generated/sklearn.metrics.mean_squared_error.html.

Art. 14 GDPR (n.d.) – Information to be provided where personal data have not been obtained from the data subject. Gen. Data Prot. Regul. GDPR.

Art. 22 GDPR (n.d.) – Automated individual decision-making, including profiling. Gen. Data Prot. Regul. GDPR.

Art. 5 GDPR (n.d.) – Principles relating to processing of personal data. Gen. Data Prot. Regul. GDPR.

Art. 7 GDPR (n.d.) – Conditions for consent. Gen. Data Prot. Regul. GDPR.

Assisted Living-prosjektet. In: Assist. Living-Prosjektet. n.d.. https://assistedlivingweb.wordpress.com/.

Barth S, de Jong MDT. The privacy paradox—investigating discrepancies between expressed privacy concerns and actual online behavior—a systematic literature review. Telemat Inform. 2017;34:1038–58.

Boise L, Wild K, Mattek N, Ruhl M, Dodge HH, Kaye J. Willingness of older adults to share data and privacy concerns after exposure to unobtrusive in-home monitoring. Gerontechnology. 2013;11:428–35.

Caine K (2009) Visual sensing devices in home-care systems. In: Proc. First ACM Workshop Secur. Priv. Med. Home-Care Syst. ACM, pp 61–62.

Chan M, Campo E, Estève D. Assessment of activity of elderly people using a home monitoring system. Int J Rehabil Res. 2005;28:69–76.

Coughlin KW. Medical decision-making in paediatrics: infancy to adolescence. Paediatr Child Health. 2018;23:138–46.

Hammer B, Hofmann D, Schleif F-M, Zhu X. Learning vector quantization for (dis-)similarities. Neurocomputing Amst. 2014;131:43–51.

iRobot®: Robot vacuum and mop. n.d.. http://www-origin9.irobot.com/.

Junestrand S. Being private and public at home. Sweden: Stockholm; 2004.

Lawton PM. Aging and performance of home tasks. Hum Factors. 1990;32:527–36.

Lincoln S. 'My bedroom is me': young people, private space, consumption and the family home 2015. pp 87–106.

Lymberis A, Paradiso R (2008) Smart fabrics and interactive textile enabling wearable personal applications: R&D state of the art and future challenges. 2008 30th Annu Int Conf IEEE Eng Med Biol Soc 5270–5273.

Magjarevic R. Home care technologies for ambient assisted living. In: 11th Mediterr. Conf. Med. Biomed. Eng. Comput. Berlin, Heidelberg: Springer Berlin Heidelberg; 2007. p. 397–400.

Malone TB, Kirkpatrick MJ, Herman RP, Creedon MA, Cohen-Mansfield J, Dutra LA. Electronic memory aids for community-dwelling elderly persons: attitudes, preferences, and potential utilization. J Appl Gerontol. 2005;24:3–20.

Mayo Clinic. Parkinson's disease—Symptoms and causes. In: Mayo Clin. n.d.. https://www.mayo-clinic.org/diseases-conditions/parkinsons-disease/symptoms-causes/syc-20376055.

Nick M, Becker M. A hybrid approach to intelligent living assistance. In: 7th Int. Conf. Hybrid Intell. Syst. HIS 2007 2007. pp 283–289.

Norberg PA, Horne DR, Horne DA. The privacy paradox: personal information disclosure intentions versus behaviors. J Consum Aff. 2007;41:100–26.

Palumbo F, Ullberg J, Stimec A, Furfari F, Karlsson L, Coradeschi S. Sensor network infrastructure for a home care monitoring system. Sensors. 2014;14:3833–60.

Pedregosa F, Varoquaux G, Gramfort A, et al. Scikit-learn: machine learning in python. J Mach Learn Res. 2011;12:2825.

Pounds-Cornish A, Holmes A. The iDorm—a practical deployment of grid technology. In: 2nd IEEEACM Int. Symp. Clust. Comput. Grid CCGRID02. IEEE, 2002; 470–470.

Rashidi P, Mihailidis A. A survey on ambient-assisted living tools for older adults. IEEE J Biomed Health Inform. 2013;17:579–90.

Smarr C-A, Fausset CB, Rogers WA (2011) Understanding the Potential for Robot Assistance for Older Adults in the Home Environment.

Socha R, Kogut B. Urban video surveillance as a tool to improve security in public spaces. Sustain Basel Switz. 2020;12:6210.

Thorstensen E (2018) Privacy and future consent in smart homes as assisted living technologies. In: Hum. Asp. IT Aged Popul. Appl. Health Assist. Entertain. Springer International Publishing, Cham, pp 415–433.

Vollmer N (2020) Recital 46 EU general data protection regulation (EU-GDPR). https://www.privacy-regulation.eu/en/recital-46-GDPR.htm.

Chapter 12
Detecting Personal Health Mentions from Social Media Using Supervised Machine Learning

Zhijun Yin, Congning Ni, Daniel Fabbri, S. Trent Rosenbloom, and Bradley Malin

Abstract Traditional methods for collecting data in support of clinical research include prospectively collected surveys, retrospective analyses of existing medical records, and a combination of the two. However, these resources are limited in how comprehensively their content covers an individual's life. Non-traditional information domains (e.g., online forums and social media) have the potential to supplement the view of an individual's health. In this chapter, we investigate how people disclose their own or others' health status over a broad range of health issues on

Z. Yin (✉) · D. Fabbri
Department of Computer Science, Vanderbilt University, Nashville, TN, USA

Department of Biomedical Informatics, Vanderbilt University Medical Center, Nashville, TN, USA
e-mail: zhijun.yin@vumc.org; daniel.fabbri@vumc.org

C. Ni
Department of Computer Science, Vanderbilt University, Nashville, TN, USA
e-mail: congning.ni@vanderbilt.edu

S. T. Rosenbloom
Department of Biomedical Informatics, Vanderbilt University Medical Center, Nashville, TN, USA

Department of Medicine, Vanderbilt University Medical Center, Nashville, TN, USA

Department of Pediatrics, Vanderbilt University Medical Center, Nashville, TN, USA

School of Nursing, Vanderbilt University, Nashville, TN, USA
e-mail: trent.rosenbloom@vumc.org

B. Malin
Department of Computer Science, Vanderbilt University, Nashville, TN, USA

Department of Biomedical Informatics, Vanderbilt University Medical Center, Nashville, TN, USA

Department of Biostatistics, Vanderbilt University Medical Center, Nashville, TN, USA
e-mail: b.malin@vumc.org

© The Author(s), under exclusive license to Springer Nature Switzerland AG 2022
P.-Y. S. Hsueh et al. (eds.), *Personal Health Informatics*, Cognitive Informatics in Biomedicine and Healthcare, https://doi.org/10.1007/978-3-031-07696-1_12

Twitter. We applied both traditional and deep learning-based machine learning models effectively to detect such online personal health status mentions. We collected more than 250 million tweets via the Twitter streaming API over a two-month period in 2014 and focused on 34 high-impact health issues that were selected based on the guidance from the Medical Expenditure Panel Survey. We created a labeled corpus of over three thousand tweets via a survey, administered over Amazon Mechanical Turk, that documents when terms correspond to mentions of personal health issues or an alternative (e.g., a metaphor). We found that Twitter users disclosed personal health status for all of the investigated health issues and personal health status was disclosed over 50% of the time for 11 out of 34 (33%) investigated health issues. We also found that the disclosure rate, as well as the likelihood that people disclose their own versus other people's health status, were dependent on the health issue in a statistically significant manner ($p < 0.001$). While models based on traditional machine learning frameworks built upon bag-of-word features led to decent performance (AUC = 0.810), models based on deep learning significantly boosted performance (AUC =0.885).

Keywords Consumer health · Information retrieval · Machine learning · Social media · Natural language processing · Health status mention detection

Learning Objective
1. Understand the health status disclosure about self and others on Twitter
2. Learn Twitter data collection, annotation design and deployment, and result analysis
3. Learn to apply both traditional and deep learning-based machine learnings for health mention detection
4. Learn sensitivity analysis on the impact of the training dataset on the model performance

Introduction

Traditional methods for collecting data in support of clinical research include prospectively collected surveys (e.g., (Garratt et al. 1993)), retrospective analyses of existing medical records (e.g., (Samsa et al. 2000; Williams et al. 2000)), and a combination of the two (e.g., (Quam et al. 1993)). Numerous computerized approaches to data collection have emerged, with traditional surveys for health research moving onto the Internet (Eysenbach and Wyatt 2002) and increasingly widespread adoption of electronic medical records (EMRs) that can be mined to investigate a wide range of phenotypes (Coorevits et al. 2013; Jensen et al. 2012; Rea et al. 2012). At the same time, these approaches tend to focus only on a medically-centric worldview, and they may provide only a partial view of a patient's life. Recognizing this limitation, investigators believe that that data contributed through non-traditional domains, such as mobile applications (Estrin 2014; Kumar et al. 2013; Tomlinson et al. 2013) and online forums where patients self-report on their status (Riedl and Riedl 2013; Wicks et al. 2014; Yin et al. 2017; Slemon et al. 2021), will help provide a more complete view of an individual's health and population-based health trends. Particularly, during the COVID-19 pandemic, online environments have been gained popularity for sharing personal health status with high social stigma (Slemon et al. 2021; Brewer et al. 2021).

An increasing number of studies demonstrate that the data disseminated via social media platforms, such as Twitter, can inform health-related investigations. For instance, these studies have shown that such data can be mined to model aggregate trends about health (e.g., detection of statistically significant adverse effects of pharmaceuticals (Bian et al. 2012; Mukherjee et al. 2014; Pappa and Stergioulas 2019; Josc 2020)). Recent investigations have also demonstrated that an individual's health status can be corroborated by the statements they publish over social media platforms (e.g., confirmation of flu diagnoses (Daughton et al. 2020; Ljubic et al. 2019)). Despite the power of such investigations, they are limited in that the associated approaches do not filter data from social media streams for any arbitrary health-related concept.

The objective of this chapter is to investigate how people disclose their own or others' health status over a broad range of health issues on a specific social media platform, namely Twitter, and apply both traditional and deep learning-based machine learning models to effectively detect such online personal health status mentions.

Our research is based on 250 million tweets, collected via the Twitter streaming API over a two-month period in 2014. We specifically focus on 34 high-impact health issues, which were selected based on the guidance from the Medical Expenditure Panel Survey. These include certain high impact health issues investigated in the Medical Expenditure Panel Survey (Medical Expenditure Panel Survey Home 2015), such as arthritis, asthma, bronchitis, cancer, diabetes, hypertension, and stroke. We created a labeled corpus of several thousand tweets via a survey, administered over Amazon Mechanical Turk (MT), that documents when terms correspond to mentions of personal health issues or an alternative (e.g., a metaphor). We show that the likelihood an individual self-discloses is dependent on the health issues that are communicated. For example, personal health status is revealed more than 50% for 11 of the 34 health issues. For certain health issues (e.g., allergies, bronchitis, insomnia, migraines, and ulcers), people are more likely to disclose their own health status, while for other health issues (e.g., Alzheimer's, Down syndrome, leukemia, miscarriage, and Parkinson's), people are more likely to disclose another person's status. Our experiments on building health status mention detection classifiers show that while the traditional machine learning models built upon bag-of-word features led to a decent performance (AUC = 0.80), deep learning-based approaches boosted model performance (AUC =0.88).

Related Work

Social Media and Health Research

Various investigations have demonstrated that social media can be successfully leveraged to (1) enable individuals to discuss their health status, (2) influence an individual's health behavior and (3) support the analysis of aggregate trends around health activities.

First, a certain portion of studies have focused on the extent to which, as well as how, social media enables self-reports of health information. Hale et al. (Hale et al. 2014) showed that users discuss their health conditions on public Facebook pages, but recognized that such pages tend to be overly general to attract users to contribute to a discussion. However, Bodnar and colleagues (Bodnar et al. 2014) found that individuals who use social media discuss certain ailments with high accuracy on Twitter. Specifically, this study demonstrated that college students tend to talk about their influenza diagnosis and associated symptoms. More generally, Paul et al. (Paul and Dredze 2014) performed latent topic model discovery over self-reported health status in Twitter to detect complex and potentially novel phenotypes. It has further been shown that some Twitter users reveal genome sequencing results (in relation to ancestry information according to 23andme.com services) over Twitter (Olejnik et al. 2014). Recently, as the rapid development of deep learning framework, it was shown that convolutional neural network (CNN) can be applied to effectively identify personal heath mentions from Twitter (Wang et al. 2020).

Second, there is a growing body of evidence to suggest that social media can influence an individual's health behavior. In certain cases, exploitation of social media can bring about negative health behaviors. For instance, based on discussions about prescription abuse over Twitter, it was observed that social media may aggravate such problems (Hanson et al. 2013a; Hanson et al. 2013b; Primack et al. 2019). In a similar vein, a content analysis of tweets, in association with the demographics of the followers of marijuana Twitter handles, showed that social media may allure young people to establish substance use patterns. Wilson et al. also argued that social media enables more individuals to be involved in an anti-vaccination movement (Lamb et al. 2013). However, it was also shown that social media can encourage more positive changes in health behavior. Notably, it was shown that increasing communications with smokers on social media can promote free cessation services (Duke et al. 2014; Luo et al. 2021). Moreover, Cobb and colleagues (Cobb et al. 2014) developed a Facebook application that was able to track the significant elements of an intervention on smoke cessation. It was also found that the design and realization of a community opinion leader model may mitigate the spread of HIV (Jaganath et al. 2011) and address the impact of COVID-19 (Quinn 2020).

Third, social media can be mined to identify and characterize aggregate trends with respect to health activities. For instance, it was shown that flu trends can be effectively extracted from Twitter using standard machine learning strategies

(Aramaki et al. 2011; Xue et al. 2019). More specifically, the analysis of daily tweets across a major metropolitan region (e.g., New York) can enable the prediction of which health issues are currently influencing the health of the public (Nagar et al. 2014). Meanwhile, Nagel et al. (Nagel et al. 2013) showed that both the keywords chosen to filter and create subgroups of tweets affected prediction accuracy. Beyond health status, it has been illustrated that the rare or unknown side-effects of drugs can be discovered through sentiment analysis over Twitter (Mukherjee et al. 2014).

Though social media can support a wide array of health-related investigations, there are a number of hurdles to making the associated methodologies scalable. As Curtis and colleagues (Curtis 2014) point out, for instance, insufficient procedures for protecting participants' privacy were one of the challenges to recruiting members from social media to conduct HIV research. In addition, it was revealed that the unreliability of big data and continuous changes of search algorithms contributed to failures in the Google Flu Trends program (Lazer et al. 2014).

This work presented in this chapter differs from the aforementioned studies in that we focus on personal health status disclosure on Twitter and aimed to detect mentions of a broad range of health issues.

Classification on Social Media

To mine health-related information from social media, it is critical to develop an automated classifier. However, tweets are constrained in size and, thus, are composed of limited content. Consequentially, it is essential to define and select discriminative features to support automated health status detection. In certain studies, tweets were enriched with features by referencing external sources, such as Wikipedia (Gattani et al. 2013; Yang et al. 2014), to improve topic modeling, but their generality hamper them in the support of personal health mention detection.

Research has shown that punctuation, emoji characters, hashtags, and the @username designation, and text (including n-grams of words or characters (Banerjee et al. 2009)) from the webpage referenced by the URL in a tweet, can form meaningful features for classification purposes (Gattani et al. 2013; Davidov et al. 2010; Sriram et al. 2010). Features generated using natural language processing tools, such as part of speech tags and dependencies between terms were also successfully incorporated as features in social media classifiers (Lamb et al. 2013; Banerjee et al. 2012). Recently, other more advanced models were developed to efficiently identify personal health mentions. These models included, but were not limited to, figurative usage detection with CNN-based methods (Iyer et al. 2019), permutation-based word representation learning (Khan et al. 2020), and based on transformer and decision tree (Lee et al. 2020). In this chapter, we applied both traditional machine learning models and deep learning-based model to show they perform in personal health mention detection tasks on Twitter.

Method

The Personal Health Status Mention Problem

To formalize the problem, we define the notions of personal health status and personal health mention.

- Definition 1 (Personal Health Status) The condition of a specific person regarding a health issue or symptom.
- Definition 2 (Personal Health Mention) A statement of personal health status in social media.

These definitions focus on the health information of the individuals who are potentially identifiable. For instance, tweets such as "my father is cancer free for ten years", "I have to do chemo tomorrow" and "my little cousin has leukemia" are representatives of personal health mentions. By contrast, "Local charity doing great work to help cancer patients" is not a personal health mention because the subject is a group of people as opposed to a specific person.

We treat the problem of personal health mention detection as binary classification. We say a tweet is positive if it reveals personal health status and negative otherwise. For example, two MT masters assigned positive labels to each of the first three tweets in Table 12.1 (details in Method Section). Yet a term associated with a health issue can be uttered on Twitter for many other reasons, such as in a metaphorical sense, to express a viewpoint about a health issue in general, or to

Table 12.1 Examples of tweets related to health issues and the labels obtained through the MT survey (Banerjee et al. 2009)

Tweet	Label via MT	
Positive	Master 1	Master 2
I'm suffering from schizophrenia and a little bit of insomnia.	Author	Author
Prayers for my dad would be appreciated. He has lymphoma. Thanks for the support everyone.	Relative	Relative
didn't she have a miscarriage like 3 days ago?	Someone else	Someone else
Negative		
you're gonna give Viv a heart attack	Metaphor	Metaphor
Even after Bill Gates relentless support and millions of dollars Poured into Malaria research, we are not successful.	Viewpoint	Viewpoint
Praying I don't have pneumonia	Worry	Worry
Ambiguous		
Cheerios say she'll never have to worry about dieting. Too bad with 2:1 sodium to cal, she'll have to worry about high blood pressure.	Metaphor	Someone else
Yooo soo i walk out my apt and here this girl screaming for help. Apparently, she kneed her testicular cancer bf in the nuts repeatedly.	Metaphor	Someone else
Memorial find. 10% of your bills went to leukemia and lymphoma research. When amber was around she brightened everyone's day in one way.	Viewpoint	Someone else

communicate a worry. The next three tweets in Table 12.1 provide examples of these reasons respectively.

Given their brevity, tweets often have limited context. Consequentially, assigning a class label to a tweet is substantially more challenging than detecting if a given tweet communicates status of the author. The last three tweets in Table 12.1 illustrates this observation, where MT masters assigned different option labels to the same tweet.

In this chapter, we study how people disclose personal health statuses on Twitter and present a personal health mentions detection system for Twitter stream. Specifically, we decompose this investigation into the following four hypotheses:

- H1: People discuss personal health status on Twitter.
- H2: Personal health status disclosure rate is health issue dependent.
- H3: The likelihood that people disclose their own versus other people's personal health status is health issue dependent.
- H4: Personal health status mention classifiers that are based on deep learning models are more scalable than those traditional models working on bag-of-word features.

Construction of a Health Mention Corpus

To create a labeled corpus of health status mentions, we solicited annotators through MT. Specifically, we randomly selected 100 tweets for each of the 34 health issues (see Fig. 12.1), and set up a survey for labeling a corpus on MT. For each tweet, we directed two MT masters to select the best of seven options that describes how the tweet uses the health issue:

1. *Author*. The tweet discloses the health status of the author. (e.g., going to get my last chemo treatment)
2. *Relative or friend*. The tweet discloses the health status of the author's family members or friends. (e.g., my uncle just found out he has cancer; my friend Tom has been cancer free for 4 years)
3. *Someone else*. The tweet discloses the health status of someone else, excluding the author, the author's family members and friends. (e.g., She has hypertension; Donald Sterling Is Battling Cancer)
4. *Metaphor*. The tweet uses the health issue as a metaphor (e.g., he is a cancer; the game makes me high blood pressure)
5. *Viewpoint*. The tweet expresses a viewpoint on the health issue, or some kind of support to general patients with the health issue (excluding those specific persons mentioned in option 1, 2 and 3). (e.g., I think cancer is horrible; Guys I'm #feelingnuts raising awareness for testicular cancer I'm nominating; Breast Cancer Awareness Month is JUST around the corner)
6. *Worry*. The tweet expresses a worry about the health issue. (e.g., I hope I don't get cancer by using my cell phone)
7. *N/A*. None of the above

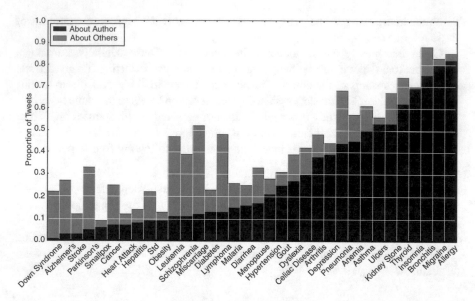

Fig. 12.1 The extent to which people tweet about themselves versus others when disclosing personal health status. Note that this is a *stacked bar* chart, such that the sum of the author and others proportions corresponds to the overall proportion of positive instances (Yin et al. 2015)

These options represent the common usage of most health issues. In this study, the positive class includes the labels of *author*, *relative or friend*, and *someone else*. The negative class consists of labels for *metaphor*, *viewpoint* and *worry*. Table 12.1 provides examples of tweets and the labels supplied by the MT masters. The last option label, *N/A*, which means none of the above, is also treated as a negative label in this investigation because it was observed (by the authors) that such labels were generally negative. For instance, these include tweets with job related information, which is spam that has nothing to do with a personal health mention. Each tweet that received conflicted labels from the two MT masters was labeled by a third MT master to break the tie.

Health Mention Classifiers

We consider two groups of classification models. The first group of classifiers consists of four common traditional machine learning models: logistic regression (LR), random forest (RFC), k-nearest-neighbors (KNN), and support vector machines within linear kernels (SVC). Previous investigations verified the effectiveness of such classifiers (Lamb et al. 2013), (Gattani et al. 2013; Davidov et al. 2010; Sriram et al. 2010; Banerjee et al. 2012). We applied their implementation in the *sklearn* package (version 0.24) in our experiments.

For these models, we proposed to use the following types of features:

- Linguistic categories extracted by using Linguistic Inquiry and Word Count (LIWC). LIWC is a popular tool that is applied in computational social science to extract linguistic categories as features to learn a broad range of topics, including but are not limited to mental health.
- Bag-of-word features with word count as feature values.
- Bag-of-word features with term frequency inverse document frequency (TFIDF) as feature values. TFIDF is a classic statistic in natural language processing to quantify the importance of word to a document in a data corpus. A higher TFIDF value in a tweet suggests the related word is more likely to differentiate this tweet from tweets in the data corpus.
- N-gram characters ($2 \leq N \leq 5$) with TFIDF as feature values.

The second group of classifiers consists of deep learning-based models. The past decade has witnessed dramatic advances in deep learning and its application in image, video and natural language processing (NLP) (Zhang et al. 2018). Particularly, in NLP, how to effectively capture the semantic information, context, or sequential patterns within the language into machine learning models is a key to improve model performance. For example, word2vec is a static low dimensional representation learning technique that can capture the word semantic (Mikolov et al. 2013). However, a limitation of such static representation learning is that each term can only have a unique embedding vector no matter what context it is in. By contrast, the transformer, or other models built upon its components, such as Bidirectional Encoder Representations from Transformers (BERT) (Devlin et al. 2018), can effectively capture the dynamic context information. For example, BERT is designed to pre-train deep bidirectional representations in the unlabeled text by jointly performing conditional preprocessing on the left and right contexts of all layers (Wicks et al. 2014).

We apply four deep learning classifiers based on Long Short-Term Memory network (LSTM) and BERT, and implement these models using PyTorch (version 1.4.0) and transformers (version 3.5.1).

- A Long Short-Term Memory model with one hot representation of each tweet (LSTM-One-Hot). LSTM is a recurrent neural network (RNN) model which aims to mitigate the vanishing gradient issues and capture long-distance dependency.
- An LSTM with word2vec representation of each tweet (LSTM-Word2vec). In this model, we replaced the input of the LSTM-One-Hot model with the word2vec representation of each term in a tweet. Comparing one-hot sparse representation, word2vec representation can be applied to measure the semantic similarity between two words by calculating the cosine similarity of their related vectors, which may lead to a better model performance. In this study, we adopted the Google pre-trained word2vec, *word2vec-google-news-300*, to build vector representation of each term in a tweet.
- A Bi-directional LSTM model with attention using word2vec features (Bi-LSTM- Attention). Attention is a mechanism to improve model performance in RNN models (Vaswani et al. 2017). In this study, we used the last hidden state to

compute the attention scores with the previous hidden states in a LSTM model and feed the weighted average of the hidden states into another fully connected neural network to make the prediction.

- BERT Fine-Tuning Model (BERT-Fine-Tuning). While BERT model can be used to generate vector presentation for each tweet, which can be used to train traditional machine learning models, a common application of BERT is to re-fine all the model parameters together with the downstream classification task. In this study, we used Google pretrain BERT model, *bert-base-uncased*, and refine the model with the health mention detection task.

Performance Measures

To assess model performance, we rely upon accuracy, precision, recall, F1 and area under ROC (AUC). In our setting, Accuracy corresponds to the proportion of the tweets classified correctly. Precision corresponds to the proportion of tweets classified as positive that are in fact positive. Recall corresponds to the fraction of real positive tweets that are classified as positive. F1 is a balanced measure between precision and recall which is defined as 2 * precision * recall / (precision + recall). It should be noted that the accuracy, precision, recall and F1 are measured based on a default decision boundary of 0.5. In other words, a tweet will be classified as positive class if the predicted probability is above 0.5. Otherwise, it will be classified as negative class. AUC measures the overall performance of models.

Experimental Methodology

For each experiment, we stratify the tweets and generate 10 train-test sets. In doing so, (1) each set preserves the proportion of samples for each positive (negative) class and (2) the data is partitioned, such that we train on 80% of the tweets while we test on the remaining 20%. To control the comparison, the size of the training set for each compared classifier is equivalent. We use paired a t-test to compare model performance at a significance level of 0.05.

Results

Dataset

We used the Twitter streaming API to filter for tweets between May 7, 2014 and July 23, 2014 that were (1) published in the contiguous United States according to their geolocation and (2) written in the English language only. A total of 261,468,446 tweets were subject to a filter composed of keywords for 34 health issues (Yin et al. 2015), resulting in 281, 357 tweets (0.11%) for further investigation.

Table 12.2 Strength of agreement in labeling 34 health issues (100 tweets for each health issues)

Strength	Good (0.61–0.80)	Moderate (0.41–0.60)	Fair (0.21–0.40)	Poor (<0.20)
Health issues	15	14	5	1

The annotation was performed on MT in 2014, and the strength of agreement (based on Kappa scores) between two annotators are summarized in Table 12.2. The results confirmed the reliability of the MT masters' tasks.

How People Disclose Personal Health Status on Twitter

To demonstrate the opportunities for a personal health mention detection system, we investigate H1, H2 and H3. We chose 100 tweets at random for each of the 34 health issues as shown along the x-axis of Fig. 12.1, to generate the gold standard dataset. These health issues are based on common and high impact health issues as defined by the Medical Expenditure Panel Survey (Medical Expenditure Panel Survey Home 2015).

Figure 12.1 illustrates how often people disclose their own health status as opposed to other individuals' status. The black bar, "About Author", represents the proportion of positive tweets with the author label. The gray bar, "About Others", represents the proportion of positive tweets with the label relative or friends and someone else. For a specific health issue, the sum of the two values is equal to the proportion of positive tweets for this health issue. For example, 40% of the tweets about miscarriages (40 out of 100) disclosed other people's status, while only 12% (12 out of 100) disclosed the author's status (such that 52% of the tweets (52 out of 100) were positive instances).

To test hypothesis H2 (personal health status disclosure rate) and H3 (who the disclosure is about), we define the following null hypotheses:

- $H2_o$: The rate of positive and negative tweets is independent of the health issues.
- $H3_o$: The rate of tweets disclosing the author's health status and others' health status is independent of the health issues.

To test these hypotheses, we used the gold standard dataset, which (due to randomness) represents 100 samples from each of the 34 distributions regarding how people disclose health status. To test H2, we applied a Chi-square test on the number of positive tweets and the number of negative tweets in each health issue samples. To test hypothesis H3, we applied a Spearman Correlation test on the rate of tweets disclosing the author's health status and the rate of tweets disclosing the others' health status. We set the α level of significance to 0.05.

The analysis yielded several notable findings related to the first three hypotheses.

- People disclose personal health status on Twitter for a range of health issues (H1): The disclosure rate for each of the 34 health issues is greater than 9%. There are 29 health issues with disclosure rates greater than 20% and 11 health issues with disclosure rates greater than 50%. The latter group includes allergies,

anemia, arthritis, asthma, bronchitis, insomnia, kidney stones, migraines, miscarriages, pneumonia, thyroid problems, and ulcers.

- Health status disclosure rate is dependent on the health issue, $\chi 2$ (33, $N = 100$) $= 697$, $p < 0.001$: For instance, more than 80% of the tweets about migraines and allergies communicate personal health status. By contrast, only ~10% of tweets about obesity and heart attacks communicate personal health status. Bronchitis exhibits the largest proportion of tweets (88 out of 100) that disclose personal health status, while smallpox exhibits the smallest proportion (9 out of 100).
- The likelihood that people disclose their own versus other people's health status is dependent on the health issue, $Z = -5.745$, $p < 0.001$: For instance, 69% of tweets about insomnia (69 out of 100) disclose the author's personal health statuses compared, while only 1% (1 out of 100) disclose another person's status. By contrast, 1% of the tweets for Down syndrome (1 out of 100) disclose the author's status, while 21% (21 out of 100) disclose another person's status.

Classification Results

While each health issue has a different percentage of health mention tweets, the dataset is relatively balanced when all of the labeled tweets are merged together. We applied these 3400 annotated tweets to build and test each proposed classifier. Table 12.3 shows the model performance of traditional machine learning models. From the table, it can be seen that character n-gram features with TFIDF values results in the best performance in all of the measures. Particularly, with character n-gram features, LR has the largest average performance in accuracy (0.750), F1 (0.688), and AUC (0.810), RFC has the largest average precision (0.741), and SVC has the largest recall (0.662).

While there are less than 100 semantic features extracted using LIWC, RFC with such features has weaker but quite similar model performance (e.g., AUC = 0.800) with RFC with character n-gram features. However, it should be noted that accuracy, precision, recall and F1 are measured under a default decision boundary of 0.50, and a different decision boundary will lead to different results (e.g., a higher precision but lower recall).

Table 12.4 shows the performance of the deep learning-based models. The BERT Fine-Tuning model achieves the best performance and the smallest variance on all of the measures ($p < 0.001$) when comparing with other deep learning-based models. It also outperforms all the traditional model learning models in each measure ($p < 0.001$). Additionally, Bi-LSTM-Attention outperforms the traditional models in AUC ($p = 0.002$), F1 ($p < 0.001$), and recall ($p < 0.001$). However, it does not statistically outperform the traditional models in accuracy and has a lower precision ($p < 0.001$).

Table 12.3 The performance of the traditional models. The best performance in each measure is highlighted using bold font

Model	Measure	LIWC	Word Count	Word TF-IDF	Character N-Gram TFIDF
LR	Accuracy	0.723 (0.011)	0.718 (0.013)	0.715 (0.016)	**0.750 (0.007)**
	Precision	0.689 (0.020)	0.683 (0.019)	0.675 (0.021)	0.720 (0.016)
	Recall	0.618 (0.028)	0.607 (0.020)	0.616 (0.030)	0.659 (0.022)
	F1	0.651 (0.016)	0.643 (0.016)	0.644 (0.023)	**0.688 (0.010)**
	AUC	0.791 (0.012)	0.776 (0.019)	0.775 (0.017)	**0.810 (0.007)**
RFC	Accuracy	0.732 (0.012)	0.701 (0.019)	0.707 (0.019)	0.745 (0.010)
	Precision	0.716 (0.020)	0.651 (0.03)	0.661 (0.028)	**0.741 (0.022)**
	Recall	0.599 (0.024)	0.620 (0.025)	0.614 (0.024)	0.602 (0.020)
	F1	0.652 (0.018)	0.634 (0.021)	0.637 (0.021)	0.664 (0.013)
	AUC	0.800 (0.009)	0.751 (0.016)	0.754 (0.019)	0.810 (0.014)
KNN	Accuracy	0.660 (0.025)	0.684 (0.020)	0.690 (0.022)	0.711 (0.016)
	Precision	0.597 (0.031)	0.648 (0.036)	0.650 (0.033)	**0.670 (0.023)**
	Recall	0.575 (0.035)	0.540 (0.032)	0.564 (0.03)	0.611 (0.023)
	F1	0.585 (0.032)	0.588 (0.023)	0.604 (0.026)	0.639 (0.020)
	AUC	0.704 (0.027)	0.722 (0.024)	0.731 (0.029)	0.764 (0.015)
SVC	Accuracy	0.629 (0.056)	0.719 (0.013)	0.713 (0.015)	0.745 (0.010)
	Precision	0.667 (0.095)	0.683 (0.018)	0.673 (0.02)	0.709 (0.017)
	Recall	0.386 (0.268)	0.610 (0.023)	0.611 (0.027)	**0.662 (0.022)**
	F1	0.416 (0.175)	0.644 (0.018)	0.640 (0.021)	0.685 (0.013)
	AUC	0.716 (0.039)	0.775 (0.018)	0.774 (0.017)	0.806 (0.008)

Table 12.4 The performance of the deep learning-based models

Model	Accuracy	Precision	Recall	F1	AUC
LSTM-One-Hot	0.742 (0.012)	0.686 (0.022)	0.708 (0.032)	0.696 (0.014)	0.813 (0.012)
LSTM-Word2vec	0.740 (0.010)	0.695 (0.026)	0.680 (0.036)	0.686 (0.012)	0.814 (0.010)
Bi-LSTM-Attention	0.754 (0.013)	0.689 (0.030)	0.758 (0.046)	0.720 (0.012)	0.829 (0.008)
BERT-Fine-Tuning	**0.813 (0.009)**	**0.781 (0.011)**	**0.769 (0.023)**	**0.775 (0.013)**	**0.885 (0.011)**

Sensitivity Analysis

Figure 12.2 shows how the model performance change with different sizes of training data. Here, we use Logistic regression and BERT Fine-Tuning as examples to show the number of training tweets will affect model performance. From the figure, we can observe that Logistic Regression reaches the largest mean of AUC between 1000 and 1500 training tweets. After that its performance drops a little bit but not significantly. By contrast, the BERT Fine-Tuning model experiences two turning points at 500 and 1500 training tweets, respectively. However, unlike the Logistic Regression, the BERT Fine-Tunning model still has consistent performance increase in a moderate rate as the number of training tweets surpasses 1500. This suggests that our annotated data is sufficient to train a traditional machine learning model well. While the performance of deep learning-based models might be improved by

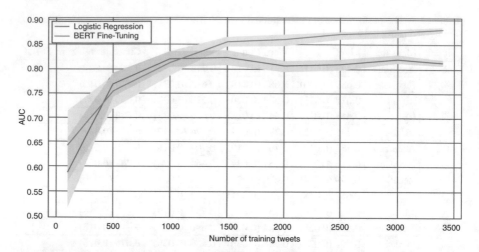

Fig. 12.2 AUC of the Logistic Regression and BERT Fine-Tuning models with different numbers of training tweets. The shaded area shows the one standard deviation of the AUC. The AUCs are collected from the 10 training-test data splits

bringing additional labeled data, the marginal benefits are expected to be limited, considering the cost of data annotation.

Discussion

Principal Findings

There are several notable findings from this investigation. First, Twitter users disclose the health status of themselves and others. Second, the health status disclosure rate appears to depend on the health issue. Third, how people disclose their own and other people's health status may also be health issue dependent. Fourth, tweets related with a small group of health issues can train a scalable classifier to detect health mentions on Twitter streams.

The traditional classification model results show that character n-grams features help build better models than word features. This may be because character n-grams are less sensitive than words to the noisy tweets where misspellings are not uncommon. While semantic features extracted using LIWC, from the perspective of dimension reduction, compress the information communicated in each tweet much more than the thousands of raw words or n-gram features, the models built upon LIWC features achieve similar performance as the models built upon words or n-gram features. This suggests that the semantic categories matter in recognizing health mentions. Our experiments on building models to detect health mentions in tweets adds the evidence that deep learning-based model, especially transfer learning using BERT, improve the performance of text classification. With over three thousand annotated tweets, Bi-LSTM with attention model did not substantially outperform standard LSTM models.

Impact on Health-Related Research

According to this investigation, roughly 44% of the tweets containing health issue keywords disclose personal health status. We believe there is a potential for information to assist healthcare professionals in learning about their patients or their patients' family medical history, information often missing in the EMRs. This indicates that social media platforms, such as Twitter contains huge amount of personal health care related information that may complement traditional EMRs in research and practice. We recognize that we must still verify the veracity of such data, but the opportunity exists, nonetheless.

Limitations

We wish to highlight several limitations of this investigation. First, two parameters to extract tweets from Twitter streams require configuration: (1) the set of keywords invoked in the filter and (2) the geolocation applied to discover tweets. Compared to keywords, geolocation can filter tweets disseminated by authoritative organizations (due to the absence of "coordinates" and "place" information in these tweets), such as the American Cancer Society, and thus greatly reduce noise. However, it should be noted that invoking such a filter can also exclude the tweets of individuals who choose not to disclose their location. A second limitation exists in the survey provided to the MT masters for labeling the corpus. Specifically, we assumed the N/A option was a member of the negative class, but this could be an incorrect assumption in certain instances. Third, this investigation was restricted to only 34 health-related issues, which is clearly only a sample of all possible health issues. The keywords filter service can be enhanced by integrating a laymen health vocabulary (Vydiswaran et al. 2014). Given that this study shows there is (1) high variability in the rate at which people tweet about a certain health issue and (2) to whom the statement of health issue corresponds, it will be critical to investigate how these methods fare in the context of other health issues. Finally, each of our annotation task relied on two independent annotators and a third annotator if there was a conflict existing in labels from the first two annotators. It has been shown that the optimal number of annotators to obtain reliable results may be around ten (Carvalho et al. 2016), and the quality of annotation results can be improved by providing additional training to annotators (Jha et al. 2010; Sabou et al. 2014; Simperl 2015; Gadiraju et al. 2015; Hube et al. 2019). While the average inner annotator agreement in our data show that these might not be a critical issue to this task, future studies should investigate whether such an empirical value is still valid in health mention labeling tasks.

Future Work

We envision several opportunities for extending this work. First, we believe the scalability of the classifier may be improved by determining the minimal set of health issues and features (e.g., more complicated grammar features). Second, while deep learning-based models prove to be effective in capturing the language context within a single tweet, we anticipate that the performance of the classifier could be improved by accounting for other context, such as dialogue, relationships in the network, and profile information as new supplemental features. Third, the model performance could be improved by continuing to train BERT model with a large number of unlabeled tweets before fine-tuning it. Finally, while the rate that health status is disclosed for the author versus other individuals is dependent upon the considered health issue, further investigation is required to determine what drives this disparity. We suspect, for instance, that it may be dependent on the sensitivity and severity of health issues, but this is only a conjecture.

Conclusions

In this chapter, we show that health status mentions can be effectively detected from Twitter using machine learning, especially deep learning, algorithms. At the same time, we illustrate that the information communicated through such mentions can disclose the health status of the authors and other individuals at a wide range of rates. Our findings set the stage to build a scalable system to efficiently extract such health mentions from online environments to make them useful in practice.

Acknowledgements This research was sponsored in part by grants from the National Science Foundation (CCF-0424422) and the Patient Centered Outcomes Research Institute (CDRN-1306-04869). The authors would like to thank the members of the Mid-South Clinical Data Research Network for useful discussions during the development of this research.

> **Clinical Pearls**
> 1. People disclose not only their health conditions but also the health status of other people, suggesting the challenge of privacy protection in online environments and the necessity of considering both self- and other-health status disclosure when using such data for accurate public health surveillance.
> 2. Deep learning-based models, especially those based on large pre-trained language models, can be applied to handle health mention detection effectively.

Review Questions

1. Does a deep learning-based model consistently outperform a traditional model in short text classification (e.g., health mention detection on Twitter)?
2. Does the rate of self-health status disclosure depend on disease?

Answers

1. It depends. When the training dataset is not large, RNN-based models (e.g., vanilla RNN or Attention-based RNN) can hardly beat the traditional models (e.g., random forest, SVM, or logistic regression). However, BERT fine-tuning is exceptional. This deep learning model fine-tunes the learned context from a much larger data corpus to better classify health status on a small dataset.
2. Yes. Depend on the disease. For example, people tend to disclose their health status for common health issues like allergies and insomnia. By contrast, people tend to disclose others' health status for severe diseases such as Alzheimer's disease and heart attack.

References

Aramaki E, Maskawa S, and Morita M. Twitter catches the flu: detecting influenza epidemics using Twitter. in *Proceedings of the 2011 Conference on empirical methods in natural language processing*, 2011, pp. 1568–1576.

Banerjee N, Chakraborty D, Joshi A, Mittal S, Rai A, and Ravindran B. Towards analyzing micro-blogs for detection and classification of real-time intentions. 2012.

Banerjee N *et al.* User interests in social media sites: an exploration with micro blogs. in *Proceedings of the 18th ACM conference on Information and knowledge management*, 2009, pp. 1823–1826.

Bian J., Topaloglu U, and Yu F. Towards large-scale twitter mining for drug-related adverse events. 2012, https://doi.org/10.1145/2389707.2389713.

Bodnar T, Barclay VC, Ram N, Tucker C S, and Salathé M. On the ground validation of online diagnosis with Twitter and medical records. 2014, doi: https://doi.org/10.1145/2567948.2579272.

Brewer G *et al.* Experiences of mental distress during COVID-19: thematic analysis of discussion forum posts for anxiety, depression, and obsessive-compulsive disorder. *Illness, Cris. \& Loss*, p. 10541373211023952, 2021.

Carvalho A, Dimitrov S, Larson K. How many crowdsourced workers should a requester hire? Ann Math Artif Intell. 2016;78(1):45–72.

Cobb NK, Jacobs MA, Saul J, Wileyto EP, and Graham AL. Diffusion of an evidence-based smoking cessation intervention through Facebook: a randomised controlled trial study protocol. vol. 4, no. 1, p. e004089, 2014, doi: https://doi.org/10.1136/bmjopen-2013-004089.

Coorevits P *et al.*. Electronic health records: new opportunities for clinical research. vol. 274, no. 6, pp. 547–560, 2013, doi: https://doi.org/10.1111/joim.12119.

Curtis BL. Social networking and online recruiting for {HIV} research: ethical challenges. vol. 9, no. 1, pp. 58–70, 2014, doi: https://doi.org/10.1525/jer.2014.9.1.58.

Daughton AR, Chunara R, Paul MJ. Comparison of social media, syndromic surveillance, and microbiologic acute respiratory infection data: observational study. JMIR Public Health Surveill. 2020;6(2):e14986.

Davidov D, Tsur O, and Rappoport A. Semi-supervised recognition of sarcasm in Twitter and Amazon. in *Proceedings of the fourteenth conference on computational natural language learning*, 2010, pp. 107–116.

Devlin J, Chang M-W, Lee K, and Toutanova K. Bert: pre-training of deep bidirectional transformers for language understanding. *arXiv Prepr. arXiv1810.04805*, 2018.

Duke JC, Hansen H, Kim AE, Curry L, and Allen J. The use of social media by state tobacco
control programs to promote smoking cessation: a cross-sectional study. vol. 16, no. 7, p. e169,
2014, doi: https://doi.org/10.2196/jmir.3430.

D. Estrin. Small data, where n = me. vol. 57, no. 4, pp. 32–34, 2014, doi: 10.1145/2580944.

Eysenbach G and Wyatt J. Using the internet for surveys and health research," vol. 4, no. 2, p. e13,
2002, doi: https://doi.org/10.2196/jmir.4.2.e13.

Gadiraju U, Fetahu B, and Kawase R. Training workers for improving performance in crowdsourcing microtasks. in *European Conference on Technology Enhanced Learning*, 2015, 100–114.

Garratt AM, Ruta DA, Abdalla MI, Buckingham JK, and Russell IT. The {SF}36 health survey
questionnaire: an outcome measure suitable for routine use within the {NHS}? vol. 306, no.
6890, pp. 1440–1444, 1993, doi: https://doi.org/10.1136/bmj.306.6890.1440.

A. Gattani *et al.*, "Entity extraction, linking, classification, and tagging for social media," vol. 6,
no. 11, pp. 1126–1137, Aug. 2013, doi: https://doi.org/10.14778/2536222.2536237.

Hale TM, Pathipati AS, Zan S, and Jethwani K. Representation of health conditions on facebook:
content analysis and evaluation of user engagement. vol. 16, no. 8, p. e182, 2014, doi: https://
doi.org/10.2196/jmir.3275.

Hanson CL, Burton SH, Giraud-Carrier C, West JH, Barnes MD, and Hansen B. Tweaking and
tweeting: exploring twitter for nonmedical use of a psychostimulant drug (Adderall) Among
College Students. vol. 15, no. 4, p. e62, 2013a, doi: https://doi.org/10.2196/jmir.2503.

Hanson CL, Cannon B, Burton S, and Giraud-Carrier C. An exploration of social circles and prescription drug abuse through twitter. vol. 15, no. 9, p. e189, 2013b, doi: https://doi.org/10.2196/
jmir.2741.

Hube C, Fetahu B, and Gadiraju U. Understanding and mitigating worker biases in the crowd-
sourced collection of subjective judgments. in *Proceedings of the 2019 CHI Conference on
Human Factors in Computing Systems*, 2019, pp. 1–12.

Iyer A, Joshi A, Karimi S, Sparks R, and Paris C. Figurative usage detection of symptom words to
improve personal health mention detection. *arXiv Prepr. arXiv1906.05466*, 2019.

Jaganath D, Gill HK, Cohen AC, and Young SD. Harnessing Online Peer Education ({HOPE}):
Integrating C-{POL} and social media to train peer leaders in {HIV} prevention. vol. 24, no. 5,
pp. 593–600, 2011, doi: https://doi.org/10.1080/09540121.2011.630355.

Jensen PB, Jensen LJ, and Brunak S. Mining electronic health records: towards better research
applications and clinical care. vol. 13, no. 6, pp. 395–405, 2012, doi: https://doi.org/10.1038/
nrg3208.

Jha M, Andreas J, Thadani K, Rosenthal S, and McKeown K. Corpus creation for new genres: A
crowdsourced approach to PP attachment. in *Proceedings of the NAACL HLT 2010 workshop
on creating speech and language data with Amazon's mechanical turk*, 2010, pp. 13–20.

Jose J. Communication on drug safety-related matters to patients: is it even more significant in this
digital era? London, England: SAGE Publications Sage UK; 2020.

Khan PI, Razzak I, Dengel A, and Ahmed S. Improving personal health mention detection on
twitter using permutation based word representation learning. in *International Conference on
Neural Information Processing*, 2020, pp. 776–785.

S. Kumar *et al.*. Mobile health technology evaluation. vol. 45, no. 2, pp. 228–236, 2013, doi:
https://doi.org/10.1016/j.amepre.2013.03.017.

Lamb A, Paul M, and Dredze M. Separating fact from fear: tracking flu infections on twitter. in
*Proceedings of the 2013 Conference of the North American Chapter of the Association for
Computational Linguistics: Human Language Technologies*, 2013, pp. 789–795.

Lazer D, Kennedy R, King G, and Vespignani A. The parable of google flu: traps in big data
analysis. vol. 343, no. 6176, pp. 1203–1205, 2014, doi: https://doi.org/10.1126/science.
1248506.

Lee L-H, Chen P-H, Kao H-C, Hung T-C, Lee P-L, and Shyu K-K. Medication mention detection
in tweets using ELECTRA transformers and decision trees. in *Proceedings of the Fifth Social
Media Mining for Health Applications Workshop \& Shared Task*, 2020, pp. 131–133.

Ljubic B, Gligorijevic D, Gligorijevic J, Pavlovski M, Obradovic Z. Social network analysis for better understanding of influenza. J Biomed Inform. 2019;93:103161.

Luo T, et al. Using social media for smoking cessation interventions: a systematic review. Perspect Public Health. 2021;141(1):50–63.

Medical Expenditure Panel Survey Home (2015). https://meps.ahrq.gov/mepsweb/ (accessed Aug. 31, 2021).

Mikolov T, Sutskever I, Chen K, Corrado GS, and Dean J. Distributed representations of words and phrases and their compositionality. in *Advances in neural information processing systems*, 2013, pp. 3111–3119.

Mukherjee S, Weikum G, and Danescu-Niculescu-Mizil C. People on drugs: credibility of user statements in health communities. in *Proceedings of the 20th ACM SIGKDD international conference on Knowledge discovery and data mining*, 2014, pp. 65–74.

Nagar R, et al. A case study of the New York City 2012–2013 influenza season with daily geo-coded twitter data from temporal and spatiotemporal perspectives. vol. 16, no. 10, p. e236, 2014, doi: https://doi.org/10.2196/jmir.3416.

Nagel AC, et al. The complex relationship of realspace events and messages in cyberspace: case study of influenza and pertussis using tweets. vol. 15, no. 10, p. e237, 2013, doi: https://doi.org/10.2196/jmir.2705.

Olejnik L, Kutrowska A, Castelluccia C. I'M 2.8% Neanderthal - The beginning of genetic exhibitionism? In: Workshop on Genome Privacy. July 2014 Presented at: Workshop on Genome Privacy, 14th Privacy Enhancing Technologies Symposium PETS 2014 At: Amsterdam, Netherlands.

Pappa D, Stergioulas LK. Harnessing social media data for pharmacovigilance: a review of current state of the art, challenges and future directions. Int J Data Sci Anal. 2019;8(2):113–35.

Paul MJ and Dredze M. Discovering health topics in social media using topic models. vol. 9, no. 8, p. e103408, 2014, doi: https://doi.org/10.1371/journal.pone.0103408.

Primack BA, Karim SA, Shensa A, Bowman N, Knight J, Sidani JE. Positive and negative experiences on social media and perceived social isolation. Am J Health Promot. 2019;33(6):859–68.

Quam L, Ellis LBM, Venus P, Clouse J, Taylor CG, and Leatherman S. Using claims data for epidemiologic research. vol. 31, no. 6, pp. 498–507, 1993, doi: https://doi.org/10.1097/00005650-199306000-00003.

Quinn KG. Applying the popular opinion leader intervention for HIV to COVID-19. AIDS Behav. 2020;24(12):3291–4.

Rea S, et al. Building a robust, scalable and standards-driven infrastructure for secondary use of {EHR} data: The {SHARPn} project. vol. 45, no. 4, pp. 763–771, 2012, doi: https://doi.org/10.1016/j.jbi.2012.01.009.

Riedl J, Riedl E. Crowdsourcing medical research. vol. 46, no. 1, pp. 89–92, 2013, doi: https://doi.org/10.1109/mc.2013.15.

Sabou M, Bontcheva K, Derczynski L, and Scharl A. Corpus annotation through crowdsourcing: towards best practice guidelines. in *LREC*, 2014, pp. 859–866.

Samsa GP, et al. Quality of anticoagulation management among patients with atrial fibrillation. vol. 160, no. 7, p. 967, 2000, doi: https://doi.org/10.1001/archinte.160.7.967.

Simperl E. How to use crowdsourcing effectively: guidelines and examples. Lib Q. 2015;25(1)

Slemon A, McAuliffe C, Goodyear T, McGuinness L., Shaffer E, and Jenkins EK. Reddit users' experiences of suicidal thoughts during the COVID-19 pandemic: a qualitative analysis of r/Covid19_support Posts. *Front Public Health*, p. 1175, 2021.

Sriram B, Fuhry D, Demir E, Ferhatosmanoglu H, Demirbas M. Short text classification in twitter to improve information filtering; 2010. https://doi.org/10.1145/1835449.1835643.

Tomlinson M, Rotheram-Borus MJ, Swartz L, and Tsai AC. Scaling up {mHealth}: where is the evidence?. vol. 10, no. 2, p. e1001382, 2013, doi: https://doi.org/10.1371/journal.pmed.1001382.

Vaswani A, et al. Attention is all you need. in *Advances in neural information processing systems*, 2017, pp. 5998–6008.

Vydiswaran VGV, Mei Q, Hanauer DA, and Zheng K. Mining consumer health vocabulary from community-generated text. in *AMIA Annual Symposium Proceedings*, 2014, vol. 2014, p. 1150.

Wang Y, Li X, and Mo DY. Personal health mention identification from tweets using convolutional neural network. in *2020 IEEE International Conference on Industrial Engineering and Engineering Management (IEEM)*, 2020, pp. 650–654.

Wicks P, Vaughan T, and Heywood J. Subjects no more: what happens when trial participants realize they hold the power?. vol. 348, no. jan28 9, pp. g368--g368, 2014, doi: https://doi.org/10.1136/bmj.g368.

Williams LS, Yilmaz EY, and Lopez-Yunez AM. Retrospective assessment of initial stroke severity with the {NIH} Stroke Scale. vol. 31, no. 4, pp. 858–862, 2000, doi: https://doi.org/10.1161/01.str.31.4.858.

Xue H, Bai Y, Hu H, Liang H. Regional level influenza study based on twitter and machine learning method. PLoS One. 2019;14(4):e0215600.

Yang S-H, Kolcz A, Schlaikjer A, Gupta P. Large-scale high-precision topic modeling on twitter; 2014. https://doi.org/10.1145/2623330.2623336.

Yin Z, Fabbri D, Rosenbloom ST, and Malin B. A scalable framework to detect personal health mentions on twitter. vol. 17, no. 6, p. e138, 2015, doi: https://doi.org/10.2196/jmir.4305.

Yin Z, Malin B, Warner J, Hsueh P-Y, and Chen C-H. The power of the patient voice: learning indicators of treatment adherence from an online breast cancer forum. in *Proceedings of the International AAAI Conference on Web and Social Media*, 2017, vol. 11, no. 1.

Zhang R, Li W, and Mo T. Review of deep learning. *arXiv Prepr. arXiv1804.01653*, 2018.

Chapter 13
Common Data Models (CDMs): The Basic Building Blocks for Fostering Public Health Surveillance and Population Health Research Using Distributed Data Networks (DDNs)

Pradeep S. B. Podila

Abstract Data is considered as a valued asset due to its inherent nature to shed light on key information and pave pathways for actionable intelligence or insights. About 80% of the information collected during healthcare visits is documented in electronic format within the electronic health records (EHRs). The timely availability of the data captured with EHRs for use by hospitals, federal or state entities, and local public health agencies (LPHAs) is key component for chalking out strategic visioning and planning, and for public/population health efforts. But the rate at which the data is growing is many fold greater than the rate at which it could be shared outside of the healthcare entity where it was generated due to privacy and security concerns. In addition, healthcare also deals with an infinite array of vulnerabilities such as phishing attacks, ransomware attacks, malware attacks and thefts of laptops and electronic devices with patient identifiable information (PII) or protected health information (PHI).

Due to these concerns, and the way information is stored within different systems or databases across healthcare organizations makes it even more challenging to share data for multi-institutional collaborations. A possible solution to address this multi-dimensional challenge is conforming organizational data to a common format, known as a Common Data Model (CDM). This chapter sheds light on the concept of CDM, its key principles, and highlights the ways in which such models can help support health services research and public health surveillance.

Keywords Common Data Model · Data Governance · Distributed Data Network · Distributed Health Data Network · Electronic Health Records · Privacy · Security

P. S. B. Podila (✉)
Methodist Le Bonheur Healthcare, Memphis, TN, USA

© The Author(s), under exclusive license to Springer Nature Switzerland AG 2022
P.-Y. S. Hsueh et al. (eds.), *Personal Health Informatics*, Cognitive Informatics in Biomedicine and Healthcare, https://doi.org/10.1007/978-3-031-07696-1_13

Learning Objectives
1. A detailed introduction to Common Data Models (CDMs).
2. A step-by-step guidance on the process by which potential participating sites or members of a DDN could build CDMs.
3. Highlight the governance policies and their significance in fostering the public and population health efforts.
4. Share specific examples from the most popular Distributed Health Data Networks (DHDNs) like HSCRN, OMOP, PCORnet etc.,

Introduction

The wide spread adoption (Magnuson and Dixon 2020) of electronic health records (EHR) supported by the federal initiatives and explosion in the use of the consumer electronics like wearables and smart devices has resulted in the continuous generation of electronic health data. EHRs allow for the systematic collection and management of an individual's health information in a form that can be shared across health care settings and can help inform public health. About 80% of the information collected during healthcare visits is currently documented in electronic format within EHRs. For example, EHRs contain many key variables that can help with public health emergencies (e.g., influenza pandemics, terrorist attacks). Although EHRs have their own shortcomings they can support with data for studies that inform key public health decisions during the times of emergencies and outbreaks.

For example, a timely availability of such data assets for use by hospitals, federal or state entities, and public health agencies (PHAs) is key component for chalking out healthcare/public health strategic visioning and planning preventative and public/population health efforts; and emergency preparedness activities during pandemics such as severe acute respiratory syndrome coronavirus 2 (SARS-CoV-2) i.e., COVID-19. Hence, the utilization of a large number of records from multiple healthcare entities could help fill gaps and provide mission-critical answers to physicians, care givers, researchers, administrators, public health officials, and the general public to better chalk out the strategies.

Data as the Organizational Asset

Data is considered as a valued asset by many organizations due to its inherent nature to help unearth nuggets of key information and pave pathways for actionable intelligence or insights. Hence, it can also be referred to as the *currency* of the modern world (or) as the *new earth* as unless explored valuable resources such as minerals, and fertile lands for crops which are essential for the existence and survival of the humans could not be easily found. The ability to deftly tap into resources to draw insights from data can serve as the ultimate deciding factor as to whether an organization succeeds or fails in meeting the expectations of its stakeholders or customer base or end users.

Discordance between Data Growth and Data Sharing

The data generated or captured by healthcare organizations or hospital systems has many uses. It helps the organization where it has been originally collected for carrying out day-to-day business or operations as well as for supporting community services, population health efforts and health services research. In addition to that, such data also serves as a great resource for governmental organizations such as the federal or state or local public health agencies to better understand the needs of the population in those focused regions as well as to build disease registries to track the progress of conditions such as diabetes, hypertension, cardiovascular disease, cancer, stroke, and health vulnerabilities. In other words, the utility of healthcare data goes beyond assisting the parent organization in generating revenue ($) by adding value from a societal aspect.

But the rate at which the data is growing due to the multitude of touchpoints and devices that capture the key information during an individual's healthcare encounter is *many fold greater* than the rate at which it could be shared outside of the healthcare entity where it was generated for health services research/population health and/or public health research and surveillance purposes. This is due to the sensitivity that comes with the healthcare data. *Data security* has become the number one priority for healthcare organizations, especially in the wake of an increased number of hacking episodes, ransomware attacks, and high profile data breaches. In addition to this, healthcare also deals with an infinite array of vulnerabilities such as phishing attacks, malware attacks and thefts of laptops and electronic devices with patient identifiable information (PII) or protected health information (PHI). This has made federal government bring in more stringent rules to protect the information of an individual.

In the United States, the Health Insurance Portability and Accountability Act (HIPAA) signed into law in August 1996 has led to the development of HIPAA Privacy Rule (2003) and HIPAA Security Rule (2005). The Security Rule and the Health Information Technology for Economic and Clinical Health Act (HITECH) of 2009 comes with a very long list of necessary technical safeguards for organizations storing PII/PHI in addition to data transmission, security authentication protocols, access controls, audit checks and integrity checks to ensure information is not tampered with. In spite of all such efforts, the fallibility of humans (staff members) in handling sensitive information such as PII or PHI and adhering to best practices can complicate matters by resulting in security breaches. Due to this healthcare institutes and hospital systems have been so used to keeping their institutional data close to their chest and always go through serious considerations and essential data governance protocols and procedures such as - business associate agreements (BAAs) or data use agreements (DUAs) or data sharing agreements (DSAs) before sharing any sensitive or non-sensitive institutional information outside of their institutional boundaries.

Alleviating the Concerns of Data Owners

The U.S. Department of Health and Human Services (HHS) stressed the importance of increasing access to population-level data sources by integrating data systems to drive health planning and research. Establishing Distributed Data Network (DDN) infrastructures have been proposed as tools to support—(1) health services research, (2) evaluation of interventions and comparative effectiveness and patient-centered outcomes research (CE/PCOR), and (3) public health surveillance. DDNs have been gaining momentum due to the increased concerns related to data sharing, privacy, and governance. They are a paradigm shift (Popovic 2015) in health data sharing. Data is not centralized within a DDN; rather, it resides behind the firewalls of the participating organizations or disparate data sources within the network. They exist based on the presumption that participating organizations have standardized their in-house or organizational-level data to a single data schema known as a common data model (CDM). Let's take a look at the concept of a data model (DM) before taking a deep-dive into a CDM.

Data Models (DMs) and their Critical Building Blocks

Data Models (DMs) serve as organizational mechanisms for simplifying complex operational activities or research questions by providing a structure to the data. They are considered as the fundamentals for good database design and can be used broadly to represent either a *database schema or a CDM*. They are made up of *entities* i.e., *objects* or *concepts* related to the data that needs to be tracked and eventually become a *table* or *tables* in a *database*. In other words, the *table* of a database is a physical construct, whereas an *entity* is a logical construct and they are both expressions of the same *concept*. This does not necessarily imply that there is a 1:1 mapping between *entities (objects or concepts)* and *tables*. For example, in one instance, a single *entity* might require multiple *tables* to capture entity-related data, whereas in another instance a single *table* might combine data about multiple *entities*. *Tables* consist of rows and columns. They are uniquely named within a database and contain related data to facilitate operations, such as queries that use unique *table* names to extract specific data to answer the question of interest.

DMs are created by a process called *data modeling*. Data modeling is a step often performed during the software application design and development or whenever changes are to be made to the data elements within a database to support the real-world operational environment or research questions (PopMedNet n.d.). It occurs at three levels—(i) conceptual, (ii) logical, and (iii) physical. The complexity increases from conceptual to logical to physical, and is highlighted in the below table along with the steps that occur at each of these levels (Table 13.1).

For example, let us say we have a database called 'FREQUENT_FLYERS' with multiple *tables*. Frequent Flyers are those patients who have high utilization of a hospital's Emergency Department. Such patient population is sometimes referred to as super-utilizers. For simplicity, let's assume it has two tables named PATIENT and ENCOUNTER to help evaluate the healthcare utilization characteristics of patients over time. The *three* levels of DMs are explained in Figs. 13.1, 13.2, and 13.3 below. The *conceptual DM* for the example database 'FREQUENT_FLYERS' in Fig. 13.1 highlights the operational question of interest i.e., healthcare utilization of patients over time.

The *logical DM* in Fig. 13.2 highlights the *attributes* (columns or data variables) supported by both the *tables* (PATIENT and ENCOUNTER) and the *relationships* between the *attributes*.

The *logical DM* in Fig. 13.3 delves into the details of the *constraints* of *attributes* and the type of *relationship* i.e., One-to-Many (1: M) that exists between the *tables*

Table 13.1 The three levels of Data Models

Data Model (DM) Level	Purpose (What does this define?)	Features
Conceptual	**WHAT** the DM contains?	Identifies the high-level entities and relationships among them.
Logical	**HOW** the DM should be implemented without getting into the specifics of the database? Management system (DBMS) i.e., Oracle or Microsoft SQL or Microsoft access etc.,	1. Identifies: (a) all entities and relationships among them. (b) Attributes for all entities, and specifies keys (primary key (PK) and foreign key (FK)). 2. Applies normalization i.e., a technique to minimize data redundancy.
Physical	**HOW** the DM will be implemented using a specific DBMS?	1. Transforms: (a) Entities into tables, (b) Attributes into columns, and (c) Relationships into foreign keys. 2. Specifies constraints, and defines the exact data types, lengths and default values for the columns.

Fig. 13.1 Conceptual DM of FREQUENT_FLYERS database: Highlights "WHAT the DM contains?"

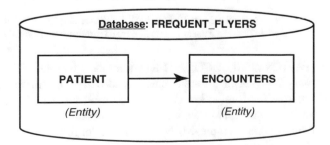

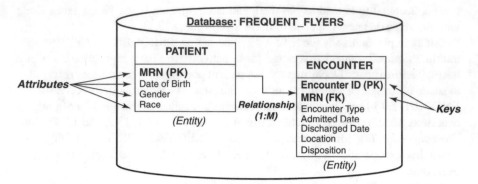

Fig. 13.2 Logical DM of FREQUENT_FLYERS database: Highlights "HOW the DM should be implemented?" without getting into specifics of database management system (DBMS)

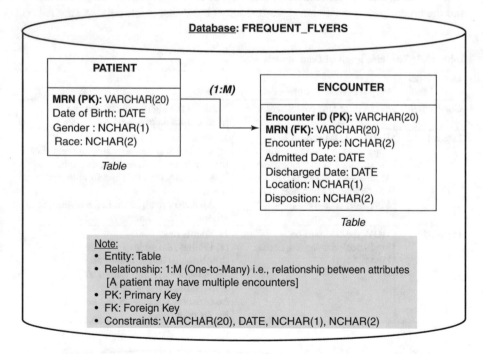

Fig. 13.3 Physical DM of FREQUENT_FLYERS database: Highlights "HOW the DM will be implemented?" using a specific database management system (DBMS)

(PATIENT and ENCOUNTER) within the FREQUENT_FLYERS database. A primary key (PK) is a used to uniquely identify a column or data variable in the table whereas the foreign key (FK) is a column (data variable) or a set of columns (data variables) in a table whose values correspond to the values of the PK in another table. In this example, MRN is a unique identifier for a patient within the healthcare system and does not change with multiple encounters whereas, the same patient is assigned unique ENCOUNTER_ID for each healthcare interaction with the hospital system to help capture the medical reason that led to the visit. It is also important to note that, MRN which is a PK field cannot have NULL values. The data type VARCHAR (20) for MRN implies that the maximum allowable characters for this field are up to 20. NCHAR stores fixed length of Unicode characters. Similarly, a data type of NCHAR (1) for Gender implies that M is used for Male, F for Female, O for Other and N for Unknown/Missing; and NCHAR (2) for Race implies that AA is used for Black or African American, W for White or Caucasian, H for Hispanic.

Attributes are also known as *columns* or *fields* and they help describe the characteristics of the entity. For example, the *attributes* listed in the PATIENT table— MRN, Date of Birth, Gender, and Race help describe the demographic data for each patient. Similarly, the *attributes* listed in the ENCOUNTER table—Encounter ID, MRN, Encounter Type, Admitted Date, Discharged Date, Location, and Disposition help describe the encounters of patients over time. Some patients may have only one encounter, while others have more than one (i.e., there exists an association among entities). This association is known as a *relationship* and there are three types of relationships – One to Many (1: M), Many to Many (M: M), and One to One (1:1).

Some of the attributes represent *domains* and have a set of possible values, also known as *value sets*. For example, the *domain* "Gender" has several value sets like: Male (M), Female (F), and Unknown (UNK) whereas the *domain* "Race" has values sets including: African American (AA), Caucasian (C), Hispanic (H), Asian (A), and Other (O). Finally, *constraints* are restrictions or rules placed on data. They help ensure data integrity (i.e., accuracy and reliability of data) in the database by regulating the type of data that goes into a table. For example, MRN is a unique, patient-level identifier that links a patient with his/her medical record and a constraint of NOT NULL is placed on this field to ensure that this column cannot have a null value.

Establishing the Necessity (Public/Population Health Needs) for Common Data Models (CDMs)

Prevalent cases – All individuals living with the health outcome of interest within a specified timeframe, regardless of when that person was diagnosed or developed the health outcome (Vaccine Safety Datalink (VSD) n.d.).

Prevalence – The proportion of a population living with a specific health outcome within a specified timeframe (Vaccine Safety Datalink (VSD) n.d.).

Numerator of Prevalence – The number of unique individuals with the condition of interest.

Denominator of Prevalence – The total population in the region.

Estimating the burden (or prevalence) of a disease condition is pivotal for both public health agencies and healthcare organizations to strategize their future chronic disease prevention and health promotion activities, plan disaster management, and allocate resources in times of both planned (annual flu seasons) and unplanned emergencies (pandemics such as COVID-19). But, given the nature of healthcare, an individual although a resident of a particular ZIP Code or geographical region in times of medical emergencies may have healthcare encounters at other healthcare systems outside of his/her geographical region. As the information of an individual is captured across different healthcare systems, it opens many challenges such as – (1) lack of common interoperability standards across systems, (2) small sample sizes which may not better represent current trends or predict future trends, and (3) heavy ask on the time and resources for the time it takes to develop agreements to facilitate data sharing.

Let us consider an example to understand the challenges that come in the context of estimating the prevalence of a chronic disease condition in a geographical region. In the Fig. 13.4 below, let the square represent a hypothetical city with 3 geographical regions (Region – 1, Region – 2, and Region – 3) separated by dotted lines. Organization # 1, Organization # 2, and Organization # 3 are hospitals within these three geographical regions. (Organization # 1 is a part of a large healthcare system with 5 hospitals across region - 1, Organization # 2 is a standalone hospital, and Organization # 3 is a clinic that offers psychiatric counseling and health promotion services for diabetic patients. Let's complicate and make this example as real-world as possible, by assuming that these 3 hospitals are on different Electronic Health Record (EHR) systems – Organization # 1 (Cerner Millennium), Organization # 2 (Epic), and Organization # 3 (GE Centricity).

Let us look at an example patient named John Doe. John is a male resident of Region—1 born on October 11, 1970 with multiple chronic conditions (MCCs) such as diabetes mellitus, and hypertension. Due to the nature of the MCCs, John is a superutilizer of healthcare resources and had five encounters across these three

Fig. 13.4 Hypothetical city with 3 regions and 3 hospital systems

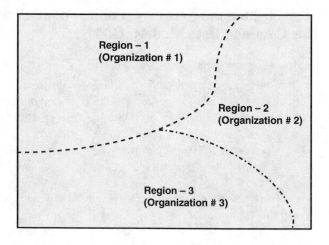

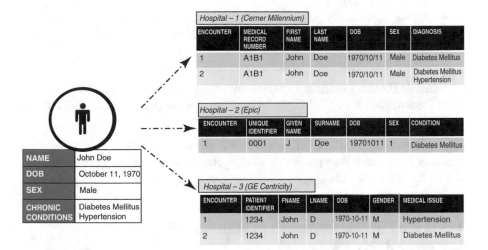

Fig. 13.5 Example patient John Doe's Healthcare encounters across the three hospital systems

hospitals within the region during 2021. Refer to Fig. 13.5. Due to the lack of a unique patient identifier (Medical Record Number) for individuals across the nation and a lack of a common EHR vendor across the three hospitals within the region the information of the same individual was captured in different ways i.e., data elements and data codings within the individual EHR database systems.

A summary of the data element and coding differences were presented below.

- **Unique Patient Identifier:** This information was documented as: MEDICAL RECORD NUMBER (A1B1) at Organization # 1 vs. UNIQUE IDENTIFIER (0001) at Organization # 2 vs. PATIENT IDENTIFIER (1234) at Organization # 3.
- **First Name:** This information was documented as: FIRST NAME (John) at Organization # 1 vs. GIVEN NAME (J) at Organization # 2 vs. FNAME (John) at Organization # 3.
- **Last Name:** This information was documented as: LAST NAME (Doe) at Organization # 1 vs. SURNAME (Doe) at Organization # 2 vs. LNAME (D) at Organization # 3.
- **Date of Birth:** This information was documented as: DOB across the 3 organizations.

  - Although, the *date of birth* data element was documented as DOB across all the three organizations the codings at the respective organizations were different i.e., DOB = 1970/10/11 at Organization # 1, DOB = 19,701,011 at Organization # 2, and DOB = 1970-10-11 at Organization # 3.

- **Sex or Gender:** This information was documented as: SEX (Male) at Organization # 1 vs. SEX (1) at Organization # 2 vs. GENDER (M) at Organization # 3.

- Although, the *sex or gender* data element was documented as SEX at both the Organization # 1 and 2; the codings at the respective organizations were different i.e., SEX = Male at Organization # 1 whereas it was documented as SEX = 1 at Organization # 2.

- **Chronic Disease Condition:** This information was documented as: DIAGNOSIS at Organization # 1 vs. MEDICAL ISSUE at Organization # 2 vs. CONDITION at Organization # 3.

Due to these complexities, it makes it very difficult to accurately identify the unique count of individuals for a particular disease condition i.e., the numerator variable within the prevalence calculation.

What is a Possible Approach to address this Interoperability Challenge?

A possible solution to address this multi-dimensionality challenge is conforming to a common format. Let us look at a simple analogy to better understand the proposed solution to address the challenge at hand. To make the electrical appliances from different regions such as "India", "Israel" and "China" work within "North America", a *universal power adapter* would be required. Please refer to Fig. 13.6. Similarly, Common Data Models (CDMs) serve as the "universal power adapter" to ensure that the information stored within siloed systems or databases could be seamlessly accessed by easing the interoperability related communication challenges.

Fig. 13.6 Universal power adapter Example

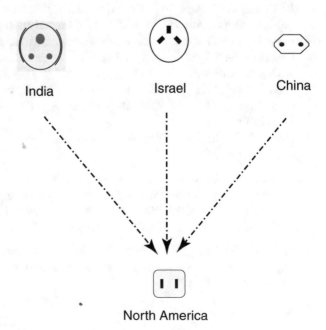

India

Israel

China

North America

Common Data Models (CDMs): Definition, History, Utility, and Steps in the Process

Definition   A CDM aims to standardize the *logical DM* infrastructure highlighted in Fig. 13.2 so that **many related applications** can operate on the **same shared data**. So, Microsoft Corporation defines a CDM as "*a standard and extensible collection of schemas (entities, attributes, relationships) that represents business concepts and activities with well-defined semantics, to facilitate data interoperability.*"

History   The popular CDM in healthcare dates back to 1990. It was a collaborative project between the National Immunization Program (NIP) and the U.S. Centers for Disease Control and Prevention (CDC). This effort helped establish a CDM called the Vaccine Safety Datalink (VSD) Shared Data Network (SDN) with several large Health Maintenance Organizations (HMOs) to investigate the safety of vaccines (Vaccine Safety Datalink (VSD) n.d.).

Utility   A CDM is a way of organizing data into a standard structure and an essential task for multi-organizational collaborative research. The concept behind this approach is to transform data contained within those individual participating institutions databases into a common format (or DM) as well as a common representation (terminologies, vocabularies, coding schemes), and then perform systematic analyses using a library of standard analytic routines (using a platform of choice such as—SAS, R, Python) that have been written based on the common format.

Distributed Data Networks (DDNs) or Distributed Health Data Networks (DHDNs) are those networks where a few similar entities (such as hospitals) or diverse entities (hospitals, federally qualified health centers (FQHCs), primary care clinics) collaborate and share/pool their data for surveillance or research purposes using a CDM. A few examples of healthcare-related DDNs or DHDNs are—Food and Drug Administration (FDA) Mini-Sentinel, The National Patient-Centered Clinical Research Network (PCORnet), Health Care Systems Research Network (HCSRN) (formerly Health Maintenance Organization (HMO) Research Network (HMORN)), and Observational Medical Outcomes Partnership (OMOP) CDM from Observational Health Data Sciences and Informatics (OHDSI). While PCORnet CDM focuses on bringing together data and resources to patient-reported outcomes to support CE/PCOR, OMOP CDM allows users for the systematic analysis of disparate observational databases. We will take a look at these CDMs in the latter part of this book chapter along with the data tables within these models.

Steps in the Process   Conforming to a CDM ensures that standardized applications and methods can be executed by distributing a query or code using a platform maintained by the hub or linkage unit in order to generate aggregated results from pooled data from participating organizations.

Let us revisit our earlier example from the lens of a (see Fig. 13.7) DDN or DHDN with 3 diverse organizations (Organization # 1, Organization #2, and

Organization # 3). These organizations come together as a collaborative to support the patient population in the geographic region to address their physical and mental wellbeing while maintaining the full control on their institutional data. The *administrative, technical*, and *operational* steps required to bring this process to fruition are:

Administrative Process:

(i) As a part of the overall DDN governance process, the organizations develop a charter with agreed upon governance (policies, procedures, and guidelines) that would need to be followed in order to support the research questions that could be explored as a part of this multi-organizational or multi-institutional collaborative.

(ii) Following the governance process, the collaborative formed works with a team of researchers to help identify more than a few research questions that would serve as use-cases to test the utility of the CDM developed. *For example, a research question could be estimation of racial and gender disparities among patients with Non-Alcoholic Fatty Liver Disease (NAFLD) within the region.*

Technical Process:

(i) Data elements that would need to be considered in order to explore the data to find valuable insights would be proposed by the Information Systems (IS) departments at each of these three institutions.

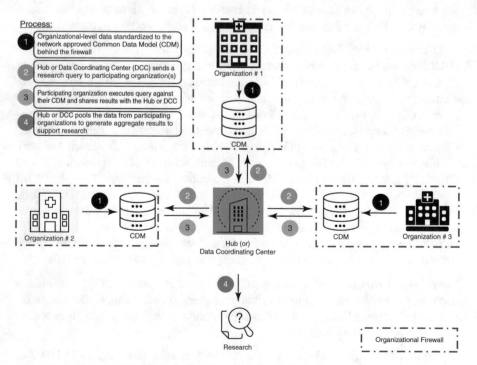

Fig. 13.7 Distributed Data Network (DDN) or Distributed Health Data Network (DHDN)

(ii) A subgroup consisting of IS and business experts is formed to help share with each other as to how these data elements are documented within each of their systems so that a CDM standard for the collaborative could be proposed to the research team.

(iii) After going through a rigorous iterative process, the subgroup and the research team would finalize the proposed CDM to the governance body.

Operational Processs:

(i) The IS Implementation Teams at the respective organizations would help develop the CDM instance at the individual organizations.

(ii) Organizational data is conformed to the CDM approved by the multi-institutional collaborative.

Now, let us revisit the enhanced version of example shared in the earlier section by looking at Fig. 13.8 to understand how the CDM looks like in that example. A crosswalk of individual organizational data elements and their mirror within the CDM are presented for the consumption of the readers in Table 13.2.

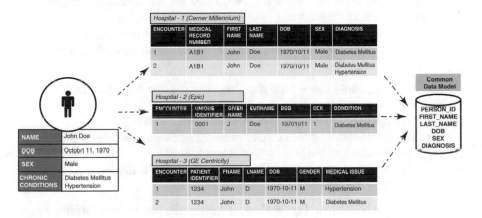

Fig. 13.8 Distributed data network (DDN) or distributed health data network (DHDN)

Table 13.2 Crosswalk of individual organizational data elements against common data model (CDM)

Domain/Data Concept	Data Element (Organization # 1)	Data Element (Organization # 2)	Data Element (Organization # 3)	Data Element within the CDM
Unique patient identifier	MEDICAL RECORD NUMBER	UNIQUE IDENTIFIER	PATIENT IDENTIFIER	PERSON_ID
First Name	FIRST NAME	GIVEN NAME	FNAME	FIRST_NAME
Last Name	LAST NAME	SURNAME	LNAME	LAST_NAME
Date of birth	DOB	DOB	DOB	DOB
Sex or gender	SEX	SEX	GENDER	SEX
Chronic disease condition	DIAGNOSIS	CONDITION	MEDICAL ISSUE	DIAGNOSIS

(iii) A neutral institute such as an Academic Institute or a Public Health Agency serves as a Data Coordinating Center or Hub or Linkage Unit to facilitate the operations in a *federated approach* i.e., the sensitive data remains behind the firewalls of participating organizations whereas an informatics platform is used to query minimum necessary information. A scalable and extensible open-source informatics platform such as PopMedNet designed by Department of Population Medicine at Harvard Medical School and Harvard Pilgrim Healthcare Institute installed at the Data Coordinating Center will assist with the operation of DDNs (PopMedNet n.d.). The PopMedNet Client sends the query related to the approved research question to the participating organizations.

(iv) Participating organization(s) executes the query using PopMedNet Client against their respective institutional CDMs and shares results with the Hub or Data Coordinating Center.

(v) Data Coordinating Center pools the results from participating organizations to generate aggregates which includes - overall sample size and distribution by key stratifications such as age group, race, gender, ethnicity, geographical spread. This information will be shared with the researchers.

Let us assume, researchers requested for aggregate results from participating institutes of this DDN for on NAFLD patient population. The results would look something like below:

- Overall sample size = 1400 patients (Organization # 1 – 525; Organization # 2 – 475; and Organization # 3 – 400)
- Age distribution: <65 years = 35%; 65+ years = 65%
- Race distribution: African American = 72%; Caucasian = 20%; other = 8%
- Gender distribution: Male = 78%; Female = 22%
- Geographical distribution: Region – 1 = 45%; Region – 2 = 33%; Region – 3 = 22%

(vi) The researchers would then evaluate if the sample size provides the necessary statistical power required to proceed further with the research effort.

(vii) If the researchers decide to proceed further, and if the research requires access to patient level detail then additional agreements would need to be worked out for such data access.

Key Principles related to CDMs

Usually, the principles that govern the DDNs organically evolve over time and most often by learning from the best practices identified during the development and implementation of: (1) current DDN (i.e., internal knowledge management) and (2) other DDNs (i.e., external knowledge management). *Data governance* (policy framework that ensures smooth flow of operations incl., data management) and *data provenance* (historical record of data and its origins) are two most important pillars when it comes to the management of DDNs. While the former refers to what kind of data goes into the CDM and how it needs to be handled, the latter refers to the lineage or origin of a data element or a concept from other implemented DDNs. The following are a few principles related to CDMs:

1. **Alleviate Privacy and Security Concerns. The concerns that usually come with privacy and security aspects of health data is alleviated by the *federated nature of the operational mechanism*.** The federated approach is the ability of individual participating institutes to develop the CDM behind the institutes firewall so that no individualized data is exposed to the external organizations. By doing this, more participants would be encouraged to become a part of the collaborative so that the breadth and depth of the research questions could be expanded. In our earlier example, we have considered three organizations – a large healthcare system, a standalone hospital, and a psychiatric clinic. Now, if a fourth participant such as a pharmacy joins the collaborative then the research questions could be expanded to identify the healthcare utilization in patients with non-adherence to a strict psychiatric medication regimen.
2. **A Clear Primary Purpose** (Ross et al. 2014). The primary purpose of the data populated within the CDM should be bound by a clear goal or approach. For example, is to—(a) foster collaborative research, (b) monitor disease surveillance, and (c) improve patient outcomes by drawing inferences from the knowledge gained from the pooling of the data from multiple participating institutions.
3. **A Strict Adherence to Institutional Governance Policies.** The CDM and any related tools should strictly adhere to the governance rules set forth by the institution where it has been implemented by following the guidelines set forth by respective organization's Institutional Review Board (IRB) and any other federal/state privacy and data sharing regulations.
4. **Agnostic to source data systems** (Ross et al. 2014). The CDM should be agnostic to source data systems as they are defined by data concepts rather than data sources.
5. **Flexible and extensible to accommodate multiple institutes.** The CDM should be flexible and extensible to accommodate the interests and data sources of a wide range of participating institutions.
6. **Ability to easily adapt or clone.** The empty shells of the CDMs can be made available to the public or other institutions so that they could easily adapt or clone to meet their respective organizational needs or while onboarding to an existing collaborative.

How do the CDMs foster Public Health Surveillance/ Population Health Efforts?

The CDMs includes data from EHRs i.e., clinical, pharmacy, and laboratory information and financial information systems or EMRs i.e., physician offices, clinics. The data can include inpatient, observation, emergency, and outpatient encounters along with medication data, lab data, and vital signs; and conforms to standards such as - ICD-9-CM/ICD-10-CM codes, NDC, LOINC, and SNOMED. In this section, let us take a look at a few scenarios to highlight how the CDMs can help foster both public heath surveillance and population health efforts.

1. **Test ground for use cases.** The CDMs serve as ground for developing test use cases to identify patient populations or groups with disease conditions of interest.
2. **Estimate the burden of disease conditions.** For example, let us say a geographic region contained four diverse healthcare systems, and three of them who have a collective market share area (MSA) of 80 percent in the region have come together as a part of a DDN to collaborate on research efforts. By pooling the data from these three hospitals using their CDMs, a better estimate of the burden or prevalence of chronic disease conditions within the same geographical region could be identified.
3. **Increase the sample size of rare disease conditions.** As CDMs can pool the data from diverse organizations, they can really help researchers by increasing the sample size of individuals with rare disease conditions so that better treatment strategies could be developed.
4. **Assist public health agencies with surveillance efforts.** The prevalence estimates generated using CDMs could help inform the public health agencies in strategizing their localized preventative efforts.
5. **Perform external validation of prior studies.** As CDMs pool the data from multiple organizations, sometimes the research questions that have been solved by organizations in a different region could be tested for external validation purposes to reconfirm the results.

Most Popular CDMs

This section provides a brief introduction to the most popular CDMs along with their focus areas or domains as highlighted by the tables within those data models.

Vaccine Safety Datalink (VSD) Shared Data Network (SDN) (Vaccine Safety Datalink (VSD) n.d.)

The Vaccine Safety Datalink (VSD) started in 1990 is a collaborative project between CDC's Immunization Safety Office and nine health care organizations listed below that use EHR data to monitor safety of vaccines and conduct studies about rare and serious adverse events following immunization:

1. Kaiser Permanente Washington, Seattle, Washington
2. Harvard Pilgrim Health Care Institute, Boston, Massachusetts
3. HealthPartners Institute, Minneapolis, Minnesota
4. Kaiser Permanente Northwest, Portland, Oregon
5. Kaiser Permanente Northern California, Oakland, California
6. Kaiser Permanente Colorado, Denver, Colorado
7. Denver Health, Denver, Colorado
8. Marshfield Clinic Research Institute, Marshfield, Wisconsin
9. Kaiser Permanente Southern California, Los Angeles, California.

The VSD conducts vaccine safety studies based on questions or concerns raised from the medical literature and reports to the Vaccine Adverse Event Reporting System (VAERS). VAERS is the early warning system in the United States that monitors the safety of vaccines after they are authorized or licensed for use by the U.S. Food and Drug Administration (FDA) and co-managed by CDC and FDA (Vaccine Safety Datalink (VSD) n.d.). This system helps ensure that vaccines in circulation are safe for the general public. In order to capture this information, the CDM for this system contains three main tables listed below (Table 13.3).

Health Care Systems Research Network (HCSRN) VDW (HCSRN n.d.)

The Health Maintenance Organization Research Network (HMORN) was formed back in 1994 to better translate research findings into practice. This was later morphed into HCSRN. Currently, this supports healthcare systems in additional to Health Maintenance Organizations (HMOs) and supports the development of grant proposals, planning out preliminary studies and identifying potential subjects for research projects. In order to capture this information, the CDM for this system contains *twelve* main tables listed below (Table 13.4).

Table 13.3 VSD SDN Common Data Model

Data Table	Description of the Data Table
ENROLLMENT	Details of enrollment of the individual for vaccination
UTILIZATION	Details pertaining to the dose and type of administration
VACCINES	Details of the vaccine(s) administered

Table 13.4 HCSRN VDW Common Data Model

Data Table	Description of the Data Table
DEMOGRAPHICS	Demographic records of individual patients
ENROLLMENT	Enrollment (insurance) details of the patients with HMOs
ENCOUNTERS	Health delivery encounters of patients
DIAGNOSES	Diagnoses or medical conditions documented during encounters
PROCEDURES	Procedures performed during encounters
PROVIDER	Details of the medical staff i.e., physician performing the procedure
TUMOR	Details of the tumor including reporting of cancers to registries
PHARMACY	Details of the medications
VITAL SIGNS	Details of the vital signs documented during the encounters
LAB RESULTS	Details of the lab results ordered during the encounters
DEATH	Information related to the cause of the death and death date
EVER NDC	Details related to drug codes

Table 13.5 i2b2 Common Data Model

Data Table	Description of the Data Table
DEMOGRAPHICS	Demographic records of individual patients
DEATH	Information related to the cause of the death and death date
ENROLLMENT	Enrollment (insurance) details of the patients
SOCIAL HISTORY	Information related to tobacco, and alcohol consumption
LAB	Labs ordered during the patient encounters
VITAL SIGNS	Details of the vital signs documented during the encounters
PHARMACY	Details of the medications
UTILIZATION	Health delivery encounters of patients
TUMORS	Details of the Tumors including reporting of cancers to registries
CENSUS	Details related to geographical locations of the patients
LANGUAGE	Details related to language spoken by the patients

Informatics for Integrating Biology and the Bedside (i2b2) CDM (Weeks and Pardee 2019; Anon. n.d.-a)

Partners Healthcare System and Harvard Medical School have collaborated to create the i2b2 CDM. This is a data model combined with a web-based interface for querying and inspecting data. The *eleven* most common domains used in this model are highlighted in the table below (Table 13.5).

Food and Drug Administration (FDA) Sentinel (Weeks and Pardee 2019)

The focus of this effort is to monitor drug safety and repurposed the names used within the HCSRN VDW (Table 13.6).

The National Patient-Centered Clinical Research Network (PCORnet) CDM (Weeks and Pardee 2019; PCORnet n.d.)

The PCORnet CDM is supported by all networks in the Patient Centered Outcomes Research Institute (PCORI). It is derived from the Mini-Sentinel data model and over 80 institutions have transformed their data into this model. PCORnet focuses on bringing together data and resources to support CE/PCOR. The PCORnet CDM v4.1 consists of 19 *tables* listed below with 355 *attributes* (data elements or variables) available to support research (Table 13.7).

Observational Medical Outcomes Partnership (OMOP) CDM (OMOP n.d.)

The goal of OMOP was to create a warehouse for studying the effects of medical products. This CDM contains 16 Clinical Event tables, 10 Vocabulary tables, 2 metadata tables, 4 health system data tables, 2 health economics data tables, 3 standardized derived elements, and 2 Results schema tables (Tables 13.8, 13.9, 13.10, 13.11, 13.12, 13.13).

Table 13.6 FDA Sentinel VDW

Data Table	Description of the Data Table
DEMOGRAPHICS	Demographic records of individual patients
DEATH	Information related to the cause of the death and death date
ENROLLMENT	Enrollment (insurance) details of the patients
LAB	Labs ordered during the patient encounters
VITAL SIGNS	Details of the vital signs documented during the encounters
PHARMACY	Details of the medications
UTILIZATION	Health delivery encounters of patients

Table 13.7 PCORnet common data model

Data Table	Description of the Data Table	# Attributes
DEMOGRAPHIC	Demographics record of individual patients	16
ENROLLMENT	Insurance enrollment information	5
ENCOUNTER	Healthcare delivery interactions	31
DIAGNOSIS	Diagnosis codes as a result of diagnostic processes and medical coding within healthcare delivery	19
PROCEDURES	Procedure codes such as surgical procedures and lab orders delivered within a healthcare context	14
VITAL	Captures vital signs such as height, weight, systolic, and diastolic blood pressure that directly measure an individual's current state of attributes	21
DISPENSING	Prescriptions filled through a community, mail-order or hospital pharmacy	14
LAB_RESULT_CM	Stores quantitative and qualitative measurements from blood and other body specimens	31
CONDITION	The patient's medical history and current state may both be represented	14
PRO_CM	Store responses to patient-reported outcome measures (PROs) or questionnaires	26
PRESCRIBING	Provider orders for medication dispensing and/or administration	30
PCORNET_TRIAL	Patients who are enrolled in PCORnet clinical trials and PCORnet studies	8
DEATH	Reported mortality information for patients	5
DEATH_CAUSE	The individual causes associated with a reported death	6
MED_ADMIN	Records of medications administered to patients by healthcare providers	20
PROVIDER	Data about the providers who are involved in the care processes	6
OBS_CLIN	Standardized qualitative and quantitative clinical observations about a patient	20
OBS_GEN	Table to store everything else	20
HARVEST	Attributes associated with the specific PCORnet DataMart implementation, including data refreshes	49

Table 13.8 OMOP clinical data tables

Clinical data tables: The following data tables capture the demographic, clinical, and lab related domains during the interaction of patients with the healthcare system for medical attention

PERSON	DRUG_EXPOSURE	NOTE
OBSERVATION_PERIOD	PROCEDURE_OCCURENCE	NOTE_NLP
VISIT_OCCURENCE	DEVICE_EXPOSURE	SPECIMEN
VISIT_DETAIL	MEASUREMENT	FACT_RELATIONSHIP
CONDITION_OCCURENCE	OBSERVATION	SURVEY_CONDUCT

Table 13.9   Health system data tables

Health system data tables: The following data tables capture the details relevant to healthcare provider such as—location of the provider, details of the provider etc.,			
LOCATION	LOCATION_HISTORY	CARE_SITE	PROVIDER

Table 13.10   OMOP health economic data tables

Health economic data tables: The following data tables capture the insurance details such as payer plan and the cost associated with the healthcare encounter.	
PAYER_PLAN_PERIOD	COST

Table 13.11   OMOP standardized derived elements data tables

Standardized derived elements: The following tables capture the derived data elements such as drug, dosage, and condition details		
DRUG_ERA	DOSE_ERA	CONDITION_ERA

Table 13.12   OMOP meta data tables

Metadata tables: The following tables capture the metadata related information.	
METADATA	CDM_SOURCE

Table 13.13   OMOP vocabulary tables

Vocabulary tables: The following tables capture the information related to the vocabulary such as SNOMED, LOINC etc.,		
CONCEPT	CONCEPT_RELATIONSHIP	SOURCE_TO_CONCEPT_MAP
VOCABULARY	RELATIONSHIP	DRUG_STRENGTH
DOMAIN	CONCEPT_SYNONYM	COHORT_DEFINITION
CONCEPT_CLASS	CONCEPT_ANCESTOR	

Real-world Examples of the Applications of CDM

The data captured by the partners within a network (DDN or DHDN) using the same CDM can be used to answer important patient outcome related research questions. This section highlights an example that focuses on the utility of CDMs in capturing patient reported outcomes. The PCORnet CDM contains a data table called "PRO_CM" which stores responses to patient-reported outcome measures (PROs) or questionnaires.

The implementation of Patient-Reported Outcomes Measurement (PROM) in routine clinical practice for heart failure patients is a study that came out the PaTH Network (PaTH Network n.d.) that contained 3 clinical sites (Vanderbilt University, Duke University, and University of Pittsburgh) at two PCORnet networks. The PROM data was collected by the research team using the EHR systems after conducting interviews with patients using 3 questionnaires—(1) Kansas City Cardiomyopathy Questionnaire (KCCQ-12) which focuses on heart failure symptoms, (2) Patient-Reported Outcomes Measurement Information System (PROMIS) Global Health Scale which focuses on general health issues, and (3) Patient Health Questionnaire (PHQ-2) which focuses on depression (Anon. n.d.-b). The collected data was later incorporated into the PCORnet CDM. The PopMedNet query ran against the CDMs of the three participating clinical sites identified 1054 patients who completed the 3 questionnaires from 2019-2020 (PaTH Network n.d.; Anon. n.d.-b). The team compared patient characteristics of these patients against 3126 patients who did not complete PROM questionnaires across the two clinical sites to understand the association of the PROM scores and patient's demographics and comorbid conditions. It was noticed that the patients who completed PROM questionnaires were significantly younger than those who did not complete the PROM questionnaires. Such information would be helpful to understand the patients' perspectives and implement strategies in place to collect such information in the future.

Limitations

The CDMs do have their own limitations—(1) they are limited to the data generated by the participating institutes collected as a part of their day-to-day business and operations, (2) the local data documentation practices at individual DDN participating sites may not be resolved using standardized CDMs, and (3) ongoing maintenance of a DDN requires dedicated resources such as human capital, time, and quality checks in order to refresh the data at regular intervals.

Conclusion

The data collected by various organizations is growing due to the availability of computing resources at relatively low costs. CDMs are great mechanism to help alleviate the growing concerns of healthcare institutions when it comes to sharing their data with external entities for collaborative efforts due to privacy and security concerns. While the CDMs are a great way to foster multi-organizational data, they are also a great resource for fostering Cross-Network Directory Service (CNDS) i.e., collaboration of different DDNs as well as diverse systems capturing data within the same organization by means of Inter-institutional Research Infrastructure (IIRI).

Review Questions

1. **What is a Common Data Model (CDM)?**
   Answer: Microsoft Corporation defines a Common Data Model (CDM) as "*a standard and extensible collection of schemas (entities, attributes, relationships)*

that represents business concepts and activities with well-defined semantics, to facilitate data interoperability."

2. **By means of structured process outline the operational steps for getting the aggregate results generated using a CDM in a Distributed Health Data Network (DHDN).**
   Answer:

   (i) The IS departments at the respective organizations help developed the CDM instance at the individual organizations.
   (ii) Organizational data is conformed to the CDM approved by the collaborative.
   (iii) Researchers submit their research question request to the neutral institute such as an academic institute or a Public Health Agency which serves as a Data Coordinating Center
   (iv) Data Coordinating Center using a scalable and extensible open-source informatics platform such as PopMedNet sends the query requests to participating organizations in the Distributed Data Network.
   (v) Participating organization(s) executes the query using PopMedNet Client against their respective institutional CDMs and shares results with the Data Coordinating Center.
   (vi) Data Coordinating Center pools the results from participating organizations to generate aggregates which includes - overall sample size and distribution by key stratifications such as age group, race, gender, ethnicity, geographical spread.
   (vii) Finally, this information will be shared with the researchers to assess whether the sample size has the necessary statistical power to move forward with the research effort.

3. **Outline the key principles related to CDMs.**
   Answer: There are 6 key principles that highlight the importance of CDMs.

   (i) **Alleviate Privacy and Security Concerns.** The concerns that usually come with privacy and security aspects of health data is alleviated by the federated nature of the operational mechanism. The federated approach is the ability of individual participating institutes to develop the CDM behind their institutes firewall so that no individualized data (PII or PHI) is exposed outside of the organization.
   (ii) **A Clear Primary Purpose.** The primary purpose of the data populated within the CDM should be bound by a clear goal or approach.
   (iii) **A Strict Adherence to Institutional Governance Policies.** The CDM and any related tools should strictly adhere to the governance rules set forth by the institution where it has been implemented by following the guidelines set forth by respective organization's Institutional Review Board (IRB) and any other federal/state privacy and data sharing regulations.
   (iv) **Agnostic to source data systems.** The CDM should be agnostic to source data systems as they are defined by data concepts rather than data sources.

(v) **Flexible and extensible to accommodate multiple institutes.** The CDM should be flexible and extensible to accommodate the interests and data sources of a wide range of participating institutions.

(vi) **Ability to easily adapt or clone.** The empty shells of the CDMs can be made available to the public or other institutions so that they could easily adapt or clone to meet their respective organizational needs or while onboarding to an existing collaborative.

4. **What is your major take away after comparing the i2b2 and FDA's Sentinel CDMs.**

Answer: There are 6 domains that are common to both the i2b2 and FDA's Sentinel CDMs. They are: DEMOGRAPHICS, DEATH, ENROLLMENT, LAB, VITAL SIGNS, PHARMACY, and UTILIZATION.

References

Anon. n.d.-a Informatics for integrating biology and the bedside (i2b2). https://www.i2b2.org/

Anon. n.d.-b Using PCORnet to track patient-reported symptoms of heart failure. Retrieved from: https://www.pcori.org/research-results/2018/using-pcornet-track-patient-reported-symptoms-heart-failure

HCSRN. n.d.. Retrieved from: https://www.hcsrn.org/en/Tools%20&%20Materials/VDW/

Magnuson JA, Dixon BE. Public health informatics: an introduction. In: Public health informatics and information systems. Cham: Springer; 2020. p. 3–16.

OMOP. n.d.. https://ohdsi.github.io/CommonDataModel/cdm60.html#Changes_in_v60

PaTH Network. n.d.. https://www.pathnetwork.org/Research/Implementation_Patient_Reported_Outcomes_Measurement_Routine_Clinical_Practice_Heart_Failure_Patients_PCORnet.html

PCORnet. n.d.. Retrieved from: https://pcornet.org/wp-content/uploads/2020/12/PCORnet-Common-Data-Model-v60-2020_10_221.pdf

PopMedNet. n.d. Retried from: https://www.popmednet.org/

Popovic JR. Distributed data networks: a paradigm shift in data sharing and healthcare analytics (2015). https://www.pharmasug.org/proceedings/2015/HA/PharmaSUG-2015-HA07.pdf.

Ross T, Ng D, Brown JS, Pardee R, Hornbrook MC, Hart G; and Steiner JF "The HMO Research Network Virtual Data Warehouse: A Public Data Model to Support Collaboration," eGEMs (Generating Evidence & Methods to improve patient outcomes): 2014 Vol. 2: Iss. 1, Article 2.

Vaccine Safety Datalink (VSD). n.d.. Retrieved from: https://www.cdc.gov/vaccinesafety/ensuringsafety/monitoring/vsd/index.html#objectives

Weeks J, & Pardee R. Learning to share health care data: a brief timeline of influential common data models and distributed health data networks in U.S. Health Care Research. EGEMS (Washington, DC), 2019 7(1), 4. https://doi.org/10.5334/egems.279.

Part III
Methods for Patient-centric Design

Chapter 14
Person-Centered Design Methods for Citizen Science

Robin R. Austin and Cecilia X. Wang

Abstract The growth of patient involvement in health care has grown exponentially. Health information technology (HIT) has enabled the ability to provide a valuable way to gain access to vital health information. HIT has enabled the quantified self-movement, the ability to track and trend personal health information. This has further increased the interest in citizen science, involvement of public participation in research or in collaboration with research. Increased complexity of patient care makes engaging patients in their own care all the more important. Electronic health information (eHealth) or digital health has the potential to improve quality of care, increase patient engagement, and provide opportunities for self-management of diseases. In today's healthcare environment, it is vital for individuals to be active participants in their care but also in the design of that care to facilitate clinical decisions. This chapter will focus on the broad overview of citizen science, person-centered design, and specific methodologies used in person-centered design. Person-centered design uses methods to ensure that the needs of the patient, as a whole person and an equal partner in their care are included within the design team. Current programs, national initiatives, and valuable resources will be discussed. This chapter will enable the learner to examine various design methods and models to guide person-centered design for citizen science.

Keywords Patient-centered care · Participatory design · Co-creation design processes · Electronic health literacy · Citizen science · Design methods

R. R. Austin (✉)
School of Nursing, University of Minnesota, Twin Cities, Minneapolis, MN, USA
e-mail: quis0026@umn.edu

C. X. Wang
College of Design, University of Minnesota, Minneapolis, MN, USA
e-mail: ceciw@umn.edu

© The Author(s), under exclusive license to Springer Nature
Switzerland AG 2022
P.-Y. S. Hsueh et al. (eds.), *Personal Health Informatics*, Cognitive Informatics in Biomedicine and Healthcare, https://doi.org/10.1007/978-3-031-07696-1_14

Learning Objectives
1. Examine person-centered design methodology through the lens of citizen science
2. Develop guiding principles for authentic inclusive co-designing processes
3. Explore design thinking methods inform person-centered design methods
4. Assess guide/checklist for person-centered design methods

The growth of patient engagement coupled with emerging digital technologies and the quantified-self movement have paved the way for citizen science as a growing worldwide phenomenon.(Petersen 2018; Wang et al. 2015) Citizen science, also called public participation or participation action research, is a research method conducted, in-part of whole, by non-scientists.(Gura 2013; Steven et al. 2019; Petersen et al. 2021) Digital technologies, such as mobile health applications (mHealth apps) have enabled improved capabilities for patients to easily and effectively connect with researchers and become engaged in the scientific community. The citizen science movement is catalyzed by citizens' wanting to be actively involved in a scientific processes and provides a valuable tool in offering contributions to solve needed health questions.(Van Vliet and Moore 2016; Bonney et al. 2016) As more informed patients and citizens' are seeking answers to health-related questions, more defined co-creative design methods are needed. Person-centered design uses methods to ensure that the needs of the patient, as a whole person and an equal partner in their care are included within the design team.(Kildea et al. 2019) Further person-centered design methods can aid in establishing a process and structure to facilitate an inclusive and respectful environment.

The purpose of this chapter is to enable the learner to examine various design methods to guide person-centered design for citizen science research. This chapter provides an overview of establishing guiding principles to facilitate co-creative alignment of multiple-stakeholder involvement and use of design-thinking methods to provide structure and rigor to the design process.

Citizen Science

Citizen Science, also known as community science, crowd science, crowd-sourced science, civic science, or volunteer monitoring is scientific research conducted in whole, part, or partnership with amateur scientists (Hinckson et al. 2017; Evans 2016). Citizen science has been described as public participation research or participatory action research whose outcomes often advance scientific research and increasing the publics understanding of science.(Petersen et al. 2021; Den Broeder et al. 2016) Ten principles of Citizen Science were established to provide an

Table 14.1 Citizen science resources

Resource	Description
Citizenscience.gov	CitizenScience.gov is an official government website designed to accelerate the use of crowdsourcing and citizen science across the U.S. government
CitiSci.org	CitSci.org supports your research by providing tools and resources that allow you to customize your scientific procedure—All in one location on the internet.
Citizen Science Alliance (CSA) Citizensciencealliance.org	The Citizen Science Alliance (CSA) is a collaboration of scientists, software developers and educators who collectively develop, manage and utilize internet-based citizen science projects in order to further science itself, and the public understanding of both science and of the scientific process.
The Citizen Science Association (CSA)	The Citizen Science Association (CSA) is a member-driven organization that connects people from a wide range of experiences around one shared purpose: Advancing knowledge through research and monitoring done by, for, and with members of the public.
Citscibio.org	NIH sponsored online collaboration space for the growing and virtually dispersed biomedical citizen science resources, projects, references, methods, and communities to be discovered and engaged by interested stakeholders.
Biocurious.org	BioCurious is a community that includes people from many different backgrounds to participate in science. Projects are driven by whoever wants to show up and participate.
Makerfaire.Com	This is a convention of do-it-yourself participants from various backgrounds with interests in robotics, computers, arts, crafts and hacker culture
Nationofmakers.us	Non profit supporting American's maker organizations through community building, resource sharing, and advocacy.
Openingpathways.org	Collaboration between patients and traditional researchers to explore the process of research and innovation in healthcare. Each project the patient serves as the Principle Investigator. This is supported by the RWJF.
Publiclab.org	Public Lab is a community and non-profit democratizing science to address environmental issues that affect people.
Scistarter.com	Online citizen science hub searchable by location, topic, age, and level. Projects are registered by individual project leaders through partnerships with federal agencies.
Zooninverse.org	Platform for people-powered research to enable research that would not be possible, or practical. This research is made possible by volunteers to assist professional researchers.

overview to understand about involving citizen scientists in the research process. (Robinson et al. 2018) Citizen science is a rapidly expanding field and requires active participation of the public in scientific research projects.(Den Broeder et al. 2016) Several citizen science project, resources, and organizations can be found online, see Citizen Science Resources (Table 14.1).

What Is Person-Centered Design?

Person-centered design is a process where by the design team works to ensure that the needs of the patient are taken into consideration as a whole person and an equal partner in their care rather than simply a passive recipient, are foremost (Kildea et al. 2019). A Whole-person perspective includes and values the understanding that a person's environment where they live and work, psychosocial and physical aspects, and health behaviors can impact overall health.(Sminkey 2015; Carter et al. 2015) Therefore a person-centered approach to design approach focuses on multiple aspects of a persons' life versus only focusing on a single aspect. Rigorous methods and design processes are needed in person-centered citizen science research to ensure all voices are heard and represented.(Petersen 2018).

Methods

In this section we explore person-centered design methods for citizen science. These methods fall into two main categories: Guiding principles and design-thinking processes. Guiding principles are value-driven and fundamental to inclusive and equitable citizen science collaboration (Vandekerckhove et al. 2020; Hoadley 2018). Design-thinking processes provide key steps in the co-creative design journey. Using design-thinking processes can inform methodological research strategies and have potential to add rigor to the overall design process (Vandekerckhove et al. 2020).

Guiding Principles

Guiding principles of co-creative design for citizen science encompass personal beliefs and values that are used to guide the design process throughout its life in all circumstances, irrespective of changes in its goals, strategies or type of work (King et al. 2019; Dick 2017).

In this section, we provide an example of guiding principles. It is recommended to establish guiding principles before research or design processes take place. It is also recommended to discuss with all stakeholders up front and possibly throughout the design process. The principles provide the necessary support for inclusion, to ensure voices are to be heard throughout the deign process, and honor agency among the group (Vandekerckhove et al. 2020). Guiding principles should be seen as a complement to research principles rather than replace. We provide an example of guiding principles that are informed by the generative design process and include: (1) Democracy; (2) Mutual learning; (3) Tacit or latent knowledge; and (4) Collective creativity (see Table 14.2) (Vandekerckhove et al. 2020).

Table 14.2 Guiding principles

Guiding principles	Definition
Democracy	All members (citizen scientists and researchers) are equal partners of the design team
Mutual Learning	Establish respectful for learning and acknowledgement all participants can learn from each other
Tacit or latent knowledge	Subtle knowledge that is not always apparent and may require deeper observation or introspection
Collective creativity	Everyone considered creative and part of the process. Collective creativity can be stronger than individuality in co-design

Establishing guiding principles from the beginning of any project can establish boundaries and help to define the collective purpose and partnership within a group. With clear guiding principles established it is time to move to the design phase.

Person-Centered Design-Thinking Methods

Design methods, specifically design thinking, are tools used to guide the design process and provide a systematic method for each step along the way. There are several methods to draw from but not limited to community-based participatory methods, informatics design processes, design thinking, person-centered design methods or a hybrid of many methods for a specific or unique project.

The purpose of design-thinking methods are to create an established pathway to reach the end result such as a new mobile health application, co-participatory research study, or simple electronic health data collection prototype. Choosing the right method is dependent on several factors such as motivations of the team and the need to match the method to the question. Drawing from person-centered design methods to ensure that the needs of the patient, as a whole person and an equal partner in their care are included within the design team.(Kildea et al. 2019)

Empathic Design

Leonard and Rayport's empathic design would entail "techniques require exceptional collaborative skills, open-mindedness, interview and observation skills, and inquisitiveness. The use of visual information entails an understanding of the user. In short, build a new observation in user's familiar contexts (Leonard and Rayport 1997). Of course, we cannot experience the way others experience, but with supportive tools, we can attempt to get as close as possible and without pre-judgment and preconceived ideas.

Empathic design is a collaboration of tools to facilitate the design team obtains a deeper understanding of the problem and stakeholders they are designing for. It requires designers to uncover user's emotional and physical needs and how users see, understand, and interact with the world around them to manage their interactive behaviors and build a better experience. Empathic design is not concerned with facts about users but more about their desires and motivations. For instance, why the outpatient prefers to get instructions before the CT/MRI scan.

"Empathies" is the *first* stage of the Design Thinking process. The following stages can be summarized as research, ideation, and refinement. The goal is to gather an in-depth empathic understanding of users and the problem context. In order to interpret the user's experience and motivations, empathic design thinking involves observing, empathizing with all the relevant stakeholders, and stepping into their physical environment to have a holistic understanding of the challenges. The most commonly used empathic design methods,

- Set up a beginner's mindset
- Ask What-How-Why
- Design and conduct interviews with empathy
- Use personal photo and video journals
- Engage with all the relevant stakeholders
- Stories tell-and-capture
- Use journey map

Human-Centered Design-Thinking Process

Apart from creating an innovative culture, institutions need to know how to proceed: fully understand a problem and then solve it by creating something relevant for their customers or stakeholders. The "designer's way of thinking" has been identified as a fruitful approach to user-centered innovation (Duanne and Martin 2006).

Design Thinking (DT) is a systemic design methodology that provides a solution-based approach to frame and solves problems (Chasanidou et al. 2015; Ferreira et al. 2015). The problems designers and design researchers face are more complex or ill-defined by tackling the human-centered needs involved. Understanding these three stages of human-centered empathic design thinking will enable anyone to apply design thinking methods to frame and solve problems that occur every day.

Design thinking is a non-linear, iterative process that teams use to build an empathic understanding of users, create anticipates, reframe problems and create innovative solutions to facility behavior and get a better experience. The three stages of Design Thinking are as follows: Research, Ideation, and Refinement. Let us take a closer look at the three different stages of Design Thinking (Fig. 14.1).

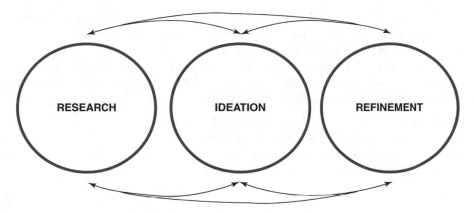

Fig. 14.1 Design thinking process

Research Phase

Design thinking research systematically studies all the relevant stakeholders and their requirements, adding contexts and collecting insights to design thinking processes. It is the steppingstone towards defining the requirements for the product are about to design. Design researchers adopt various methods to uncover problems and design opportunities. Doing so, they reveal valuable information which can feed into the design process.

Research is an essential step across the entire design thinking process. It will most likely happen every time a new idea is framed or improve existing ones. The primary value of the pre-development research phase is defining the initial direction that the product/service will take moving forward. The majority outcome from the research phase includes:

- Who are the stakeholders, what are their relationships?
- What are the stakeholders trying to achieve and desire?
- What are the pain points, and how to solve these problems?
- Who are the competitors?

Ideation Phase

The goal of ideation is to create ideas that the team can test with stakeholders then cut down into the most suitable, most practical, and innovative solutions. More specifically, ideation is interested in the activity whereby designers are exteriorizing stakeholder's internal mental images, engaging in a conversation of the sort with them. By widening the solution scope, the design team will look beyond the usual methods of solving problems to find better, more elegant, and satisfying solutions to problems that affect a user's experience of a product or service.

The Ideation stage often follows the research stages with significant overlap. Understanding the user, interpreting data/information, and frame/reframe the problem(s) and ideation drive the generation of solutions.

The methods the design team incorporates in the two stages are overlapping as well. For example, co-creation activities and usability tests are often used in both of these stages. Ideation will help the design team,

- Mapping stakeholder and bring together perspectives
- Increase the innovation potential of solutions
- Uncover unexpected areas of innovation.
- Create volume and variety in innovation options

Refinement Phase

This stage helps the design team to develop ideas and concepts and deliver them to stakeholders. Once the team or designer is confident that the proposed solution will work for users after research and ideate, the project transitions into build and launch mode. For the designer, this can involve producing high-fertility prototype for the development team, or working with a visual designer, and generally being involved during the implementation phase to ensure that the design intent is being carried through to the final product. This can mean providing feedback to the development team or doing usability testing on beta versions of a product to check that interactions are as intended. The main focus of this phase is to,

- Develop, incorporating early end-user consideration as much as possible.
- Test and debug.
- Deploy.

In addition to the design-thinking methods just explored, it may be beneficial to review the Patient Centered Outcomes Research Institute (PCORI) Criterion for patient and stakeholder engagement for funded research.(PCORI Institute 2019) These criterion can be used to guide co-participation for patient and stakeholder engagement and be used to inform research and projects (Table 14.3).

Putting it all Together

We created this chapter to serve as a guide for person-centered participatory design. The methods presented in this chapter only scratch the surface for available options to select from and to aid in the design process. We have created recommendations for putting it all together and to inform the design process.

Table 14.3 Checklist for co-creative design

Topic	Detailed question
Can the team provide a well-justified description of how various stakeholders will be included in research activities?	Does the study/project include the right individuals (e.g., patients, caregivers, clinicians, policy makers, hospital and health system representatives, payers, purchasers, industry, researchers, and training institutions) to ensure that the projects will be carried out successfully?
Can the team show evidence of active engagement among scientists, patients, and other stakeholders throughout the research process (e.g., formulating questions, identifying outcomes, monitoring the study, disseminating, and implementing)?	Is the frequency and level of patient and stakeholder involvement sufficient to support the study goals?
What is the proposed engagement or co-design approach appropriate and tailored to the study?	Check methods to engage participants in authentic and aligns with the study design. If not, perhaps a pre-planning meeting with co-design team to revisit strategies and ensure team is in alignment with methods.
What are the roles and the decision-making authority of all study partners described clearly?	Clearly identify roles and responsibilities of all stakeholders and decision makers early in the process. Provide a dedicated time to re-assess the project within the design process to pause and re-evaluate the structure if needed.
Are the organizational structures and resources appropriate to engage patients and stakeholders throughout the project?	What additional steps can be done to ensure inclusive open environment?

Recommendation #1: First, establish guiding principles for the entire team and throughout the design process. This can serve to guide the team and establish mutual respect and trust from the beginning. As stated earlier, establish a process to pause and reassess principles, overall process, and methods to provide an opportunity to adjust as needed. This may serve well if there are new stakeholders brought in throughout the process.

Recommendation #2: Next, begin with the end product or deliverable in mind. Beginning with the end in mind can provide a pathway for the design process. This will also serve to include all stakeholders with a clear vision of the end goal.

Recommendation #3: Last, keep and open mind. While we have provided methods to structure the design process, holding too rigid can stifle the creative process. There is a balance between structured processes and allowing creativity and flow of ideas. Due to the nature of the co-creative participatory design, many multiple stakeholders with differing intentions can be part of the process. Keeping an open mind enables an inclusive environment, which is essential for person-centered design methodology.

Conclusions

Citizen science has led to knowledge discovery and exciting new collaborations to improve health and healthcare for all. Citizen science is a growing mechanism and pathway for non-researchers to be included in the research process. Guiding principles can serve to foster an inclusive and respective environment for co-created design. Using co-creative design methods provide structure to the process and ensure all voices can be included. This chapter provides examples of person-centered design methods to aid in development and sustainability of citizen science research collaboration.

Clinical Pearls
- Begin with the end in mind
- Include patients/citizen scientists early and throughout the design process
- Honor agency within the individual, family, or community

Review Questions
1. What is the main concept of person-centered design?

   A. The patient is part of the process but only as a passive participant to listen to the design team.
   B. Focuses on multiple aspects of a person's life versus a single component or aspect.
   C. Rigorous methods are not needed as all stakeholders can speak up equally at any time
   D. Patients are not equal members of the design team as the main researcher has the final say in all matters related to design.

2. Of the three phases in design thinking, which phase focuses on creating ideas the team can test with stakeholders?

   A. Research
   B. Creative
   C. Prospective
   D. Ideation

Answers
Question 1: B is the correct answer. The person-centered design focuses on the whole-person and takes multiple aspects of the person into account.

   A. Incorrect answer. The patient is an equal partner in the design process.
   C. Incorrect answer. Rigorous methods are needed to ensure all stakeholders, including patients, have a voice within the design process.
   D. Incorrect answer. Patients are equal partners in the deign process.

Question 2: D is the correct answer. Ideation is the process in create ideas that the team can test with stakeholders then cut down into the most suitable, most practical, and innovative solutions

A. Not correct. Research phase defining the requirements for the product are about to design.
B. Not correct. Refinement phase helps the design team to develop ideas and concepts and deliver them to stakeholders
C. Not Correct. Prospective phase is not a phase.

References

Bonney R, Phillips TB, Ballard HL, Enck JW. Can citizen science enhance public understanding of science? Public Underst Sci. 2016;25(1):2–16. https://doi.org/10.1177/0963662515607406.

Carter J, Zawalski S, Sminkey PV, Christopherson B. Assessing the whole person: case managers take a holistic approach to physical and mental health. Prof Case Manag. 2015;20(3):140 6. https://doi.org/10.1097/NCM.0000000000000087.

Chasanidou D, Gasparini AA, Lee E. Design thinking methods and tools for innovation. Cham: Springer; 2015. https://doi.org/10.1007/978-3-319-20886-2_2.

Den Broeder L, Devilee J, Van Oers H, Schuit AJ, Wagemakers A. Citizen science for public health. Health Promot Int. 2016:daw086. https://doi.org/10.1093/heapro/daw086.

Dick DM. Rethinking the way we do research: the benefits of community-engaged, citizen science approaches and nontraditional collaborators. Alcohol Clin Exp Res. 2017;41(11):1849–56. https://doi.org/10.1111/acer.13492.

Duanne D, Martin R. Design thinking and how it will change management education: an interview and discussion. Acad Manag Learn Educ. 2006;5(4):512–23.

Evans B. Barbarians at the gate: consumer-driven health data commons and the transformaiton of citizen science Am J Law Med. 2016;70(12):773–9. https://doi.org/10.1097/OGX.0000000000000256.Prenatal.

Ferreira FK, Song EH, Gomes H, Garcia EB, Ferreira LM. New mindset in scientific method in the health field: design thinking. Clinics. 2015;70(12):770–2. https://doi.org/10.6061/clinics/2015(12)01.

Gura T. Citizen science: amateur experts. Nature. 2013;496(7444):259–61. https://doi.org/10.1038/nj7444-259a.

Hinckson E, Schneider M, Winter SJ, et al. Citizen science applied to building healthier community environments: advancing the field through shared construct and measurement development. Int J Behav Nutr Phys Act. 2017;14(1):1–13. https://doi.org/10.1186/s12966-017-0588-6.

Hoadley, C. (2018). Designing citizen science projects (Whitepaper commissioned by the National Academy of Sciences Committee on Public Participation in Science). 2009:1–13.

Kildea J, Battista J, Cabral B, et al. Design and development of a person-centered patient portal using participatory stakeholder co-design. J Med Internet Res. 2019;21(2):1–17. https://doi.org/10.2196/11371.

King AC, Winter SJ, Chrisinger BW, Hua J, Banchoff AW. Maximizing the promise of citizen science to advance health and prevent disease. Prev Med (Baltim). 2019;119(December 2018):44–7. S0091743518303955.

Leonard D, Rayport JF. Spark innovation through empathic design. Harvard business review. 1997;75:102–15.

PCORI Institute. PCORI methodology report. 2019. https://www.pcori.org/research-results/about-our-research/research-methodology/pcori-methodology-report.

Petersen C. Patient informaticians: turning patient voice into patient action. JAMIA Open. 2018;1(May):130–5. https://doi.org/10.1093/jamiaopen/ooy014.

Petersen C, Austin RR, Backonja U, et al. Citizen science to further precision medicine: from vision to implementation. JAMIA Open. 2021;3:1. https://doi.org/10.1093/JAMIAOPEN/OOZ060.

Robinson L, West S, Bonn A, Ansine J. Ten principles of citizen science. In: Hecker S, Haklay M, Bowser A, Makuch Z, Vogel J, Bonn A, editors. Citizien science: innovation in open science, society, and policy. UCL Press; 2018. p. 1–23.

Sminkey PV. The "whole-person" approach : understanding the connection between physical and mental health. Prof Case Manag. 2015;20(3):154–5. https://doi.org/10.1097/NCM.0000000000000094.

Steven R, Barnes M, Garnett S, et al. Aligning citizen science with best practice: threatened species conservation in Australia. Conserv Sci Pract. 2019;1(10) https://doi.org/10.1111/csp2.100.

Van Vliet K, Moore C. Citizen science initiatives: engaging the public and demystifying science. J Microbiol Biol Educ. 2016;17(1):13–6. https://doi.org/10.1128/jmbe.v17i1.1019.

Vandekerckhove P, Ma DM, Bramer WM, De Bont AA. Generative participatory design methodology to develop electronic health interventions: systematic literature review. J Med Internet Res. 2020;22(4):1–18. https://doi.org/10.2196/13780.

Wang Y, Kaplan N, Newman G, Scarpino R. CitSci.org: a new model for managing, documenting, and sharing citizen science data. PLoS Biol. 2015;13(10):1–5. https://doi.org/10.1371/journal.pbio.1002280.

Chapter 15
Leveraging Library and Information Science to Discover Consumer Health Informatics Research

Christie L. Martin, Elizabeth V. Weinfurter, Kristine M. Alpi, and Scott Sittig

Abstract The field of consumer health informatics (CHI) is constantly evolving. The literature that supports CHI includes a broad scope of expertise and disciplines, which makes discovering relevant literature a challenge. Through a library and information science lens, we provide foundational familiarity with the structures of information discovery systems and considerations that impact the discovery of CHI literature. We outline the steps included in the design and execution phases of a CHI-related literature search. We also provide an example search using wearable technologies and a case in point that illustrates how terminologies differ across databases. We describe the importance of operationalizing elements of a research question and strategically combining search terms in a query to enhance the findability of CHI literature. The reader will gain a database-agnostic understanding of the structures and factors relevant to the retrieval of CHI literature, which should be particularly useful as the field of CHI and the tools for retrieving literature continuously change.

Keywords Controlled vocabulary · Consumer health informatics · Databases
Literature searching · Subject headings · Wearable technology

C. L. Martin (✉)
School of Nursing, University of Minnesota, Minneapolis, MN, USA
e-mail: mart1026@umn.edu

E. V. Weinfurter
Health Sciences Library, University of Minnesota, Minneapolis, MN, USA

K. M. Alpi
OHSU Library and Department of Medical Informatics & Clinical Epidemiology, Oregon Health & Science University, Portland, OR, USA

S. Sittig
College of Nursing and Allied Health Professions, University of Louisiana at Lafayette, Lafayette, LA, USA

© The Author(s), under exclusive license to Springer Nature
Switzerland AG 2022
P.-Y. S. Hsueh et al. (eds.), *Personal Health Informatics*, Cognitive Informatics in Biomedicine and Healthcare, https://doi.org/10.1007/978-3-031-07696-1_15

Learning Objectives
1. Become familiar with the wide scope of content and expertise that comprises the consumer health informatics literature.
2. Outline the steps included in the design and execution phases of a consumer health informatics-related literature search to find relevant articles in health and engineering databases.
3. Understand the role of search terms (keywords, phrases, and subject headings) used to enhance the findability of consumer health informatics literature within a specific context (e.g., wearable technologies).

Introduction

Identifying and retrieving the knowledge base of consumer health informatics (CHI) is a foundational skill for all learners and researchers engaging with informatics literature. This chapter offers a framework relevant to those who would benefit from a systematic and efficient approach to searching CHI literature. Consumer health informatics is a rapidly evolving subdiscipline of health informatics that requires ongoing learning about new terminology and system search strategies. According to the American Medical Informatics Association (AMIA),

> *Consumer Health Informatics is the field devoted to informatics from multiple consumer or patient views. These include patient-focused informatics, health literacy and consumer education. ...Consumer informatics stands at the crossroads of other disciplines, such as nursing informatics, public health, health promotion, health education, library science, and communication science* (American Medical Informatics Association n.d.).

Consumer health informatics research is always within the context of human health and often pursued by multidisciplinary teams of professionals, including varied health care experts, engineers, computer and data scientists, librarians, economists, designers, sports scientists, community organizers, and consumer advocates. Although CHI research has been around for several decades (United States General Accounting Office 1996, p.1), it has evolved. Published work is varied and can include basic science studies on textiles and materials, proof-of-concept work with healthy research participants, feasibility studies in the patient population of interest, and dissemination (or direct-to-consumer marketing) of commercial products. The professional discipline of the lead author and the type or stage of the CHI research often determine the preferred place of publication, such as engineering or computer science journals for proof-of-concept work, or health discipline or informatics journals for outcome studies. Recent CHI research investigates consumer electronic technologies, such as wearables, mobile health devices, and sensors to support consumers for the purposes mentioned above. These latter technologies are myriad and rapidly changing, making it difficult for researchers to locate relevant literature[1] due to the widely varied terminology that is inconsistently applied in *electronic databases*, or information discovery sources.

Successful literature retrieval is not exclusive to searching databases but instead consists of strategically designing and executing a literature search. The ***design phase of a literature search*** involves formulating a research question and operationalizing the question's elements. The ***execution phase of a literature search*** consists of a database query that utilizes ***search terms*** (keywords, phrases, and subject headings) representing these elements as concepts. The design phase is the most critical component of the literature retrieval process.

This chapter lays the groundwork that will allow researchers at all levels to make informed and mindful decisions about designing and executing CHI literature searches. We have written this chapter for readers coming from any background. Our goal is to create a shared understanding of the typical structure of databases and techniques used to search literature; knowledge that is often skipped over in a rush to focus on the logistics of searching a particular database. In addition to this conceptual foundation, we also aim to provide practical guidance for retrieving literature regardless of where it is published or electronically stored. To this end, we detail designing and executing a literature search, provide an executed literature search exemplar, and illustrate insights from our own research on how database terms relate to the language used by the author(s). This chapter does not extend beyond knowledge discovery, but to learn more you may consult one of the many resources detailing different literature review processes in their entirety (Aromataris and Munn 2020; Garrard 2017; Higgins et al. 2021).

Designing a Literature Search

Consult with Information and Library Scientists

Information scientists (e.g., library scientists, informationists, or librarians), herein librarians, are specially trained and experienced in searching the literature and are important collaborators on projects that depend on a thorough review of the literature. Involving librarians early in the search process is critical. Each database has slightly different features and functions that constantly change. Librarians can advise on the current best practices for challenging research topics and on the intricacies of databases. Developing a database-agnostic foundational knowledge with the help of a librarian can serve researchers throughout their careers despite database changes or the advent of new resources. Additionally, and more importantly, librarians can help facilitate the best approach to scoping the literature, starting with drafting a research question. Academic institutions almost always employ

---

[1] We are using "literature" as a catch-all term for journal articles, books and chapters, dissertations, conference proceedings, standards of practice, etc.

professional librarians with specialized knowledge, but if you are not based at an institution with librarians, you can consult the Network of the National Library of Medicine Member Directory at https://nnlm.gov/membership/directory for a referral to a health sciences library or visit your local public library.

Draft a Research Question

Before executing a search query in a database, you should think critically about the foundational component of the design phase, which includes organizing information and ideas in the format of a research question. There are many ways to collect and organize information and ideas to prepare for a search; they all share two common goals: (1) identifying the essential elements in your research question and (2) determining the relative priority of these elements.

Research is iterative, and each step reveals new information that helps refine the research question and approach. The approach will vary depending on your goal. For example, your goal might be to find specific CHI-related exemplars or broadly explore the CHI literature. A different goal might be to find all relevant literature on a CHI topic for a patent or grant application or to ask an evidence-based question about a CHI intervention.

There are several frameworks used to develop evidence-based, searchable questions. Clinicians and informatics researchers, especially those trained in nursing and allied health, often use the *PICO(T) format* to search for evidence surrounding topics of therapy and prevention, diagnosis, etiology, and prognosis. PICO(T) is a mnemonic with the following *PICO(T) elements*: P (problem or patient/population); I (intervention); C (comparison); O (outcome); and T (time frame). Depending on the question, the C and the T may be implied as the current standard of care and timeframe and may be important to screening eligible literature once it is retrieved; these elements are often not included when executing a search, as you will see in the *Exemplar Literature Search* section below (Riva et al. 2012).

Drafting a PICO(T) question is the first step in framing a problem to be explored efficiently and effectively. Ideally, in the case of "consumer health informatics," each of the three elements (i.e., "consumer," "health," "informatics") would fit uniformly into the PICO(T) format: "consumer" would correspond with P (problem or patient/population), "health" might correspond with either P (problem) or O (outcome), and "informatics" would likely correspond with I (intervention). While informaticians can use the PICO(T) format to draft CHI-related research questions, there is great value in expanding the concepts representing these elements beyond using the words "consumer health informatics" because these elements are too broad in scope. Instead, you should conceptualize precise PICO(T) elements to comprise a specific research question. For example, you might ask: In adults (P) with asthma (P), are wearable devices (I) effective at helping them self-manage their symptoms (O)? To illustrate the sequence of steps in the design and execution stages of searching the literature, we will continue to use this PICO.

Operationalize Elements

After formulating a research question, you should operationalize or define each element of interest before combining them into a search query (discussed in the *Executing a Literature Search* section). To operationalize, first extract each element from your research question (i.e., "adults," "asthma," "wearable devices," "self-management") and then conceptualize the elements and all synonymous elements. For example, when operationalizing the element "adult," you might consider the particular age category (e.g., "college-aged" or "older adults, 65+") or their place of residence (e.g., "rural" or "urban"). The former may impact the adult's ability to interface with the wearable, and the latter may affect their access to mobile health technologies or the air quality or asthma management. When operationalizing the element "wearables," you might consider synonyms like "activity tracker," "Fitbit," "smartwatch," etc. If, for example, your intended audience includes persons unfamiliar with informatics or wearable technologies, you may choose elements that are easier to understand (e.g., "iPhone" or "mobile app").

Prioritize Elements

After operationalizing the elements of your research question, consider which elements are most important. A common mistake in designing your literature search is to put search terms (keywords, phrases, and/or subject headings) for *all* of the elements or concepts of your research question into your database. This approach is usually overly specific and may not yield any literature. Ideally, you would use a high-level approach that starts with a few essential elements. Are you most interested in your specific population and willing to broaden the intervention and outcomes? Or is a particular intervention your highest priority? It is critical to determine which elements of your question are of the highest priority and necessary for your database query. It is also important to decide which elements to narrow down or broaden out conceptually when executing a literature search. A librarian can assist with the vital task of prioritizing elements and considering concept combinations, the latter of which is described next.

Executing a Literature Search

Consider Concept Combinations

Next, you will incorporate the elements of your research question into the execution phase of the literature search. In the first step of this phase, you typically combine elements as concepts with *Boolean operators*: AND (narrows down), OR (broadens out), NOT (excludes). These operators are used to combine search terms, such as keywords, phrases, and subject headings. After isolating and operationalizing the elements in your research question, you will determine the concepts of the highest priority and use **_Boolean logic_** to combine concepts that best align with the search terms and the research question. Next, you will place these combinations into the database search query. For example,

> AND (narrows down): wearables AND asthma
> > OR (broadens out): wearables OR mobile apps
> > NOT (excludes): asthma NOT exercise-induced asthma

We provide additional examples of Boolean logic within a search query in the *Exemplar Literature Search* section.

Choose Relevant Databases

Information relevant to CHI is broadly available online. Therefore, a CHI topic exploration might start with a search of Google Scholar to get an idea of what is available and how a topic is discussed. However, Google Scholar covers a different depth and breadth of literature than other databases and does not allow the sophisticated and reproducible search methodologies discussed later in this chapter. A researcher will not be able to fully characterize and the impact of Google Scholar's search algorithm on retrieval. Google Scholar also does not offer the level of search precision available in more highly structured databases. It is an important tool for researchers but knowing when to use it is key. See Table 15.1 for a list of databases selected for their relevance to CHI literature searches and their characteristics (i.e., topics covered, content/type covered, years covered, and controlled vocabulary status).

As previously stated, literature pertinent to your CHI research question may have been published in a wide variety of journals, requiring you to search multiple discipline-specific databases. If you are interested in the health implications of the technology in a patient or consumer population, you may focus solely on the health literature. The single largest database comprising health literature is PubMed/MEDLINE, which contains over 32 million citations as of 2021 and is free to search at https://www.pubmed.gov (National Library of Medicine: National Center for Biotechnology Information 2021).

PubMed/MEDLINE includes some engineering literature, such as selected publications of the Institute of Electrical and Electronics Engineers (IEEE), to provide exposure to earlier technology research and development literature. There is overlap in the topics and content covered across the databases in Table 15.1. We give an example of this overlap within the context of "wearables" in the *Case in Point* section.

Few journals focus specifically on CHI or personal health/pervasive computing, and minimal terminology clearly identifies these areas. Thus, when querying a wide

Table 15.1 Selected databases relevant to CHI literature searches and their characteristics

Database name	Topics covered	Content/type covered	Years covered	Controlled vocabulary
PubMed/ MEDLINE	Health and Biomedical Sciences	Primarily journal articles	1946-present[a]	Medical subject headings (MeSH)
Cumulative index to nursing and allied health literature (CINAHL)	Nursing/ Allied health	Journal articles, books and chapters, nursing dissertations, selected conference proceedings, standards of practice, legal cases, and other document types	1982-present	CINAHL terms
Compendex	Engineering/ computer science	Journal articles, conference proceedings, reports, and monographs (books)	1884-present	Main headings
INSPEC	Engineering/ computer science	Journal articles, conference proceedings, and reports	1896-present	Controlled/ subject terms
IEEE Xplore (Institute of Electrical and Electronics Engineers)	Engineering/ computer science	Journal articles, conference proceedings, books, and standards published by the IEEE and its publishing partners	1988-present	IEEE terms, as well as INSPEC controlled terms[b]
Google scholar	All scholarly topics	Scholarly articles, theses and dissertations, patents, legal cases	Always changing	None
Scopus	All scholarly topics	Journal articles	1968-present[c,d]	Varies[e]
Web of science	All scholarly topics	Journal articles, book chapters, proceedings[c]	1900-present[c,f]	Varies[e]

[a] 1946-present consistently, with the ability to query earlier articles
[b] MeSH terms for 14 IEEE biomedical-related titles
[c] Varies by subscription
[d] Articles date back to as early as 1788
[e] Records include terms from the source database; keywords are generated from words in titles/abstracts/references
[f] Articles may date back earlier than 1900

range of literature, it is essential to use various search terms. The most challenging part of conceptualizing CHI is ascertaining whether the consumer is engaged in their own health or with the technology. In general, the technology and engineering journals typically do not report on the clinical outcomes of patients using the technology or, if they do, this literature may not use language that reflects the individual's engagement with the devices. Many of the databases that include this literature augment the author-provided keywords and phrases used to index the articles by applying database-specific vocabulary to categorize the content. Several databases have additional strategies for using the author-provided keywords and phrases as well as words in the title, abstract, full text, or references of the article (discussed in more detail in the next section).

If you are searching a database for the first time, consult a librarian or review the user guide provided by the database producer to ensure you understand the database structure and its search fields. Librarians can also provide input on choosing the most appropriate database(s) and search terms. Once you have successfully located literature in one database, you may want to query another database. Since each database queries literature slightly differently, consider consulting a librarian to assist you with translating the search terms appropriately. Finally, be certain to document your search strategy to ensure reproducibility or meet the requirements for search documentation if you are performing any type of scoping or systematic review.

Understand the Difference Between Keyword and Subject Heading Queries

Once you draft your research question, operationalize and prioritize your elements, consider concept combinations, and choose the desired database(s), you are ready to execute a database search query. The bridge between designing and executing a literature search lies in understanding how information sources are structured and queried.

There are two main ways to execute a database query. You can execute a **keyword query**, which retrieves literature by looking for an exact match for a word or phrase used by the author(s) and/or a **subject heading query**, which retrieves literature by using controlled vocabularies or concepts assigned by the database as metadata. **Metadata** is data that describes other data. In this case, it is the data attached to an article in a database. Metadata can be created by humans, by an automated process involving machine learning and natural language processing, or by combining the two processes (whereby humans curate the terms to be used automatically, or they approve terms originally suggested by automated approaches). Subject heading queries, described in the *Subject Heading Queries* section, capture literature related to a specific concept regardless of the exact words the author(s) use since this metadata describes the author-provided language in a standardized way. Most scholarly databases have some system of subject headings, though this type of controlled vocabulary varies in depth and specificity.

Knowing the characteristics of the database, including its keyword search capabilities and subject heading structure, is an integral part of decision-making when constructing a solid search strategy. We generally recommend searching all fields since author keywords and other relevant terms may be in fields other than the abstract, such as the "Other Terms" field in the PubMed/MEDLINE database. However, search strategies focused on keywords across all fields may reduce opportunities to fully use the features in the hierarchy of vocabularies discussed in the following sections of this chapter. A comprehensive search likely uses OR statements to combine keyword and subject headings for maximal sensitivity in identifying relevant literature.

Keyword Queries

When conducting a keyword query to identify articles using a search term, databases work in various ways. At its simplest, a keyword query picks up an exact match for words as used by the author(s). For example, querying "wearable devices" will retrieve articles using that exact phrase but will not retrieve articles with the word "wearables" or "wearable device." A keyword query for "asthma" will not retrieve articles with the word "asthmatic." When used in a query, these slight variations of search terms representing the same concept are called *term variants*. To yield multiple term variants, most databases allow for the truncation of keyword queries. *Truncation* comprises a symbol (most often the *) representing a stem, or portion, of a search term. For example, querying "asthma*" will retrieve "asthma" as well as "asthmatic," "asthmatics," etc. Truncation only works at the end of a term, not at the beginning or internally. Some databases also allow for an internal *wildcard character*, which comprises a character ("?") and represents the absence or presence of a portion of a search term, which can be helpful for international spelling variants. For example, "digitali?ation" would retrieve the words "digitalization" or "digitalisation." Regardless of the keyword query options allowed by a database, you should consult your librarian to help you consider slight variations of terms.

It is also important to know how a database handles *phrase searching*, a type of keyword query that searches for two or more search terms exactly as entered into the query. To execute a phrase search, databases often require you to use quotation marks to group words together in a query; for example, "wearable devices." If you do not use the quotation marks, querying the term 'wearable devices' may query both of the words individually (e.g., devices that are not wearable). Some databases allow for *adjacency searching*, searching for two words located within a specified number of words from each other. For search terms with variants that cannot be included with a simple truncation, you can use adjacency searching to allow for more flexibility while still keeping the search terms within context. For example, to execute a query for "symptom clusters" that allows for this type of flexibility, you could query "symptom* adj4 cluster*," which would retrieve the words "symptom cluster," "symptom clusters," "cluster of symptoms," "symptoms that are clustered," etc.

An additional consideration when executing keyword queries is knowing *where* the database looks for the words in your search query. Most scholarly databases do not search the full text of an article. Instead, a query often uses article metadata and author-provided data (e.g., title, abstract, author(s), etc.). For example, a default keyword query usually looks for keyword matches in the title, abstract, and metadata. You could instead choose to only query words in the title of the article to retrieve literature with higher relevance. When executing a keyword query, it is vital to consider term variants, *where* in the literature the database searches for the author(s)' words, and whether there is any database-specific syntax for truncation, wild cards, phrase searching, etc. Databases sometimes allow for greater specificity when executing a query by enabling you to place **search limits**, or filters (e.g., language, range of dates), on your query.

Clinical Pearl 1: Keyword Searching in PubMed Have you ever felt as if you had seen a paper with a particular word or phrase in the title or abstract before, but when you query that phrase in PubMed, you are unable to retrieve any articles? For reasons of response time and search demand, PubMed cannot search *all* of the individual words and phrases in the title and abstract of the millions of records in real-time. Instead, it searches a pre-generated phrase index of the most commonly occurring phrases. You may need to use a commercial version of MEDLINE (such as Ovid Medline) that allows for word and adjacency searching.

Subject Heading Queries

A *subject heading* is a standardized term for a concept within a *controlled vocabulary*, which is a list of subject headings that represents concepts in a standardized way. Controlled vocabulary often exists in a *taxonomy*, or hierarchical classification system, used by a database. Subject headings are components of a system of controlled vocabulary (e.g., Medical Subject Headings) developed for a discipline, usually specific to a single database (see the "Controlled Vocabulary" column in Table 15.1). As previously stated, subject heading queries retrieve literature using concepts rather than exact matches of words used by the author(s). For example, you might not know to include the search terms "fitness tracker" and "smartwatch" when searching "wearables." When literature is added to a database, subject headings are identified and applied to the *article records* as metadata to describe the article's content in a standardized way making the literature retrieval more efficient. In this way, metadata application is similar to, and different from, using hashtags when posting on social media. The application of hashtags and metadata differs in that the person interfacing with social media "controls" using the hashtags, while the database "controls" the subject headings on the backend. While the creation of subject headings by humans takes time and can be subject to human error, a subject heading query has the benefit of inherent human judgment, especially since the context has already been considered. On the other hand, keyword queries are dependent on the sophistication of the database and the search engine itself. You would execute a keyword query when literature has yet to be indexed with subject headings.

Medical Subject Headings (MeSH) terms are among the most highly developed subject headings used in PubMed/MEDLINE, the primary database used to retrieve

CHI literature. The United States National Library of Medicine created MeSH terms in the 1960s to facilitate literature discovery in the life sciences (National Library of Medicine 1960). With the advent of electronic databases, queries quickly became more accessible and highly complex. Still, the underlying structure utilizing MeSH terms to facilitate the discovery of literature persists to this day. Given the enormous volume of literature that requires controlled vocabulary, the National Library of Medicine has its own indexing initiative (National Institutes of Health: U.S. National Library of Medicine 2018; National Institutes of Health: U.S. National Library of Medicine 2019).

Clinical Pearl 2: PubMed vs. MEDLINE vs. Ovid? The MEDLINE database is the National Library of Medicine's primary bibliographic database containing more than 27 million references to journal articles in life and health sciences fields. MEDLINE records have Medical Subject Headings attached. You can search MEDLINE using many electronic databases, including the free version (PubMed) or commercially available versions (Ovid Medline, EBSCO Medline, Scopus, and more). Each method used to search MEDLINE contains slightly different search options and additional material, but the core MEDLINE database is the same. Talk to a librarian for details on a specific method of searching MEDLINE.

See Fig. 15.1 for the CHI MeSH term found in PubMed/MEDLINE. Subject headings are particularly useful for CHI-related queries, given the broad scope of the CHI discipline. Countless keywords can describe CHI, which makes a comprehensive keyword query nearly impossible. However, with its associated subheadings (i.e., economics, ethics, etc.), as seen in Fig. 15.1, a subject heading query can capture concepts represented by a wide variety of keywords and phrases.

The CHI MeSH term displayed in Fig. 15.1 highlights two beneficial features of subject headings. First, the ability to narrow down to a specific facet of the topic by choosing the desired "subheadings" (i.e., economics, ethics, methods, etc.) under "PubMed search builder options." Second, the ability to restrict, or focus, to a "MeSH Major Topic," which leverages the aforementioned human judgment

---

Consumer Health Informatics
The field devoted in Informatics from multiple consumer or patient views.
Year introduced: 2018

PubMed search builder options
Subheadings:

☐ economics   ☐ organization and administration   ☐ statistics and numerical data
☐ ethics   ☐ standards   ☐ trends
☐ methods

☐ Restrict to MeSH Major Topic.
☐ Do not include MeSH terms found below this term in the MeSH hierarchy.

Fig. 15.1 Consumer health informatics term display from the MeSH Database, PubMed, 2021 (National Center for Biotechnology Information, U.S. National Library of Medicine 2018a)

inherent in subject headings to retrieve articles where this MeSH term is one of the top concepts in an article. Focusing can be a powerful tool in cases where you seek clear examples of CHI literature rather than literature where CHI might be a less important concept.

The CHI MeSH term example also highlights the weaknesses of a subject heading. As seen in Fig. 15.1, PubMed/MEDLINE added the CHI MeSH term to the database taxonomy in 2018, and this evolution is typical with emerging concepts. It is essential to understand that the "Year introduced" date (Fig. 15.1) means that this subject heading will not reliably yield literature before 2018, limiting the discovery of literature. A subject heading will not usually be added to the taxonomy until a critical mass of literature or a concept has emerged as essential and well-defined. Thus, long periods of time may pass before a relevant subject heading is available to researchers executing literature searches; some concepts may not ever be deemed necessary enough to create a subject heading.

See Fig. 15.2, which displays the MeSH term "Consumer Health Informatics" within a conceptual hierarchy. Taxonomies are often organized within a *conceptual hierarchy*, or a multilevel structure that arranges concepts in relation to similar concepts. As previously stated, subject headings (e.g., MeSH terms) exist within a taxonomy or conceptual hierarchy. Thus, the structure of a conceptual hierarchy provides the context for the concepts you query. Similar to the CHI MeSH term example above, the conceptual hierarchy also offers additional options for refining or focusing your query. To include the narrower concepts related to the selected subject heading in a query, databases typically provide a function called *explode*. In the example below, searching the subject heading "Medical Informatics" with the explode option would include in the query the subject headings "Health Information Exchange," "Medical Informatics Applications," and "Medical Informatics Computing," as well as any narrower terms included under those three subject

All MeSH Categories
      Information Science Category
          Information Science
            Informatics
                Cheminformatics
                Computational Biology
                Consumer Health Informatics
                Dental Informatics
                Medical Informatics
                    Health Information Exchange
                    Medical Informatics Applications +
                    Medical Informatics Computing +
              Nursing Informatics
              Public Health Informatics

Fig. 15.2 Display of "Consumer Health Informatics" MeSH term within a conceptual hierarchy (National Center for Biotechnology Information, U.S. National Library of Medicine 2005)

All MeSH Categories
    Analytical, Diagnostic and Therapeutic Techniques and Equipment Category
        Equipment and Supplies
            Electrical Equipment and Supplies
                Wearable Electronic Devices
                    Fitness Trackers
                    Hearing Aids
                    Smart Glasses

Fig. 15.3 Display of "Wearable Electronic Devices" MeSH term within a conceptual hierarchy (National Center for Biotechnology Information, U.S. National Library of Medicine 2018b)

headings (as denoted by the +). The conceptual hierarchy and the explode option allow for easy retrieval of a large concept group in ways that are not possible with a keyword query. Consult your librarian if you need assistance with focusing your query.

See Fig. 15.3, which displays the "Wearable Electronic Devices" MeSH term within a conceptual hierarchy. The PICO question we presented earlier presumes that, as a McSH term, "Wearable Technologies" are a specific type of "Consumer Health Informatics" intervention. However, within the MeSH taxonomy, a wearable device is conceptualized as "Wearable Electronic Devices" and is placed into the conceptual hierarchy under "Electrical Equipment and Supplies," as shown in Fig. 15.3. The exemplars in Fig. 15.2 and Fig. 15.3 highlight the subtle differences in organizing subject headings within conceptual hierarchies and the importance of including different subject headings, or aspects of controlled vocabulary, to precisely capture relevant literature. A strong execution strategy will utilize multiple ways to retrieve literature that consists of the concepts of your research question.

Keyword Versus Subject Heading Queries: What Is the Optimal Balance?

As stated above, there are strengths and weaknesses to subject heading queries, and there is no *best way* to execute a query. In general, an effective query will use both keywords and subject headings to diversify the methods and types of literature retrieval. The execution phase of a literature search is typically shaped by the goals laid out in the planning phase. If you are in the early stages of your research project, you should ask yourself what you are trying to accomplish. Are you looking for exemplars on a topic or trying to get a sense of what is out there? Or, are you doing a systematic review or otherwise attempting to retrieve as much literature as possible? If your goal is the former, you may not need to include many term variants or even query multiple databases because you would be okay with not retrieving *all* of the literature. If your goal is the latter, you will need to do a much more comprehensive search and query multiple databases. Sometimes, you may execute a search using a **hedge**, a combination of keywords and subject headings that others have developed to retrieve literature on a concept (see the *Case in Point* section for an example of a hedge).

Every search involves a sort of cost-benefit analysis, where the cost is the amount of work that goes into screening the retrieved literature to determine what literature is relevant. The benefit is the amount of directly relevant literature retrieved. There is no magic bullet that will result in a perfect literature retrieval. The advantage of increased confidence that you are not missing relevant literature usually comes at the cost of needing to screen more literature that may not be relevant. For example, if you conduct a systematic review, you might have to screen thousands of articles only to find a small quantity of literature pertinent to your research question. Executing a search like the latter would thus not be an effective strategy if you did not need to find vast amounts of literature on a topic. To help you determine the correct approach to executing your search, you should think realistically about the goals and deadlines of your literature search and consider a time-cost analysis based on your availability.

Information scientists often describe the breadth of a query in terms of sensitivity and specificity. A **sensitive query** yields *many* 'false positives' but should capture the majority of relevant literature. A **specific query** yields *few* 'false positives' and thus may miss literature, but the literature retrieved will be mostly relevant. Thinking about what literature is essential to retrieve will help you determine which database features to use to achieve your goals. For example, suppose you want to execute a specific query that yields mostly relevant literature that is easy to screen. You could use just a few search terms that match the author-provided words in a "title," or you could use the "major subject heading" search field. In this case, you would be okay with the chance of not retrieving *all* relevant literature, likely because you do not want to spend a lot of time screening through irrelevant literature or because you only need a few articles. If, on the other hand, you want to execute a sensitive query, you could include many term variants to increase your confidence that you are not missing important information. In this case, you are less likely to miss literature, and you would be okay spending more time screening the literature. Another important consideration is that the search query is not the only way you will retrieve relevant literature. Screening the cited references in the articles will help you discover other relevant literature, which in turn will inform revisions to your search query.

Clinical Pearl 3: The Complexity of Screening Literature Discovering literature that speaks to consumer engagement is complex since many databases look for your search terms only in the title, abstract, subject headings, or other metadata rather than in the full text. The amount of literature where consumers are clearly identified as active participants in their health and with the technology is less than you might expect and not always apparent from the language used in the title, abstract, or metadata. Screening lists of results to determine which ones are related to consumer engagement is a normal part of the search process.

Exemplar Literature Search

Now that you have a better sense of the considerations and logistics that go into a successful literature search, we will apply that knowledge to the example PICO question we introduced above by building upon it with more specific details in our new PICO question: In urban American Indian adults aged 65+ with asthma (P), are wearable devices (I) more effective than usual analog care (C) for self-management of symptoms (O)?

Identify the Research Question In urban American Indian adults aged 65+ with asthma (P), are wearable devices (I) more effective than usual analog care (C) for self-management of symptoms (O)?

Establish the Research Goal For this scenario, which assumes that you are in the early stages of research, the purpose of our research question is to better understand the scope of the literature on the topic and to discover the different ways the topic is approached in existing literature.

Determine What Database Is Best Suited for Executing Your Literature Search The clinical focus of the question makes PubMed/MEDLINE the most relevant database from which to start. The scope is the discipline of health sciences, and the audience is healthcare providers and health informaticians.

Understand How to Best Execute Your Keyword and Subject Heading Queries Know how to use PubMed/MEDLINE's advanced search features (Boolean combinations, search limits, subject headings, major MeSH terms, etc.) to yield relevant literature. Read the database's training material or consult a librarian if needed.

Now that the pre-work is completed, it is time to execute a query. The PICO format creates a good starting point, but you will need to think more specifically about operationalizing the elements and determining which concepts are your highest priority. As described in the *Executing a Literature Search* section, you should start by using Boolean logic to combine elements to reflect your search priorities.

P: "adults with asthma," "American Indians," "urban populations," "age 65+"
I: "wearable devices"
C: "usual care"
O: "self-management of symptoms"

Your first query, which looks for exactly what you want, might be:

(American Indians AND older adults AND urban populations AND asthma AND
wearable devices AND self-management)

This query will likely not retrieve many (if any) articles relevant to your topic, given the specificity of the query. In this case, you could either broaden or drop specific terms in your subsequent query, depending on the most important concepts. For example, you could broaden your concepts to include other types of technology used by the population of interest by expanding your list of technology terms:

(American Indians AND older adults AND urban populations AND asthma AND (wearable devices OR smartphone apps OR mobile health OR smart watches OR mobile phones) AND self-management)

Alternatively, you could broaden the population by excluding the terms "urban populations" and "age 65+":

(American Indians AND asthma AND (wearable devices OR smartphone apps OR mobile health OR smartwatches OR mobile phones) AND self-management)

You could also drop concepts from the search entirely or combine terms after determining if it is necessary to include each of the concepts of the combination into the query. For example, the combination of "asthma" and "wearable device" implies that the wearer is managing their own symptoms, so "self-management" likely does not need to be included in the query as seen below:

(American Indians AND asthma AND (wearable devices OR smartphone apps OR mobile health OR smart watches OR mobile phones)

Remember that articles about "self-management" will still be included in the retrieved literature with this broad literature search strategy, as you will discover them while screening the literature. Of note, a search query retrieves relevant literature as long as you utilize search terms pertinent to your research question (in essence, it is like knowing how to ask for the things you want). At this point, you will have already operationalized your elements and combined and prioritized your concepts (like "asthma," "American Indians," etc.) in a manner that should yield a reasonable amount of literature to screen. Yet, it is important to remain flexible as you may need to use additional search terms to discover different or more literature that best answers your question.

You can also broaden out concepts in whatever way that makes sense for your end goal. For example, if you are most interested in the diseases that are being managed by the technology, you could consider broadening to other chronic diseases:

(American Indians AND (asthma OR diabetes OR COPD) AND (wearable devices OR smartphone apps OR mobile health OR smart watches OR mobile phones)

Thinking about different versions of the PICO question will help you identify and articulate the most essential concepts. As you try different combinations of concepts and analyze the types of literature retrieved, you will learn more about the literature (and more about the database retrieval process), informing you how to refine future queries if needed. This iterative process of designing and executing a literature search and analyzing retrieved literature continues until you have a well-defined research question and have distilled your search strategy to yield the most relevant literature.

Case in Point

See Fig. 15.4 for our search strategy developed for a pilot study to comprehensively retrieve literature focused on "wearable devices" in PubMed/MEDLINE. We share this exemplar hedge from our own CHI research to illustrate the complexities of executing a query and retrieving relevant CHI literature. Since our goal was to retrieve any literature about "wearable devices," we developed a highly inclusive strategy. The "wearable devices" search strategy in Fig. 15.4, as designed for PubMed/MEDLINE, illustrates the complexity of vocabulary and practical implications of constructing a search on a CHI topic.

See Table 15.2 for our pilot's single-article citation with terminology from the author(s) and PubMed/MEDLINE, INSPEC, and Compendex databases. See Table 15.3 for our pilot's systematic review citation with terminology from the author(s) and PubMed/MEDLINE, CINAHL, INSPEC, and Compendex databases. As previously discussed, CHI topics are often published for audiences in many different disciplines. Thus, depending on the goal of your literature search, you may need to query literature in more than one database. Terminologies are sometimes discipline-specific, and different databases often have distinct search options and syntax. As part of our pilot study, we analyzed how various databases represented a single article (Table 15.2) and a systematic review article (Table 15.3) using

Search: ("fitness trackers"[MeSH Terms] OR ("fitness"[All Fields] AND "trackers"[All Fields]) OR "fitness trackers"[All Fields]) OR "fitness tracker"[All Fields] OR "fitness app*"[All Fields] OR "fitness devices"[All Fields] OR "digital compass"[All Fields] OR (fitness[All Fields] AND "band"[All Fields]) OR "smart watch"[All Fields] OR (smartwatch[All Fields] OR smartwatch's[All Fields] OR smartwatches[All Fields] OR smartwatches'[All Fields]) OR ("fitness trackers"[MeSH Terms] OR ("fitness"[All Fields] AND "trackers"[All Fields]) OR "fitness trackers"[All Fields] OR ("activity"[All Fields] AND "trackers"[All Fields]) OR "activity trackers"[All Fields]) OR "activity tracker"[All Fields] OR "activity monitor"[All Fields] OR "activity monitors"[All Fields] OR ("wearable electronic devices"[MeSH Terms] OR "wearable computing" OR "wearable health technologies" OR "wearable medical devices" OR "body attached sensor" OR ((wearable* or wrist or wrist-* or watch or watch-* or pendant or pendants) AND (accelerometer* OR altimeter OR barometer OR pedometer OR accelerometry OR actigraph* OR polysomnography OR "activity monitoring" OR "activity recognition" OR self track* OR track* OR remote sensing OR "wearable sensors" OR chronobiology OR nudge OR reminder OR "ambient assist*"))) OR ("apple watch"[All Fields] OR "Fit Bit"[All Fields] OR FitBit[All Fields] OR (Garmin[All Fields] AND Forerunner[All Fields]) OR (Garmin[All Fields] AND Vivoactive[All Fields]) OR "Garmin Vivofit"[All Fields] OR Garmin[All Fields] OR (Garmin[All Fields] AND Vivosmart[All Fields]) OR (Huawei[All Fields] AND "fit"[All Fields]) OR ("map"[All Fields] AND My[All Fields] AND Run[All Fields]) OR (Misfit[All Fields] AND Ray[All Fields]) OR "Misfit Shine"[All Fields] OR (Moov[All Fields] AND Now[All Fields]) OR (Nike[All Fields] AND plus[All Fields]) OR (Nokia[All Fields] AND Go[All Fields]) OR (Nokia[All Fields] AND "steel"[All Fields]) OR ("polar"[All Fields] AND (A360[All Fields] OR "RS800"[All Fields] OR watch[All Fields])) OR (Samsung[All Fields] AND Gear[All Fields]) OR (TomTom[All Fields] AND Spark[All Fields]) OR (Under[All Fields] AND Armour[All Fields] AND "band"[All Fields]) OR Vfit[All Fields] OR FuelBand[All Fields] OR MapMyRun[All Fields] OR Moov[All Fields] OR Nike+[All Fields] OR MyFitnessPal OR "Nike Training" OR Plyo OR MapMyRide)

Fig. 15.4 Search strategy developed for a pilot study aiming to comprehensively retrieve literature focused on "Wearable Devices" in PubMed/MEDLINE

Table 15.2 Pilot single-article citation with terminology from the author and PubMed/MEDLINE, INSPEC, and Compendex Databases (Chen et al. 2017). Terminology similarly used across databases is bolded

Author	PubMed/ MEDLINE	INSPEC	Compendex
Author keywords: • **Biosensor** • **Fuzzy theory** • **Heat stroke** • **Wearable devices**	*MeSH terms:* • Body temperature • Exercise • Galvanic skin response • **Heat stroke** • Humans • **Wearable electronic devices**	*Controlled/subject terms:* • **Body sensor networks** • Cardiology • **Fuzzy set theory** • Medical information systems • Medical signal processing • Patient monitoring • Risk analysis • Risk management • **Sensors** • Skin • Telemedicine *Uncontrolled terms:* • Heartbeat • Early notification ability • **Wearable heat-stroke-detection device** • Dangerous situation • Heat stroke detection • **Wearable device**[a]	*Main heading:* • **Wearable technology** • *Controlled/subject terms:* • **Biosensors** • Electrophysiology *Uncontrolled terms:* • Body temperature • Dangerous situations • Design and development • Functional components • **Fuzzy theory** • Galvanic skin response • **Heat stroke** • **Wearable devices**[a]

[a] Same terminology as author keywords

different terminologies. The results illustrate the diversity of vocabulary and audiences that informatics researchers must consider when designing their research approach.

The depth of terms in a particular domain is usually associated with the type of database and its intended audience. Health databases provide many terms related to health topics and few terms related to technology, while engineering databases primarily provide technology terms. In both citations illustrated in the tables, the engineering databases assign fewer controlled terms and more system-generated uncontrolled terms to enhance retrieval. Using Table 15.3 as an example, the author keywords represent a mix of spelling variations for the technology (smartwatch and smart watch), high-level terms to represent the type of consumer or patient engagement (health intervention), and terms to describe the paper at a high level (systematic review and translational research). The author keywords in the first column also appear in the Compendex uncontrolled terms. Comparing the wearable technology terms across databases, the engineering databases INSPEC and Compendex have similarities and differences. Both databases have the term "watches," but INSPEC also uses "intelligent sensors," and Compendex also uses "wearable computers" to represent related concepts. The health database PubMed/MEDLINE uses "wearable electronic devices" and "wearable sensors." These nuances support our recommendation that to search optimally across distinct domain databases requires some customization of the search term choices.

Table 15.3 Pilot systematic review citation with terminology from the author and PubMed/MEDLINE, CINAHL, INSPEC, and Compendex Databases (Reeder and David 2016). Terminology specific to "Wearable Technologies" is bolded

Author	PubMed/MEDLINE	CINAHL	INSPEC	Compendex
Author keywords: • Health intervention • **Smart watch** • **Smartwatch** • Systematic review • Translational research	*MeSH terms:* • Clinical trials as topic • Communication • Diabetes mellitus/therapy • Health status • Humans • Parkinson disease/therapy • Self care* • Surveys and questionnaires • **Wearable electronic devices**[a] *Publication types:* • Review • Systematic review	*Major subjects:* • **Wearable sensors** • Monitoring, physiologic – methods • Health behavior – evaluation • Wellness *Minor subjects:* • Human • Pubmed • Embase • Systematic review • Heart rate – evaluation • Diabetes mellitus • Speech therapy – evaluation • Physical activity – evaluation • Surveys • Patient compliance *Publication types:* • Article • Research • Systematic review	*Controlled/subject terms:* • Cardiology • Diseases • Health care • **Intelligent sensors** • Medical disorder • Patient monitoring • **Watches** *Uncontrolled terms:* • **Smart watch** • Self-monitoring • Personal activity • Bidirectional communication • Health care providers • PubMed libraries • Embase libraries • IEEE XPlore libraries • ACM digital libraries • Demographics • Device features • Watch applications • Activity monitoring • Heart rate monitoring • Speech therapy adherence • Diabetes self-management • Seizure detection • Tremors • Scratching • Eating • Medication-taking behaviors • Parkinson's disease • Epilepsy	*Main heading:* • **Wearable computers** *Controlled/subject terms:* • Digital libraries • Intensive care units • Patient monitoring • Patient treatment • **Watches** *Uncontrolled terms:* • Bi-directional communication • Diabetes self-management • Health care providers • Health interventions[a] • Heart-rate monitoring • Smartwatch[a] • Systematic review[a] • Translational research[a]

[a]Same terminology as author keywords

*MeSH Major Topic

Conclusion

The field of CHI is rapidly evolving as new types of digital health technologies are developed and the push toward patient engagement and empowerment increases. Improving the ability of researchers to discover relevant CHI literature to enhance the science is essential. With the ever-evolving incorporation of new digital health technologies into engineering and health databases, researchers must plan their literature search design and execution phases. As discussed in this chapter, there are many considerations when conducting a CHI-related literature search. With the ever-changing field of CHI, we recommend that new and established researchers work with librarians when formulating research questions and when executing database queries. This collaboration is critical when working on systematic reviews and meta-analyses covering specific CHI topics to ensure that you have retrieved all relevant literature.

Acknowledgments We recognize Dr. Robin Austin for her contributions to the conceptualization of this project, Jennifer Wells for her work on developing the wearables terms search hedge used in the wearables pilot study, and Dr. Rachel Wong for her confirmation of author keywords in the pilot study.

Question
Describe how consumer health informatics, and specifically patient participation, could be utilized as an element of your searchable PICO(T) question.

Answer
- P – the (patient/population) is the consumer or the (problem) is the health-related issue
- I/C – the intervention or comparison engages the patient or intentionally does not engage the patient
- O – the outcome has to be health-related and important to the patient
- T – the timeframe has to be feasible for the patient

Question
Describe the difference between a keyword query and a subject heading query.

Answer
In a keyword query, the database looks for an exact match for the word or phrase as used by the author(s); in a subject heading query, the database uses controlled vocabulary, based on concepts, to retrieve literature.

Question
Give one or more reasons that a search in CINAHL for wearable electronic devices would retrieve a different number of consumer-oriented articles than discoverable via PubMed/MEDLINE.

Answer
CINAHL focuses on nursing and allied health literature and therefore has a narrower disciplinary scope than PubMed/MEDLINE; The search term in CINAHL is "wearable sensors" whereas the Medical Subject Heading in PubMed/MEDLINE is "wearable electronic devices"; PubMed also covers many more journals than CINAHL.

Glossary

Adjacency searching A type of query that searches for two words located within a specified number of words from each other

Article record Essential details of the article (e.g., title, abstract, authors, etc.); often included in the article metadata

Boolean logic Used to combine concepts to be placed into the database search query; utilizes Boolean operators (AND, OR, NOT)

Boolean operators Commands used to combine elements of a research question: AND (narrows down), OR (broadens out), NOT (excludes)

Conceptual hierarchy A multilevel structure that arranges concepts in relation to similar concepts

Controlled vocabulary A list of subject headings that represents concepts in a standardized way

Design phase of a literature search The phase of a literature search that involves formulating a research question and operationalizing the question's elements

Electronic databases Information discovery sources

Execution phase of a literature search The phase of a literature search that involves putting search terms (keywords, phrases, and subject headings) representing the elements of a research question into a database query

Explode A database function that includes the narrower concepts related to the selected subject heading in a query

Hedge A combination of keywords and subject headings developed to retrieve literature on a concept

Information scientists Library scientists, informationists, or librarians

Keyword query A database query that looks for an exact match for the word or phrase as used by the author(s)

Metadata Data that describes other data; the data (usually subject headings) attached to an article in a database

Phrase searching A type of keyword query that searches for two or more search terms exactly as entered into the query

PICO(T) element A component of a PICO(T)-formatted question: P (problem or patient/population); I (intervention); C (comparison); O (outcome); and T (time frame)

PICO(T) format A framework used to develop evidence-based, searchable research questions that is often used by clinicians and informatics researchers

Search limits Filters (e.g., language, range of dates) used in a database query

Search terms Keywords, phrases, and subject headings that represent elements of a research question and are utilized in a database query

Sensitive query A database query that yields *many* 'false positives' but should capture the majority of relevant literature

Specific query A database query that yields *few* 'false positives' and thus may miss literature, but the literature retrieved will be mostly relevant

Subject heading A standardized term for a concept

Subject heading query A database query that uses controlled vocabulary (i.e., subject headings), instead of only relying on exact words as used by the author(s)

Taxonomy A hierarchical classification system

Term variant A slight variation of search terms used in a database query representing the same concept

Truncation A stem, or portion, of a search term that is often represented with an asterisk

Wildcard character A character that represents the absence or presence of a portion of a search term

References

American Medical Informatics Association. Consumer Health Information. n.d.. https://www.amia.org/applications-informatics/consumer-health-informatics Accessed online 7 April 2021.

Aromataris E, Munn Z (Editors). *JBI manual for evidence synthesis*. JBI, 2020. https://synthesis-manual.jbi.global. https://doi.org/10.46658/JBIMES-20-01.

Chen ST, Lin SS, Lan CW, Hsu HY. Design and development of a wearable device for heat stroke detection. Sensors (Basel). 2017;18(1):17. https://doi.org/10.3390/s18010017.

Garrard J. Health sciences literature review made easy: the matrix method. Burlington, MA: Jones and Bartlett Learning; 2017.

Higgins JPT, Thomas J, Chandler J, Cumpston M, Li T, Page MJ, Welch VA (editors). *Cochrane handbook for systematic reviews of interventions version 6.2* (updated February 2021). Cochrane, 2021. www.training.cochrane.org/handbook.

National Center for Biotechnology Information, U.S. National Library of Medicine. Informatics [MeSH browser entry]. Bethesda, MD: National Library of Medicine; 2005. [updated 2021]. https://www.ncbi.nlm.nih.gov/mesh/68048088 Accessed online 30 April 2021

National Center for Biotechnology Information, U.S. National Library of Medicine. Consumer health informatics [MeSH browser entry]. Bethesda, MD: National Library of Medicine; 2018a. [updated 2021]. https://www.ncbi.nlm.nih.gov/mesh/2023337 Accessed online 30 April 2021

National Center for Biotechnology Information, U.S. National Library of Medicine. Wearable electronic devices [MeSH Browser entry]. Bethesda, MD: National Library of Medicine; 2018b. [updated 2021]. https://www.ncbi.nlm.nih.gov/mesh/2023539 Accessed online 30 April 2021

National Institutes of Health: U.S. National Library of Medicine. Incorporating values for indexing method in MEDLINE/PubMed XML. NLM Tech Bull [Internet]. 2018;423:e2. https://www.nlm.nih.gov/pubs/techbull/ja18/ja18_indexing_method.html Accessed online 30 April 2021

National Institutes of Health: U.S. National Library of Medicine. Indexing initiative: NLM medical text indexer (MTI) [internet]. Bethesda, MD: U.S. National Library of Medicine; 2019. [updated 30 May 2019]. https://ii.nlm.nih.gov/MTI/ Accessed online 30 April 2021

National Library of Medicine. Medical subject headings: Main headings, subheadings, and cross references used in the index medicus and the national library of medicine catalog [internet]. Bethesda, MD: National Library of Medicine; 1960. [updated 2018]. https://www.nlm.nih.gov/hmd/collections/digital/MeSH/mesh.html Accessed online 30 April 2021

National Library of Medicine: National Center for Biotechnology Information. PubMed.gov [Online database]. Bethesda, MD: National Library of Medicine; 2021. [updated 2021]. https://pubmed.ncbi.nlm.nih.gov/ Accessed online 30 April 2021

Reeder B, David A. Health at hand: a systematic review of smart watch uses for health and wellness. J Biomed Inform. 2016;63:269–76. https://doi.org/10.1016/j.jbi.2016.09.001.

Riva JJ, Malik KM, Burnie SJ, Endicott AR, Busse JW. What is your research question? An introduction to the PICOT format for clinicians. J Can Chiropr Assoc. 2012;56(3):167–71.

United States General Accounting Office. Testimony before the subcommittee on human resources and intergovernmental relations committee on government reform and oversight, house of representatives. Consumer health informatics: emerging issues. Washington, D.C.: United States General Accounting Office; 1996. 26 July . Page 1. https://www.gao.gov/products/t--aimd-96-134 Accessed online 30 April 2021

Chapter 16
Ecosystem of Patient-Centered Research and Information System Design

Pei-Yun Sabrina Hsueh

Abstract With healthcare costs rising year by year, one of the well-known issues modern health systems contends is the need to move from reactive to preventive care. However, prior public health studies show that clinical factors contribute to only 30-40% of a person's health determinants. Meanwhile, patient-centered factors dominate the rest. These include genetic and environmental, social, and behavioral factors. Therefore, understanding these patient-centered factors is the key, and the most significant healthcare opportunity thus lies in better integrating patient understanding into the workflow for patient-centered care. The introduction of AI/ML technologies has brought a promise for enhancing precision patient understanding. Still, they have also incurred new problems such as inherent data-driven bias that must be combated to ensure AI fairness and health equity.

Recently, more investments have been placed on the technology-enabled democratization of patient-centered care, starting from collecting patient-generated health data (PGHD) and powered through the generation of real-world evidence (RWE). Meanwhile, multiple catalysts, including a series of health reform regulations, have been fueling this field. Herein emerges an ecosystem around the idea of reinventing health systems with a deeper level of patient understanding. This ecosystem comprises many traditional healthcare players, such as health systems, payers, and national organizations. It also includes many untraditional players, such as researchers leading patient engagement and patient-centered research studies and health consumers who serve versatile roles such as patient advocates and citizen scientists. Moreover, tech and retail giants, pharmaceutical companies, and healthcare startups are also exploring multiple pathways to impact.

To realize the potential of this multi-stakeholder ecosystem, we first review the barriers each of them is facing in this chapter. Then, as each stakeholder is responsible for one part of the integrated patient-centered care practice, we examine the case studies and lessons learned from each perspective regarding the inclusion of

P.-Y. S. Hsueh (✉)
Bayesian Health Inc., New York, NY, USA
e-mail: pyhsueh@berkeley.edu

© The Author(s), under exclusive license to Springer Nature
Switzerland AG 2022
P.-Y. S. Hsueh et al. (eds.), *Personal Health Informatics*, Cognitive Informatics
in Biomedicine and Healthcare, https://doi.org/10.1007/978-3-031-07696-1_16

patients in the research and information system design process. Critical use cases describe the best practice for incorporating PGHD-based RWE into healthcare delivery and clinical pharmacology. Based on the lessons learned from the case studies, this chapter summarizes challenges and future opportunities wherein health AI could help identify actionable insights to improve outcomes through patient-centered research and information system design. Finally, it is worth noting that this chapter reports on the learnings from a series of workshops organized between 2015 and 2020. This series of workshops gathered leading researchers, citizen scientists, and patient/caregiver advocates across multiple professional societies, including the American Medical Informatics Association (AMIA), the International Medical Informatics Association (IMIA), and the Association of Computing Machinery (ACM).

Keywords Citizen science · Patient-generated health data · Patient-reported outcome · Patient-centered care · Health AI · Proactive care · Precision healthcare Healthcare ecosystem

Learning Objectives for the Chapter
- Understand the evolution of the emerging health ecosystem to support patient-centered care system design and patient-led research
- Identify the critical barriers across technical, organizational, and collaboration issues to patient-centered research and patient-centered system design
- Characterize the lifecycle of the process across the patient-centered design from planning to design to deployment to evaluation
- Discuss the advantages and disadvantages of the vital design methodology frameworks
- Help formulate strategies for user engagement, innovation, dataflow, visualization, and workflow modeling for patient-assistive tooling

Overview

With the healthcare costs rising annually and the baby boomer generation entering their retirement age, the health spending as a percentage of GDP in the US has increased from 5.5% in 1960 to almost 18% in 2019 (NHE Fact Sheet | CMS n.d.). Over the years, healthcare systems have deployed a variety of strategies to control costs and improve outcomes. However, these efforts did not stop the increase in health spending; instead, the spending is projected to reach $6 trillion by 2027 at a rate of 5.5 percent of increase annually in the next decade. In addition, according to data from the Organization for Economic Co-operation and Development (OECD) and the report from Kaiser Family Foundation, the US lags behind other developed countries in many major health quality indicators, such as the rates of all-cause mortality, premature death, death amenable to healthcare, and disease burden (Sisko et al. 2019). Almost 75 percent of US healthcare spending (83% for Medicaid and 96% for Medicare) is tied to treatments for patients with chronic conditions (Galea and Maani 2020). In comparison, preventative services constitute only three percent.

These statistics point to a systematic flaw in the former strategies and the need for new levers to control costs and improve outcomes. Such new levers include moving toward value-based care from fee-for-service financially and providing support for incorporating patient-specific clinical decisions at both the system and technology levels. All the new levers require a better understanding of patient-centered health determinants.

Therefore, it is essential to enable a deeper patient understanding of our health systems and leverage such knowledge in the workflow for patient-centered care. Prior public health studies show that clinical factors contribute to only 30–40% of a person's health determinants. At the same time, patient-centered factors dominate the rest. These factors range from genetic to environmental, social, and behavioral factors (Raghupathi and Raghupathi 2018; Hsueh et al. 2018). Thus, even if two patients come into the hospital with the same clinical conditions, the interventions that would work for them could be quite different, depending on their behavioral patterns and the likelihood of engaging in preventive care measures. Our work in care management has shown that it is possible to leverage the estimation of individual differences in the probability of being engaged for health goal attainment (McGinnis et al. 2017). Thus, adequate adaptive clinical decision support (CDS) would need to include a patient-centered care ecosystem that together could help offer a precision understanding of patient-centered factors (Tuomilehto et al. 2009).

In many other industries, Artificial Intelligence and Machine Learning (AI/ML) technologies have played an essential role in the ecosystem to power various recommendation systems with a precision understanding of person-centric factors. Recent innovations in AI/ML have also started showing promise in imaging and signal detection tasks in the healthcare industry (Petersen et al. 2021). For example, they can now detect congestive heart failure (CHF) with almost perfect accuracy. As a result, there has been a rising expectation that proactive, informed, patient-centered care, i.e., the future of clinical care, can be enabled with the AI/ML innovations. However, new challenges have also emerged when applying AI/ML technologies in the healthcare industry (Matheny et al. 2019; Bates et al. 2021; Bica et al. 2020). This chapter talks about this from two perspectives: clinical care and clinical pharmacology.

First, in clinical care, commercial AI/ML algorithms implemented in practice have been found to introduce bias from their predictions, which favor groups that often access hospital services rather than those who need them most (Wong et al. 2021; Singh et al. 2020a). The inherent bias comes from the fact that the algorithms are trained based on "ground truth" as defined by labels assigned by doctors. By matching the ground-truth labels produced in healthcare practice, algorithms inherit the implicit human bias, contributing to disparate health outcomes in marginalized populations (Bates et al. 2020; Obermeyer and Topol 2021; Chen et al. 2019).

Take pain assessment in knee osteoarthritis patients for example. Previous research has found a low correlation between self-reported pain assessment and radiographic severity (Ibrahim 2021). Yet, in current practice, the Kellgren–Lawrence grade (KLG), a commonly used grading system developed from data of coal miners in the UK in the 1950s, is used to determine the radiographic severity of knee osteoarthritis. As a result, it has led to the "pain gap" between black and white patients. Take breast cancer as another example. Pierson et al. (2021) shows that black women are more likely to develop aggressive triple-negative tumors and are often diagnosed later in life at more advanced stages of the disease. Moreover, implicit data-driven bias could propagate even more broadly when applying models trained from health data blindly. Second, in clinical pharmacology, the most critical issue is to provide external validity to randomized controlled trials (RCTs) by applying Real-World Evidence (RWE) generated from electronic health records (Rothwell et al. 2016; Frieden 2017). Unfortunately, RCTs are often conducted with strict inclusion criteria in a traditional setting, making its findings hard to generalizable beyond the study population. This limitation, in turn, made individual treatment tricky, as each patient's subpopulation can be under-represented in the study population.

Hence, this chapter describes the caveats in forming a healthy ecosystem to overcome these limitations as observed from the two perspectives. The gist of the ecosystem approach is to prevent problems of introducing implicit data-driven bias into clinical care and clinical pharmacology. We need to engage health ecosystem stakeholders in an industry standard-setting movement with the goal of an eventual AI governance mechanism. These industry standards would be necessary to monitor post-ai implementation efficiency and diagnostic accuracy, detect underlying data and concept bias and drifts in the widely deployed AI/ML models and maintain health equity and fairness (Finlayson et al. 2021; Joaquin Quiñonero-candela et al. 2009; Park et al. 2021). Moreover, to improve the external validity of RCTs and determine individual treatments, multiple national-level government authorities have encouraged the inclusion of broader inclusion criteria. Meanwhile, academia and the industry are partnering to develop theoretical underpinning and the applications of models (Bica et al. 2021) and the collection of real-world data (RWD) for supporting the generation of RWE (Reading et al. 2018; Fröhlich et al. 2018).

This chapter reports on the findings from a series of workshops organized between 2015 and 2020. This series of workshops are organized with leading researchers, citizen scientists, and patient/caregiver advocates across the American Medical Informatics Association (AMIA), the International Medical Informatics Association (IMIA), and the Association of Computing Machinery (ACM). We look back at the trend of the last decade to identify the driving forces behind citizen science, electronic patient-reported outcome (ePRO), patient-generated health data (PGHD), and the evolution of the personal health informatics infrastructure tooling as the basis of patient-centered care.

From Precision Medicine to Precision Care

In precision medicine, the key idea for improving patient understanding is to search for person-specific genetic variants and other biomarkers in patients' molecular profiles. Physicians can then use the identified patient-specific factors to determine which treatment plan is more effective for a given patient. For example, in the Biomarker-integrated Approaches of Targeted Therapy for Lung Cancer Elimination (BATTLE) clinical trial (Rashdan and Gerber 2016) for non-small lung cancer patients, researchers found the optimal chemotherapeutic agent seen by a specimen of the patient's tumor biopsy. In recent years, more large-scale clinical trials have evolved to incorporate the precision medicine principle. Examples include NCI-MATCH Trial (Colwell J. 2016) and ASCO TAPUR trial (ASCO 2016; Schuetze et al. 2021).

In real-world applications, such methods do not need to be limited to searching for biomarkers. Modern health systems can also use these methods to understand other patient-specific social, environmental, and behavioral factors. Furthermore, academia and the industry partners are working together to identify targeted treatments given the incremental patient understanding during the trials. Finally, health systems have also started to work with researchers to develop precision health applications to assist with care planning.

Besides the methodological breakthroughs in improving patient understanding, new financial levers also emerged in the past decade. One well-known lever is value-based care, designed to help move the needle from reactive to preventive care. Many countries have implemented payment structure reforms to turn traditional reimbursement models from fee-for-service to value-based care (Long 2017). Health economics studies estimated that the reform could help save a quarter of US health spending (West et al. 1997). Multiple catalysts have been fueling this field on the path to realizing its potential. For example, the Department of Health and Human Services (HHS) announced that it intended to link half of all traditional Medicare payments to a value-based reimbursement model. In practice, several health regulations enabled bundle payments under the Affordable Care Act (West et al. 1997; Health Information Technology for Economic and Clinical Health (HITECH) Act 2009; The 21st Century Cures Act 2016; The Interoperability and Patient Access final rule (CMS-9115-F) 2020). Under this bundled payment structure, healthcare providers assume accountability for the quality and cost of care delivered during a predetermined episode of care from initiation to 90 days of post-acute care. In recent years, Medicare and Medicaid expenditures switched from fee-for-service to value-based reimbursement contracts and bundled payment initiatives. In contrast, the percentage of commercial payments shrunk from 42% to 35% (Black et al. 2018).

Another financial lever currently under experimentation is the alternative payment (APM) model, a subcategory of value-based purchasing initiatives. This lever would help shift financial incentives further from volume by linking provider payments to quality and total cost of care results (Bundled Payments for Care Improvement (BPCI) Initiative: General Information | CMS Innovation Center n.d.). The Medicare Access and CHIP Reauthorization Act (MACRA) framework support the 2015 HHS announcement that focuses on APMs for quality care improvements (Brown and Crapo 2014).

While it is the beginning of providers investigating the switch to value-based care, the transition is not easy for many organizations. Only when we can improve patient understanding and leverage the financial lever at the same time will we be able to control healthcare spending due to preventable health conditions. In addition, the switch would require many players in the ecosystem to participate in observing impacts. For instance, the successful implementation of value-based reimbursement models requires extensive data analytics capabilities, population health management programs, and the ability to use the Electronic Health Record (EHR) systems for documentation and reporting.

The Emerging Ecosystem

First, we review the role and the barriers each of the ecosystem stakeholders are facing. Then, as each stakeholder is responsible for one part of the integrated patient-centered care practice, we examine the lessons learned from each perspective regarding the inclusion of patients in the research and information system design process. We then identify critical use cases that illustrate the best practice for incorporating PGHD-based Evidence into healthcare delivery. Finally, we summarize the common challenges with an additional focus on future opportunities wherein health AI could help identify actionable insights to improve outcomes through patient-centered research and information system design.

Patients and Caregivers

In recent years, one significant trend has been the involvement of patients and caregivers in advancing science and health information system design. On the one hand, many patients and caregivers are willing to share but do not technically have their data under control. On the other hand, health organizations are hesitant to communicate the data back to patients due to the risk of a data breach, negotiating costs, and technical compatibility and security difficulties. Neither are academic researchers incentivized to share, while the funding scheme does not directly support sharing. As the middle ground, in recent years, we have observed the emergence of the data industry (including both startups and technology giants), which aims to serve as the bridge to connect patients and health organizations. The data industry is still pivoting on its business model and evolving its role in the process of data democratization due to the complexity of the regulatory space.

Currently, as no single force has complete control over this middle layer, the most common ways to communicate PGHD back to the health organizations include

(1) having the patient outcomes documented with health system-initiated ePRO tools and (2) having patients wear passive sensors to record patient behaviors. Given the lack of integration into clinical care flow, the benefits of involving patients and caregivers directly in an informed clinical care flow so far are still a promise to be realized. While the field is still evolving, some best practices have emerged to demonstrate the benefits of the primary and secondary use of PGHD in their sub-fields in consumer health informatics (Hsueh et al. 2017a; Lai et al. 2017). These subfields include but are not limited to augmenting shared care plans for care coordination for patients with multiple conditions, informing chronic and cancer care, evaluating personal informatics tools in adaptive trials, and integrating patient-centered understanding of omics-data for clinical research. In (Hsueh et al. 2017), we have summarized the best practices in these subfields and put the secondary use of PGHD and its overarching themes such as privacy, interpretability, interoperability, utility, and ethics. In addition, the recent advancement of telehealth during the Covid-19 pandemic has significantly pushed all related technologies.

Citizen Scientists

Beyond the scope of patient-generated health data, there are also groups of citizen scientists contributing to the generation of scientific questions by sharing their data. Citizens can generate answers to population health questions of interest to both patients and the healthcare system and offers an opportunity to empower marginalized groups, such as sexual and gender minorities, to shape scientific inquiry through participation. The above-mentioned technological advances, changing reimbursement models, and innovative informed consent approaches are all driving a shift in power dynamics within healthcare, affording greater integration of citizen scientists' work into research and clinical care (Petersen et al. 2020).

Pro Research Network and Community-Based Participation

To further break the walls between patients and health organizations, the National Institute of Health (NIH) has developed the 10-year PROMIS (Patient-Reported Outcomes Measurement Information System) roadmap (AHRQ n.d.) to propose next-generation patient-reported outcome measures (PROMs) in more than 70 domains, such as pain, fatigue, physical functioning, emotional distress, and social role participation that significantly impact patients' quality of life across a variety of chronic diseases. In addition, there also exist validated self-administrative proxy PROs, including PROMIS, NeuroQoL, ASCQ-Me, and NIH Toolkit.

During the Covid-19 pandemic, Covid19-related PROs are also captured from the community, leveraging the structure of community-based participatory research (CBPR) (Israel et al. 1998). Using the CBPR model, community members, organizational representatives, and academic researchers work together in all aspects of the research process with shared responsibility and ownership. This model integrates knowledge gained through both interventions and policy change.

While using the ePRO tooling or sensors through the facilitation of CBPR is promising, this approach often requires a high integration with EHR and is not easy to achieve. The growing use of electronic patient-reported outcomes (ePROs) (Austin et al. 2020) in clinical care requires change across the health system. Health system stakeholders considering initiating or expanding ePROs for care delivery must invest in the integration, education, and behavioral change initiatives, following the best practice guidelines or toolkits from prior work (Austin et al. 2021).

The Partnership Between Private and Public Organizations

Driven by prior success in using RWD for comparative effectiveness studies, multiple stakeholders have started to integrate ePRO tools with EHR, aiming to demonstrate the value of PGHD-based RWE. The "linked" data collection would serve as a powerful tool to fuel clinical care and research, quality improvement, population health, and public health. Therefore, many private and public organizations have geared up to provide funding support. This ecosystem includes not only pharmaceutical companies but also government agencies such as the NIH, Agency for Healthcare Research and Quality (AHRQ), Patient-Centered Outcomes Research Institute (PCORI), Centers for Medicare and Medicaid Services (CMS), and the Office of the National Coordinator for Health Information Technology (ONC).

Health Systems

Among all the stakeholders, health systems are the ones that hold multiple incentives to participate in the creation of such a patient-centered care ecosystem. To name a few, the switch from fee-for-service to value-based care is one, and the expansion to include the home health care model is another.

As mentioned in the introduction of this chapter, governments worldwide have been providing incentives for the switch to a value-based care model. Since home health services have been proven to be highly cost-effective while achieving the same patient outcomes, many government payment structures would include the coverage of home health services. For example, in the U.S., Medicare reimbursements provide value-based care for improved patient outcomes. In addition, health systems have been looking into expansion into home health services to lower the total cost of care.

In addition, the increased prevalence of lifestyle diseases and other target diseases requiring long-term care, such as Alzheimer's disease and dementia, has also been fueling the health systems' expansion to home health services. Meanwhile, the improved awareness of the importance of in-home care and the technological advance in self-care devices, such as heart rate monitors, oxygen therapy devices, and blood glucose monitors, have also improved the efficiency and effectiveness of home care.

Besides financial incentives, health systems also have technological incentives to work in their favor: the Fast Healthcare Interoperability Resource (FHIR) framework (- FHIR v4.0.1 n.d.) has matured enough lately to help providers implement APIs that create, read, update, and delete (CRUD) FHIR resource data for authorized applications. Health systems can leverage the API framework to implement clinical decision tools based upon an individual patient's status as indicated by their EHR data. In population health management, the use of FHIR Bulk Data Access (Flat FHIR) APIs can also help streamline the process and simplify the interfaces.

By leveraging the technological advance in API, health systems are also better positioned today to improve clinical decision-making. For example, the APIs enable precision patient understanding by integrating consumer devices to collect PGHD, defined as health-related data created, recorded, or gathered by or from patients (or family members or other caregivers) to help address a health concern. Similarly, health systems are also better positioned to incorporate a wide range of ePRO and PGHD data sources through patient API in other use cases, such as shared decision making, patient safety, and clinical trials.

Payers

Payers, who set health service rates and process claims, play a significant role in the ecosystem to facilitate the increase of a deeper level of patient understanding in support of the new financial levers. Major payers such as health plan providers, Medicare, and Medicaid, have high incentives to use patient understanding to design care programs that can help improve the outcomes of vulnerable higher-risk populations. Some AI applications applied have been preventing claim fraud, reducing provider burden, and enhancing care program integrity. With more data streams related to patient-reported outcomes integrated into the ecosystems, we now have an opportunity to measure healthcare quality and reflect patient outcomes more accurately. CMS has further pushed for a common set of measurement tools to help curate patient information such as health-related quality of life, symptoms and symptom burdens (e.g., pain, fatigue), health behaviors (e.g., smoking, diet, exercise) (CMS 2021). By integrating PROM data with the claims data that reflect the results of evaluation by health care professionals from the patient encounter, the ecosystems now have a chance to assess the commonalities and discrepancies between the different values and limitations.

Regulation Authorities

The Food and Drug Administration (FDA) has also recently deepened its engagement in this area. Specifically, the goal of the FDA is to guard the safety and effectiveness of drugs, biologics, and medical devices. Meanwhile, the FDA also provides guiding principles for regulating Software as a Medical Devices (SaMD), based on its intent to treat, diagnose, cure, mitigate, or prevent disease or other conditions. As of 2021, the FDA has approved more than 60 SaMD applications (Benjamens et al. 2020). Examples include AI/ML algorithms in computer-aided detection software that analyze Magnetic Resonance Imaging images or signals from smartphones to detect and diagnose a stroke or breast cancer (Muehlematter et al. 2021a).

The Agency has published a series of updates on the guiding principles and called for comments and proposals in this area (Artificial Intelligence and Machine Learning in Software as a Medical Device | FDA n.d.; Good Machine Learning Practice for Medical Device Development: Guiding Principles | FDA n.d.; FDA 2019). The AI/ML-Based SaMD Action Plan (Artificial Intelligence and Machine Learning in Software as a Medical Device | FDA n.d.) was released in 2018, followed up by the Good Machine Learning Practice for Medical Device Development: Guiding Principles (Good Machine Learning Practice for Medical Device Development: Guiding Principles | FDA n.d.) in 2021. These guiding principles outline how to update the predetermined change control plan and encourage standard harmonization to improve the interchangeability and transparency to end-users. In addition, the Agency has also developed Sentinel (Jillson 2021), a clinical data partner network and platform supporting the validation study of patient safety across partner sites based on common data model (CDS) standards that would allow for the test of the same hypothesis across sites.

Finally, another government authority that would become active in this ecosystem is the Federal Trade Commission (FTC). The goal of the FTC is to protect consumers and promote fair market competition. Given the potential problem that the implicit AI bias would produce adverse outcomes for health consumers, the guidance emphasizes using transparent, fair, robust, and explainable tools to the end consumers (HL7 Standards Product Brief - HL7 Version 3 Product Suite | HL7 International n.d.). The FTC has been monitoring the market movements and getting ready to take action against those organizations whose algorithms may be biased or inaccurate.

Standardization Ecosystems over Health Data Exchange

Given recent technological advances, government agencies and international not-for-profit standard-developing organizations have put forward quite a few standardization efforts. For example, Health Level Seven International (HL7), founded by the Joint Initiative Council for Global Health Informatics Standardization and members in more than 50 countries in 1987, supports the activities of health data standardization. Each country-based member organization is an ecosystem on its own, consisting of a mixture of industry, government agencies, academic institutions, and practitioners of interoperability. Together, they serve as multi-stakeholder platforms to provide standards that empower global health data interoperability. In 1989, HL7 released the HL7 v2 standard (HL7 Standards Product Brief - HL7 Version 3 Product Suite | HL7 International n.d.), reaching 95 adoption rates by providers. In 2005, HL7 further released HL7 v3 standards to enact the Consolidated Clinical Document Architecture (CCDA) (HL7 Standards Product Brief - HL7 Version 2 Product Suite | HL7 International n.d.). Under the ecosystem-supported efforts, any providers that adopt HL7 standards can securely access and use health data across multiple data sources, such as electronic health records (EHR) systems, lab information systems (LIS), imaging services, and billing systems.

Since 2011, HL7 pushed forward the FHIR framework (Index - FHIR v4.0.1 n.d.) as an alternative to the original HL7 v2 and v3 standards to improve interoperability and data exchange. The transition to the FHIR framework would enable data manipulation with web technologies, e.g., Representational State Transfer (RESTful) web service, making it easier for health systems and clinicians to share health data. In addition, the Substitutable Medical Apps, Reusable Technologies (SMART) Health IT project created the SMART on FHIR API, including not only FHIR but also OAuth2 and OpenID Connect, to enable developers to write an app once and run it anywhere in the healthcare system.

On Apr 21, 2020, HHS filed the CMS and the ONC Interoperability final rules under the 21 Century Cure Act (Federal Register 2020; 21st Century Cures Act 2016; Information Blocking and the ONC Health IT Certification Program 2020). In particular, the 2020 ONC Cures Act Final Rule requires using FHIR Release 4 as part of its new certification criterion in 45 CFR 170.315(g) (10), Standardized API for Patient and Population Services. During the Covid19 pandemic, HHS updated the deadlines for full compliance. Health IT vendors must provide customers with upgraded API technology certified under this new certification criterion no later than Dec 31, 2022 (21st Century Cures Act 2016; Information Blocking and the ONC Health IT Certification Program 2020).

While adopting the new standards is catching up, many providers are still using the legacy systems with the earlier standards to consume data. Yet not all the standards are backward compatible. Therefore, healthcare providers must translate between different standards in the foreseeable future, including HL7 v2, HL7 v3, CCDA, and FHIR. From the ecosystem point of view, it is beneficial to have more and more EHR systems supporting the creation of FHIR profiles, value sets, and other conformance resources. In addition, SMART on FHIR has also accelerated the development of a robust ecosystem of EHR-agnostic apps. Together, these trends have significantly lowered innovation barriers by applying third-party applications to process and analyze data.

Standardization Ecosystems over Health Knowledge

In the past few decades, many public and private organizations are also pushing for the enablement of secondary use of health data through standardizing biomedical terminologies and ontologies. These standards include but are not limited to the Systematized Nomenclature of Medicine Clinical Terms (SNOMED CT) (SNOMED n.d.), the Logical Observation Identifiers, Names, and Codes (LOINC®) (LOINC n.d.), RxNorm in the US (Nelson et al. 2011), the NHS Dictionary of medicines and devices (dm + d) in the UK (NHS Business Service Authority 2018), and the Australian Medicines Terminology (AMT) in Australia (Australian Digital Health Agency 2018).

The government plays a significant role in this standardization movement in the ecosystem. First, as the standardization efforts are multi-year, it is better off to be led by specialized institutions with the mission of acquiring, organizing, preserving, and providing access to curated knowledge. Take the US as an example. National Library of Medicine (NLM) is carrying out a mission to enable biomedical research, support health care and public health, and promote healthy behavior. In addition, the US government has further established programs such as the Meaningful Use incentive program to ensure compliance by the providers. These programs have created the growth of many EHR systems, and the adoption of these standard terminologies and ontologies by these EHR systems has formed the basis of broader adoption in the clinical community.

In recent years, large-scale research networks are also playing an increasingly vital role to help in the development of a common data model (CDM). Such networks include: the National Patient-Centered Clinical Research Network's PCORnet (Collins et al. 2014), the Observational Health Data Sciences and Informatics (OHDSI) research group (Hripcsak et al. 2015), and the FDA's Mini-Sentinel (Platt et al. 2018). For example, OHDSI has developed the Observational Medical Outcomes Partnership (OMOP) common data model in clinical data warehouses internationally. The recent development has all pointed toward positive signs of progress (Petersen et al. 2021; Bodenreider et al. 2018; Frazier et al. 2001).

Discussion

Overall, with the patient-oriented ecosystems growing and the curation of patient-generated health data, the accumulation of evidence has enabled clinical and wellness decision support across a wide range of specialties such as radiology, oncology, ophthalmology, critical care, and preventive care. As a result, the FDA has published action plans regulating AI/ML-Based SaMD activities and approved more than 160 medical AI products in recent years. Meanwhile, due to the sensitivity of clinical AI in producing unintended consequences such as incorrect diagnoses, unnecessary treatments, and racial disparities, there is also a growing concern on how to build safe, reliable, and trustworthy AI for adaptive clinical decision support (Adaptive CDS) systems (Petersen et al. 2021).

The growing concern has yielded an increasing body of literature exploring the methodology of estimating the impact of bias and counter strategies, including those related to the accumulation of patient-generated health data and the design of patient-centered systems (Hsueh et al. 2017a; Lai et al. 2017; Hsueh et al. 2017). However, in real-life scenarios, implementing such applications often requires experience in the trenches for how best to embed the actionable insights in clinical workflows and warrant behavioral change and sustainable adoption from clinicians (Miksad and Abernethy 2018; Reading et al. 2018). In 2021, implementation science researchers observed incidences wherein commercial algorithms have been deployed without validation (Wong et al. 2021; Aubert et al. 1998). Even the SaMD applications with FDA clearance have been criticized for insufficient transparency of the metadata associated with the dataset used for validation and not having an external validation mechanism (Singh et al. 2020b).

The healthcare ecosystems need to draw on the best practice examples to fulfill the potential of applying health AI to ensure a patient-centered view on patient safety in adaptive CDS systems (Bates et al. 2020; Hsueh et al. 2017; Muehlematter et al. 2021b; Dickson et al. 2021; Park et al. 2020; Turner Lee 2018; Romei and Ruggieri 2013; Vokinger et al. 2021). More AI evaluation frameworks are currently being experimented with in the ongoing trials or real-world evidence veneration studies that are expected to lead us to the next level of understanding toward a systematic framework.

There is also a growing concern about health equity issues in this rising domain (Wilkinson et al. 2016; Gichoya et al. 2021). Having a more robust ecosystem built around a set of industry standards that hold up to the rigor needed to keep the field thriving in the years to come. Our own work in care management has shown the potential of leveraging the heterogeneous sources of data to gauge individual patients' propensity to respond and tailor for their individual care plans (Hsueh et al. 2018; Graffigna et al. 2015). Many others have also proposed the behavioral engagement and change framework to incorporate what is needed in the individual plan for a more successful implementation of care coordination programs (Hekler et al. 2020; Narayanan and Georgiou 2013; Brown et al. 2012). In addition, the public health programs can also leverage the use of heterogeneous patient-centered data sources as a panel to help with continuous surveys in a cost-effective fashion (Diaz et al. 2016).

The Opportunities and Common Challenges Facing the Ecosystem

With the ecosystem stakeholders identified, common issues have also emerged. Therefore, we need to check on the challenges facing stakeholders of the patient-centered ecosystems to further investigate the solutions. In this chapter, we followed our framework set up in Petersen et al. (2020) to categorize these common issues and discuss the challenges facing the whole ecosystem. The remaining chapter will address the challenges from three perspectives: technical, organization, and collaboration challenges.

Technical Challenges

First, the increasing focus on health AI bias and health equity have brought more discussion in the ecosystems about how to collectively mitigate data-driven bias and apply the FAIR (findable, accessible, interoperable, and reusable) principle on the frontier of healthcare applications. The key is enabling a common set of industry standards for measuring and reporting potential data-driven bias and evaluation metrics for post-implementation model monitoring.

Second, the primary benefit of forming the health ecosystems around the patient-centered health data is to create a distributed network in which data from multiple sites are transformed into a CDM. The common CDM would allow for research studies to be conducted on a more diverse set of subpopulations. This would enable the measurement of health data bias and concept drift, and the development of risk-mitigating modeling strategies. There are typically three ways to construct such a network. Table 16.1 illustrates the example of each approach.

In addition to building networks for hypothesis testing, the ecosystems can also assist in the curation of large-scale quality datasets that are fit-for-purposes. This requires the development of a data provenance mechanism that can enable the tracking of subpopulations wherein the curated data were originally from and their associated metadata.

Last but not least, another set of technical challenges arises around the patient-centered design of the health IT system. When applying the application in real world settings, the users do not know which app will be helpful at which point in their workflow. While the design is all well-intended, there need to be additional technology components such as SMART on FHIR and Clinical Decision Support Hooks (CDS Hooks) to help the users (e.g., clinicians) to learn which app to launch in what context and receive relevant information at the point of care within their clinical workflows in EHR. The regulators in the ecosystem also

Table 16.1 Three Approaches that support conducting research via a common CDM

Approach	Example
Through a centralized network managed by a single business entity	Veterans Health Administration owned by U.S. Department of Veterans Affairs
Through a hybrid distributed model that supports a centralized repository of a combined data set	National Syndromic Surveillance System BioSense 2.0 owned by U.S. CDC
Through enabling research hypothesis testing against networks of data systems, with heterogenous data structured and managed by multiple owners	Sentinel system operated by U.S. FDA OHDSI

need to play their role in providing incentives for compliance checking. This is to ensure the production of safe, reliable, and trustworthy AI for Adaptive CDS systems.

Organizational Challenges

Beyond the technical challenges, each participating organization in the ecosystem is also facing questions such as how health systems can ensure value for patients in the use of PGHD (e.g., ePRO) in the health system design? In addition, how can health systems drive cultural changes towards a continuous learning environment? If our ecosystems can answer these questions, there would be a high potential to help move the needle of healthcare from reactive to proactive and improve health quality and patient outcomes. However, these questions also pose more organizational challenges for the ecosystem.

First, each ecosystem partner needs to tackle the social-technical challenge to enhance trust and relationship with the adoption of the patient-centered applications or PGHD-driven evidence for CDS. This would include behavioral change mechanisms from both the organization and patient side: On the one hand, the organization needs to increase the accessibility for patients and ease the burden of documentation for clinicians in the constrained EHR environment. On the other side, the organization also needs to implement data governance mechanisms for providing privacy safeguards and to design engagement tools to increase trust and patient autonomy.

Second, each ecosystem partner needs to find ways that can increase its organization's emphasis on the importance of patients' role in science and involving patients early in the design process of patient access and use of tools. In addition, as all organizations have their own bottom lines to be covered, it is necessary to understand how patient outcome and experience improvement can tie to the financial return on investment (ROI). If there is no direct ROI can be improved, the organization needs to at least demonstrate the value of patient-powered research. In turn, the relationship can help strengthen the need for the additional investment in improving patient-centeredness and establishing shared goals around patients and their outcomes.

Last but not least, on this front, the ecosystem also needs to look beyond the health system level to tackle the challenges by creating external drivers from the whole ecosystem level. In recent years, we have observed that the discussion of ethics and equity has contributed to the uptake of a more rigorous evaluation framework and scrutiny of the fairness of healthcare AI applications and healthcare practice in general. As we learned from the AI bias study, the AI algorithm bias are often coming from the health practice where the data were generated from in the first place. This collective effort would require a partnership between Health IT and governance leadership, as well as c-suite leadership driving culture buy-in and dedicated resources for change and process management. This would only work when the incentives from the stakeholders are all aligned to establish routines that center around the mission and vision for patient-centered care.

Collaboration Challenges

While the patient-centered care ecosystem approach shows a high potential to improve the precision understanding of patients, one significant barrier is the lack of participatory design methods that would work well with patients in the loop directly for workflow re-design.

Moreover, fast technological progress calls for a societal debate and decision-making process on a multitude of challenges: (1) how privacy is transformed by the new workflow; (2) how new data modalities and clinical data should be interpreted in the new workflow; (3) how to explain the data-driven insights to facilitate the development of patient-centered services; and (4) how to provide a risk assessment framework to evaluate the potential threats against new benefits and enable fact-based discussions. The ecosystem partners would need to work together on answering these questions.

In addition, innovations need to be balanced with what needs to happen on the ground in the realities of care delivery and live with the constraints such as time pressure and funding. In addition, sandbox environments are also needed to provide patient safety safeguards before the collaboration challenges are addressed. This part of challenges is especially challenging when the use of data raises ethical concerns, particularly around data quality and characteristics, representation, as well as potential bias.

Conclusion and Future Direction

Recent development of the patient-centric care ecosystem has started to facilitate a wide spectrum of clinical use cases, ranging from clinical decision support to patient safety to healthcare quality improvement. With the consumer and in-home care devices maturing and data API technical framework maturing, the ecosystem can further empower patients to decide which route their data will take depending on the quality of service they receive. This development is in early stages, but it marks an exciting development in healthcare to shift from a compartmentalized provider-centric model to a democratized patient-driven service care model.

Another exciting opportunity to improve healthcare based on the ecosystem development is through the recent advances in AI/ML for healthcare. However, the translation of research techniques to effective clinical deployment presents a new frontier for clinical and machine learning research. Thus, the ecosystem needs to work on a set of industrial standards to push forward robust, prospective clinical evaluation for ensuring AI systems to produce effective and clinically applicable performance metrics that go beyond measures of technical accuracy. This is essential for including how health AI affects the quality of care, the care variation in practice, the documentation burden on clinicians and, most importantly, patient outcomes.

Beyond the industrial standards for evaluation, the ecosystem is also posed to help bring about a distributed network for large-scale hypothesis testing and curate fit-for-purposes quality datasets. The would be essential for any future health applications to understand the applicability and potential bias and fitting to unintended confounders in its target sub-populations, as well as enabling the comparison of new algorithms against benchmarks. Ecosystem partners who are developing health AI tools can use the ecosystem-supported networks to further assess potential unintended consequences against the FAIR principles of good machine learning practice.

Further tackling the common challenges of the ecosystem partners from the three perspectives—technical, organizational, and collaborative challenges—would help us ensure that the precision patient understanding is supported by the development of technical standards (such as CDM, CDS Hooks and all the data interoperability standards), patient co-design methods, privacy and data provenance safeguards, governance mechanism, interpretable explanation work, and so on. Therefore, the ecosystem could be fully utilized to understand how best to help leverage the abundance of PGHD and ePRO data to enrich our clinical understanding and feedback to care delivery models supported by the development of thoughtful regulatory frameworks.

The importance of this direction is paramount under the COVID-19 pandemic when critical responses are essential with the additional time and resource constraints imposed. There have been new activities that can now be captured through reimbursable codes, such as virtual visits and vaccine administration. We need to ensure these new care delivery models are coded and billed to align providers and payers for a timely response. During the Covid-19 era, there was also an outcry for the lack of public health infrastructure support. Therefore, it is important to figure out how to remove the barriers to tackling preventive care, including rebuilding public health infrastructure and nurturing underinvestment in this area. While the prior proof-of-concept studies have demonstrated the benefits of having such a patient-centered ecosystem for addressing various care needs in clinical use cases, there have been huge missing opportunities around the needs on the patient side.

There are still a few methodological gaps to be overcome. First, patient-centered factors are undefined in practice. We need to start from scratch to understand what makes sense to be included. Second, the theoretical models and co-design methods are usually very high-level, and the patient-generated health data that may contain signals are generally quite noisy whose quality needs additional processing. The big gap in-between needs our efforts to develop methods and keep putting them into practice to learn more about applying person-level precision understanding to build precision health applications for tomorrow's medicine.

The fundamental goal of all the efforts would be to enable an RWE validation platform through a distributed network of partner sites on a platform using the same shared data model. Similar platforms have been developed for patient-safety post-market surveillance. For example, the FDA's Sentinel platform could help send a patient-report research hypothesis about patient safety to multiple sites for external validity verification. This could help eliminate the need to conduct a separate patient-safety study, save resources, and obtain answers to the research hypothesis with the needed statistical rigor.

In the future, with the ecosystem partners on board, the ecosystems can also help push forward industrial standards to use a standard set of metadata for the data repository and a common set of metrics for AI bias measurement and post-implementation evaluation. In the wake of interoperability and data blocking rules that went into effect in 2020, the ecosystem is in an ever-better position to empower innovative applications that were previously impossible when each ecosystem partner was working in silos. Examples include the development of a collaborative filtering recommender system for patient treatment preference; the enablement of N-of-1 trials based on patient phenotypes (including all the factors beyond clinical understanding); the recommendation of care plans that would enable higher compliance rates; and the design of health promotion programs that are genuinely based on patient preferences and needs. We expect the ecosystems to be the foundation for realizing the potential for integrating data science with science of care at the point of need.

Review Questions

1. What is the percentage of clinical factors contributing to a person's health determinants?
2. What are the other categories of factors that contribute to a person's health determinants?
3. What financial levers drive the development of precision patient understanding methods for moving the health systems from reactive to proactive?
4. Who are the potential ecosystem partners and stakeholders to enable a proactive health system that can provide precision patient understanding?
5. What are the cross-stakeholder initiatives important for leveraging the ecosystem's private-public partnership?
6. What are the common technical challenges for ensuring fairness principles?

Answers

1. **30-40%**
2. Genetic, Environmental, behavioral, social factors
3. Value-based care, APM.
4. Patients/Caregivers, citizen scientists, pharmaceutical companies, health tech startups, government agencies, standardization bodies.
5. Real-world evidence validation platform and fairness principles for AI/ML practice.

References

American Society of Clinical Oncology (ASCO). Testing the use of Food and Drug Administration (FDA) approved drugs that target a specific abnormality in a tumor gene in people with advanced stage cancer (TAPUR). NCT02693535. First posted 2016; Last update posted 2022.

Agency for Healthcare Research and Quality (AHRQ). Developing design principles to integrate patient-reported outcomes (PROs) into clinical practice through health information technology: data, user experience, and workflow requirements for PRO dashboards | Digital Healthcare Research. (n.d.). Retrieved May 8, 2021, https://digital.ahrq.gov/ahrq-funded-projects/developing-design-principles-integrate-patient-reported-outcomes-pros-clinical

FDA. Proposed regulatory framework for modifications to artificial intelligence/machine learning (AI/ML)-based software as a medical device (SaMD)-discussion paper and request for feedback (2019). Retrieved Aug 16, 2021, https://www.fda.gov/downloads/medicaldevices/deviceregulationandguidance/guidancedocuments/ucm514737.pdf

Dickson B, et al. Algorithmic bias detection and mitigation: best practices and policies to reduce consumer harms. Brookings Institute, 2020. Retrieved Aug 29, 2021, https://www.brookings.edu/research/algorithmic-bias-detection-and-mitigation-best-practices-and-policies-to-reduce-consumer-harms/

Artificial Intelligence and Machine Learning in Software as a Medical Device | FDA. (n.d.). Retrieved July 16, 2019, https://www.fda.gov/medical-devices/software-medical-device-samd/artificial-intelligence-and-machine-learning-software-medical-device

Aubert RE, Herman WH, Waters J, Moore W, Sutton D, Peterson BL, Bailey CM, Koplan JP. Nurse case management to improve glycemic control in diabetic patients in a health maintenance organization: a randomized, controlled trial. Ann Intern Med. 1998;129(8):605–12.

Austin E, LeRouge C, Hartzler AL, Segal C, Lavallee DC. Capturing the patient voice: implementing patient-reported outcomes across the health system. Qual Life Res. 2020;29(2):347–55.

Austin EJ, LeRouge C, Lee JR, Segal C, Sangameswaran S, Heim J, Lober WB, Hartzler AL, Lavallee DC. A learning health systems approach to integrating electronic patient-reported outcomes across the health care organization. Learn Health Syst. 2021;5:4.

Australian Digital Health Agency. (2018). Australian Medicines Terminology.

Bates DW, Auerbach A, Schulam P, Wright A, Saria S. Reporting and implementing interventions involving machine learning and artificial intelligence. Ann Intern Med. 2020;172(11):137–44.

Bates DW, Levine D, Syrowatka A, Kuznetsova M, Jean K, Craig T, Rui A, Jackson GP, Rhee K. The potential of artificial intelligence to improve patient safety: a scoping review. NPJ Digit Med. 2021;4(1):54.

Benjamens S, Dhunnoo P, Meskó B. The state of artificial intelligence-based FDA-approved medical devices and algorithms: an online database. NPJ Digit Med. 2020;3(1):1–8.

Bica I, Alaa AM, Lambert C, van der Schaar M. From real-world patient data to individualized treatment effects using machine learning: current and future methods to address underlying challenges. Clin Pharmacol Ther. 2020;1:87–100.

Bica I, Alaa AM, Lambert C, van der Schaar M. From real-world patient data to individualized treatment effects using machine learning: current and future methods to address underlying challenges. Clin Pharmacol Ther. 2021;109(1):87–100.

Black JR, Hulkower RL, and Ramanathan T. Health information blocking: responses under the 21st century cures act. In Public Health Reports (Vol. 133, Issue 5, pp. 610–613). 2018 SAGE Publications Ltd.

Bodenreider O, Cornet R, Vreeman DJ. Recent developments in clinical terminologies—SNOMED CT, LOINC, and RxNorm. Yearb Med Inform. 2018;27(1):129.

Brown B, Crapo J. The key to transitioning from fee-for-service to value-based reimbursement. New Engl J Med Catal. 2014.

Brown RS, Peikes D, Peterson G, Schore J, Razafindrakoto CM. Six features of Medicare coordinated care demonstration programs that cut hospital admissions of high-risk patients. Health Aff. 2012;31(6):1156–66.

Bundled Payments for Care Improvement (BPCI) Initiative: General Information | CMS Innovation Center. (n.d.). https://innovation.cms.gov/innovation-models/bundled-payments

Chen IY, Szolovits P, Ghassemi M. Can AI help reduce disparities in general medical and mental health care? AMA J Ethics. 2019;21(2):167–79.

CMS. Supplemental material to the CMS MMS blueprint patient-reported outcome measures. 2021. Retrieved from https://mmshub.cms.gov/blueprint-measure-lifecycle-overview.

Collins FS, Hudson KL, Briggs JP, Lauer MS. PCORnet: turning a dream into reality. J Am Med Inform Assoc. 2014;21(04):576–7.

Colwell J. NCI-MATCH trial draws strong interest. Cancer Discov. 2016;6:334.

Diaz F, Gamon M, Hofman JM, Kıcıman E, Rothschild D. Online and social media data as an imperfect continuous panel survey. PLoS One. 2016;11(1):e0145406.

Federal Register: Medicare and medicaid programs; patient protection and affordable care act; Interoperability and patient access for medicare advantage organization and medicaid managed care plans, state medicaid agencies, CHIP Agencies and CHIP managed care entities, issuers of qualified health plans on the federally-facilitated exchanges, and health care providers. 2020. Retrieved November 28, 2021, from https://www.federalregister.gov/documents/2020/05/01/2020-05050/medicare-and-medicaid-programs-patient-protection-and-affordable-care-act-interoperability-and

Finlayson SG, Subbaswamy A, Singh K, Bowers J, Kupke A, Zittrain J, Kohane IS, Saria S. The clinician and dataset shift in artificial intelligence. N Engl J Med. 2021;385:283–6.

Frazier P, Rossi-Mori A, Dolin RH, Alschuler L, Huff SM. The creation of an ontology of clinical document names. Stud Health Technol Inform. 2001;84(Pt 1):94–8.

Frieden TR. Evidence for health decision making—beyond randomized, controlled trials. N Engl J Med. 2017;377:465–75.

Fröhlich H, Balling R, Beerenwinkel N, Kohlbacher O, Kumar S, Lengauer T, Maathuis MH, Moreau Y, Murphy SA, Przytycka TM, Rebhan M, Röst H, Schuppert A, Schwab M, Spang R, Stekhoven D, Sun J, Weber A, Ziemek D, Zupan B. From hype to reality: data science enabling personalized medicine. BMC Med. 2018;16(1):150.

Galea S, Maani N. The cost of preventable disease in the USA. Lancet Public Health. 2020;5(10):513–4. Elsevier Ltd

Gichoya JW, McCoy LG, Celi LA, Ghassemi M. Equity in essence: a call for operationalising fairness in machine learning for healthcare. BMJ Health Care Inf. 2021;28(1):e100289.

Good Machine Learning Practice for Medical Device Development: Guiding Principles | FDA. (n.d.). Retrieved October 28, 2021, from https://www.fda.gov/medical-devices/software-medical-device-samd/good-machine-learning-practice-medical-device-development-guiding-principles?utm_medium=email&utm_source=govdelivery

Graffigna G, Barello S, Bonanomi A, Lozza E. Measuring patient engagement: development and psychometric properties of the patient health engagement (PHE) scale. Front Psychol. 2015;6:274.

Health Information Technology for Economic and Clinical Health (HITECH) Act, Title XIII of Division A and Title IV of Division B of the American Recovery and Reinvestment Act of 2009 (ARRA), Pub. L. No. 111-5, 123 Stat. 226 (Feb. 17, 2009), codified at 42 USC §§300jj et seq.; §§17901 et seq.

Hekler E, Tiro JA, Hunter CM, Nebeker C. Precision health: the role of the social and behavioral sciences in advancing the vision. Ann Behav Med. 2020;54(11):805–26.

HL7 Standards Product Brief—HL7 Version 2 Product Suite | HL7 International. (n.d.). Retrieved April 28, 2021, http://www.hl7.org/implement/standards/product_brief.cfm?product_id=185

HL7 Standards Product Brief - HL7 Version 3 Product Suite | HL7 International. (n.d.). Retrieved April 28, 2021, https://www.hl7.org/implement/standards/product_brief.cfm?product_id=186

Hripcsak G, Duke JD, Shah NH, Reich CG, Huser V, Schuemie MJ, et al. Observational health data sciences and informatics (OHDSI): opportunities for observational researchers. Stud Health Technol Inform. 2015;2015(216):574–8.

Hsueh PS, Cheung Y, Dey S, Kim KK, Martin-Sanchez FJ, Petersen SK, Wetter T. Added value from secondary use of person generated health data in consumer health informatics. Yearb Med Inform. 2017a;26(01):160–71. https://doi.org/10.15265/IY-2017-009.

Hsueh PS, Das S, Maduri C, Kelly K. Learning to personalize from practice: a real world evidence approach of care plan personalization based on differential patient Behavioral responses in care management records. AMIA Ann Symp Proc. 2018;2018:592–601.

Hsueh PS, Dey S, Das S, & Wetter T. Making sense of patient-generated health data for interpretable patient-centered care: The transition from "More" to "Better." Stud Health Technol Inform. 2017;245:113–17.

Ibrahim SA. Artificial intelligence for disparities in knee pain assessment. Nat Med. 2021;27(1):22–3.

FHIR v4.0.1. (n.d.). Retrieved April 28, 2021., https://www.hl7.org/fhir/

Information Blocking and the ONC Health IT Certification Program: Extension of compliance dates and timeframes in response to the COVID-19 public health emergency. 85 FR 70064. 2020. https://www.federalregister.gov/documents/2020/11/04/2020-24376/information-blocking-and-the-onc-health-it-certification-program-extension-of-compliance-dates-and

Israel BA, Schulz AJ, Parker EA, Becker AB. Review of community-based research: assessing partnership approaches to improve public health. Annu Rev Public Health. 1998;19:173–202.

Jillson E. Aiming for truth, fairness, and equity in your company's use of AI. Federal Trade Commission, Retrieved April 19, 2021, https://www.ftc.gov/news-events/blogs/business-blog/2021/04/aiming-truth-fairness-equity-your-companys-use-ai.

Joaquin Quiñonero-candela EB, Sugiyama M, Schwaighofer A, Lawrence ND. Dataset shift in machine learning (Neural Information Processing), MIT Press, 2009.

Lai AM, Hsueh P-YS, Choi YK, Austin RR. Present and future trends in consumer health informatics and patient-generated health data. Yearb Med Inform. 2017;26(01):152–9.

Long PV, editor. Effective care for high-need patients: opportunities for improving outcomes, value, and health. National Academy Of Medicine; 2017.

Matheny ME, Whicher D, Thadaney Israni S. Artificial intelligence in health care. JAMA. 2019;323(6):509–10.

McGinnis JM, Williams-Russo P, Knickman JR. The case for more active policy attention to health promotion. Health Affair. 2017;21(2):78–93.

Miksad RA, Abernethy AP. Harnessing the power of real-world evidence (RWE): a checklist to ensure regulatory-grade data quality. Clin Pharmacol Ther. 2018;103(2):202–5.

Muehlematter UJ, Daniore P, Vokinger KN. Approval of artificial intelligence and machine learning-based medical devices in the USA and Europe (2015–20): a comparative analysis. Lancet Digit Health. 2021a;3(3):e195–203.

Muehlematter UJ, Daniore P, Vokinger KN. Approval of artificial intelligence and machine learning-based medical devices in the USA and Europe (2015–20): a comparative analysis. Lancet Digit Health. 2021b;3(3):e195–203.

Narayanan S, Georgiou PG. Behavioral signal processing: deriving human behavioral informatics from speech and language. Proc IEEE. 2013;101(5):1203–33.

Nelson SJ, Zeng K, Kilbourne J, Powell T, Moore R. Normalized names for clinical drugs: RxNorm at 6 years. J Am Med Inform Assoc. 2011;18(4):441–8.

NHE Fact Sheet | CMS. (n.d.). Retrieved June 7, 2021, from https://www.cms.gov/Research-Statistics-Data-and-Systems/Statistics-Trends-and-Reports/NationalHealthExpendData/NHE-Fact-Sheet

NHS Business Service Authority. (2018). Dictionary of medicines and devices.

Obermeyer Z, Topol EJ. Artificial intelligence, bias, and patients' perspectives. Lancet. 2021;397(10289):2038. https://doi.org/10.1016/S0140-6736(21)01152-1.

Office of the National Coordinator for Health Information Technology (ONC). 21st century cures act: interoperability, information blocking, and the ONC Health IT certification program. 85 FR 25642. In effect 2016. https://www.healthit.gov/curesrule/overview/oncs-cures-act-final-rule-highlighted-regulatory-dates.

Park Y, Hu J, Singh M, Sylla I, Dankwa-Mullan I, Koski E, Das AK. Comparison of methods to reduce bias from clinical prediction models of postpartum depression. JAMA Netw Open. 2021;4(4):e213909.

Park Y, Jackson GP, Foreman MA, Gruen D, Hu J, Das AK. Evaluating artificial intelligence in medicine: phases of clinical research. JAMIA Open. 2020;3(3):326–31.

Petersen C, Austin RR, Backonja U, Campos H, Chung AE, Hekler EB, Hsueh P-YS, Kim KK, Pho A, Salmi L, Solomonides A, Valdez RS. Citizen science to further precision medicine: from vision to implementation. JAMIA Open. 2020;3(1):2–8.

Petersen C, Smith J, Freimuth RR, Goodman KW, Jackson GP, Kannry J, Liu H, Madhavan S, Madhavan S, Sittig DF, Wright A. Recommendations for the safe, effective use of adaptive CDS in the US healthcare system: an AMIA position paper. J Am Med Inform Assoc. 2021;28(4):677–84.

Pierson E, Cutler DM, Leskovec J, Mullainathan S, Obermeyer Z. An algorithmic approach to reducing unexplained pain disparities in underserved populations. Nat Med. 2021;27(1):136–40.

Platt R, Brown JS, Robb M, McClellan M, Ball R, Nguyen MD, Sherman RE. The FDA sentinel initiative - an evolving National Resource. N Engl J Med. 2018;379(22):2091–3.

Raghupathi W, Raghupathi V. An empirical study of chronic diseases in the United States: a visual analytics approach to public health. Int J Environ Res Public Health. 2018;15:3.

Rashdan S, Gerber DE. Going into BATTLE: umbrella and basket clinical trials to accelerate the study of biomarker-based therapies. Ann Transl Med. 2016;4:24.

Reading MJ, Merrill JA. Converging and diverging needs between patients and providers who are collecting and using patient-generated health data: an integrative review. J Am Med Inform Assoc. 2018;25(6):759–771.

Romei A, Ruggieri S. Discrimination data analysis: a multi-disciplinary bibliography. Stud Appl Philos Epistemol Rational Ethics. 2013;3:109–35.

Rothwell LE, Greene JA, Podolsky SH, Jones DS. Assessing the gold standard — lessons from the history of RCTs. N Engl J Med. 2016;374:2175–81.

Schuetze S, Rothe M, Mangat PK, et al. Palbociclib (P) in patients (pts) with soft tissue sarcoma (STS) with CDK4 amplification: results from the Targeted Agent and Profiling Utilization Registry (TAPUR) study. J Clin Oncol. 2021;39(suppl 15):11565. https://doi.org/10.1200/JCO.2021.39.15_suppl.11565.

Singh K, Valley TS, Tang S, Li BY, Kamran F, Sjoding MW, Wiens J, Otles E, Donnelly JP, Wei MY, McBride JP, Cao J, Penoza C, Ayanian JZ, Nallamothu BK. Evaluating a widely implemented proprietary deterioration index model among hospitalized COVID-19 patients. Ann Am Thorac Soc. 2020a;18(7):1129–37.

Singh K, Valley TS, Tang S, Li BY, Kamran F, Sjoding MW, Wiens J, Otles E, Donnelly JP, Wei MY, McBride JP, Cao J, Penoza C, Ayanian JZ, & Nallamothu BK. Evaluating a widely implemented proprietary deterioration index model among hospitalized COVID-19 patients. Annals of the American Thoracic Society 2020b.

Sisko AM, Keehan SP, Poisal JA, Cuckler GA, Smith SD, Madison AJ, Rennie KE, Hardesty JC. National health expenditure projections, 2018–27: economic and demographic trends drive spending and enrollment growth. Health Aff. 2019;38(3):491–501.

SNOMED Clinical Terms® (SNOMED CT®). (n.d.). Retrieved Apr. 29, 2021, https://www.nlm.nih.gov/research/umls/Snomed/snomed_main_old.html

The Interoperability and Patient Access final rule (CMS-9115-F), published May 1, 2020,

Tuomilehto J, Lindström J, Eriksson G, Valle T, Hämäläinen H, Ilanne-Parikka P, Keinänen-Kiukaanniemi S, Laakso M, Louheranta A, Rastas M, Salminen V. Prevention of type 2 diabetes mellitus by changes in lifestyle among subjects with impaired glucose tolerance. N Engl J Med. 2009;344(18):1343–50.

Turner Lee N. Detecting racial bias in algorithms and machine learning. J Inf Commun Ethics Soc. 2018;16(3):252–60.

Vokinger KN, Feuerriegel S, Kesselheim AS. Mitigating bias in machine learning for medicine. Commun Med. 2021 1:1. 2021;1(1):1–3.

West JA, Miller NH, Parker KM, Senneca D, Ghandour G, Clark M, Greenwald G, Heller RS, Fowler MB, DeBusk RF. A comprehensive management system for heart failure improves clinical outcomes and reduces medical resource utilization. Am J Cardiol. 1997;79(1):58–63.

What LOINC is – LOINC. (n.d.). Retrieved Apr. 29, 2021, from https://loinc.org/get-started/what-loinc-is/

Wilkinson MD, Dumontier M, Aalbersberg IJ, Appleton G, Axton M, Baak A, Blomberg N, Boiten JW, da Silva Santos LB, Bourne PE, Bouwman J, Brookes AJ, Clark T, Crosas M, Dillo I, Dumon O, Edmunds S, Evelo CT, Finkers R, et al. The FAIR guiding principles for scientific data management and stewardship. Scientific Data. 2016;3.

Wong A, Otles E, Donnelly JP, Krumm A, McCullough J, DeTroyer-Cooley O, Pestrue J, Phillips M, Konye J, Penoza C, Ghous M, Singh K. External validation of a widely implemented proprietary sepsis prediction model in hospitalized patients. JAMA Intern Med. 2021;181(8):1065–70.

Chapter 17
Personalizing Research: Involving, Inviting, and Engaging Patient Researchers

Dana Lewis

Abstract There are many benefits to engaging and involving patients in traditional, researcher-led research, ranging from improved recruitment and increased enrollment to accelerating and facilitating the implementation of research outcomes. Researchers, however, may not be aware of when and where they can involve patients (people with lived healthcare experience) in research or what the benefits may be of improving patient engagement in the research process or of expanding patient involvement to other research stages. This chapter seeks to highlight the benefits and opportunities of engaging patients in traditional research and provide practical suggestions for inviting or recruiting patients for participation in research, whether or not there is an established patient and public involvement (PPI) program. This includes tips for developing a productive working relationship and culture between researchers and the patients involved in research. There are also many patients themselves conducting research, and often without the benefits, resources, and opportunities made available to traditional researchers. Traditional researchers should identify and recognize researchers who have emerged from non-traditional paths who are driving and engaging in their own research, and provide support and resources where appropriate to foster further patient-driven research. This investment can lead to collaboration opportunities for additional highly relevant and effective research studies with traditional researchers in the future. This chapter provides examples of patient researchers and offers tools to support traditional researchers who want to support patient-led research efforts and improve their ability to successfully engage patient stakeholders in their own research.

Keywords Patient engagement · Patient research · Patient-driven research Patient researcher · Patient-led research · Patient-centered care · Stakeholder engagement · Patient outcomes · Patient-centered outcomes · Patient and service

D. Lewis (✉)
OpenAPS, Seattle, WA, USA
e-mail: Dana@OpenAPS.org

© The Author(s), under exclusive license to Springer Nature   353
Switzerland AG 2022
P.-Y. S. Hsueh et al. (eds.), *Personal Health Informatics*, Cognitive Informatics
in Biomedicine and Healthcare, https://doi.org/10.1007/978-3-031-07696-1_17

user engagement · Patient stakeholder · Empowered patients · E-patients
Patient and public involvement · PPI

Learning Objectives
- Identify one of the benefits of having patients involved in or engaged in traditional research
- Describe the distinction between patients engaging in traditional, researcher-led research and patient-driven research
- Identify two or more ways to invite patients into existing or proposed research projects
- Identify two or more ways that a traditional researcher could support patients in their own research endeavors

Overview

There are many benefits to engaging and involving patients in traditional, researcher-led research, ranging from improved recruitment and increased enrollment to accelerating and facilitating the implementation of research outcomes. Traditional researchers, however, may not be aware of when and where they can involve patients (people with lived healthcare experience) in research or what the benefits may be of improving patient engagement in the research process or of expanding patient involvement to other research stages. This chapter seeks to highlight the benefits and opportunities of engaging patients in traditional research and provide practical suggestions for inviting or recruiting patients for participation in research, whether or not there is an established patient and public involvement (PPI) program. This includes tips for developing a productive working relationship and culture between researchers and the patients involved in research. There are also many patients themselves conducting research, and often without the benefits, resources, and opportunities made available to traditional researchers. Traditional researchers should identify and recognize researchers who have emerged from non-traditional paths who are driving and engaging in their own research, and provide support and resources where appropriate to foster further patient-driven research. This investment can lead to collaboration opportunities for additional highly relevant and effective research studies with traditional researchers in the future. This chapter provides examples of patient researchers and offers tools to support traditional researchers who want to support patient-led research efforts and improve their ability to successfully engage patient stakeholders in their own research.

Involving Patients In Research Has Many Benefits

Patients have increasingly been involved in research in recent years. Some of this is driven by mandates from funders, such as from the Patient Centered Outcomes Research Institute (PCORI) who both fund research and also strive to have research guided by patients and carers or care partners (PCORI 2020). Funders may require researchers to involve patients. Additionally, there may be established or past patient and public involvement (PPI) initiatives (Greenhalgh et al. 2019) at your organization, where researchers can leverage organizational learning around partnering with patients in research.

Researchers who haven't yet partnered with patients, or whose involvement of patients was limited to the minimum required by funder mandates, may not be aware of the benefits of more fully involving patients in research—of which there are many (Petersen 2018).

Researchers may perceive that they should add patients to research projects after a project has been funded and the project has commenced. But there are also many earlier opportunities to engage patients in research throughout the entire research process. Patient engagement from the earliest stages of research, beginning with defining key research questions, protocol development, and even the grant writing stage, can contribute to increasing study enrollment rates and identifying relevant outcome measures (Domecq et al. 2014).

Another name for this is "participatory research". It's increasingly being recognized as a value-add to improve the relevance of studies for the communities being studied, in addition to improving accuracy of data interpretation and increasing the likelihood of a community adopting any resulting intervention (Decker et al. 2010). Whether you think of the communities participating as "patients", or as representing more general subgroups such as women, increasing participatory research can accelerate the implementation of any solutions driven by research results. Which of course, likely aligns with your goals—after all, you're probably not just doing research for the sake of doing research!

Additionally, there have been studies assessing the financial impact of patient engagement in the research process. One such study looked at whether patient engagement can help avoid protocol amendments and/or improve enrollment and retention within clinical trials. It found that the cumulative impact of patient engagement activity that could likely reduce a protocol amendment would lead to a 500-fold return on any investment involved in funding the patient engagement process (Levitan et al. 2018). In one example, $100,000 toward patient engagement would yield an increase in net present value of $62MM for a pre-phase 2 project, and could expedite eventual product launches by several years.

The cost of patient engagement doesn't necessarily need to be that high. But patient engagement in research is not free: it takes additional time from both researchers and patients (who should be paid for their time and expertise).

Patients can provide benefits to the research project similar to other types of research collaborators who might contribute to or partner with you in research. Like other collaborators, it may take time to identify the right patient partner and to develop the working relationship. It's worth it: patients can challenge assumptions and improve the research, as well as increase transparency and trust within their community to engage with or participate in research (Duffett 2017). But it takes engaging patients as partners, rather than seeing them as "subjects" (Lewis 2019a), to help achieve this.

In the rest of this chapter, we'll address how you might identify new patient partners for research, how to involve them throughout the research process, and also how you might engage and support patient researchers who are driving their own research in areas that overlap with your interests and expertise.

Inviting Patients To Participate In Research—As Partners

One perspective on research is that patients are already involved in research - as subjects. There are efforts to get researchers to think about and refer to patients as active "participants", rather than passive 'subjects': many patients are highly engaged and actively seek out research studies or clinical trials. Despite ongoing efforts since the 1990s to drive this terminology change (Chalmers et al. 1999), many researchers still refer to, think of, and treat those who agree to participate in their research as "subjects".

Even when patients are thought of and treated as participants in studies, and make valuable contributions by sharing their data, information, etc., the design or process of research studies generally does not allow them to fully participate in the research process. They have no power, and no say, in the research process or the protocol as participants. At the point of enrolling patients in a research study, it's generally too late to make many changes to the protocol. While patients may have suggestions during the study, which researchers may or may not write down to take the feedback into account for future studies, the process is not generally set up to enable changes.

Achieving full participation from patients requires involving them as partners, much earlier in the research process, in order to provide the opportunity to meaningfully change, adapt, shape, and influence the research. And that's what should be done. But not all participants are ideal - or available - partners. To successfully partner with patients, you first have to identify which patients to partner with early in the research process, and this can be challenging. Which patients would even want to do this? And how do you find them and ask them to participate? Here are some suggestions.

Identifying Partners—Starting With Your Own Patients Or Past Research Participants

Once you realize that you'd like to partner with patients, it helps to know if you have a particular project where you would like to first engage patients as partners, or if you're generally trying to find patient partners for all future projects.

One of the first things you can do, if you are a clinician, is look to your own patient population. You likely have an intuitive sense of patients who are very engaged in their own care, or who have previously indicated interest in engaging with the healthcare system to improve it or fix it in some way. Patients who are willing to engage in fixing a system that is broken are often the same patients who would love to be asked to participate in a formal process (e.g. research) to improve knowledge, care delivery, and new treatments and therapies to aid themselves and their fellow patient community.

Similarly, even if you are not a clinician, you should ask around, starting with your colleagues. If you can, ask those who have already successfully engaged patient partners. If you don't know anyone at your own institution or within your own field, look to other fields. For example, oncology, psychology, and endocrinology are fields that tend to have academic and clinical researchers who are already successfully engaging patients as research partners. They can give you tips, or recommendations of patients and caregivers to reach out to.

If you are looking for patients within a specific disease space or community, there are likely non-profit organizations that you can reach out to for assistance in identifying patients who would be good candidates for becoming research partners. There may also be specific online communities (whether those are forums hosted by an organization, or groups within particular social media platforms) that you can participate in to develop relationships and identify potential patient research partners. This can be especially effective when you are planning to work on a project that is for a rare disease or a narrow subset within a more common disease space.

Proactively Recruiting Patients

Don't hesitate to look on social media for patient research partners. In fact, if you're already active on social media, you likely have already digitally engaged with patients who may be great research partners for you. Once you start looking, you'll likely find many excellent candidates. Don't be afraid to ask out loud and look for recommendations - from other researchers and also from patients—about who might be interested in engaging in research.

Ideally, if you are on social media, you already have relationships with a variety of others on social media, including patients. If not, it's a good idea to open your eyes to the potential of developing relationships with patients and care partners, in addition to fellow traditional academic or clinical researchers. As mentioned in the introduction, patients can contribute significantly to research at all stages, and that includes discussions in social media about the opportunities, challenges, and pitfalls of different research topics and strategies.

Any patient who has voluntarily engaged in or responded to any content you've shared about past research may be open to engaging in conversation to determine whether they would be interested in getting involved in future research. Sometimes, patients may not be aware of what "getting involved with research" would mean and seem initially hesitant. Being prepared to discuss the types of activities you would recommend their involvement in, and being prepared to discuss your research ideas to make the research feel more concrete, could help.

In general, you can proactively recruit patients by talking about your experience engaging with patient researchers in the past; engaging patients in discussions about your research in general; and by indicating that you're actively looking for patient partners for future work.

Ask Patients How They'd Like To Be Involved In Research

It's important to ask patients how they'd like to be involved in research, of course. Depending on your past experiences or your funding mechanism, there may be specific roles, amounts of time, and ways to engage in research that you have in mind. If so, you can share those with the potential patient partner and discuss it with them. If not, you can also ask them how they might want to be involved in research.

They may not know, especially if they've not previously been involved in research partnerships before, how they can be involved, or what they'd like to do. In that case, you can share some ideas you have for how to include them.

It's important to assess their availability in terms of time commitment, and to be up front and clear with them about how much time (minimum) you think a project and/or role will involve. Some patients may want to be involved, but not have the time required for a particular project. Or maybe they are a great fit and don't have time, but you can adapt the project timeline to better fit in with their schedules. In other cases, they may be willing and able to spend more time on a project, in which case it is also important to have transparent (and early) conversations about funding and compensation for their time and contributions. It's important to keep in mind that individuals who have more time to devote to research may also be in various positions of privilege. Consider how you can adapt or design your project to include people with varied schedules and levels of availability for side projects in addition to their primary work.

In some cases, you may be inviting patients early enough in the research process where there is no funding, because your project hasn't been funded yet. It's important to be transparent with patient research partners if this is the case, and also initiate the conversation about the budgeting process and what you would recommend for funding their time and including it within the research proposal, so that their efforts are compensated if the project does receive funding.

Now that you have read this chapter, you should also begin building a pipeline of funding, so that you do have a bucket of funding that could be used to fund patient partners' work that falls out of the traditional research process, such as for the efforts with brainstorming projects and writing grants, even if a grant ultimately doesn't receive funding. Remember that you are likely being paid a salary for your role that covers your time for the funding seeking process for research; however, patient partners are often volunteering their time - for free. There can be other benefits (Smith et al. 2019) they receive as a result of participating in this process, but it's important to be cognizant of this fact and when possible, recognize their contributions with funding of some kind—and if not, find other ways to honor and acknowledge their contributions to your work.

Involving Patients In Prospective Or Existing Research Projects

As mentioned earlier in the chapter, don't wait until you've received funding for a project to engage patients in your research. Ideally, don't even wait for writing an initial proposal to engage patients! If you've already developed relationships with patient partners, you can begin involving patient partners in your research process at the ideation stage. Invite your patient partners to be involved and contribute in the creation and design of the study, ranging from defining the relevant outcomes to designing recruitment materials.

In some cases, you may have a clear idea of what the research study is. If so, you can invite patient or partner involvement with guardrails of what the defined project is. There are still many areas where patient partners can contribute and add value to the research process, even when there is already a clear research idea involved.

Don't feel like you need to have everything figured out before involving patient partners. Involve them early in conversations: they likely have their own ideas that are relevant to the patient community that you may not have thought of; or they can participate in a brainstorm with all of the research collaborators to iterate on the project topic and design.

You may not have funding to cover patient partner time at this stage and are instead writing funding for them into the budget for a research project. If so, be up front and involve patients in determining what is an appropriate budget line item for their contributions in context of the amount of work and contribution to a project. Share a realistic timeline about the research application and funding process, and make sure to communicate whether they should expect to hear back from you within weeks, months, or up to a year.

And importantly, if a grant or research proposal is submitted and it is turned down or funding is not awarded: make sure to tell your patient partner the outcome and any next steps (such as re-submitting). Don't "ghost" a patient partner or require them to email months later looking to find out what happened with a project. If you wouldn't do it to a traditional research partner or collaborator such as a co-PI or contributor on your project, make sure you don't do it to a patient partner, either.

Relationship Building And Culture Setting Is Important

The relationships you develop with patient partners in research are important. It is critical to recognize that there are power imbalances within the healthcare system, and this power imbalance definitely transfers over to the research process as well. Especially if you are a clinical researcher - and more so if a patient partner for research is an actual patient - there are existing hierarchies and power structures that will also flow into the research relationship and process.

The first thing to do is to recognize—and vocalize—this fact. Addressing the power dynamics up front and establishing a culture of partnership can go a long way in developing relationships and effective collaborations with patient partners in research. It may take several times of bringing this up and finding ways to reinforce it (gently) before patient partners in research truly feel comfortable engaging and contributing equitably in a research project. Be aware of not only the healthcare dynamics in play (e.g. the hierarchy where patients are typically in the bottom and powerless), but also other systemic biases that may be influencing a patient partner's comfort level in speaking up.

Speaking up and challenging the system is hard. It's hard when you're a patient and you want your doctor or researcher to "like" and respect you. It's not an equal playing field like it potentially is for a traditional collaborator or co-principal investigator on your project. But, developing a strong and open relationship between researcher and patient partner can go a long way for improving the opportunity to equitably contribute to a research project, now or in future research projects.

Sometimes, this may involve the researcher playing "defense" and course-correcting other traditional researchers or stakeholders on the project who may not be aware that they are overwhelming or 'running over' the patient partner. This can include interrupting and stopping if they interrupt a patient partner, and returning the "floor space" back to patient partners to be able to finish what they are saying. It can involve creating different ways for patients to contribute feedback to a stage of research: consider not only inviting verbal contributions in a meeting, but perhaps by involving them in discussions over email or collaborating on an online document that allows equitable participation in different formats where there is less pressure to perform or speak up on the spot in an environment where they are not fully comfortable (yet).

Additionally, you could consider creating different feedback checkpoints across the life of a project with your patient research partners. Build it in as a milestone during and near the end of a project. Add it to an agenda item for specific meetings. Or, think about strategies like creating an anonymous survey that can be filled out at any time by patient research partners to give feedback on how things are going. The more opportunities and channels for feedback there are, the more likely you are to receive feedback about how things are going and when things might need course-correcting, without having to wait until it's too late (such as when a project is over, or someone chooses to leave the project) to be able to address any concerns.

When you look to recruit a new patient research partner, you should ask them if they've previously participated in research. You can ask what they liked - and didn't like - about the process and experience, and what they're hoping to get out of this new partnership or project.

In general, if you set clear expectations for the roles of patient partners and how they could and should contribute, you can check back against those expectations and see if there are any structural barriers - or personality behaviors from other team members - that are blocking participation and contributions from patient partners.

Setting Expectations Matters For Everyone Involved

Wherever possible, set clear expectations up front. The more clear that you are - whether that's about the role of a patient research partner compared to the role of other team members, or about the research topic or the stage of the research project - the easier things will be, and the easier it will be to address any situation that's contributing to blocking patient partners from meeting those expectations.

Patient research partners can contribute to a variety of roles in research, when invited and equipped to do so. They can help with study development and identifying relevant outcomes for the study. They can aid in designing study recruitment materials and also assist in actively recruiting participants for the research study (Vogsen et al. 2020). They can also help with data analysis after the research study concludes. And they can help with planning dissemination and participating in dissemination efforts. This can include patient-written blog posts, social media posts, videos, and/or presentations. Patient partners can also help "translate" research findings for multiple audiences, making sure to create materials and summaries of the research that can be read by patients and caregivers, or used in mainstream media outreach, in addition to supporting the traditional forms of dissemination researchers may traditionally prioritize such as scientific conference presentations or journal publications.

Setting expectations for patients invites discussion around whether patient partners feel equipped to participate in those roles or components of a project. In some cases, team culture may need adjusting to allow for equitable contributions from patient research partners. In other cases, patient research partners may not yet have the skills to contribute to an area where you would like their involvement.

You can help them learn as they go through the process like an apprenticeship ('learn on the job') if they are willing to give it a try, or you may realize that you want to recruit additional patient research partners with specific skill sets.

Or, you can offer more formal training and support to patient research partners to help them grow new skills and contribute to your and other research projects in additional ways. For example, some academic medical centers often provide (or require) patient partners access to web-based courses (CITI 2021) on the subjects of research ethics and compliance.

Training And Skill-Building For Patient Partners In Research

Patients may be identified for participating in research for one or more reasons. Perhaps they have been willing to share their own story or experiences; maybe they have raised awareness or funding for their disease; and likely they have already begun looking to help address problems for their larger community or communities. Depending on their background and other experiences, they may have a professional background where they have the relevant skills needed to contribute to any phase or type of research. Other patients may not have the same background or training, and would benefit from additional training or support to develop skills specific to being a patient research partner. Patient partners often learn 'on the job' and with 'trial by fire' on their first project, but there are other programs that exist to aid patients in gaining research skills that you could proactively suggest that patient partners look into, and/or recommend they participate in before you recruit them for a specific project.

For example, the International Association for Study of Lung Cancer (IASLC) created the STARS program for "Supportive Training for Advocates on Research & Science". They recruit patients and caregivers with personal experiences in cancer to become "patient research advocates". The STARS program involves education and training related to cancer research, enabling participants to subsequently improve research relevance, quality, and dissemination (Davis 2021).

Such a specific program may not yet exist in your research area for you to point patient research partners to, but if not, you may be able to reach out to disease-focused organization related to your area of study and help them develop a program, make existing resources more widely available, and/or tailor existing resources to help patients in their specific subject area learn how to engage in the research process.

PCORI has resources for both patient research partners as well as researchers seeking to engage patient partners (Anon. 2021), and many other resource lists exist (CIHR 2020) to support patient research partners and researchers. Patient partners themselves also often create their own resources and contribute to the literature to support future patient research partners. Liz Salmi, for example, works to make it easier or patients to participate in research (Salmi 2020) and aids in supporting patient partnership development (Kwan et al. 2019).

The perfect resource may not yet exist for your research area, so if you're working with patient research partners already, it's worth asking: what materials could you and your patient research partners develop to better help other researchers and patient research partners in the future? What you've learned by partnering together is likely very valuable to other patient research partners and researchers, and could (and maybe should) be shared in addition to your own research outcomes. Consider sharing them in the traditional literature (and especially in an open access journal where possible), on your website, on social media, and also by presenting at relevant conferences – or all of the above.

Engaging Patient Researchers Who Are Driving Their Own Research

Patients may want to contribute to research in a variety of ways, up to and including performing research on their own.

Some may feel that the only way to "steer the ship" is by leading research themselves, because they see a need that is not currently being met by existing academic and/or clinical researchers. Others may feel like the area of research they want to focus on has been de-prioritized or deemed not relevant by funders or other organizations. As a result, they may seek to get involved at the ultimate level of becoming researchers themselves.

One great example of this is Sara Riggare who has "made the management of my own disease the topic of research", conducting a doctoral degree in self-tracking and personal science for Parkinson's disease, and considers herself a "patient researcher" (Riggare 2020). She has contributed to participatory design in Parkinson's research (Serrano et al. 2015), n – 1 placebo-controlled studies (Riggare et al. 2017), patient-initiated self-tracking (Riggare and Hägglund 2018), and more.

She is not the only example of patients who switched into research fields. Sonia Vallabh and her husband, Eric Vallabh Minikel, changed careers after Sonia's mom passed away from a rare prion disease and Sonia found out that she inherited the same mutation (Bichell 2017). They pursued PhDs from Harvard Medical School in Biological and Biomedical Sciences and now have a plan for developing a preventative drug for prion diseases (Minikel n.d.).

On the other hand, there are some patients who happen to be professional researchers (of any kind) who pivot to health research as a result of their own or a family member's diagnosis and facing barriers to treatment or access to health data or information. Stephen Keating (Hosny et al. 2018) is one such example: he temporarily changed his affiliation at MIT while a PhD candidate in order to access his own brain tumor DNA as a researcher after he was previously denied access as a research participant (Bobe et al. 2019).

Similarly, Matt Might has a PhD in computer science and taught as a professor of computer science and pharmaceutical chemistry. He evolved his work to focus on precision medicine after his family did the research to determine the molecular cause of a new rare disease that their son was experiencing (Longshore n.d.).

But patients don't have to be PhDs, MDs, or otherwise serving as professional, traditional researchers - while also happening to be a patient - in order to lead research as a patient.

Some patient researchers have convened under non-profit organizations. For example, "ROS1ders" is a non-profit public benefit corporation bringing together an international group of patients and family members dealing with ROS1+ cancer (The ROS1ders 2021). Noting that the pace of research and drug delivery 'will not be fast enough to save us all' (Freeman-Daily n.d.), they work to collaboratively expedite and initiate research that previously was not done because of the perceived size of the relevant patient population. While raising funds for existing research is always a need in most disease areas, the ROS1ders group wanted to explore options for partnering to develop and conduct projects that specifically addressed unmet needs in ROS1 diagnosis and treatment, as well as prioritize and research questions that are most important to patients (Sustaining and Accelerating Research for ROS1+ Cancer 2021).

I can also speak from my own experience, where a background in health communications intersected with my open source work to make a closed loop "artificial pancreas" or "automated insulin delivery system"(Lewis 2019b), and led me to conducting research myself as an independent researcher (Lewis and Leibrand 2016). Like health technology development's slow timeline, I observed that it takes many years before academic or clinical researchers would pick up research or focus on the innovations created within and by individuals in the diabetes community. As a result, I began publishing the first literature on the open source diabetes innovations and launched research studies (Lewis 2018a; Melmer et al. 2019; Grant et al. 2021; Asarani et al. 2020) in partnership with the community, laying the groundwork for future research studies by traditional researchers, including a randomized control trial (Burnside et al. 2020) based on the open source technology that I helped create.

While presenting my independent research at a conference, I met and developed relationships with a group of new collaborators who really helped me better understand the opportunities for traditional researchers to support patient researchers (Lewis 2018b). This encounter began somewhat unproductively - because they suggested running an observational trial on the community. But, that's not what the community needed. When I told them so, they pivoted to ask the question, *"What can we do to help? What do you need?"*, and it opened up a productive conversation and relationship where we were able to collaborate on a grant (Lewis 2017)—with myself as the lead scientific PI driving the project (Lewis 2018c)—and successive collaborations (Pine et al. 2020).

If You Want To Support Patient Researchers, First Ask: "How Can I Help?"

If you are looking to go from engaging patients in your own research to supporting and encouraging their own research: first ask, *"How can I help?"* and think through what resources and support that you could provide. This could be mentorship and support as they navigate grant writing and the grant making process, if they're going down that path. It could be collaborative authorship with them on scientific papers and/or presentations at scientific conferences—if they desire such support. You could help them gain funding for their efforts, or otherwise support them, without taking over and making it "your" research - unless you're invited to do so.

It's helpful to be aware of and clear about your intentions, and first determine whether you should best help from afar, such as with public support and promotion of their work; aid in networking and linking them in to your communities; or by identifying and funneling resource opportunities their way. Or, you could provide hands-on support to their research. But first, ask.

Instead of viewing patient researchers as people who work "outside of the system" or "don't know what they're doing", your perspective may change if you consider their fresh take to traditional research as a benefit. They may not have the same levels of expertise in working with academia that you do, but that means often they have fresh ideas or see opportunities to do things differently. You can encourage and support novice and established patient researchers the same way you might mentor and support other early career researchers such as PhD students, post-docs, and other new career researchers in various roles:

- You can help patient researchers develop and identify resources to fund their work, if it needs funding.
- You can cite their work, when relevant.
- You can mentor them about the research itself, the process of scientific publications and/or scientific conferences, and other "system" elements where there is no guidebook and unspoken rules of the road that are the 'hidden curriculum (Mahood 2011)' of the research world.
- You can also provide resources such as access to journals or articles, access to scientific conferences, and access - and explicit invitations - to meetings.
- You can advocate for an affordable "patient membership" level for inclusion to professional societies, as well as patient scholarship or funded patient involvement programs to attend research and healthcare conferences.
- You can make a seat for them at the table and make sure patient voices - as researchers and as patients—are included in relevant conversations.

While you may not have the expertise or desire to contribute directly to the research project a patient is leading, if you are interested in supporting their work, you could also consider housing their work by providing fiscal sponsorship through your organization. For patient researchers who do not have an "academic home" or who do not do their work out of a non-profit organization or similar organization set up to manage grants, they are often unable to be grant funded as individuals. However, they can receive grants as a PI with co-PI's at universities, so that the university handles the grant funding and they can continue to do the work (often as a subcontractor or consultant into the grant, to receive their own funding for their time on the project). This can be immensely helpful (Lewis 2019c), especially if you are already established as a grant-funded researcher and you are comfortable working with your university administrators to receive and process grants. There is a lot of red tape (paperwork) in receiving a grant, and by taking on that work, it frees the patient researcher to focus on the research and not having to work 'the system'.

But, each patient researcher may want or need different types or levels of support: including none at all. The best way to find out what they need is to develop relationships with them and to ask. They may not know offhand what they need, but by offering ideas and having a positive relationship established, you may be able to identify over time the best way to successfully collaborate and advance their work, in addition to all the ways that patient partners can also empower and support your own research.

Conclusion

You can play a role in increasing the number of patients partnering in research, by inviting and engaging them in your own research efforts; creating materials to support other researchers to successfully engage patients in the research process; and also supporting patients who are researchers in their own right. Patients can and should be involved at every stage of research, and will provide immense value to the work, to the research team, and to the ultimate recipients of research: the patient community themselves.

Clinical Pearls
1. You may think you are ready to partner with patients, but do you know how to get started? Do you have any existing relationships with patients? You can use the Opening Pathways Partner Readiness Quiz to assess your readiness to equitably partner with patients and ensure that you and your patient stakeholder research partner have a strong start. See https://partner.openingpathways.org/quiz as a resource. You can also save your answers and review or share them with your potential patient stakeholder research partner to help you further your relationship.
2. Based on this chapter, you now have a few ways to identify patients who can partner with you on research. But one key step is developing an open relationship that allows for feedback in both directions so that you can collaborate effectively. One thing you can do is ask patients who have previously had research engagement what did NOT go well in other projects. Developing a list of "to don't" in your design criteria to work to not do can be as effective as having a to-do list.
3. Be an active partner ally to patients by improving the culture of research overall. Coach, mentor and support your colleagues and fellow researchers and help them become better partners for engaging patients in research. If a patient speaks up and voices a problem with research or the research

process - whether it is your work or someone else's - support them in their efforts to improve the culture and process of research.

4. There are other tools such as the PCORI Engagement Rubric (Sheridan et al. 2017) and the 7Ps of Stakeholder Engagement (Concannon et al. 2012) for evaluating additional methods for stakeholder engagement and evaluating patients as research partners and evaluating benefits of patient contributions to research. If you need more resources or rationale for engaging patients in research, ask the patient community!

Chapter Review Question & Answers

1. Imagine that you have a research project where you would like to apply for funding, and the funder mandates that you have a patient involved in your research project. At what stage do you involve a patient in your project, and how would you do so?
2. You are at a scientific conference and observe a patient giving a presentation about their own research or project. They're not a traditional researcher - they don't have a PhD or have a day job as a researcher. You want to offer your help with their research. What do you offer when you approach them?

Answers

1. You should try to involve a patient as soon as you have a project identified and before you write and submit your grant application. You might want to start networking with patients to identify potential research partners even before you have a specific project idea. If you can identify the right patient, you'll want to give them the opportunity to contribute ideas and feedback to the project proposal, so it is important to identify them and incorporate them into the research team as soon as possible - don't wait until after you have received funding or after you have submitted a funding application. It is also important to establish any patient partner as a team member and to be clear about the role you would like them to play, and provide feedback and specifically invite their participation if they seem shy or unsure of how to contribute when you expect their contributions.
2. You can approach patient researchers and share your enthusiasm and support for their work, first and foremost. You can ask what direction their research is heading next, and whether they have any blockers that they might want help addressing (such as funding, funding infrastructure such as where to house a grant, or knowledge about how to navigate the research system and processes). If they have a clear need, you may want to offer your direct help - but only if you know you can and will follow through on the offer. Otherwise, you can offer to keep in touch and develop a relationship where you could assist in future, if a need arises.

References

Asarani NA, Reynolds AN, Elbalshy M, Burnside M, de Bock M, Lewis DM, Wheeler BJ. Efficacy, safety, and user experience of DIY or open-source artificial pancreas systems: a systematic review. Acta Diabetol. 2020; https://doi.org/10.1007/s00592-020-01623-4.

Bichell RE. A couple's quest to stop a rare disease before it takes one of them. In: NPR. https://www.npr.org/sections/health-shots/2017/06/19/527795512/a-couples-quest-to-stop-a-rare-disease-before-it-takes-one-of-them. Accessed 13 Apr 2021 2017.

Bobe J et al. Privacy and agency are critical to a flourishing biomedical research enterprise: misconceptions about the role of CLIA (December 6, 2019). Florida Law Review Forum, Forthcoming, Available at SSRN: https://ssrn.com/abstract=3499923

Burnside M, Lewis D, Crocket H, Wilson R, Williman J, Jefferies C, Paul R, Wheeler BJ, de Bock M. CREATE (community deRivEd AutomaTEd insulin delivery) trial. Randomised parallel arm open label clinical trial comparing automated insulin delivery using a mobile controller (AnyDANA-loop) with an open-source algorithm with sensor augmented pump therapy in type 1 diabetes. J Diabetes Metab Disord. 2020;19:1615–29.

Chalmers I, Jackson W, Carvel D. People are "participants" in research. BMJ. 1999;318:–1141.

CIHR. Patient engagement in research resources. In: CIHR. https://cihr-irsc.gc.ca/e/51916.html. 2020 Accessed 9 Apr 2021.

CITI Program Individual learners. In: CITI Program. https://about.citiprogram.org/en/individual-learners/. Accessed 11 Aug 2021.

Concannon TW, Meissner P, Grunbaum JA, et al. A new taxonomy for stakeholder engagement in patient-centered outcomes research. J Gen Intern Med. 2012;27:985–91. https://doi.org/10.1007/s11606-012-2037-1.

Davis LE. Program trains patient research advocates to be STARS. In: IASLC. https://www.iaslc.org/iaslc-news/ilcn/program-trains-patient-research-advocates-be-stars. 2021. Accessed 9 Apr 2021.

Decker M, Hemmerling A, Lankoande F. Women front and center: the opportunities of involving women in participatory Health Research worldwide. J Women's Health. 2010;19:2109–14.

Domecq JP, Prutsky G, Elraiyah T, et al. Patient engagement in research: a systematic review. BMC Health Serv Res. 2014; https://doi.org/10.1186/1472-6963-14-89.

Duffett L. Patient engagement: what partnering with patient in research is all about. Thromb Res. 2017;150:113–20.

Freeman-Daily J. ROS1ders Patient group promotes research. In: National Cancer Institute. n.d.. https://www.cancer.gov/about-nci/organization/ccg/blog/2017/ros1-patient-driven-research. Accessed 13 Apr 2021.

Grant AD, Lewis DM, Kriegsfeld LJ. Multi-timescale rhythmicity of blood glucose and insulin delivery reveals key advantages of hybrid closed loop therapy. J Diabetes Sci Technol. 2021; 193229682199482

Greenhalgh T, Hinton L, Finlay T, Macfarlane A, Fahy N, Clyde B, Chant A. Frameworks for supporting patient and public involvement in research: systematic review and co-design pilot. Health Expect. 2019;22:785–801.

Hosny A, Keating SJ, Dilley JD, et al. From improved diagnostics to presurgical planning: high-resolution functionally graded multimaterial 3D printing of biomedical tomographic data sets. 3D Printing and Additive Manufacturing. 2018;5:103–13.

Kwan B, Salmi L, Saria MG, Otis-Green S. Stakeholder partnership development for brain cancer palliative care research: research priorities and unmet needs. In: Annals of Behavioral Medicine 2019 Mar 1 (Vol. 53, pp. S545-S545).

Levitan B, Getz K, Eisenstein EL, Goldberg M, Harker M, Hesterlee S, Patrick-Lake B, Roberts JN, DiMasi J. Assessing the financial value of patient engagement: a quantitative approach from CTTI's patient groups and clinical trials project. Ther Innov Regul Sci. 2018;52:220–9.

Lewis D. Opening pathways for discovery, research, and innovation in health and healthcare. In: DIYPS.org. https://diyps.org/2017/09/15/opening-pathways-for-discovery-research-and-innovation-in-health-and-healthcare/. Accessed 13 Apr 2021 2017.

Lewis D. History and perspective on DIY closed looping. J Diabetes Sci Technol. 2018a;13:790–3.

Lewis D. What I want to tell others doing patient-driven work. In: Opening Pathways. http://openingpathways.org/what-I-want-to-share-with-others-doing-patient-driven-work. Accessed 13 Apr 2021 2018b.

Lewis D. First Lessons learned as a patient PI. In: Opening Pathways. http://openingpathways.org/first-lessons-learned-as-patient-PI. Accessed 13 Apr 2021 2018c.

Lewis D. Patient in the cage. In: Opening Pathways. http://openingpathways.org/patient-in-the-cage. Accessed 9 Apr 2021 2019a.

Lewis D. Automated Insulin Delivery: How artificial pancreas "closed loop" systems can aid you in living with diabetes. 2019b.

Lewis D. Reflecting on the life of the Opening Pathways grant. In: Opening Pathways. http://openingpathways.org/reflecting-on-life-of-opening-pathways-grant. Accessed 13 Apr 2021. 2019c.

Lewis D, Leibrand S. Real-world use of open source artificial pancreas systems. J Diabetes Sci Technol. 2016;10:1411.

Longshore J. Codebreaker: A deeply personal quest made Matthew Might a leader in precision medicine and brought him to UAB. In: Home—The University of Alabama at Birmingham. n.d.. https://www.uab.edu/medicine/magazine/178-codebreaker-adeeply-personal-quest-made-matthew-might-a-leader-in-precision-medicine-and-brought-him-to-uab. Accessed 13 Apr 2021.

Mahood SC. Medical education: beware the hidden curriculum. Can Fam Physician. 2011;57:983–5.

Melmer A, Züger T, Lewis DM, Leibrand S, Stettler C, Laimer M. Glycaemic control in individuals with type 1 diabetes using an open source artificial pancreas system (OpenAPS). Diabetes Obes Metab. 2019;21:2333–7.

Minikel EV. About. In: CureFFI.org. http://www.cureffi.org/about/. Accessed 13 Apr 2021.

PCORI. In: Engagement resources. 2021. https://www.pcori.org/engagement/engagement-resources. Accessed 9 Apr 2021.

PCORI. Vision & mission. In: PCORI. https://www.pcori.org/about-us/our-vision-mission. Accessed 9 Apr 2021 2020.

Petersen C. Patient informaticians: turning patient voice into patient action. JAMIA Open. 2018;1(2):130–5. https://doi.org/10.1093/jamiaopen/ooy014.

Pine KH, Hinrichs MM, Wang J, Lewis D, Johnston E. How checks enable more impactful community engagement. Communications of the ACM. 2020.

Riggare S. Patient researchers—the missing link? Nat Med. 2020;26:1507.

Riggare S, Hägglund M. Precision medicine in Parkinson's disease—exploring patient-initiated self-tracking. J Parkinsons Dis. 2018;8:441–6.

Riggare S, Unruh K, Sturr J, Domingos J, Stamford J, Svenningsson P, Hägglund M. Patient-driven N-of-1 in Parkinson's disease. Methods Inf Med. 2017; https://doi.org/10.3414/me16-02-0040.

Salmi L. Making it easier to participate in research: a patient's perspective. In: Clinical Cancer Research. 2020 Jun 1 (Vol. 26, No. 12, pp. 17-17).

Serrano JA, Larsen F, Isaacs T, et al. Participatory design in Parkinson's research with focus on the symptomatic domains to be measured. J Parkinsons Dis. 2015;5:187–96.

Sheridan S, Schrandt S, Forsythe L, Hilliard TS, Paez KA, Advisory panel on patient engagement (2013 inaugural panel). The PCORI engagement rubric: promising practices for partnering in research. Ann Fam Med. 2017;15(2):165–70. https://doi.org/10.1370/afm.2042. PMID: 28289118; PMCID: PMC5348236

Smith E, Bélisle-Pipon J-C, Resnik D. Patients as research partners; how to value their perceptions, contribution and labor? Citizen Science: Theory and Practice. 2019. doi: https://doi.org/10.5334/cstp.184.

Sustaining and accelerating research for ROS1+ Cancer (March 31, 2021). Accessed 13 Appr 2021.

The ROS1ders. https://ros1cancer.com/. Accessed 13 Apr 2021.

Vogsen M, Geneser S, Rasmussen ML, et al. Learning from patient involvement in a clinical study analyzing PET/CT in women with advanced breast cancer. Res Involv Engagem. 2020;6:1. https://doi.org/10.1186/s40900-019-0174-y.

Chapter 18
User-Centered Development and Evaluation of Patient-Facing Visualizations of Health Information

Meghan Reading Turchioe and Ruth Masterson Creber

Abstract User-centered design is a design philosophy in which the end user is the expert and their goals and needs drive the design process. The end user is deeply integrated into the design process, from the early conceptualizations of a visualization through iterative design cycles and ultimately the implementation of interactive interfaces that include visualization. This approach is crucial when designing visualizations oriented towards patients displaying their personal health data—patient-facing visualizations—to ensure that visualizations are comprehended by target patient populations, who may have unique sociocultural backgrounds and needs with respect to health literacy, numeracy, and graph literacy. As personal health information is returned to patients at an increasing rate through patient portals and other mobile health technology, well-designed visualizations can improve comprehension of health information and reduce anxiety, confusion, and potentially unsafe responses. In this chapter, we provide suggestions for best practices for user-centered design of patient-facing visualizations, including selecting a framework to guide the design process, gathering requirements to understand the end user, and conducting rigorous evaluation studies. To illustrate many of these best practices, we provide a detailed case study describing the development of *mi.Symptoms*, a mobile health application that uses patient-facing visualizations to support symptom self-monitoring of symptoms for older adults with heart failure. The visualizations used in *mi.Symptoms* were developed through a set of iterative design activities to determine desired content as well as features and functions to increase usability of a symptom monitoring application for older adults.

Keywords User-centered design · Data visualization · Personal health information
Mobile health · Consumer health information · Culturally appropriate technology

M. R. Turchioe (✉) · R. M. Creber
School of Nursing, Columbia University, New York, NY, USA
e-mail: mr3554@cumc.columbia.edu; rm3284@cumc.columbia.edu

© The Author(s), under exclusive license to Springer Nature
Switzerland AG 2022
P.-Y. S. Hsueh et al. (eds.), *Personal Health Informatics*, Cognitive Informatics
in Biomedicine and Healthcare, https://doi.org/10.1007/978-3-031-07696-1_18

Learning Objectives
- Identify unique attributes of patient-facing visualizations and current challenges associated with designing these types of visualizations.
- Describe the user-centered design process and its importance when designing patient-facing visualizations.
- Describe qualitative and quantitative approaches to gathering requirements from end users prior to development of patient-facing visualizations.
- Identify key outcome measures, sampling strategies, and study designs to be considered when designing rigorous evaluation studies.
- Apply the principles of user-centered design to a case study describing the iterative process of developing an interface for a patient-facing mobile health technology that features data visualizations.

Introduction

Personal health information is being returned to patients in a variety of different formats from different devices (2016 Program Requirements. https://www.cms.gov/Regulations-and-Guidance/Legislation/EHRIncentivePrograms/2016ProgramRequ irements; Oh et al. 2005; Mishra et al. 2019; Jeevanandan and Nøhr 2020; Baumhauer 2017; Cortez et al. 2018; Lai et al. 2017). A variety of national initiatives, including Meaningful Use Stage 2 (Centers for Medicare and Medicaid Services 2012), which gives patients access to their medical results, and OpenNotes (Wolff et al. 2017) which gives patient's access to their medical notes, have both given patients more access to their medical record information. At the same time, patients have access to their own patient-generated health data, including patient-reported outcomes (PROs), through smartphone mobile health (mHealth) apps and wearables (Cortez et al. 2018; Lai et al. 2017). The overall purpose of returning this health information to patients is to increase patient knowledge of their health conditions, engagement with managing their disease or condition, and ultimately to support positive behavior change.

A significant challenge related to the return of patient information is that many patients struggle to comprehend their personal health data when it is represented as raw data or with medical jargon.

Displaying raw results, without interpretation or contextualization, makes it accessible only to the most well-educated and health-literate patients who are informed about the specific outcome measures that are being used. This is important because a high proportion of U.S. adults have low health literacy; the U.S. Department of Education has estimated that only 12% of U.S. adults have proficient health literacy (U.S. Department of Health and Human Services (HHS) 2009). Returning data in a format that supports comprehension represents an opportunity for the patient to become a more active participant in their own health. Providing health information in an inaccessible format can drive intervention-generated inequity, a phenomenon in which well-intentioned interventions worsen existing health disparities, rather than reduce them (Veinot et al. 2018; Lorenc et al. 2013; Hart 1971).

Many healthcare professionals are reluctant to give patients direct access to their health data without interpretation due to concerns about poor comprehension, risk perception, and misunderstandings that could cause anxiety or a potentially dangerous response (Lai et al. 2017; Reading and Merrill 2018). Given the potential for misunderstanding, many healthcare professionals prefer to directly deliver medical results and information to patients so they can provide necessary interpretation and contextualization (Sanger et al. 2016; Cohen et al. 2016; Cheng et al. 2015). Despite the direct provision of health information between a patient and healthcare processional being ideal, the sheer volume of patient data often makes this infeasible. Therefore, it is imperative to be intentional about supporting patients to comprehend their own health information.

Defining Patient-Facing Visualizations

Visualizations are defined as the representation of information using graphs or images (Fekete et al. 2008; Hawley et al. 2008; Solomon et al. 2016; Zikmund-Fisher et al. 2017). The human brain can perceive even small differences in the size, shape, color, and spatial position of objects and build cognitive maps based on these perceived differences, making visualizations powerful tools for communication (Chen 2017). Visualizations are often used to aid in the interpretation of health-related information (Grossman et al. 2018; Woods et al. 2016; Few 2013). When visualizations are oriented towards patients by displaying their personal health data, they are called *patient-facing visualizations*. The most common types of patient-facing visualizations are described in Fig. 18.1; these include visual paragraphs, icons, number lines, body maps, radar graphs, scatterplots, line graphs, and bar graphs. It is important to note that the names of different patient-facing visualizations may vary by field. Therefore, it is most useful to refer to images or descriptions rather than names of visualizations.

There are many reasons that patient-facing visualizations have become widely used. Studies have shown that visualizations have helped patients understand their laboratory test results (Solomon et al. 2016; Zikmund-Fisher et al. 2014, 2017; Morrow et al. 2017), different treatment options available to them (Hawley et al. 2008; Zikmund-Fisher et al. 2008a, b; Vogt and Marteau 2012), and personal risk for certain health conditions which improves their medical decision making (Hawley et al. 2008; Wegier and Shaffer 2017; Stone et al. 2017; Siegrist et al. 2008). In addition, visualizations help patients who may lack an in-depth understanding of medical concepts and jargon to better interpret and contextualize health data. For example, colors can communicate when data is outside of normal ranges better than written text or numbers (Arcia et al. 2015). Designers can use shades and tints to create additional discrimination between colors for colorblind users to be able to detect differences. Colorblind filters can be used to ensure adequate contrast

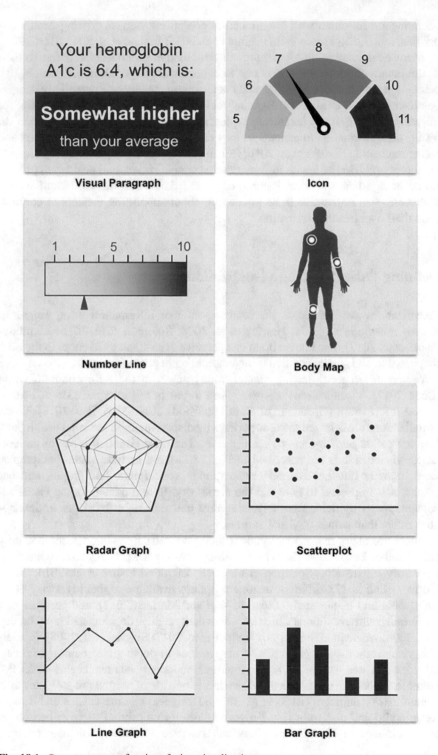

Fig. 18.1 Common types of patient-facing visualizations

between colors, especially the most common forms of colorblindness: red-green and blue-yellow (National Eye Institute (NEI) 2019). As more technologies are being developed to deliver personal health information to patients, including patient portals, mobile applications, and wearable devices, visualizations are a clear and effective way to communicate the most salient information while focusing attention away from granular and non-clinically significant changes in the data (i.e., noise) (Grossman et al. 2018).

Patient-facing visualizations are still relatively new compared to visualizations of health data created for research or medical communities. As a result, there are still many challenges that the design, human-computer interaction, and informatics communities are facing when designing these types of visualizations. Patients use different cognitive processes to interpret and contextualize health data because their mental models of disease processes usually differ from researchers and clinicians with advanced knowledge of statistics and medicine (Mamykina et al. 2016; Garcia-Retamero and Cokely 2017). Some health-related information is inherently statistically complex; for example, the widely used Patient-Reported Outcomes Measurement Information System (PROMIS) reports patient-reported outcomes as T-scores with standard deviations. Interpretation of the scales, and comparison of scores between scales, is a major challenge for patients (Snyder et al. 2012).

There is also wide variation in numeracy and graph literacy among patients. As much as 40% of the U.S. population has poor graph literacy, meaning they have difficulty interpreting information presented graphically (Galesic and Garcia-Retamero 2011). However line graphs have been the most commonly used patient-facing visualization to date (Snyder et al. 2017; Brundage et al. 2015; Smith et al. 2016; Arcia et al. 2018; Tolbert et al. 2018; Turchioe et al. 2019a). Therefore, those developing patient-facing visualizations are now beginning to explore options beyond graphs (Turchioe et al. 2020). Patients may also have varying levels of health literacy and may have cognitive impairment due to disease- or age-related processes, which influences comprehension of visualizations (Turchioe et al. 2020). Interpretation of visualizations, particularly the meaning attributed to a specific color or icon, also varies by sociocultural backgrounds. Finally, visualizations that can be quickly and easily interpreted in real-world circumstances, in which patients may be distracted or have limited time to view and comprehend information, is an important consideration; many studies evaluate visualizations in controlled, laboratory-based settings only when patients have more time to study and understand the information being presented (Snyder et al. 2017; Brundage et al. 2015; Smith et al. 2016; Arcia et al. 2018; Tolbert et al. 2018; Sun and May 2013).

Importance of User-Centered Design and Evaluation

Because of the challenges of designing visualizations that patients can understand and interpret accurately, user-centered design is a critically important activity. *User-centered design* is a design philosophy in which the goals and needs of the end user, or in this case the patient viewing a visualization, drive the design process; the end user is the expert (Saffer 2010). User-centered design involves a set of activities and approaches that are iterative in nature; designs are created, evaluated by end users, modified based on the feedback and evaluated again. In this way, the end user is deeply integrated into the design process, from the early conceptualizations of a visualization through the implementation of interactive interfaces that include visualization. These activities are crucial to ensure that visualizations are comprehended by target patient populations, who may have unique socio-cultural backgrounds and needs with respect to health literacy, numeracy, and graph literacy.

Although it is an essential element in the development of highly effective patient-facing visualizations, user-centered design is not always done. A recent systematic review of patient-facing visualizations found that nearly half of the articles reviewed did not conduct an evaluation with patients or describe patient involvement in the design process (Turchioe et al. 2019a). Moreover, of the studies that did evaluate visualizations, a wide range of methods and outcomes measures were used. While there is an absence of clear standards, in this chapter we offer suggestions for best practices for conducting user-centered design of patient-facing visualizations.

Best Practices for User-Centered Design

Suggestion 1: Selecting a Framework

Depending on the purpose of the consumer health informatics tool, we recommend starting with a user-centered design framework and health behavior change model to inform the user-centered design process. If specific patient-reported outcomes (PROs) are measured in the CHI tool, we also recommend documentation of a specific measurement model for the specific PRO measure, as reported by the International Society for Quality of Life Research (ISOQOL) (Reeve et al. 2013). If the goal of the tool is to promote health behavior change, a health behavior change model can guide design choices. Commonly employed behavior change models include, but are not limited to, the Health Belief Model, Theory of Reasoned Action, Stages of Change Model, and Self-Determination Theory. For example, one study mapped different features of a mobile application for self-monitoring of Type 2 diabetes to different levels of intrinsic motivation to self-monitor based on Self-Determination Theory (Turchioe et al. 2019b).

There are also several general user-centered design frameworks; each have similar components, including iterative processes for designing, testing, and revising, with each iteration incorporating prior feedback into the next design iteration. Also, core to the UCD process is incorporating specific behavior change or technology acceptance models to help ensure visualizations and CHI tools involving visualizations align with user behaviors. One example of a user-centered design framework

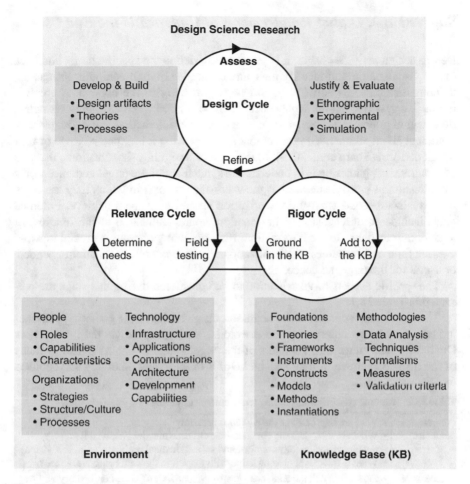

Fig. 18.2   The Information System Research (ISR) framework

is the Information System Research (ISR) framework (Fig. 18.2). The ISR framework includes three distinct cycles: Relevance, Rigor, and Design. In the relevance cycle, the needs of the end users and the contexts of use are explored. In the rigor cycle, relevant literature and fundamental theories are consulted, and additional studies developing theories, frameworks, instruments, or methods are conducted to contribute to the knowledge base as appropriate. In the design cycle, iterative design, development, and evaluation activities are conducted to create and refine prototypes with extensive end user feedback. Other frameworks also exist for specific contexts of user-centered design. For example, the International Patient Decision Aid Standards (IPDAS) Collaboration has created detailed processes for engaging end users in decision aid design (International Patient Decision Aid Standards (IPDAS) Collaboration 2013).

Suggestion 2: Gather Requirements to Understand the End User

Before design activities begin, it is important to define the specific target audience of the visualization and identify their unique needs. Human-computer interaction communities call this activity *requirements gathering* in the context of creating interactive systems, but the same concept can be applied when designing visualizations within interactive systems. In human-computer interaction, a *requirement* is a statement about an intended product that specifies what it is expected to do or how it will perform (Sharp et al. 2019). In the case of designing visualizations, the goal of requirements gathering is to understand as much about the target audience of the visualization as possible, as well as the ways and contexts in which they are using the visualization and what the visualization should help them achieve. Potential goals include comprehension of information, contextualization of information, or an action in response to the information. Requirement gathering is crucial to avoid wasting time and resources on visualizations that are not effective, comprehended, or useful for the target audience.

The specific aspects of visualization to be considered during this stage are presented in Table 18.1.

There are many approaches for requirements gathering. Data gathering activities include qualitative interviews, observations, and quantitative data collection. Qualitative interviews with members of the target audience can help answer many of the questions above. It may also be helpful to interview other key stakeholders

Table 18.1 Example considerations during requirements gathering

Target audience	• Who are they? Define the audience precisely • What are their defining characteristics? These may include health literacy, numeracy, technology comfort, and salient medical problems (e.g., low vision) • What is their level of knowledge with respect to the data being visualized?
Contexts of use	• How often will the audience view the visualization? Working memory will be lower with less frequent viewing and therefore require more support to engage with and understand the visualization • How much time will the audience have to view, comprehend, and synthesize information being presented? • How will the visualization be displayed? If electronically, how will screen size (mobile phones, tablets, laptops, and desktop computers) impact design choices? • What are salient characteristics (if any) of the physical environment in which the audience will view the visualization? Light levels, noise, distractions, and the physical presence of others nearby who can provide assistance may influence comprehension and overall engagement with a visualization
Data being visualized	• What kinds of data need to be visualized—categorical or continuous; longitudinal or cross-sectional? • How much detail in the data is important to show versus data summaries? • Are there privacy concerns or sensitive information that may need to be displayed with more nuance? • Will the data update or refresh over time? If so, is it important to differentiate data collected or extracted at different times?

with important perspectives about contexts of use and the needs of the target audience; for example, healthcare providers who routinely deliver certain types of health data to patients may have important insights about how patients comprehend and use these data. Observations of the target audience viewing and interacting with the visualization may be useful when the context of use, and particularly the physical environment, is unique and expected to substantially influence how an individual engages with a visualization.

There are also several quantitative measures that are beneficial to measure as they provide useful context about the target audience. Constructs that relate directly to the comprehension of information in a visualization include health literacy (Chew et al. 2004), numeracy (McNaughton et al. 2015), and graph literacy (Galesic and Garcia-Retamero 2011; Okan et al. 2019), which can all be measured using brief screening tools. Additionally, there are validated scales objectively assessing cognitive status, such as the Montreal Cognitive Assessment or MoCA (Nasreddine et al. 2005), and the self-identified presence of physical, hearing-related, or visual disabilities can also be ascertained ((ISO), International Organization for Standardization 2014). Finally, it may be important to quantify technology experience, including computer ownership, smartphone ownership, and Internet access and use (Masterson Creber et al. 2019; Creber et al. 2016a), if the visualization will be accessed electronically.

After data is collected, it can be analyzed and translated into requirements for the visualization. The process of translating requirements is also best served by involvement with the target audience and other stakeholders. After an initial set of requirements are generated, they can be discussed and iterated upon with the target audience.

One important challenge that has been broadly described in the literature is engaging a wide range of end users. Typically, the most engaged end users are the easiest to recruit for requirements gathering studies, which can result in designs that are only usable to the most engaged individuals. A critical area for future work is developing strategies to involve individuals who may be less likely to proactively engage in technologies for health management, but who could potentially benefit from them the most if used. One promising approach is leveraging the infrastructure of stakeholder engagement boards and community-based participatory research studies that have already conducted intense outreach and engagement within a specific community or group of individuals. For example, one study leveraged the community-based study, "Washington Heights Initiative Community-based Comparative Effectiveness Research," to recruit low-income Latino adults with multiple chronic conditions for design sessions when creating a self-monitoring application (Turchioe et al. 2019b; Reading Turchioe et al. 2020a). However, strategies for involving less engaged end users is an important problem deserving more attention in future work.

Suggestion 3: Apply Rigor in Designing Evaluation Studies

After visualizations are designed, they must be rigorously tested with the target audience through evaluation studies. The purpose of evaluation studies is to show that a visualization achieves its goals. Evaluation studies may also highlight opportunities to improve visualizations, and the revised visualizations are again evaluated. In this way, design and evaluation activities are tightly interconnected and iterative in nature.

Once the visualization goals are clearly defined, objective measures can be selected to quantify the effectiveness of the visualization in meeting the goals. Many times, evaluation studies ask the target audience which visualizations they prefer. Ways of measuring preferences include asking participants to select their favorite visualization out of a series or identify which aspects of a visualization they like most and least. While preferences provide important insights for design, they should not be the only outcome measure or used as a proxy for comprehension. In fact, studies have found that patients often prefer visualizations that they do not objectively understand (Turchioe et al. 2020; Brewer et al. 2012). Therefore, it is important to measure objective outcomes, as well. Some important objective outcomes to consider measuring, along with validated scales used to measure these outcomes, are described in Table 18.2.

There are different strategies for sampling participants for evaluation studies, which should also be selected based on the target audience and visualization goals. Online samples can be recruited through platforms such as Prolific (Palan and Schitter 2018; Peer et al. 2017) and Amazon Mechanical Turk (Strickland and Stoops 2019; Mortensen and Hughes 2018). These platforms allow for visualizations to be tested with extremely large sample sizes, and are ideal for visualizations intended for more general audiences. For example, these platforms have been used to test different visualizations displaying laboratory test results (Zikmund-Fisher et al. 2017), which is relevant for nearly all individuals who receive healthcare. While some sites allow segmentation by demographic characteristics and geographic location, in general, it is difficult to recruit a very specific type of sample on these sites (for example, older adults or patients with a specific disease). Therefore, in other cases, it may be desirable to recruit a more targeted population. Strategic recruitment depends on the key characteristics of the target audience; for example, if the audience is patients with a specific disease, recruitment can take place in healthcare settings (including clinics or inpatient areas) that treat that disease. A downside to this approach is that sample sizes will be limited, as recruitment will take more time and resources compared to online samples.

When multiple versions or types of visualization will be evaluated in a study, counterbalancing is a helpful strategy to reduce bias in the results. *Counterbalancing* involves systematically randomizing the order and information contained in each visualization. This is important to reduce *order effects*—the order of the visualizations having an effect on outcomes. Participants may learn more information as they view each subsequent visualization, making comprehension appear to be higher for

Table 18.2 Objective evaluation study outcome measures

Construct	Rationale for inclusion	Example measurement tools	
		Instrument	Questions/measurement
Comprehension	Participants' objective comprehension of a visualization is necessary so it can inform their decision-making. Preferences cannot be used as a proxy for objective comprehension (Turchioe et al. 2020; Brewer et al. 2012)	Adapted ISO 9186 comprehension protocol ((ISO), International Organization for Standardization 2014; Rn et al. 2019)	How would you explain what this means to a loved one?
		Response time (Brewer et al. 2012)	Viewing time between seeing the visualization and answering the comprehension question
Risk perception	Appropriate when visualizations show risk information. Risk perception mediates relationships between comprehension of visualizations and behavioral intention, and is influenced by an individual's numeracy levels (Zikmund-Fisher et al. 2008a; Garcia-Retamero and Cokely 2011)	Subjective risk perception questionnaire (Zikmund-Fisher et al. 2008a; Garcia-Retamero and Cokely 2011)	Three items asking about the perceived likelihood, seriousness, and concern for the worsening health condition
		Objective risk perception (Zikmund-Fisher et al. 2008a)	Two items measuring gist recall (remembering the gist of the visualization; ex: Values were worsening) and verbatim recall (remembering the key data; ex: Score dropped from 8 to 3) after visualization is removed from view
Behavioral intention	Appropriate when intention to act in response to a visualization is a goal	Adapted ISO 9186 comprehension protocol ((ISO), International Organization for Standardization 2014; Rn et al. 2019)	How likely would you be to do something in response to this visualization?

visualizations shown later in the sequence. A simple example of a study design using counterbalancing is provided in Fig. 18.3. In this example, each subsequent participant is shown a set of visualizations in a different order. The information in the visualizations can also be systematically randomized if it is thought to influence the outcomes being measured. For instance, in one study, both the type of visualization and direction (worsening, improving, or staying the same) of patient-reported outcomes scores being visualized were randomized (Turchioe et al. 2020).

Fig. 18.3 Example study design using counterbalancing

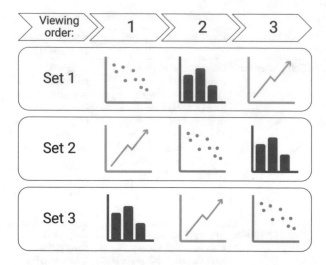

Randomization can also be employed through "A/B" testing, a rapid experimentation process intended to quickly identify optimal designs (Austrian et al. 2021). In A/B testing, two variants of the same application or web page are quickly deployed to different subsamples of the same target population, and outcome metrics of interest are gathered and compared. The two variants may be very different in a number of respects, or very similar with minor feature differences between them. The variant which performs the best on specified outcomes is modified and tested again. Multiple, rapid rounds of A/B testing are usually conducted until the outcomes are satisfactory; the best performing variant is then deployed more permanently. A/B testing is an ideal option for tools in which real-world endpoints, such as number of logins to a patient portal or messages to the care team, are most useful in assessing designs.

Case Study: User-Centered Design of a Mobile Application to Support Older Adults with Routine Symptom Monitoring

Here we present an in-depth case study intended to illustrate the user-centered design process from initial conception of the need for a mobile application through feasibility testing with the near-final application. The rationale for selecting a guiding design framework, specific data gathering methods, and design choices are described. By describing the process in detail, we aim to illustrate how to apply the concepts described above in an example context. Different contexts and use cases of patient-facing visualizations will call for different guiding frameworks and data collection methods.

Overview

mi.Symptoms is a mobile health (mHealth) application that uses patient-facing visualizations to support symptom self-monitoring of symptoms for older adults with heart failure, a highly prevalent condition in which symptom monitoring is important to reduce hospital admissions and improve outcomes (Riegel et al. 2011). This was an important problem to address because disparities in mHealth application use still exist among older adults. Advanced age and associated limited technology literacy, in addition to socioeconomic disparities, can be barriers to using mHealth to support symptom reporting, monitoring, and self-care management (Mishra et al. 2019). Older adults with chronic conditions may be unable or unwilling to take advantage of new technologies to monitor and manage symptoms that are not tailored to their needs (Creber et al. 2016b). Overall, accessibility of mobile applications for older adults, including mobile responsiveness and system response times, is a major concern in the field. Most mobile applications typically do not incorporate design principles to enhance accessibility for older adults (Jeevanandan and Nøhr 2020). This makes tailoring of mHealth applications to older adult populations through user-centered design critically important (Veinot et al. 2018; Creber et al. 2016c).

The visualizations used in *mi.Symptoms* were developed through a set of iterative design activities to determine desired content as well as features and functions to increase usability of a symptom monitoring application for older adults. Its development was guided by the three cycles of the ISR framework: Relevance, Rigor, and Design (Hevner 2007; Schnall et al. 2016).Across the Relevance and Design Cycles, multiple user-centered design methods were applied and older adult users were incorporated into each stage of development (Table 18.3). In the Relevance Cycle, pertinent symptoms, methods for the measurement of symptoms, and the optimal clinical location for measurement (inpatient setting, outpatient setting, or home) were identified. In the Rigor Cycle, features currently offered in mHealth apps were identified in a systematic review of existing commercially available applications. Across four Design Cycles, rapid iteration between prototyping the designs, refining the artifacts, and evaluating the prototypes based on end-user feedback took place.

Relevance Cycle

Structured surveys, semi-structured interviews, and field testing were used to identify pertinent symptoms, tools, and needs for reporting. Both global and disease-specific symptom measures were included in *mi.Symptoms*. For global measures, ten standardized Patient-Reported Outcome Measurement Information System

Table 18.3 Activities in the relevance, rigor and design cycles

Sample	Method	Purpose
Relevance cycle: Connects the *environment* and *design science research*		
Patients (n = 13), Health care providers (n = 11)	Semi-structured interviews	Identify pertinent symptoms and tools for measurement and needs among older adults (Grossman et al. 2018)
Rigor cycle: Connects *design science research* with a scientific *Knowledge Base*		
mHealth apps	Review of mHealth apps	Identify features available in commercially available mHealth apps by doing a review of the domain for older adults (Creber et al. 2016b)
Design cycle: Connects *develop and build* and *justify and evaluate* artifacts		
Patients (n = 13), Health care providers (n = 11)	**Phase I** Individual design sessions	Identify design features for symptom reporting and communication with healthcare providers among older adults (Grossman et al. 2018)
Patients (n = 168)	**Phase II** Usability	Evaluate usability for reporting physical and psychological symptoms (Baik et al. 2019; Reading Turchioe et al. 2020b; Masterson Creber et al. 2017)
Patients (n = 40)	**Phase III** Comprehension	Evaluate comprehension of summary visualizations (Turchioe et al. 2020)
Expert clinicians and informaticians (n = 7)	**Phase IV** Heuristic evaluation	Provide feedback on the content and examine usability heuristics with expert clinicians and informaticians

(PROMIS) short-form questionnaires were selected because they are freely available and not disease specific, thus capturing non-cardiac specific symptoms that are common across multiple chronic conditions. PROMIS questionnaires are linguistically validated in multiple languages and understandable at a sixth-grade reading level. To measure acute disease-specific physical symptoms, the Heart Failure Somatic Perception Scale was chosen (Jurgens et al. 2017). Semi-structured interviews with patient and healthcare provider participants were conducted to identify the most relevant symptoms to older adults: shortness of breath, swelling, pain, exercise intolerance, abdominal discomfort, fatigue, sleep disturbance, and anxiety. In addition, the literature was reviewed for pertinent design requirements for older adults and provide select themes in Table 18.4 (Zikmund-Fisher et al. 2014, 2017; Wu et al. 2013; Wynia and Osborn 2010; Zarcadoolas et al. 2013; Arcia et al. 2016).

Rigor Cycle

As previously published and summarized below (Creber et al. 2016b), a review of commercially available mobile health applications was conducted to support heart failure symptom self-monitoring. Thirteen keywords such as "heart failure," "cardiology," "heart failure and self-management," "heart failure and symptom management," were used across three mobile app stores: Apple iTunes Store, Android

Table 18.4 Design requirements for older adults and patients

Low numeracy	Low numeracy, defined as an inability to productively use quantitative health information (Wu et al. 2013), impacts a patient's ability to interpret quantitative health data and make informed decisions (Wynia and Osborn 2010). Considering low numeracy, text or simple visual displays may be optimal over graphs or tables
Older adults	When designing for older adults, researchers and others need to consider sensory and motor capabilities, and cognitive and numeracy abilities (Zarcadoolas et al. 2013). methods to improve usability in older adults include simple navigation without extensive branching, large touch-target regions with high responsiveness, large readable fonts, slower system response times (Zikmund-Fisher et al. 2014), consistent interaction patterns, verbose error messages, audio voice-overs, video content, and encouragement messages (Lyles et al. 2013)
Mobile-first	Considering the potential use of a mHealth app for outpatient self-management, patients may eventually complete surveys on personal devices at home, at work, or in public. The interface should use responsive design for viewing on various screen sizes and devices, and ensure privacy of personal identifying information
Longitudinal use	Patients may complete surveys periodically over time for self-management. The interface must change over time and with repeated use to successfully track symptoms longitudinally
High usability	To ensure use among low–technology-literacy patients and prevent socioeconomic disparities in use (Vogt and Marteau 2012), the interface must conform to usability heuristics such as visibility of system status and recovery from errors. To avoid overwhelming non-advanced users, consider placing access to advanced features in less prominent locations such as inside menus
Low health literacy	Disparities in both mHealth app and portal use have been well documented. The interface and graphics must be accessible to patients with a range of health literacy levels (Wynia and Osborn 2010; Arcia et al. 2013, 2016)

Google Play store, and Amazon Appstore. All applications were evaluated by two to four reviewers using the Mobile Application Rating Scale (Stoyanov et al. 2015), the functionality score from the IMS Institute for Healthcare Informatics report (Aitken and Gauntlett 2013), and Heart Failure Society of America guidelines for non-pharmacologic management (Lindenfeld et al. 2010). A total of 3636 apps were identified and 34 mHealth applications met the full inclusion criteria (Creber et al. 2016b). This review showed that mobile applications were generally in early stages of development, as few scored well across the domains of quality, functionality, and adherence to evidence-based guidelines. None were specifically designed for older adults (Creber et al. 2016b).

Based on this mobile application review, personal communication with experts in the field, and a summary of published literature, important design requirements for older adults were identified. The design requirements that were identified during the Rigor Cycle and the questionnaires measuring cardiac and non-cardiac symptoms identified during the Relevance Cycle were incorporated into subsequent Design Cycle activities.

Design Cycles

The purpose of the Design Cycle was to support development, evaluation, and refinement of *mi.Symptoms*. Four distinct design phases through the Design Cycles were conducted using static mock-ups (Design Phase I), interactive web-based prototypes (Design Phase II), paper-based prototypes of summary visualizations (Design Phase III), and the mobile interface (Design Phase IV).

Static (non-interactive) mock-ups were created using InDesign and PowerPoint for Design Phases I, III and IV. In Design Phase II, an interactive web-based prototype of *mi.Symptoms* was created using HTML/CSS/JavaScript for front-end development and ASP.NET as the back-end framework. Additionally, jQuery 1.12.4 was used as the JavaScript library to support older versions of Internet Explorer, which is an important consideration for our target population. From Design Phase II, specific limitations in comprehension of the summary visualizations were identified, so novel visualization formats were created and evaluated using paper-based prototypes in Design Phase III.

Design Phase I: Design Features

The objective of the first design phase was to identify design features for older adult patients with heart failure for symptom reporting and communication with healthcare providers through individual design sessions. The methods have been published and are summarized below (Grossman et al. 2018). Individual design sessions were conducted using storyboarding to detail patients' interactions with the interface and determine the necessary components. Storyboarding is a technique that involves displaying a set of illustrations shown in sequence to pre-visualize how navigation of an application will work (Truong et al. 2006). Each design session was audio-recorded, lasted 20–40 min, and covered topics on the application such as general usefulness, usefulness for patient–provider communication, helpful and unhelpful features, suggested changes, and the perceived impact of using a mHealth application to interact with their healthcare provider.

Based on the semi-structured interviews, five design themes were identified, including designing to: (1) aid comprehension, (2) return results to patients and providers, (3) support education, (4) promote communication, and (5) include multiple languages (Table 18.5) (Grossman et al. 2018).

Table 18.5 Design themes, descriptions and how they were identified (Phase 1)

Design to aid comprehension	Poor comprehension inhibited accurate symptom reporting	The interface incorporated visualizations to aid patient comprehension of symptom questions, answer choices, and results
Design to return results to patients and providers	Both patients and providers wished to track symptoms over time to aid disease management and identify missed opportunities for intervention	The interface conveyed symptom survey results to patients and providers
Design to support education	Patients described how the interface helped them associate their symptoms and underlying disease	The interface incorporated strategies to help patients strengthen connections between symptoms and the disease process and publicly available educational content developed by the American Heart Association
Design to promote communication	Patients described wanting unstructured messaging features to communicate further with their healthcare provider regarding their symptoms	The interface included an option for unstructured messaging
Design for multiple languages	Patients and providers reported the importance of the app being available in both English and Spanish in order to support comprehension	The web-app was available in English and Spanish

Design Phase II: Perceived Usability

The objective of the second design phase was to determine usability of *mi.Symptoms* for reporting physical and psychological symptoms. Each participant completed the *mi.Symptoms* application on an Apple iPad Pro. After completing *mi.Symptoms*, they were given a printout of their symptom report including their prioritized list of symptoms to communicate with their healthcare provider. Participants also completed a comprehensive demographic questionnaire, including health literacy (Chew et al. 2004), and evaluated usability by completing the Health-IT Usability Evaluation Scale (Health-ITUES) (Chen 2017) using Qualtrics survey software. To assess two key constructs related to usability, perceived usefulness and ease of use, a tailored version of the Health-ITUES (scores range from 1 to 5, lowest to highest) was used (Yen et al. 2010). For the data analysis, standard descriptive statistics of frequency, central tendency, and dispersion were applied to describe the sample characteristics, including demographics, health literacy, technology literacy, and Health-ITUES data in StataSE v13 (College Station, Texas) and R.

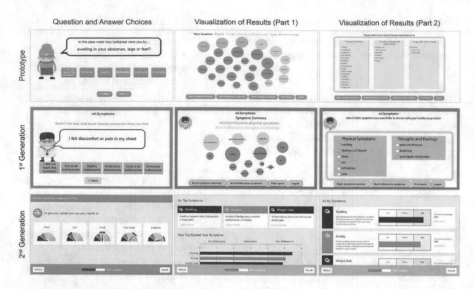

Fig. 18.4 mi.Symptoms interface and visualizations in the prototype, first and second generation web-app

In total, 168 English- and Spanish-speaking older adults with heart failure were recruited complete *mi.Symptoms* (Table 18.3, Phase II) (Reading Turchioe et al. 2020b). The visualizations in this design phase are included in Fig. 18.4. The top row is the prototype which was the first artifact described in Design Phase 1. The second row is the first Generation of mi.Symptoms that was evaluated in Design Phase 2. The third row is the second generation of mi.Symptoms that was evaluated in Design Phase 3 and 4 as a paper-based artifact.

Overall, participants were able to use *mi.Symptoms* to report complete PRO data with no missingness. The total scores for perceived usefulness and perceived ease of use measured using Health-ITUES were high, and usability scores did not significantly differ by age. These results demonstrated that it is feasible for older adults to use *mi.Symptoms* to report PROs. However, qualitative feedback on the designs from patients indicated that patients did not fully understand the summary visualizations included in *mi.Symptoms*, which led to a more in-depth, objective evaluation of summary visualization options in Design Phase III.

Design Phase III: Comprehension of Visualizations

The objective of the third design phase was to assess hospitalized patients' objective comprehension (using the International Organization for Standardization protocol) (Rn et al. 2019) of four novel summary visualizations that display longitudinal PROs: text-only, number-line, visual analogy and line graph (Turchioe et al. 2020). Each participant viewed every condition and all possible PRO changes over time

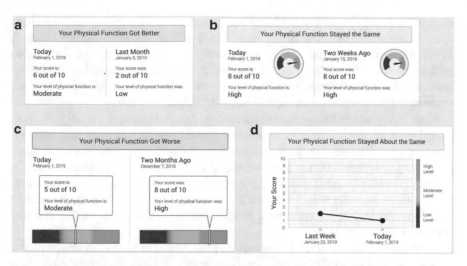

Fig. 18.5 Novel summary visualizations that display longitudinal PROs: (**a**) text-only; (**b**) text plus visual analogy; (**c**) text plus number line; (**d**) text plus line graph

(improvement, decline, no change). Further, counterbalancing was used to control for potential order effects. Participants stated their preferred condition, and we then showed them their preferred condition with PRO decline over time and assessed risk perception and behavioral intentions.

When the four novel summary visualizations (Fig. 18.5) were evaluated with 40 patient participants, 63% correctly comprehended the text-only condition and 60% comprehended the line graph condition, compared with 83% for the visual analogy and 70% for the number line conditions (Turchioe et al. 2020). Participants comprehended the visual analogy significantly better than the text-only and line graph conditions. The results support using visual analogies rather than text to display longitudinal PROs but caution against relying on graphs. Importantly 14% of participants who comprehended at least 1 condition preferred a condition that they did not comprehend. This emphasizes the importance of objectively measuring comprehension of visual formats, rather than relying on preferences as a proxy for comprehension.

Design Phase IV: Heuristic Evaluation for Mobile Interface

The objective of the fourth design phase was to collect feedback on the content of paper prototypes of *mi.Symptoms* (in contrast to the iPad interface) and examine the extent to which the proposed interface met usability heuristics for mobile devices. Paper prototypes were used in this phase to allow feedback to be directly and clearly recorded on the new designs for item-level responses and summary visualization designs for the mobile version. Participants engaged in a focus group session to discuss the prototype, and individually completed an 18-item survey that we developed based on Nielsen's usability heuristics for user interface design (Nielsen 1992). The survey included one to three binary responses to questions related to each of the heuristics. During each focus group, research team members presented paper handouts of prototype mockups, concurrent with an electronic display of the same mockups on a large screen, and asked participants to discuss the content and features that would be included as functionality in the mobile app. Participants were also given paper copies of the mockups, and were encouraged to revise the information presented by marking it up and making changes. Additional research team members were present during the session and took detailed notes. After the design session, the research team met and reviewed the usability heuristic surveys, notes, and drawings from the design session. The research team agreed on the features to include in the mobile interface with patients based on the results of the usability surveys and focus groups.

Seven informaticians and clinical experts participated in the fourth design phase, which entailed a heuristic evaluation lasting about 1 h. Findings from the heuristic evaluation, in which any score less than one indicates worse usability, were categorized by Nielsen's usability heuristics for user interface design. The lowest scores were identified in the following three categories: Visibility of system status, User Control, and Freedom and Recognition rather than recall. From the fourth design session, a total of nine changes were made for the design of the mobile interface.

Conclusion

Using the ISR framework as an organizing framework, this chapter outlines the iterative user-centered design process that was conducted to design an mHealth application to facilitate symptom monitoring. As a result of user-centered design, patients in a disadvantaged patient population with a high symptom burden, many of whom were older adults, were able to successfully use the visualization-rich interface of the *mi.Symptoms* web-application for symptom reporting and communicating with healthcare providers. This demonstrates the value of developing tools that align with the needs and preferences of targeted end-users through rigorous user-centered design.

Chapter Review Questions

Scenario: You are asked to develop a visualization displaying a type of genetic testing result to patients with a specific disease in a health system's patient portal. The goal of the visualization is to improve patient's understanding of their genetic information.

Questions

1. What is a design activity you can conduct to better understand the end user's needs before designing visualizations? Select all that apply.

   (a) Measure patients' health literacy, numeracy, and graph literacy levels.
   (b) Measure patients' objective comprehension of visualizations.
   (c) Design a study using counterbalancing to randomize the order in which visualizations are shown.
   (d) Conduct semi-structured interviews with patients to understand contexts of use and preferences for viewing health information.

2. What is the best sample of participants for an evaluation study of patient-facing visualizations?

   (a) A random sample of doctors and nurses from the health system.
   (b) A convenience sample of patients who have been diagnosed with the disease.
   (c) A random online sample recruited through a research platform such as Prolific.
   (d) A sample of internationally renowned clinicians and researchers with expertise in this type of genetic disorder.

3. Which question allows you to measure objective comprehension of the visualization?

   (a) How much do you like this visualization on a scale of 1–5?
   (b) How likely is it that your health is worsening based on this visualization?
   (c) How would you explain what this means to a loved one?
   (d) What was the gist of the visualization you just saw?

Answers

1. **(a) Measure patients' health literacy, numeracy, and graph literacy levels and (d) Conduct semi-structured interviews with patients to understand contexts of use and preferences for viewing health information.** These activities are two ways of gathering requirements. Options B and C are appropriate for evaluating visualizations after they are developed.

2. **(b) A convenience sample of patients who have been diagnosed with the disease.** While the perspectives of other stakeholders such as doctors, nurses, and experts are helpful to understand, the patients are the ultimately end users and therefore the most important group with which to conduct the evaluation study. A random online sample is unlikely to include many patients with the particular disease and is best for testing visualizations displaying more general or common health information.

3. **(c) How would you explain what this means to a loved one?** This is the objective comprehension question from the ISO 9186 protocol. Option A measures preferences, and B and D measure risk perception.

References

(ISO), International Organization for Standardization. ISO protocol 9186-1: graphical symbols—test methods—part 1: method for testing comprehensibility; 2014.

2016 Program Requirements. https://www.cms.gov/Regulations-and-Guidance/Legislation/EHRIncentivePrograms/2016ProgramRequirements. Accessed 31 Mar 2021.

Aitken M, Gauntlett C. Patient apps for improved healthcare: from novelty to mainstream. Parsippany, NJ: IMS Institute for Healthcare Informatics; 2013.

Arcia A, Bales ME, Brown W 3rd, et al. Method for the development of data visualizations for community members with varying levels of health literacy. AMIA Annu Symp Proc. 2013;2013:51–60.

Arcia A, Velez M, Bakken S. Style guide: an interdisciplinary communication tool to support the process of generating tailored infographics from electronic health data using EnTICE3. EGEMS (Wash DC). 2015;3(1):1120.

Arcia A, Suero-Tejeda N, Bales ME, et al. Sometimes more is more: iterative participatory design of infographics for engagement of community members with varying levels of health literacy. J Am Med Inform Assoc. 2016;23(1):174–83.

Arcia A, Woollen J, Bakken S. A systematic method for exploring data attributes in preparation for designing tailored infographics of patient reported outcomes. EGEMS (Wash DC). 2018;6(1):2.

Austrian J, Mendoza F, Szerencsy A, et al. Applying A/B testing to clinical decision support: rapid randomized controlled trials. J Med Internet Res. 2021;23(4):e16651.

Baik D, Reading M, Jia H, Grossman LV, Masterson CR. Measuring health status and symptom burden using a web-based mHealth application in patients with heart failure. Eur J Cardiovasc Nurs. 2019;18(4):325–31.

Baumhauer JF. Patient-reported outcomes—are they living up to their potential? N Engl J Med. 2017;377(1):6–9. https://doi.org/10.1056/nejmp1702978.

Brewer NT, Gilkey MB, Lillie SE, Hesse BW, Sheridan SL. Tables or bar graphs? Presenting test results in electronic medical records. Med Decis Making. 2012;32(4):545–53.

Brundage MD, Smith KC, Little EA, Bantug ET, Snyder CF, PRO Data Presentation Stakeholder Advisory Board. Communicating patient-reported outcome scores using graphic formats: results from a mixed-methods evaluation. Qual Life Res. 2015;24(10):2457–72.

Centers for Medicare and Medicaid Services. Electronic health records incentive program–stage 2; 2012.

Chen HM. Information visualization. Libr Technol Rep. 2017;53(3):0024–2586.

Cheng KG, Hayes GR, Hirano SH, Nagel MS, Baker D. Challenges of integrating patient-centered data into clinical workflow for care of high-risk infants. Pers Ubiquit Comput. 2015;19(1):45–57.

Chew LD, Bradley KA, Boyko EJ. Brief questions to identify patients with inadequate health literacy. Fam Med. 2004;36(8):588–94.

Cohen DJ, Keller SR, Hayes GR, Dorr DA, Ash JS, Sittig DF. Integrating patient-generated health Data into clinical care settings or clinical decision-making: lessons learned from project HealthDesign. JMIR Hum Factors. 2016;3(2):e26.

Cortez A, Hsii P, Mitchell E, Riehl V, Smith P. Conceptualizing a data infrastructure for the capture, use, and sharing of patient-generated health data in care delivery and research through 2024. Office of the National Coordinator for Health Information; 2018.

Creber RM, Prey J, Ryan B, et al. Engaging hospitalized patients in clinical care: study protocol for a pragmatic randomized controlled trial. Contemp Clin Trials. 2016a;47:165–71. https://doi.org/10.1016/j.cct.2016.01.005.

Creber RMM, Masterson Creber RM, Maurer MS, et al. Review and analysis of existing Mobile phone apps to support heart failure symptom monitoring and self-care management using the Mobile application rating scale (MARS). JMIR mHealth uHealth. 2016b;4(2):e74. https://doi.org/10.2196/mhealth.5882.

Creber RMM, Masterson Creber RM, Hickey KT, Maurer MS. Gerontechnologies for older patients with heart failure: what is the role of smartphones, tablets, and remote monitoring devices in improving symptom monitoring and self-care management? Curr Cardiovas Risk Rep. 2016c;10(10) https://doi.org/10.1007/s12170-016-0511-8.

Fekete J-D, van Wijk JJ, Stasko JT, North C. The value of information visualization. In: Kerren A, Stasko JT, Fekete J-D, North C, editors. Information visualization: human-centered issues and perspectives. Springer: Berlin; 2008. p. 1–18.

Few S. Data visualization for human perception. In: The encyclopedia of human-computer interaction. 2nd ed. 2013.

Galesic M, Garcia-Retamero R. Graph literacy: a cross-cultural comparison. Med Decis Making. 2011;31(3):444–57.

Garcia-Retamero R, Cokely ET. Effective communication of risks to young adults: using message framing and visual aids to increase condom use and STD screening. J Exp Psychol Appl. 2011;17(3):270–87.

Garcia-Retamero R, Cokely ET. Designing visual aids that promote risk literacy: a systematic review of health research and evidence-based design heuristics. Hum Fact. 2017;59(4):582–627.

Grossman LV, Feiner SK, Mitchell EG, Masterson Creber RM. Leveraging patient-reported outcomes using Data visualization. Appl Clin Inform. 2018;9(3):565–75.

Hart JT. The inverse care law. Lancet. 1971;297(7696):405–12. https://doi.org/10.1016/s0140-6736(71)92410-x.

Hawley ST, Zikmund-Fisher B, Ubel P, Jancovic A, Lucas T, Fagerlin A. The impact of the format of graphical presentation on health-related knowledge and treatment choices. Patient Educ Couns. 2008;73(3):448–55.

Hevner AR. A three cycle view of design science research. Scand J Inform Syst. 2007;19(2):4.

International Patient Decision Aid Standards (IPDAS) Collaboration. 2013. http://ipdas.ohri.ca/. Accessed 2019.

Jeevanandan N, Nøhr C. Patient-generated health data in the clinic. Stud Health Technol Inform. 2020;270:766–70.

Jurgens CY, Lee CS, Riegel B. Psychometric analysis of the heart failure somatic perception scale as a measure of patient symptom perception. J Cardiovasc Nurs. 2017;32(2):140–7.

Lai AM, Hsueh P-Y, Choi YK, Austin RR. Present and future trends in consumer health informatics and patient-generated health data. Yearb Med Inform. 2017;26(1):152.

Lindenfeld J, Albert NM, Boehmer JP. HFSA 2010 comprehensive heart failure practice guideline. J Cardiac. 2010; https://europepmc.org/article/med/20610207

Lorenc T, Petticrew M, Welch V, Tugwell P. What types of interventions generate inequalities? Evidence from systematic reviews: table 1. J Epidemiol Commun Health. 2013;67(2):190–3. https://doi.org/10.1136/jech-2012-201257.

Lyles CR, Sarkar U, Ralston JD, et al. Patient–provider communication and trust in relation to use of an online patient portal among diabetes patients: the diabetes and aging study. J Am Med Inform Assoc. 2013;20(6):1128–31.

Mamykina L, Heitkemper EM, Smaldone AM, et al. Structured scaffolding for reflection and problem solving in diabetes self-management: qualitative study of mobile diabetes detective. J Am Med Inform Assoc. 2016;23(1):129–36.

Masterson Creber R, Chen T, Wei C, Lee CS. Brief report: patient activation among urban hospitalized patients with heart failure. J Card Fail. 2017;23(11):817–20.

Masterson Creber RM, Grossman LV, Ryan B, et al. Engaging hospitalized patients with personalized health information: a randomized trial of an inpatient portal. J Am Med Inform Assoc. 2019;26(2):115–23.

McNaughton CD, Cavanaugh KL, Kripalani S, Rothman RL, Wallston KA. Validation of a short, 3-item version of the subjective numeracy scale. Med Decis Making. 2015;35(8):932–6.

Mishra VK, Hoyt RE, Wolver SE, Yoshihashi A, Banas C. Qualitative and quantitative analysis of patients' perceptions of the patient portal experience with OpenNotes. Appl Clin Inform. 2019;10(1):10–8.

Morrow D, Hasegawa-Johnson M, Huang T, et al. A multidisciplinary approach to designing and evaluating electronic medical record portal messages that support patient self-care. J Biomed Inform. 2017;69:63–74.

Mortensen K, Hughes TL. Comparing Amazon's mechanical turk platform to conventional data collection methods in the health and medical research literature. J Gen Intern Med. 2018;33(4):533–8.

Nasreddine ZS, Phillips NA, Bedirian V, et al. The Montreal cognitive assessment, MoCA: a brief screening tool for mild cognitive impairment. J Am Geriatr Soc. 2005;53(4):695–9.

National Eye Institute (NEI). Types of color blindness; 26 June 2019. https://www.nei.nih.gov/learn-about-eye-health/eye-conditions-and-diseases/color-blindness/types-color-blindness. Accessed 23 July 2021.

Nielsen J. Finding usability problems through heuristic evaluation. In: Proceedings of the SIGCHI conference on Human factors in computing systems—CHI '92; 1992. https://doi.org/10.1145/142750.142834

Oh H, Rizo C, Enkin M, Jadad A. What is eHealth (3): a systematic review of published definitions. J Med Internet Res. 2005;7(1):e110.

Okan Y, Janssen E, Galesic M, Waters EA. Using the short graph literacy scale to predict precursors of health behavior change. Med Decis Making. 2019;39(3):183–95.

Palan S, Schitter C. Prolific.Ac—a subject pool for online experiments. J Behav Exp Finan. 2018;17:22–7.

Peer E, Brandimarte L, Samat S, Acquisti A. Beyond the turk: alternative platforms for crowdsourcing behavioral research. J Exp Soc Psychol. 2017;70:153–63.

Reading MJ, Merrill JA. Converging and diverging needs between patients and providers who are collecting and using patient-generated health data: an integrative review. J Am Med Inform Assoc. 2018;25(6):759–71.

Reading Turchioe M, Burgermaster M, Mitchell EG, Desai PM, Mamykina L. Adapting the stage-based model of personal informatics for low-resource communities in the context of type 2 diabetes. J Biomed Inform. 2020a;110:103572.

Reading Turchioe M, Grossman LV, Baik D, et al. Older adults can successfully monitor symptoms using an inclusively designed mobile application. J Am Geriatr Soc. 2020b;68(6):1313–8.

Reeve BB, Wyrwich KW, Wu AW, et al. ISOQOL recommends minimum standards for patient-reported outcome measures used in patient-centered outcomes and comparative effectiveness research. Qual Life Res. 2013;22(8):1889–905.

Riegel B, Lee CS, Dickson VV, Medscape. Self care in patients with chronic heart failure. Nat Rev Cardiol. 2011;8(11):644–54.

Rn AA, Grossman LV, George M, Turchioe MR, Mangal S, Creber RMM. Modifications to the ISO 9186 method for testing comprehension of visualizations: successes and lessons learned. In: 2019 IEEE Workshop on Visual Analytics in Healthcare (VAHC); 2019. p. 41–7.

Saffer D. Designing for interaction: creating innovative applications and devices. Berkeley: New Riders; 2010.

Sanger PC, Hartzler A, Lordon RJ, et al. A patient-centered system in a provider-centered world: challenges of incorporating post-discharge wound data into practice. J Am Med Inform Assoc. 2016;23(3):514–25.

Schnall R, Rojas M, Bakken S, et al. A user-centered model for designing consumer mobile health (mHealth) applications (apps). J Biomed Inf. 2016;60:243–51. https://doi.org/10.1016/j.jbi.2016.02.002.

Sharp H, Preece J, Rogers Y. Interaction design: beyond human-computer interaction. Hoboken: Wiley; 2019.

Siegrist M, Orlow P, Keller C. The effect of graphical and numerical presentation of hypothetical prenatal diagnosis results on risk perception. Med Decis Making. 2008;28(4):567–74.

Smith KC, Brundage MD, Tolbert E, et al. Engaging stakeholders to improve presentation of patient-reported outcomes data in clinical practice. Support Care Cancer. 2016;24(10):4149–57.

Snyder CF, Aaronson NK, Choucair AK, et al. Implementing patient-reported outcomes assessment in clinical practice: a review of the options and considerations. Qual Life Res. 2012;21(8):1305–14.

Snyder CF, Smith KC, Bantug ET, et al. What do these scores mean? Presenting patient-reported outcomes data to patients and clinicians to improve interpretability. Cancer. 2017;123(10):1848–59. https://doi.org/10.1002/cncr.30530.

Solomon J, Scherer AM, Exe NL, Witteman HO, Fagerlin A, Zikmund-Fisher BJ. Is this good or bad? Redesigning visual displays of medical test results in patient portals to provide context and meaning. In: Proceedings of the 2016 CHI Conference Extended Abstracts on Human Factors in Computing Systems. CHI EA '16. Association for Computing Machinery; 2016, p. 2314–20.

Stone ER, Bruine de Bruin W, Wilkins AM, Boker EM, MacDonald GJ. Designing graphs to communicate risks: understanding how the choice of graphical format influences decision making. Risk Anal. 2017;37(4):612–28.

Stoyanov SR, Hides L, Kavanagh DJ, Zelenko O, Tjondronegoro D, Mani M. Mobile app rating scale: a new tool for assessing the quality of health mobile apps. JMIR Mhealth Uhealth. 2015;3(1):e27.

Strickland JC, Stoops WW. The use of crowdsourcing in addiction science research: Amazon mechanical turk. Exp Clin Psychopharmacol. 2019;27(1):1–18.

Sun X, May A. A comparison of field-based and lab-based experiments to evaluate user experience of personalised Mobile devices. Adv Hum Comput Interact. 2013;2013 https://doi.org/10.1155/2013/619767.

Tolbert E, Brundage M, Bantug E, et al. Picture this: presenting longitudinal patient-reported outcome research study results to patients. Med Decis Making. 2018;38(8):994–1005.

Truong KN, Hayes GR, Abowd GD. Storyboarding: an empirical determination of best practices and effective guidelines. In: Proceedings of the 6th Conference on Designing Interactive Systems. DIS '06. Association for Computing Machinery; 2006. p. 12–21.

Turchioe MR, Myers A, Isaac S, et al. A systematic review of patient-facing visualizations of personal health Data. Appl Clin Inform. 2019a;10(04):751–70. https://doi.org/10.1055/s-0039-1697592.

Turchioe MR, Heitkemper EM, Lor M, Burgermaster M, Mamykina L. Designing for engagement with self-monitoring: a user-centered approach with low-income, Latino adults with type 2 diabetes. Int J Med Inform. 2019b;130:103941.

Turchioe MR, Grossman LV, Myers AC, Baik D, Goyal P, Masterson Creber RM. Visual analogies, not graphs, increase patients' comprehension of changes in their health status. J Am Med Inform Assoc. 2020; https://doi.org/10.1093/jamia/ocz217.

U.S. Department of Health and Human Services (HHS). America's health literacy: why we need accessible health information; 2009. https://www.ahrq.gov/sites/default/files/wysiwyg/health-literacy/dhhs-2008-issue-brief.pdf

Veinot TC, Mitchell H, Ancker JS. Good intentions are not enough: how informatics interventions can worsen inequality. J Am Med Inform Assoc. 2018;25(8):1080–8. https://doi.org/10.1093/jamia/ocy052.

Vogt F, Marteau TM. Perceived effectiveness of stop smoking interventions: impact of presenting evidence using numbers, visual displays, and different timeframes. Nicotine Tob Res. 2012;14(2):200–8.

Wegier P, Shaffer VA. Aiding risk information learning through simulated experience (ARISE): using simulated outcomes to improve understanding of conditional probabilities in prenatal down syndrome screening. Patient Educ Couns. 2017;100(10):1882–9. https://doi.org/10.1016/j.pec.2017.04.016.

Wolff JL, Darer JD, Berger A, et al. Inviting patients and care partners to read doctors' notes: OpenNotes and shared access to electronic medical records. J Am Med Inform Assoc. 2017;24(e1):e166–72.

Woods SS, Evans NC, Frisbee KL. Integrating patient voices into health information for self-care and patient-clinician partnerships: veterans affairs design recommendations for patient-generated data applications. J Am Med Inform Assoc. 2016;23(3):491–5. https://doi.org/10.1093/jamia/ocv199.

Wu AW, Kharrazi H, Boulware LE, Snyder CF. Measure once, cut twice—adding patient-reported outcome measures to the electronic health record for comparative effectiveness research. J Clin Epidemiol. 2013;66(8 Suppl):S12–20.

Wynia MK, Osborn CY. Health literacy and communication quality in health care organizations. J Health Commun. 2010;15(Suppl 2):102–15.

Yen P-Y, Wantland D, Bakken S. Development of a customizable health IT usability evaluation scale. AMIA Annu Symp Proc. 2010;2010:917–21.

Zarcadoolas C, Vaughon WL, Czaja SJ, Levy J, Rockoff ML. Consumers' perceptions of patient-accessible electronic medical records. J Med Int Res. 2013;15(8):e168. https://doi.org/10.2196/jmir.2507.

Zikmund-Fisher BJ, Ubel PA, Smith DM, et al. Communicating side effect risks in a tamoxifen prophylaxis decision aid: the debiasing influence of pictographs. Patient Educ Couns. 2008a;73(2):209–14.

Zikmund-Fisher BJ, Fagerlin A, Ubel PA. Improving understanding of adjuvant therapy options by using simpler risk graphics. Cancer. 2008b;113(12):3382–90. https://doi.org/10.1002/cncr.23959.

Zikmund-Fisher BJ, Exe NL, Witteman HO. Numeracy and literacy independently predict patients' ability to identify out-of-range test results. J Med Int Res. 2014;16(8):e187. https://doi.org/10.2196/jmir.3241.

Zikmund-Fisher BJ, Scherer AM, Witteman HO, et al. Graphics help patients distinguish between urgent and non-urgent deviations in laboratory test results. J Am Med Inform Assoc. 2017;24(3):520–8.

Chapter 19
Social Determinants of Health During the COVID-19 Pandemic in the US: Precision Through Context

Marlene Camacho-Rivera, Jessica Y. Islam, Denise C. Vidot, Juan Espinoza, Panagis Galiatsatos, Anupam Sule, Vignesh Subbian, and Charisse Madlock-Brown

Abstract Within this chapter, we discuss conceptual, methodological, and logistical challenges and opportunities in incorporating social determinants of health (SDoH) into medical and health informatics research and practice. We begin by introducing key SDoH concepts and frameworks, with a focus on the social ecologi-

M. Camacho-Rivera (✉)
Department of Community Health Sciences, School of Public Health, SUNY Downstate Health Sciences University, Brooklyn, NY, USA
e-mail: marlene.camacho-rivera@downstate.edu

J. Y. Islam
Cancer Epidemiology Program, H. Lee Moffitt Cancer Center and Research Institute, Tampa, FL, USA

D. C. Vidot
School of Nursing and Health Sciences, University of Miami, Coral Gables, FL, USA

J. Espinoza
Division of General Pediatrics, Children's Hospital Los Angeles, Los Angeles, CA, USA

P. Galiatsatos
Division of Pulmonary and Critical Care Medicine, School of Medicine, The Johns Hopkins University, Baltimore, MD, USA

A. Sule
Department of Medicine, St. Joseph Mercy Oakland Hospital, Pontiac, MI, USA

V. Subbian
College of Engineering, The University of Arizona, Tucson, AZ, USA

C. Madlock-Brown
Department of Health Informatics and Information Management, Tennessee Clinical and Translational Science Institute, The University of Tennessee Health Science Center, Memphis, TN, USA

© The Author(s), under exclusive license to Springer Nature Switzerland AG 2022
P.-Y. S. Hsueh et al. (eds.), *Personal Health Informatics*, Cognitive Informatics in Biomedicine and Healthcare, https://doi.org/10.1007/978-3-031-07696-1_19

cal model as a guiding conceptual model. We present an overview of the scientific literature documenting the impacts of various SDoH measures on disparities in chronic and infectious disease outcomes. We pay considerable attention to how COVID-19 disparities have brought SDOH to light the importance of incorporating SDoH measures for public health and clinical surveillance, and policy and program-matic decision-making. We identify current approaches, as well as gaps and limita-tions in the measurement of SDoH in the existing literature. We describe potential sources of SDoH address data quality concerns and illustrate specific use-cases. Using a case study on COVID-19, we provide conceptual and methodological guid-ance on methods to incorporate SDoH measures in COVID-19 research using individual, administrative, and geographic level data. We conclude with a discus-sion of initiatives that are addressing SDOH in the context of COVID-19, discuss issues around urgency, rapid translation of research into practice, SDOH surveil-lance, and new lessons to be learned.

Keywords Social determinants of health · Health disparities · Health equity Environment · COVID-19

Learning Objectives
1. Introduce concepts and frameworks for examining social determinants of health (SDoH) SDoH broadly.
2. Present a review of the scientific literature examining SDoH.
3. Identify gaps and limitations in the measurement of SDoH in the existing literature.
4. Describe potential sources of SDoH address data quality concerns and illustrate specific use-cases.
5. Case Study: The National COVID Cohort Collaborative (N3C)—How the COVID-19 pandemic brought SDoH to the forefront of informatics.

   (a) Present a review of the scientific literature examining SDoH in the context of the COVID-19 pandemic.
   (b) Provide conceptual and methodological guidance on methods to incorporate SDoH measures in COVID-19 research using individual, administrative, and geographic level data.

Concepts and Frameworks for Examining Social Determinants of Health (SDoH)

Social determinants of health (SDoH) are the conditions in the environments where people are born, live, learn, work, play, worship, and age that affect a wide range of health, functioning, and quality-of-life outcomes and risks (Metzler 2007). SDoH can be broadly grouped into five domains: Economic stability; Education Access and Quality; Health Care Access and Quality; Neighborhood and Built Environment;

and Social and Community Context (Office of Disease Prevention and Health Promotion 2015). To understand the importance of integrating SDoH measures into medical and health informatics, it is critical to contextualize SDoH concepts into frameworks to improve individual and population health.

Within the fields of health promotion and public health, more broadly, social ecological models have been used for nearly five decades in understanding how environments influence health (Sallis et al. 2008). Social ecological models recognize individuals as embedded within larger social systems and describe the interactive characteristics of individuals and environments. Early ecological models include the work of Urie Bronfenbrenner, who articulated the ecological systems theory of child development (Brofenbrenner 1994). Bronfenbrenner argued that to study child development, it was important to not only examine the child and their immediate environment, but also the larger environment as well (Brofenbrenner and Morris 1998). A subsequent model, developed by McLeroy, Bibeau, Steckler, and Glanz would become the most adopted social ecological model within the field of public health (McLeroy et al. 1988a).

As proposed by McLeroy and colleagues, the social ecological model posits that health is not solely determined by biological factors, but instead by a collection of systems that occur at various levels (McLeroy et al. 1988a). The social ecological model articulates five levels of influence specific to individual health behaviors and outcomes: intrapersonal factors, interpersonal factors, institutional or organizational factors, community factors, and public policy (McLeroy et al. 1988b). In addition to identifying specific SDoH influences at each of these levels, social ecological models also assume that the levels of influence are interactive and reinforcing, and that SDoH factors within each level have independent, synergistic, and cumulative influences on health (Stokols 1992, 1996). Examples of SDoH measures at various levels are listed below (Fig. 19.1).

Fig. 19.1 Social Ecological Model from McLeroy et al., 1988

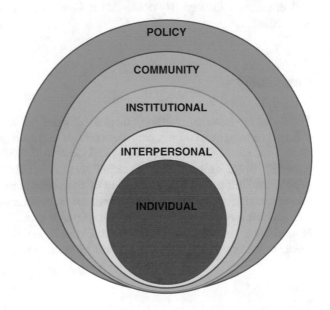

Individual

Characteristics of the individual which may influence health outcomes include biological sex assigned at birth, gender identity, race, ethnicity, age, socioeconomic status, sexual orientation, employment and occupation, and health behaviors such as smoking, alcohol, and substance use (Sutton 2004).

Interpersonal

Characteristics at the interpersonal level include formal and informal relationships with others within an individual's social network. SDoH examples include social support, social isolation, and intimate partner violence (Golden and Earp 2012).

Institutional

Institutions where individuals live, work, learn, play, and worship have an influence on their health. Examples of institutional SDoH measures where people live include homelessness, inadequate housing, or unsafe housing conditions such as exposure to mold, cockroaches, and pests (Gee and Payne-Sturges 2004). At the workplace, organizational SDoH measures include exposure to toxic substances and workplace stress (Ingram et al. 2021; Baron et al. 2014). Characteristics of healthcare institutions where individuals receive preventive, urgent, and specialty care can also have an impact on their health; these may include access to healthcare, quality of care, and disruptions in care (Ryvicker 2018; Garney et al. 2021; Martinez-Cardoso et al. 2020).

Community

The social environment within defined boundaries an individual lives in that may promote certain social norms, provide access to resources, and offer social networks (Smith and Christakis 2008; Albrecht and Goldsmith 2003; Israel 1982; Ikeda and Kawachi 2010; Goldsmith and Albrecht 2011; Ertel et al. 2009; Perkins et al. 2015). Within the built environment, location of the community, housing, transportation services, and access to health and educational facilities are important SDoH characteristics that influence individual health (Renalds et al. 2010; Jackson et al. 2013; Northridge et al. 2003; Garin et al. 2014; Evans 2003). Within the physical environment, proximity to highways, exposure to environmental hazards, and land use patterns (e.g. presence of green spaces) are examples of community-level SDoH measures (Srinivasan et al. 2003; Frank et al. 2019; Gelormino et al. 2015; Zhang et al. 2018; Bird et al. 2018).

Policy

Federal, state, or local policies play significant roles in determining health outcomes at the individual and community levels (Goldenberg et al. 2020; Bailey et al. 2017, 2021). Policies that impact allocation of funds and resources within communities, access to healthcare and other social programs, and policies that differentially impact housing, education, employment, and exposure to hazardous substances may have a profound influence on reducing or widening health and social inequities (Bailey et al. 2017; Fernández-Esquer et al. 2021; Lynch et al. 2021). Examples of such policies include redlining and racial residential segregation, The Affordable Care Act, and state-sanctioned violence through mass incarceration (Acevedo-Garcia et al. 2008; Williams and Collins 2001; National Academies of Sciences, Engineering, and Medicine et al. 2019a; Wildeman and Wang 2017; Krieger et al. 2018; Song and Kucik 2021; Singh and Wilk 2019; Hahn et al. 2018).

An understanding of social determinants of health that influence disparities will likely yield insight into a complex, multifactorial database that will span individual-, regional-, and hospital-level factors. Such an understanding of disparities, for instance, will yield appropriate resource allocation, community-based interventions and engagement, and policy. Regional-based interventions, such as health insurance access and transportation access, may help mitigate the development or management of certain common non-communicable diseases, that in turn will impact morbidity and mortality of an individual and their respective community. The insight provided in this chapter should provide an understanding of the necessity of capturing accurate sociodemographic variables, while constructing models that are grounded in an understanding of human behavior and neighborhood composition, all to create precision medical care and advocacy.

Overview of Evidence Linking SDoH and Health Outcomes

Health inequities have been identified in common pathologies in the United States, inequities that align with social and demographic variables such as race, ethnicity, and socioeconomic status (Peek et al. 2007; Diaz et al. 2021; Sullivan et al. 2021; National Academies of Sciences, Engineering, and Medicine et al. 2019b). Recognizing such disparities along social and demographic variables is significant as it may reflect variety in health behaviors, neighborhood composition, access to healthcare, quality of healthcare, and/or some or all of the above. The patterns of such inequities are complex, and at times, inconsistent, across social and demographic variables. However, taken together, there is a longstanding and significant body of literature that links social determinants of health at all levels to a variety of individual health outcomes and health inequities (National Academies of Sciences, Engineering, and Medicine et al. 2017, 2019c; Palmer et al. 2019; Kneipp et al. 2018). The following section represents a brief overview of the scientific literature linking SDoH measures to various chronic, infectious, and emerging conditions.

Cardiovascular Diseases

Cardiovascular diseases (CVD) continue to be the leading causes of death among adults within the United States, and by 2030, 40.5% of the population is projected to have some form of CVD (Bhatnagar 2017). It is generally believed that even though genetic defects underlie some infrequent forms of heart disease, most CVD is due to interactions between several gene variants and lifestyle factors. This belief is based on the results of many studies showing that, to a large extent, CVD could be prevented by maintaining a healthy lifestyle. For instance, data from the Nurses' Health Study suggest that 82% of coronary events could be prevented by maintaining a healthy lifestyle (Stampfer et al. 2000). Similarly it was found that 62% of all coronary events may have been avoided if men in the Health Professionals Follow-up Study had adhered to a low-risk lifestyle (Chiuve et al. 2008). Data combined from both these studies show that 47% of stroke in women and 35% in men could be attributed to the lack of adherence to low-risk lifestyle choices (Akesson et al. 2007). At the individual level, examples of lifestyle factors that influence CVD outcomes include diet, physical activity, and smoking. At the interpersonal level, social characteristics appear to contribute to CVD mortality risk, and the rates of CVD mortality vary across communities with different area characteristics, such as social cohesion, neighborhood identity, and stigmatization (Chaix 2009). At the community level, characteristics of built environments, from neighborhoods to cities, have been related to rates of chronic disease and mental health and risk factors such as obesity and hypertension (Frank et al. 2003a, b; Ewing et al. 2003; Juarez et al. 2020; Mauller et al. 2018). Physical activity is believed to be a critical mechanism by which built environments can affect chronic disease (Frehlich et al. 2021; Laddu et al. 2021; Lam et al. 2021; Dixon et al. 2020).

Obesity

Clear impacts of the social determinants of health can be seen with obesity disparities in the US. Meta-analyses of over 60 studies show that aspects of the built environment are positively correlated with obesity, particularly in disadvantaged groups

(Papas et al. 2007; Terrón-Pérez et al. 2021; Funderburk et al. 2020). At the community-level, the strongest evidential support was found for food stores (supermarkets instead of smaller grocery stores), places to exercise, and safety, each of these neighborhood characteristics were found to be correlated with body mass index (Pan et al. 2020; Letarte et al. 2020; Drewnowski et al. 2019; Jia et al. 2019; Hills et al. 2019). At the interpersonal level, CVD risk factors such as obesity spread through social ties; for instance, it has been reported that a person's chances of becoming obese increase by 57% is he or she had a friend who became obese within the same period (Barabási 2007) Additional social network studies, reported that if one sibling becomes obese the chances that the other would becoming obese increases by 40% (Christakis and Fowler 2007).

Healthcare Acquired Diseases

Of further interest to healthcare disparities may be those of which render a disproportionate number of persons with life-threatening, critically ill pathologies. Evidence has grown significantly in identifying that healthcare disparities exist in patients necessitating critical care and critical care resources (Grant et al. 2010). And unlike pathologies of chronicity, such as hypertension or diabetes, critical illnesses are unique in their acuity of presentation to healthcare systems and the shortened timeframe of pathology development and resulting course of treatment. Further, in a time of an infectious pandemic that may result in significant critical care resources disproportionately impacting certain populations over others, the continuum of healthcare disparities will be at the forefront. Thereby, understanding sociodemographic variables, from individual-level to contextual-level, how they impact health outcomes, how the impact healthcare and critical care utilization, warrants an assurance of accurate gathering of such data and appropriate classification as well.

One specific critical care diagnosis that aligns with healthcare disparities in a complex manner sepsis, a pathological syndrome that results from an aberrant immune response to an infection. Sepsis-related disparities along sociodemographic variables date back to a formal evaluation of diagnosis and outcomes of the syndrome based on hospital coding that spanned several decades (Martin et al. 2003). Sociodemographic variables have been identified as well, such as those aligning with race and ethnicity as well as those aligning with place of residence (Barnato et al. 2008; Galiatsatos et al. 2020). Of interest, sepsis incidence appears to occur in younger age groups in minority races, pre-dating the development of certain common morbidities, such as diabetes and hypertension, known to be risk factors for sepsis incidence and mortality. And in an opportunity to prepare for potential infectious outbreaks and global crises, insight into such sociodemographic variables may lend to more precise preparation and prognostication of populations that would be ravaged, such as we saw with SARS-CoV-2 and severe COVID-19, a syndrome that parallels sepsis.

Infectious Diseases

Public health emergencies and control of the spread of emerging diseases have been attributable to infectious diseases. Tackling the challenge of infectious disease spread and control has historically required a multifaceted approach, that expands into the concepts of social determinants of health. Contextualizing SDOH in the context of infectious disease control is vital for successful control programming due to the complex interplay between the multi-level drivers of disease, including both neighborhood-level conditions in which we live, and our ability to recover from disease on an individual-level based on economic and biological factors (Butler-Jones and Wong 2016).

Initially, the leading principles towards infectious disease control was germ theory, which provided our biological understanding of spread of infections and the foundations necessary for vaccine development and antimicrobials. Germ theory put forth by Pasteur, is based on the idea of a causal relationship between microbes, contagion, infection, and disease. The theory was largely confirmed in late 1800s by Robert Koch's the identification of Mycobacterium tuberculosis (TB), however, critics continued to question the causal role of microbes due to interindividual clinical variability in disease trajectory. For example, questions remained such as: Why do only some individuals with the same infection and disease severity die from the disease? Several biological reasons to explain interindividual variability have been put forth, such as the identification of prions and related protein misfolding disorders leading to infectious diseases not caused by microorganisms (Cashman 2015). However, with the spread of infections, such as tuberculosis (TB) and human immunodeficiency virus (HIV), in low resourced areas, the significant role of social determinants on rates of infectious disease and mortality has been appreciated.

An important example of the interplay between SDOH and infectious disease theories is the trends in TB observed in high-income settings. TB is a curable and preventable condition caused by bacteria that most often affect the lungs. TB is highly infectious and spreads from person to person through air when people with TB cough, sneeze or spit. In the eighteenth century, TB was an epidemic in Western Europe with a mortality rate as high as 900 deaths per 100,000 inhabitants per year. TB particularly affected young people, and it was dubbed "the robber of the youth." During the industrial revolution, the spread of TB was a social issue due to the higher risk of disease among those living in problematic social conditions such as the extremely deprived work settings, poorly ventilated and overcrowded housing, primitive sanitation, and other social risk factors led to the continued spread of the disease (Frith 2014). However, before the advent of successful medical therapies, incidence of TB declined in North America in the 19th and early 20th centuries. The control of TB in these areas was attributed to better housing, less overcrowding, improved nutrition and living conditions and pasteurization leading to decreased transmission risk of TB in the United States and Europe (Butler-Jones and Wong 2016; Hargreaves et al. 2011).

Currently, cases of TB continue to be inequitably distributed throughout the world: Over 95% of TB cases and deaths occur in developing or low-income countries. In 2019, the largest number of new TB cases occurred in the South East Asian region with 44%B of new cases, followed by the sub-Saharan African region with 25% of new cases. Several underlying conditions also intrinsically linked to SDOH put adults at higher risk of TB-related morbidity and mortality. For example, immunocompromised adults are at higher risk of TB, specifically people living with HIV are 18 times more likely to develop active TB. Further, people with undernutrition are 3 times more at risk of developing TB. Globally in 2019, there were 2.2 million new TB cases in 2018 that were attributable to undernutrition (Butler-Jones and Wong 2016).

Key structural determinants of TB epidemiology include global socioeconomic inequalities, high levels of population mobility, and rapid urbanization and population growth. These conditions give rise to unequal distributions of key social determinants of TB, including food insecurity and malnutrition, poor housing and environmental conditions, and financial, geographic, and cultural barriers to health care access. Those most impacted by TB reflect the distribution of these social determinants in the population (Lienhardt 2001). For example, poor ventilation and overcrowding in the home or workplaces increases the likelihood of healthy individuals being exposed to TB infection (Hill et al. 2006; Boccia et al. 2009; Baker et al. 2008). Additionally, individuals with TB symptoms such as persistent cough frequently experience significant social stigma and economic barriers that delay their contact with the health system (Elliott et al. 1993). Those diagnosed with TB faces several difficulties to obtain treatment including transport to health facilities, fear of stigmatization if they share their diagnosis with friends or family, and lack of social support to seek care when they are unwell (Somma et al. 2008) Finally, due to the close relationship between HIV and TB in many settings, notably sub-Saharan Arica, the key structural and social determinants of HIV infection also act as indirect determinants of TB risk. Efforts to control TB are characterized by interventions to improve accessibility of health systems to communities through treatment support, along with active case-finding and outreach for high-risk populations. Additionally, educational interventions to inform the public about the risk factors attributable to TB, including smoking or alcohol consumption, have been championed. Integration of HIV and TB control programs is also a major priority in many settings. Social determinants of TB are also addressed by strengthening social protection and livelihood improvement interventions to alleviate the effects of chronic poverty and malnutrition (Rothman et al. 1998; Dubos and Dubos 1987).

SARS-CoV-2 and COVID-19

On January 30, 2020, The International Health Regulations Emergency Committee of the World Health Organization (WHO) declared that the outbreak of novel coronavirus SARS-CoV-2 (COVID-19) was a "public health emergency of international concern" (Cucinotta and Vanelli 2020). By March 11th, COVID-19 was declared a global pandemic by the WHO, and the US declared a national emergency on March 13th (CDC 2020a; Sohrabi et al. 2020). The poorly coordinated public health response early in the pandemic resulted in more cases and deaths in the US than in any other country in the world (Dong et al. 2020). In the first few months of the pandemic, it became increasingly clear that Black, Latinx, and low-income communities experienced disproportionate morbidity and mortality from COVID-19 (Wortham et al. 2020; Riou et al. 2020; Webb Hooper et al. 2020). The CDC reported that between February and May 2020, Hispanic and nonwhite individuals under 65 were 2–3 times more likely to die from COVID-19 compared to their white counterparts. Mortality among these groups also far exceeded their proportion of the US population (33.9% of deaths vs. 20% of the population for Hispanics, and 40.2% of deaths vs. 23% of the US population for nonwhites) (Richardson et al. 2020; Holmes et al. 2020).

At the individual level, early emerging international and domestic evidence has identified hypertension, cardiovascular disease, obesity, and diabetes as key risk factors, aside from age, for COVID-19 incidence and mortality (Gao et al. 2020; Izcovich et al. 2020; Javanmardi et al. 2020). For example, a retrospective case series of 1591 laboratory-confirmed COVID-19 in Italy identified hypertension, cardiovascular disease, and hypercholesterolemia as the most common comorbidities among cases (Onder et al. 2020; Grasselli et al. 2020). Similar results were reported in a case series analysis of 5700 hospitalized adults in NY with confirmed COVID-19; however, after hypertension, the most common comorbidities were obesity and diabetes (Richardson et al. 2020).

At the interpersonal level, household density, crowding, and social norms around COVID-19 preventive behaviors have been independently associated with COVID-19 disparities across the US (Nafilyan et al. 2021; Milad and Bogg 2021). At the community level, geographic inequalities in COVID-19 are well documented. Neighborhood social cohesion and neighborhood racial composition has been associated with COVID-19 diagnosis and hospitalization rates, as well as neighborhood deprivation indices (Ingraham et al. 2021; CDC 2020b; Karaye and Horney 2020; Wadhera et al. 2020).

Overview of Initiatives Examining SDoH in the Context of the COVID-19 Pandemic

The COVID-19 pandemic disproportionately impacted low-income and communities of color by exacerbating existing health inequities. Healthcare access, housing, occupation, educational and income gaps, discrimination, and cultural and language differences have all been identified as factors that put these underserved communities at increased risk of COVID-19 morbidity and mortality (CDC 2020a). Certain medical conditions, like diabetes, heart disease, chronic kidney disease, asthma, and hypertension, placed individuals with COVID-19 at an increased risk for hospitalization, intubation, and death (Hussain et al. 2020; Fang et al. 2020; Izquierdo et al. 2021; Garg et al. 2020; Emami et al. 2020; The Lancet Diabetes and Endocrinology 2020; Yang et al. 2020; Mesas et al. 2020). Many of these conditions also disproportionately impact those same low-income and communities of color, and themselves are exquisitely sensitive to SDoH, further compounding the impact of COVID-19 on vulnerable communities.

In response to the pandemic, a number of data initiatives came together in order to track, quantify, and analyze the impact COVID-19. The first of these were focused on epidemiology, such as the Johns Hopkins Coronavirus Resource Center and the Institute for Health Metrics and Evaluation (Dong et al. 2020). The next wave of resources from the CDC, WHO, Google, IBM, and others aggregated public health, social, environmental, and economic data. Finally, as universities, healthcare systems, and governments cleared the necessary legal and regulatory requirements to share patient-level data, a number of rich, collaborative resources came online to enable researchers to explore clinical outcomes (Dagliati et al. 2021). Many of these are repurposed data from EHRs enriched with COVID-19 specific data, while others aggregate patient data from research studies, claims databases, and other sources. The value of these comprehensive, collaborative databases is difficult to overstate; the large number of patients and data points allow for nuanced research questions that can help better inform treatment, prevention, public health policy, and future lines of inquiry. However, it is important to acknowledge the significant technical (syntactic and semantic interoperability, access provisioning, de-identification, privacy protecting patient linkage, etc.) and regulatory (national and international data protection regulations, data use agreements) hurdles that need to be addressed in order to make these data resources available.

Gaps and Limitations in the Measurement of SDoH in the Existing Literature

Though incorporating SDoH into healthcare research can improve patient care, there are several challenges associated with measurement. For instance, a lack of consistent screening for patient-level SDoH in any given healthcare system makes identifying those who have SDoH challenging. Several screening tools exist (PREPARE, ACH-Tools). Using these tools have potential, but there are also some limitations. In a review of research published on identifying SDoH among children, researchers have found that most screeners do not ask clear questions concerning the chronicity or duration of the determinants (Sokol et al. 2019). Information on timing and duration guide interventions and referrals and affect the accuracy of reported information (Fendrich et al. 1999). Several additional features impact the measurement of SDoH with screening tools, such as the availability of the questions in the informant's language of fluency, the reading level necessary to understand each question, and how well informants can understand what is being asked. Additional parents' or caregivers' answers may be influenced by social desirability bias and fear of intervention by protective services (Feinberg et al. 2009; Falletta et al. 2018). Some screening tools were developed in conjunction with information provided by community members, experts, and/or practice experience to address this problem. The creators of the Safe Environment for Every Kid (SEEK) Parent Screening Questionnaire (PSQ) begins with a sympathetic tone towards caregivers and highlights concern for the child's safety and a willingness to assist with identified issues (Sokol et al. 2019; Van de Mortel 2008). Further research is required to investigate if including sensitive language before SDoH screening allays concerns about social desirability bias.

Research has found that standards vary in their capacity to capture specific social needs such as housing and occupation (Sokol et al. 2019; Arons et al. 2019). Arons et al. identified codes currently available across four major medical terminology systems to identify SDoH concepts that can be mapped to the six most-used SDoH screening tools (Arons et al. 2019). Those included were the NAM *Recommended Social and Behavior Domains and Measures* 2014 report, PREPARE, Center for Medicare & Medicaid Innovation's Accountability Health Communities (AHC), Health Leads, Seek, and WE Care. The authors then searched LOINC, SNOMET CT, and CPIT medical codes for the search terms. The authors found 1095 codes related to 20 SDoH domains. However, codes routinely failed to correspond to specific questions/answers in the social screening tools. The authors suggest that while their work suggests limitations in SDoH codes in medical terminologies, clinical content experts, policymakers, and informaticists will need to work together to achieve consensus on what is necessary for SDoH codes.

Missingness is a considerable issue impacting the identification and surveillance of social determinants of health and their impact (Torres et al. 2017). Though SDoH surveys are increasing in use, they are not systematically used across institutions, and information on SDoH is often missing. Without consistent screening, measurement of the prevalence of SDoH in a given healthcare system is challenging. This issue is exacerbated by the fact that disadvantaged groups often have incomplete data as they may not have the healthcare-seeking behaviors of other groups.

Additional sources of problems with measuring SDoH are associated with choosing the correct level of granularity. These data can be captured at the patient level or a range of community-level areas such as neighborhood, census block zip-code, etc. Results for the same study can vary based on the level of granularity. For instance, neighborhoods vary less in socio-economic status than a county. This can cause problems as many disadvantaged residents do not live in areas designated as disadvantaged by many measures. A study sampling 36,578 socially deprived patients from 13 states found that only 60% lived in the most deprived areas (Cottrell et al. 2020).

While detecting socially deprived areas is essential, identifying patients at social risk using area-level measures is not always appropriate. There are also several other issues with neighborhood-level measures. First, if a healthcare system uses neighborhood-level measures for targeted intervention, it is possible that neighborhood norms are not representative as those who seek care (Gottlieb et al. 2018). Alternatively, collecting and using patient data to inform interventions for the neighborhood can lead to additional issues if the patients seek within the healthcare system is not representative of the neighborhood's population.

Difficulties arise when choosing the right measure as well. Choosing summary measures vs. multivariable indices such as the social deprivation index can influence results as a multivariate measure may better capture the underlying complexity SDoH (Kolak et al. 2020). Some characteristics like discrimination and other structural barriers to adequate care are difficult to measure. Users of SDoH measures must also be aware that data processing may not always be transparent, periodicity of data collection is not consistent across measures, definitions of SDoH domains vary, and cross-region or cross-country comparisons can be challenging due to differences in collected information (Blas et al. 2016). These differences can cause research quality issues as some indices may be more up-to-date than others, and the availability of the same certain kinds of SDoH data may not be available for all areas studied. In addition to data collection, management, and integration issues, additional conceptual, ethical, and logistical challenges may prevent incorporation of SDoH data into clinical research and practice.

Additional Challenges in Incorporating SDoH Data into Clinical Practice

Clinician Viewpoint

Clinicians lack explicit and implicit training during undergraduate training or graduate clinical experience about how to empathically obtain comprehensive social data (Global Forum on Innovation in Health Professional Education, Board on Global Health, Health and Medicine Division, National Academies of Sciences, Engineering, and Medicine 2020). There is a need for training on how to establish trust and rapport to obtain this sensitive information. Implicit bias and unexplored prejudices not only influence obtaining this data but also utilization of this data when formulating a plan of care. Once data is collected, there is an opportunity to document SDoH in the EHR via ICD-10-CM Z55-Z65 codes; however, Z codes are not consistently used properly due to missing and/or incorrect data, unfamiliarity of Z codes, lack of training and clarity on the documentation of patient social needs, and lack of prioritization to collect the codes within the Z category (American Hospital Association 2021). Prioritizing the education and incorporation of comprehensive reporting of Z codes in clinical practice will increase opportunities for interpretation of SDoH of patient populations. The specific categories captured by Z-codes are listed in Table 19.1 below (PsychDB 2021).

Table 19.1 ICD-10-CM Z-code categories related to social determinants of health

Z code	Category
Z55	Problems related to education and literacy
Z56	Problems related to employment and unemployment
Z57	Occupational exposure to risk factors
Z59	Problems related to housing and economic circumstances
Z60	Problems related to social environment
Z62	Problems related to upbringing
Z63	Other problems related to primary support group, including family circumstances
Z64	Problems related to certain psychosocial circumstances
Z65	Problems related to other psychosocial circumstances

Clinicians often see patients with complex social situations as burdensome, requiring extra time and effort to provide the same standard of clinical care. The time and effort are neither reimbursed nor acknowledged. The clinician experience is compounded by a sense of frustration due to the inability to affect the root causes. The incorporation of Z code reporting and analysis may provide actionable data to begin addressing root causes of preventable negative health outcomes.

Once actionable data is available, clinicians need to be taught how to utilize it to develop optimal individualized care plans using shared decision-making and empathetic counseling. Tools to aid utilization of this data in clinical decision-making are lacking. There is a lack of understanding of the interaction between genetic and environmental factors, so even if genomic and social determinants data is available the interaction data cannot be meaningfully interpreted. Formal incentives to reward clinicians making this effort are necessary.

Patient Viewpoint

The data that is currently collected from individuals during a clinical encounter and recorded in the EHR lacks the details needed when formulating a comprehensive care plan. EHR social history structured data fields do not record all the myriad sources of healthcare disparities. Furthermore, self-reported data is subject to error and bias based on patients' perception of the utility, need, and privacy of this data. It is also influenced by the patients' ability to recall the data in the correct context. When seeking such data it is critical to ensure the patients understand the purpose and value of the data being collected. Even if the patient is willing to share the data sometimes the technical expertise required to do so may be beyond the abilities of that patient.

Healthcare Information Technology Aspect

A set of standardized measures and interoperable data sources that can reflect the neighborhood, as well as the individual and that are relevant to clinical care, is required. It is difficult to import data from external data sources into the patients health record given the lack of standardization within the healthcare information technology world and with the rest of the information technology world. When data is exchanged with public data repositories with the potential to link to individual patient's data, confidentiality and security are at risk.

Healthcare System Aspect

Some cases require interventions at the patient level while others need community level interventions. Information about other team members/organizations available to aid in the management of social issues, and when, who, and how to refer to them appropriately should be built within the EHR and presented at the point of care. Even if the data is available the tools to meaningfully use the data in organizational strategy by leaders and strong incentives to do so are missing. Although there may be a benefit in terms of healthcare costs to the society, the systems and clinicians bearing the cost of collecting, storing, and using this data may not reap the revenue benefits directly. At present healthcare organizations define their population health target group as the panel of patients assigned to them by insurance companies. These patients are from diverse communities. Defining population health catchments by geographic areas and including all the residents in that area would be more efficient but such payor plans are not yet available.

As part of our case study, we will discuss in detail the National COVID Cohort Collaborative (N3C), an initiative overseen by the National Center for Advancing Translational Sciences (NCATS) of the NIH. The objective of the N3C is to aggregate and harmonize electronic health record data across clinical organizations in the United States (Haendel et al. 2020). This initiative is possible through the novel partnership of several organizations including the Clinical and Translational Sciences Awards (CTSA) program hubs (including 60 institutions), the NCATS, the center for Data to Health (CD2H), and the scientific community. The N3C is a novel initiative as it was built in response to a public health emergency on the foundation of established, productive research communities, and their existing research resources. The primary features of N3C are national collaboration and governance, regulatory strategies, COVID-19 cohort definitions via community-developed phenotypes, data harmonization across 4 CDMs, and development of a collaborative analytics platform to support deployment of novel algorithms of data aggregated from the United States (Haendel et al. 2020). The N3C supports community-driven, reproducible, and transparent analyses with COVID-19 data, promoting rapid dissemination of results and atomic attribution and demonstrating that open science can be effectively implemented on EHR data at scale (Haendel et al. 2020).

The N3C is structured into separate workstreams including administrative and managerial efforts, namely data partnership & governance, as well as the efforts dedicated to definitions of inclusion criteria for the N3C COVID-19 cohort to support organizations in customized data export. Importantly, the N3C workstreams dedicated to specific interest areas is named Collaborative Analytics. Under this workstream, is the N3C SDOH Domain led by Drs. Charisse Madlock-Brown and Adam Wilcox. The goal of the Social Determinants of Health (SDoH) Clinical Domain Team is to evaluate the role of SDOH in the spread of COVID-19 specifically through the following areas of research: local policy around COVID-19, impact of groups experiencing resource challenges, and impact of the pandemic on inequalities (N3C 2021). The main activities carried out by the N3C SDOH domain include: (1) conducting research projects to address questions around state and county-level policy impact on disadvantaged groups and the impact on inequalities; (2) Host hackathons using the N3C |Enclave (i.e. N3C data portal) including technical training, quality control initiatives, hypothesis generation and analysis; (3) and to provide researcher support: Provide annotated bibliographies, opportunities to present related research, training on the N3C enclave, access to cleaned and transformed data for SDoH and COVID-19 research, IRB protocol support, and collaboration.

Specific research questions the N3C aims to address include:

- What are the SDoH related to vulnerability or resilience to COVID-19 incidence at the county level?
- What are the SDoH related to vulnerability or resilience to COVID-19 incidence at the patient level?
- Do SDoH factors associated with vulnerability or resilience differ by race/ethnicity?
- What are the environmental factors that impact COVID-19 incidence and outcomes?

The main barriers to carrying out these research questions include data quality and completeness concerns. As the N3C is an EHR based dataset, social determinants of health are not routinely captured in the existing N3C that has been merged through the governing institutions charged with data harmonization (Hu et al. 2017). A paucity of regular SDOH measures in the EHR may be due to a lack of available collection tools and documentation of SDOH screening processes are significant challenges for SDoH data. In the context of the N3C data resource, data missingness can arise prior to or after the data enters the harmonized data source (i.e. N3C Data Enclave), meriting evaluation for missingness at multiple levels and data processing steps. Missingness is highly dependent on data integration methods and may arise structurally from institutional data sharing hurdles or as artifacts from merging multiple data tables. The N3C SDOH Domain can leverage external data sources from studies that characterize several SDOH measures, such as 'food deserts' or other proxies for food insecurity, in certain localities. However, a major limitation to this approach is that data will not be nationally representative or cover all N3C catchment areas. Spatial features, such as U.S. postal zip codes, provide important opportunities for linkage to integrate community- or area-level determinants (e.g. % of adults without a high school degree in a zip code) of each individual captured within the N3C shared datasource.

To carry out research projects to answer these research questions, the N3C SDOH domains have identified several public datasets that can be linked to existing individual-level data available in the N3C through area-level identifiers such as county, zip code or census tract. The N3C SDOH Domain continues to evaluate data sources for their fit-for-use in potential modeling research projects. Figure 19.2 below summarizes data sources available to the Domain and what areas of research each dataset can address.

To address N3C SDOH quality concerns a number of approaches and strategies have been employed by the Domain team. These strategies have been outlined below and may inform future informatics efforts to address COVID-19 pandemic disparities or in the context of future public health emergencies in areas with the technological resources available. First, the N3C SDOH Domain has implemented a Data Quality Assessment Framework. To identify and address problems related to SDOH data quality in the N3C, the N3C SDOH Domain is taking a systematic approach to data quality assessment, based on a consensus, expert-driven framework for data quality assessment (Kahn et al. 2016). This framework provides

		Measures of Interest						
Source	Datasets	Cases and Outcomes	County Health Policies	Social and Resource Deprivation	Access to Care	Population Estimates	Shelter in Place Behaviors	Employment Type/Status
N3C	Electronic Health Records of COVID-19 positive patients	X		X	X	X		X
State-level County Health Departments	COVID-19 County Daily Status	X						
Robert Graham Center	Social Deprivation Index (SDI)			X				
USDA	Food Access Atlas			X				
State-level County Health Departments	COVID-19 Policies		X					
US Census	American Community Survey			X		X		
SafeGraph	SafeGraph Neighborhood						X	
US Census	County Business Patterns 2017					X		X
US Census	Household Pulse Survey				X		X	
Federal Communications Commission	FCC Health Maps			X	X			

Fig. 19.2 External data sources have been added to N3C to facilitate analysis. Adapted from Phuong et al. "Examining the Dynamics in Social Determinants of Health and COVID-19 patient cohort research"

guidance on assessing the quality and usability of data prior to statistical analyses. When data quality problems are identified, the Domain will perform additional assessments to determine if these deficits occur at random, or if they may result in potentially spurious findings. The Domain will use a combination of data integration and accepted statistical methods to address these deficits, thereby improving the validity of conclusions drawn from these data. As part of the framework, the following areas will be implemented to evaluate data quality in the N3C:

(a) Check for completeness (e.g.: N3C Limited Dataset quality check for zip-codes and date-shifting)
(b) Plausibility (data accuracy)
(c) Conformance (adherence to standards)
(d) Distribution checks (expected variation in data)
(e) Granularity (sufficient level of detail)
(f) Bias assessment (evaluate potential selection bias (Haneuse and Daniels 2016) and information bias)

Second, missing data is currently an issue for many COVID-19 related projects. For instance, attempts to characterize true mortality by race/ethnicity rates are hindered by missing data. Figure 19.3 shows the percent of CDC-reported COVID-19

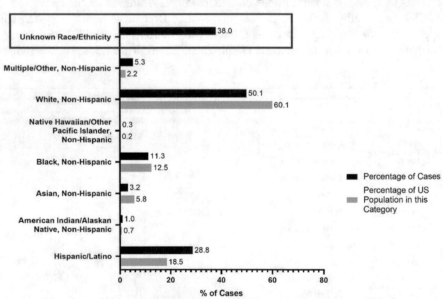

Data from 26,760,011 cases. Race/Ethnicity was available for 16,720,298 (62%) cases.

Fig. 19.3 Known COVID-19 cases and deaths in the United States broken down by race and ethnicity. Data retrieved from: https://covid.cdc.gov/covid-data-tracker/#demographics on May 31st, 2021

cases and deaths broken down by racial and ethnic categories. At first glance, these data indicate substantial differences in mortality rates across these categories. White non-Hispanics, for example, appear to represent 50% of COVID-19 cases. Important to note, however, is the high rate of missing or Unknown race and ethnicity data: 38% of cases did not have race and ethnicity reported. Without these data, it is difficult to know if conclusions regarding COVID-19 burden between racial and ethnic groups are valid. As such, efforts to assess data quality (e.g., incomplete data) and measurement and selection bias is of vital significance. By integrating multiple datasets, the N3C SDOH Domain is able to improve the validity of our statistical inference. For example, by linking these data to aggregate race and ethnicity data at the census tract level, we may be able to make inferences about the missing values, thereby improving our estimations of true case and death rates. Such work will improve our understanding of health disparities associated with COVID-19.

Third, COVID-19 testing capacity in low-resourced urban and rural settings continues to be a major point of concern (Souch and Cossman 2021). Disproportionate allocation of testing resources to the target populations results in geographic biases. To address this concern, the N3C SDOH Domain will limit counties included in analyses based on state-level testing availability evaluated through publicly available data.

Finally, the N3C SDOH Domain has engaged in discussions with N3C researchers from health systems across the US suggests that health systems have collected or could collect data on patient social and environmental determinants of health to develop a N3C Concept Map to guide data collection and harmonization across sites providing data to the N3C Enclave. This data is most commonly available from patient screening tools, or from diagnostic codes. Leveraging ongoing consortial efforts such as the SIREN Network (SIREN 2021) and the HL7 Gravity Project (HL7 International 2021), four screening tools or survey instruments were identified as the highest likelihood of adoption and implementation among clinical centers contributing to N3C: PRAPARE, AHC-Tools (Kaiser Permanente 2021), HealthLeads (Health Leads 2021), and WeCare. Prior studies have showcased the utility to understand patient population needs using PRAPARE (Cottrell et al. 2019; Billioux et al. 2017). Separately, prior efforts from the HL7 Gravity Project SDoH Connectathon have produced mappings for Food Insecurity surveys to LOINC and SNOMED CT standard concept representations. However, there remains significant challenges around concept mapping and harmonizing the provenance and semantic information collected in different screening tool versions and different language implementations.

Environmental exposures and variables (e.g., water quality, air quality, traffic density) are less commonly collected through standard clinical processes. However, clinical datasets can be enriched with environmental data by geocoding the patient's address, spatially joining it with the appropriate spatial unit (block, census tract, zip code, county), and then extracting the relevant data from a number of publicly available environmental databases. Environmental contextual data can provide additional insights on the role of the environment as a determinant of health. Place-based, contextual data should be interpreted carefully, as it is subject to the ecological fallacy—exposures with a spatial unit are not homogenous, and not all patients may be at higher risk (Gottlieb et al. 2018).

Currently, the N3C SDOH Domain has identified an initial set of SDoH features to map (i.e., housing insecurity, food insecurity, education barriers, employment/occupation status, and citizenship status), where questions and answer options have been mapped to LOINC and SNOMED CT standard encoding. Further work is needed to harmonize concepts *across* instruments, so that databases that contain patient data from different instruments can be queried, stratified and analyzed using common concepts. Separately, the group has discussed the process of data collection and anticipated biases and data collection variability that may occur before the data reaches the N3C limited dataset form. Based on the experience developing methods to harmonize concepts, we provide a number of strategies that can be implemented to improve data collection efforts (Table 19.2) (Lizzio et al. 2019).

A strength of the N3C enclave is the representation across multiple regions and multiple systems within those regions, which can increase the generalizability of the findings. Section A of Fig. 19.4 displays the number of patients in each region and the COVID trends, which vary by region indicating the importance of having national representation. Section B of the figure shows the distribution across age and race. Importantly, Fig. 19.4 shows that N3C has a much smaller proportion of missing race data.

Table 19.2 Strategies to improve data collection quality

Principle	Strategies
Minimize patient burden	Reduce overall number of questions
	Reduce overall time to completion
	Avoid redundancy: Asking patients to respond to duplicate questions or answers that that can be easily found in the chart
Minimize provider burden	Reduce time to completion
	Automation of instrument
	Allow for both remote and asynchronous administration
	Allow for patient self-reporting
	Avoid clinical delays
Maximize data collection	Design user-friendly interfaces
	Incorporate into existing workflows; minimize deviations from current practice
	Align data collection with institutional mission
	Incentivize screening (e.g., reimbursement)
Optimize for clinical, research, and quality reporting	Use single standardized forms for all patients and avoid custom questionnaires
	Perform automatic calculated scoring
	Leverage data standards, ontologies, and concept maps

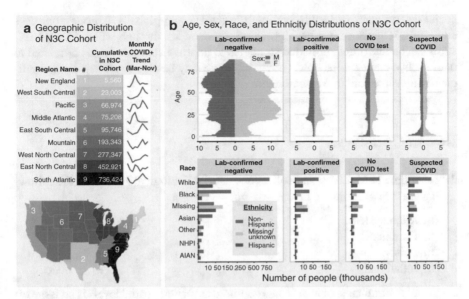

Fig. 19.4 Summary demographic statistics of data available in the N3C as of January 2021 by (**a**) U.S. Census Geographic Regions, (**b**) Age, Sex, and Ethnicity Distributions of COVID-19 Lab Positive Testing

Summary

Significant evidence documents the influence of social determinants of health on a variety of individual health outcomes and population health inequities. To improve access to and quality of healthcare, as well as design, implement, and evaluate multilevel interventions that promote the health and well-being of individuals, SDoH measures should continue to be integrated into health and medical informatics. However, several conceptual, methodological, and logistical issues challenge the improved integration of SDoH measures. Conceptually, identifying which SDoH measures are most relevant to specific health outcomes within communities of interest remains a challenge. Methodologically, issues related to missing data, granularity of available SDoH measures, and data harmonization across clinical, public health, and administrative datasets remain. Logistically, clinicians and health informaticists may have inadequate training to fully conceptualize and operationalize the contributions of SDoH measures towards health outcomes. Challenges in incentivizing clinicians and healthcare organizations towards monitoring and addressing social determinants of health within their patient catchment areas persist. However, the COVID-19 pandemic has increased attention to the importance of focusing on social determinants of health, both within the US and globally. Through our case study of N3C enclave, we have provided a framework through which SDoH measures can be integrated, provided strategies to improve common issues of related to data quality, and detailed how a novel initiative may be able to effectively and efficiently translate data into research into practice.

Review Questions

1. According to McLeroy and colleagues' Social Ecological Model, all the following are levels within the model except:

   (a) Microsystem
   (b) Community
   (c) Policy
   (d) Individual

2. Social determinants of health data captured at various spatial levels is an issue of:

   (a) Missingness
   (b) Social Desirability
   (c) Granularity
   (d) Interoperability

Answer Key

1. (a) Microsystem
2. (c) Granularity

References

Acevedo-Garcia D, Osypuk TL, McArdle N, Williams DR. Toward a policy-relevant analysis of geographic and racial/ethnic disparities in child health. Health Aff (Millwood). 2008;27(2):321–33.

Akesson A, Weismayer C, Newby PK, Wolk A. Combined effect of low-risk dietary and lifestyle behaviors in primary prevention of myocardial infarction in women. Arch Intern Med. 2007;167(19):2122–7.

Albrecht TL, Goldsmith DJ. Social support, social networks, and health. In Thompson TL, Dorsey AM, Miller KI, Parrott R. (Eds.), Handbook of health communication. Lawrence Erlbaum Associates Publishers. 2003. pp. 263–284.

American Hospital Association. ICD-10-CM coding for social determinants of health [Internet]. [cited 2021 May 31]. Available from https://www.aha.org/system/files/2018-04/value-initiative-icd-10-code-social-determinants-of-health.pdf

Arons A, DeSilvey S, Fichtenberg C, Gottlieb L. Documenting social determinants of health-related clinical activities using standardized medical vocabularies. JAMIA Open. 2019;2(1):81–8.

Bailey ZD, Krieger N, Agénor M, Graves J, Linos N, Bassett MT. Structural racism and health inequities in the USA: evidence and interventions. Lancet. 2017;389(10077):1453–63. https://doi.org/10.1016/S0140-6736(17)30569-X. PMID: 28402827.

Bailey ZD, Feldman JM, Bassett MT. How structural racism works—racist policies as a root cause of US racial health inequities. N Engl J Med. 2021;384(8):768–73.

Baker M, Das D, Venugopal K, Howden-Chapman P. Tuberculosis associated with household crowding in a developed country. J Epidemiol Community Health. 2008;62(8):715–21.

Barabási A-L. Network medicine—from obesity to the "diseasome". N Engl J Med. 2007;357(4):404–7.

Barnato AE, Alexander SL, Linde-Zwirble WT, Angus DC. Racial variation in the incidence, care, and outcomes of severe sepsis: analysis of population, patient, and hospital characteristics. Am J Respir Crit Care Med. 2008;177(3):279–84.

Baron SL, Beard S, Davis LK, Delp L, Forst L, Kidd-Taylor A, et al. Promoting integrated approaches to reducing health inequities among low-income workers: applying a social ecological framework. Am J Ind Med. 2014;57(5):539–56.

Bhatnagar A. Environmental determinants of cardiovascular disease. Circ Res. 2017;121(2):162–80.

Billioux A, Verlander K, Anthony S, et al. Standardized screening for health-related social needs in clinical settings: the accountable health communities screening tool. NAM Perspect. 2017;7(5)

Bird EL, Ige JO, Pilkington P, Pinto A, Petrokofsky C, Burgess-Allen J. Built and natural environment planning principles for promoting health: an umbrella review. BMC Public Health. 2018;18(1):930.

Blas E, Ataguba JE, Huda TM, Bao GK, Rasella D, Gerecke MR. The feasibility of measuring and monitoring social determinants of health and the relevance for policy and programme—a qualitative assessment of four countries. Glob Health Action. 2016;9:29002.

Boccia D, Hargreaves J, Ayles H, Fielding K, Simwinga M, Godfrey-Faussett P. Tuberculosis infection in Zambia: the association with relative wealth. Am J Trop Med Hyg. 2009;80(6):1004–11.

Brofenbrenner U. Ecological models of human development. International encyclopedia of education. 1994.

Brofenbrenner U, Morris P. The ecology of developmental processes. In: Handbook of child psychology, vol. 1: Theoretical models of human development; 1998.

Butler-Jones D, Wong T. Infectious disease, social determinants and the need for intersectoral action. Can Commun Dis Rep. 2016;42(S1):S1–18–S1–20.

Cashman NR. Propagated protein misfolding: new opportunities for therapeutics, new public health risk. Can Commun Dis Rep. 2015;41(8):196–9.

CDC. Coronavirus Disease 2019 (COVID-19) [Internet]. [cited 2020a May 8]. Available from https://www.cdc.gov/coronavirus/2019-ncov/index.html

CDC. COVID-19 Response Team. Geographic Differences in COVID-19 Cases, Deaths, and Incidence—United States, February 12–April 7, 2020. MMWR Morb Mortal Wkly Rep. 2020b;69(15):465–71.

Chaix B. Geographic life environments and coronary heart disease: a literature review, theoretical contributions, methodological updates, and a research agenda. Annu Rev Public Health. 2009;30:81–105.

Chiuve SE, Rexrode KM, Spiegelman D, Logroscino G, Manson JE, Rimm EB. Primary prevention of stroke by healthy lifestyle. Circulation. 2008;118(9):947–54.

Christakis NA, Fowler JH. The spread of obesity in a large social network over 32 years. N Engl J Med. 2007;357(4):370–9.

Cottrell EK, Dambrun K, Cowburn S, Mossman N, Bunce AE, Marino M, et al. Variation in electronic health record documentation of social determinants of health across a national network of community health centers. Am J Prev Med. 2019;57(6 Suppl 1):S65–73.

Cottrell EK, Hendricks M, Dambrun K, Cowburn S, Pantell M, Gold R, et al. Comparison of community-level and patient-level social risk data in a network of community health centers. JAMA Netw Open. 2020;3(10):e2016852.

Cucinotta D, Vanelli M. WHO declares COVID-19 a pandemic. Acta Biomed. 2020;91(1):157–60.

Dagliati A, Malovini A, Tibollo V, Bellazzi R. Health informatics and EHR to support clinical research in the COVID-19 pandemic: an overview. Brief Bioinform. 2021;22(2):812–22.

Diaz CL, Shah NS, Lloyd-Jones DM, Khan SS. State of the nation's cardiovascular health and targeting health equity in the United States: a narrative review. JAMA Cardiol. 2021;6(8):963–70.

Dixon BN, Ugwoaba UA, Brockmann AN, Ross KM. Associations between the built environment and dietary intake, physical activity, and obesity: a scoping review of reviews. Obes Rev. 2020;22(4):e13171.

Dong E, Du H, Gardner L. An interactive web-based dashboard to track COVID-19 in real time. Lancet Infect Dis. 2020;20(5):533–4.

Drewnowski A, Buszkiewicz J, Aggarwal A, Rose C, Gupta S, Bradshaw A. Obesity and the built environment: a reappraisal. Obesity (Silver Spring). 2019;28(1):22–30.

Dubos RJ, Dubos J. The white plague: tuberculosis, man, and society. Bookseller. 1987.

Elliott AM, Hayes RJ, Halwiindi B, Luo N, Tembo G, Pobee JO, et al. The impact of HIV on infectiousness of pulmonary tuberculosis: a community study in Zambia. AIDS. 1993;7(7):981–7.

Emami A, Javanmardi F, Pirbonyeh N, Akbari A. Prevalence of underlying diseases in hospitalized patients with COVID-19: a systematic review and Meta-analysis. Arch Acad Emerg Med. 2020;8(1):e35.

Ertel KA, Glymour MM, Berkman LF. Social networks and health: a life course perspective integrating observational and experimental evidence. J Soc Pers Relat. 2009;26(1):73–92.

Evans GW. The built environment and mental health. J Urban Health. 2003;80(4):536–55.

Ewing R, Schmid T, Killingsworth R, Zlot A, Raudenbush S. Relationship between urban sprawl and physical activity, obesity, and morbidity. Am J Health Promot. 2003;18(1):47–57.

Falletta L, Hamilton K, Fischbein R, Aultman J, Kinney B, Kenne D. Perceptions of child protective services among pregnant or recently pregnant, opioid-using women in substance abuse treatment. Child Abuse Negl. 2018;79:125–35.

Fang L, Karakiulakis G, Roth M. Are patients with hypertension and diabetes mellitus at increased risk for COVID-19 infection? Lancet Respir Med. 2020;8(4):e21.

Feinberg E, Smith MV, Naik R. Ethnically diverse mothers' views on the acceptability of screening for maternal depressive symptoms during pediatric well-child visits. J Health Care Poor Underserved. 2009;20(3):780–97.

Fendrich M, Johnson T, Wislar JS, Nageotte C. Accuracy of parent mental health service reporting: results from a reverse record-check study. J Am Acad Child Adolesc Psychiatry. 1999;38(2):147–55.

Fernández-Esquer ME, Ibekwe LN, Guerrero-Luera R, King YA, Durand CP, Atkinson JS. Structural racism and immigrant health: exploring the association between wage theft, mental health, and injury among Latino day laborers. Ethn Dis. 2021;31(Suppl 1):345–56.

Frank L, Engelke P, Schmid T. Health and community design: the impact of the built environment on physical activity. books.google.com; 2003a.

Frank L, Engelke P, Schmid T. Health and community design: the impact of the built environment on physical activity. books.google.com; 2003b.

Frank LD, Iroz-Elardo N, MacLeod KE, Hong A. Pathways from built environment to health: a conceptual framework linking behavior and exposure-based impacts. J Transp Health. 2019;12:319–35.

Frehlich L, Christie C, Ronksley P, Turin TC, Doyle-Baker P, McCormack G. The association between neighborhood built environment and health-related fitness: a systematic review protocol. JBI Evid Synth. 2021;19(9):2350–8.

Frith J. History of tuberculosis. Part 1-phthisis, consumption and the white plague. J Mil Veterans Health. 2014;22(2):29–35.

Funderburk L, Cardaci T, Fink A, Taylor K, Rohde J, Harris D. Healthy behaviors through behavioral design-obesity prevention. Int J Environ Res Public Health. 2020;17(14):5049.

Galiatsatos P, Follin A, Alghanim F, Sherry M, Sylvester C, Daniel Y, et al. The association between neighborhood socioeconomic disadvantage and readmissions for patients hospitalized with sepsis. Crit Care Med. 2020;48(6):808–14.

Gao Y-D, Ding M, Dong X, Zhang J-J, Azkur AK, Azkur D, et al. Risk factors for severe and critically ill COVID-19 patients: a review. Allergy. 2020;6(2):428–55.

Garg S, Kim L, Whitaker M, O'Halloran A, Cummings C, Holstein R, et al. Hospitalization rates and characteristics of patients hospitalized with laboratory-confirmed coronavirus disease 2019. MMWR Morb Mortal Wkly Rep. 2020;69(15):458–64.

Garin N, Olaya B, Miret M, Ayuso-Mateos JL, Power M, Bucciarelli P, et al. Built environment and elderly population health: a comprehensive literature review. Clin Pract Epidemiol Ment Health. 2014;10(1):103–15.

Garney W, Wilson K, Ajayi KV, Panjwani S, Love SM, Flores S, et al. Social-ecological barriers to access to healthcare for adolescents: a scoping review. Int J Environ Res Public Health. 2021;18(8):4138.

Gee GC, Payne-Sturges DC. Environmental health disparities: a framework integrating psychosocial and environmental concepts. Environ Health Perspect. 2004;112(17):1645–53.

Gelormino E, Melis G, Marietta C, Costa G. From built environment to health inequalities: an explanatory framework based on evidence. Prev Med Rep. 2015;4(2):737–45.

Global Forum on Innovation in Health Professional Education, Board on Global Health, Health and Medicine Division, National Academies of Sciences, Engineering, and Medicine. In: Cuff PA, Forstag EH, editors. Educating health professionals to address the social determinants of mental health: proceedings of a workshop. Washington, DC: National Academies Press; 2020.

Golden SD, Earp JAL. Social ecological approaches to individuals and their contexts: twenty years of health education & behavior health promotion interventions. Health Educ Behav. 2012;39(3):364–72.

Goldenberg T, Reisner SL, Harper GW, Gamarel KE, Stephenson R. State policies and healthcare use among transgender people in the U.S. Am J Prev Med. 2020;59(2):247–59.

Goldsmith DJ, Albrecht TL. Social support, social networks, and health. The Routledge handbook of health Communication. London: Routledge; 2011.

Gottlieb LM, Francis DE, Beck AF. Uses and misuses of patient- and neighborhood-level social determinants of health data. Perm J. 2018;22:18–078.

Grant RM, Lama JR, Anderson PL, McMahan V, Liu AY, Vargas L, et al. Preexposure chemoprophylaxis for HIV prevention in men who have sex with men. N Engl J Med. 2010;363(27):2587–99.

Grasselli G, Zangrillo A, Zanella A, Antonelli M, Cabrini L, Castelli A, et al. Baseline characteristics and outcomes of 1591 patients infected with SARS-CoV-2 admitted to ICUs of the Lombardy region, Italy. JAMA. 2020;323(16):1574–81.

Haendel MA, Chute CG, Bennett TD. The national COVID cohort collaborative (N3C): rationale, design, infrastructure, and deployment. JAMIA. 2020;28(3):427–43.

Hahn RA, Truman BI, Williams DR. Civil rights as determinants of public health and racial and ethnic health equity: health care, education, employment, and housing in the United States. SSM Popul Health. 2018;4:17–24.

Haneuse S, Daniels M. A general framework for considering selection bias in EHR-based studies: what data are observed and why? EGEMS (Wash DC). 2016;4(1):1203.

Hargreaves JR, Boccia D, Evans CA, Adato M, Petticrew M, Porter JDH. The social determinants of tuberculosis: from evidence to action. Am J Public Health. 2011;101(4):654–62.

Health Leads [Internet]. [cited 2021 May 31]. Available from: https://healthleadsusa.org/

Hill PC, Jackson-Sillah D, Donkor SA, Otu J, Adegbola RA, Lienhardt C. Risk factors for pulmonary tuberculosis: a clinic-based case control study in the Gambia. BMC Public Health. 2006;(6):156.

Hills AP, Farpour-Lambert NJ, Byrne NM. Precision medicine and healthy living: the importance of the built environment. Prog Cardiovasc Dis. 2019;62(1):34–8.

HL7 International. Gravity project [Internet]. [cited 2021 Jun 1]. Available from https://www.hl7.org/gravity/

Holmes L, Enwere M, Williams J, Ogundele B, Chavan P, Piccoli T, et al. Black-white risk differentials in COVID-19 (SARS-COV2) transmission, mortality and case fatality in the United States: translational epidemiologic perspective and challenges. Int J Environ Res Public Health. 2020;17(12):4322.

Hu Z, Melton GB, Arsoniadis EG, Wang Y, Kwaan MR, Simon GJ. Strategies for handling missing clinical data for automated surgical site infection detection from the electronic health record. J Biomed Inform. 2017;68:112–20.

Hussain A, Bhowmik B, do Vale Moreira NC. COVID-19 and diabetes: knowledge in progress. Diabetes Res Clin Pract. 2020;162:108142.

Ikeda, A., Kawachi, I. Social networks and health. In: Steptoe, A. (eds) Handbook of behavioral medicine. Springer, New York, NY. 2010. https://doi.org/10.1007/978-0-387-09488-5_18.

Ingraham NE, Purcell LN, Karam BS, Dudley RA, Usher MG, Warlick CA, et al. Racial and ethnic disparities in hospital admissions from COVID-19: determining the impact of neighborhood deprivation and primary language. J Gen Intern Med. 2021;36(11):3462–70.

Ingram M, Wolf AMA, López-Gálvez NI, Griffin SC, Beamer PI. Proposing a social ecological approach to address disparities in occupational exposures and health for low-wage and minority workers employed in small businesses. J Expo Sci Environ Epidemiol. 2021;31:404–11.

Israel BA. Social networks and health status: linking theory, research, and practice. Patient Couns Health Educ. 1982;4(2):65–79.

Izcovich A, Ragusa MA, Tortosa F, Lavena Marzio MA, Agnoletti C, Bengolea A, et al. Prognostic factors for severity and mortality in patients infected with COVID-19: a systematic review. PLoS One. 2020;15(11):e0241955.

Izquierdo JL, Almonacid C, González Y, Del Rio-Bermudez C, Ancochea J, Cárdenas R, et al. The impact of COVID-19 on patients with asthma. Eur Respir J. 2021;57(3):2003142.

Jackson RJ, Dannenberg AL, Frumkin H. Health and the built environment: 10 years after. Am J Public Health. 2013;103(9):1542–4.

Javanmardi F, Keshavarzi A, Akbari A, Emami A, Pirbonyeh N. Prevalence of underlying diseases in died cases of COVID-19: a systematic review and meta-analysis. PLoS One. 2020;15(10):e0241265.

Jia P, Zou Y, Wu Z, Zhang D, Wu T, Smith M, et al. Street connectivity, physical activity, and childhood obesity: a systematic review and meta-analysis. Obes Rev. 2019;22 Suppl 1(Suppl 1):e12943.

Juarez PD, Hood DB, Song M-A, Ramesh A. Use of an Exposome approach to understand the effects of exposures from the natural, built, and social environments on cardio-vascular disease onset, progression, and outcomes. Front Public Health. 2020;8:379.

Kahn MG, Callahan TJ, Barnard J, Bauck AE, Brown J, Davidson BN, et al. A harmonized data quality assessment terminology and framework for the secondary use of electronic health record data. EGEMS (Wash DC). 2016;4(1):1244.

Kaiser Permanente. Accountable Health Communities Health-Related Social Needs (AHC-HRSN) [Internet]. [cited 2021 Jun 1]. Available from https://sdh-tools-review.kpwashingtonresearch.org/screening-tools/accountable-health-communities-health-related-social-needs

Karaye IM, Horney JA. The impact of social vulnerability on COVID-19 in the U.S.: an analysis of spatially varying relationships. Am J Prev Med. 2020;59(3):317–25.

Kneipp SM, Schwartz TA, Drevdahl DJ, Canales MK, Santacroce S, Santos HP, et al. Trends in health disparities, health inequity, and social determinants of Health Research: a 17-year analysis of NINR, NCI, NHLBI, and NIMHD funding. Nurs Res. 2018;67(3):231–41.

Kolak M, Bhatt J, Park YH, Padrón NA, Molefe A. Quantification of neighborhood-level social determinants of health in the continental United States. JAMA Netw Open. 2020;3(1):e1919928.

Krieger N, Huynh M, Li W, Waterman PD, Van Wye G. Severe sociopolitical stressors and preterm births in New York City: 1 September 2015 to 31 August 2017. J Epidemiol Community Health. 2018;72(12):1147–52.

Laddu D, Paluch AE, LaMonte MJ. The role of the built environment in promoting movement and physical activity across the lifespan: implications for public health. Prog Cardiovasc Dis. 2021;64:33–40.

Lam TM, Vaartjes I, Grobbee DE, Karssenberg D, Lakerveld J. Associations between the built environment and obesity: an umbrella review. Int J Health Geogr. 2021;20(1):7.

Letarte L, Pomerleau S, Tchernof A, Biertho L, Waygood EOD, Lebel A. Neighbourhood effects on obesity: scoping review of time-varying outcomes and exposures in longitudinal designs. BMJ Open. 2020;10(3):e034690.

Lienhardt C. From exposure to disease: the role of environmental factors in susceptibility to and development of tuberculosis. Epidemiol Rev. 2001;23(2):288–301.

Lizzio VA, Gulledge CM, Meta F, Franovic S, Makhni EC. Using a web-based data collection platform to implement an effective electronic patient-reported outcome registry. Arthrosc Tech. 2019;8(6):e535–9.

Lynch EE, Malcoe LH, Laurent SE, Richardson J, Mitchell BC, Meier HCS. The legacy of structural racism: associations between historic redlining, current mortgage lending, and health. SSM Popul Health. 2021;14:100793.

Martin GS, Mannino DM, Eaton S, Moss M. The epidemiology of sepsis in the United States from 1979 through 2000. N Engl J Med. 2003;348(16):1546–54.

Martinez-Cardoso A, Jang W, Baig AA. Moving diabetes upstream: the social determinants of diabetes management and control among immigrants in the US. Curr Diab Rep. 2020;20(10):48.

Mauller P, Doamekpor LA, Reed C, Mfume K. Cardiovascular disease in the nation's capital: how policy and the built environment contribute to disparities in CVD risk factors in Washington, D.C. J Racial Ethn Health Disparities. 2018;6(1):1–10.

McLeroy KR, Bibeau D, Steckler A, Glanz K. An ecological perspective on health promotion programs. Health Educ Behav. 1988a;15(4):351–77.

McLeroy KR, Steckler A, Bibeau D. The social ecology of health promotion interventions. Health Educ Q. 1988b;15(4):351–77.

Mesas AE, Cavero-Redondo I, Álvarez-Bueno C, Sarriá Cabrera MA, Maffei de Andrade S, Sequí-Dominguez I, et al. Predictors of in-hospital COVID-19 mortality: a comprehensive systematic review and meta-analysis exploring differences by age, sex and health conditions. PLoS One. 2020;15(11):e0241742.

Metzler M. Social determinants of health: what, how, why, and now. Prev Chronic Dis. 2007;4(4):A85.

Milad E, Bogg T. Spring 2020 COVID-19 surge: prospective relations between demographic factors, personality traits, Social cognitions and guideline adherence, mask wearing, and symptoms in a U.S. Sample. Ann Behav Med. 2021;55(7):665–76.

N3C. Social Determinants of Health (SDoH) [Internet]. [cited 2021 Jun 1]. Available from https://covid.cd2h.org/social-determinants

Nafilyan V, Islam N, Ayoubkhani D, Gilles C, Katikireddi SV, Mathur R, et al. Ethnicity, household composition and COVID-19 mortality: a national linked data study. J R Soc Med. 2021;114(4):182–211.

National Academies of Sciences, Engineering, and Medicine, Health and Medicine Division, Board on Population Health and Public Health Practice, Committee on Community-Based Solutions to Promote Health Equity in the United States. In: Baciu A, Negussie Y, Geller A, Weinstein JN, editors. Communities in action: pathways to health equity. Washington, DC: National Academies Press; 2017.

National Academies of Sciences, Engineering, and Medicine, Health and Medicine Division; Board on Population Health and Public Health Practice, Roundtable on the Promotion of Health Equity. In: Anderson KM, Olson S, editors. The effects of incarceration and reentry on community health and well-being: proceedings of a workshop. Washington, DC: National Academies Press; 2019a.

National Academies of Sciences, Engineering, and Medicine, Health and Medicine Division; Board on Population Health and Public Health Practice, Committee on Applying Neurobiological and Socio-Behavioral Sciences from Prenatal Through Early Childhood Development: A Health Equity Approach. In: Negussie Y, Geller A, DeVoe JE, editors. Vibrant and healthy kids: aligning science, practice, and policy to advance health equity. Washington, DC: National Academies Press; 2019b.

National Academies of Sciences, Engineering, and Medicine, Health and Medicine Division, Board on Population Health and Public Health Practice. In: Alper J, Martinez RM, editors. Investing in interventions that address non-medical, health-related social needs: proceedings of a workshop. Washington, DC: National Academies Press; 2019c.

Northridge ME, Sclar ED, Biswas P. Sorting out the connections between the built environment and health: a conceptual framework for navigating pathways and planning healthy cities. J Urban Health. 2003;80(4):556–68.

Office of Disease Prevention and Health Promotion. Healthy people 2020. US Department of Health and Human Services. 2015.

Onder G, Rezza G, Brusaferro S. Case-fatality rate and characteristics of patients dying in relation to COVID-19 in Italy. JAMA. 2020;323(18):1775–6.

Palmer RC, Ismond D, Rodriquez EJ, Kaufman JS. Social determinants of health: future directions for health disparities research. Am J Public Health. 2019;109(S1):S70–1.

Pan X, Zhao L, Luo J, Li Y, Zhang L, Wu T, et al. Access to bike lanes and childhood obesity: a systematic review and meta-analysis. Obes Rev. 2020;22:e13042.

Papas MA, Alberg AJ, Ewing R, Helzlsouer KJ, Gary TL, Klassen AC. The built environment and obesity. Epidemiol Rev. 2007;29:129–43.

Peek ME, Cargill A, Huang ES. Diabetes health disparities: a systematic review of health care interventions. Med Care Res Rev. 2007;64(5 Suppl):101S–56S.

Perkins JM, Subramanian SV, Christakis NA. Social networks and health: a systematic review of sociocentric network studies in low- and middle-income countries. Soc Sci Med. 2015;125:60–78.

PsychDB. V codes (DSM-5) & Z codes (ICD-10)—PsychDB [Internet]. [cited 2021 Jun 1]. Available from https://www.psychdb.com/teaching/dsm-v-icd-z-codes#social-environment1

Renalds A, Smith TH, Hale PJ. A systematic review of built environment and health. Fam Community Health. 2010;33(1):68–78.

Richardson S, Hirsch JS, Narasimhan M, Crawford JM, McGinn T, Davidson KW, et al. Presenting characteristics, comorbidities, and outcomes among 5700 patients hospitalized with COVID-19 in the New York City area. JAMA. 2020;323(20):2052–9.

Riou M, Marcot C, Canuet M, Renaud-Picard B, Chatron E, Porzio M, et al. Clinical characteristics of and outcomes for patients with COVID-19 and comorbid lung diseases primarily hospitalized in a conventional pulmonology unit: a retrospective study. Respir Med Res. 2020;79:100801.

Rothman KJ, Adami HO, Trichopoulos D. Should the mission of epidemiology include the eradication of poverty? Lancet. 1998;352(9130):810–3.

Ryvicker M. A conceptual framework for examining healthcare access and navigation: a behavioral-ecological perspective. Soc Theory Health. 2018;16(3):224–40.

Sallis JF, Owen N, Fisher EB. Ecological models of health behavior. In Glanz K, Rimer BK, Viswanath K (Eds.), Health behavior and health education: Theory, research, and practice. Jossey-Bass. 2008. pp. 465–85.

Singh KA, Wilk AS. Affordable care act medicaid expansion and racial and ethnic disparities in access to primary care. J Health Care Poor Underserved. 2019;30(4):1543–59.

SIREN. The Neurological Emergencies Treatment Trials (NETT) Network [Internet]. [cited 2021 Jun 1]. Available from https://siren.network/

Smith KP, Christakis NA. Social networks and health. Annu Rev Sociol. 2008;34(1):405–29.

Sohrabi C, Alsafi Z, O'Neill N, Khan M, Kerwan A, Al-Jabir A, et al. World Health Organization declares global emergency: a review of the 2019 novel coronavirus (COVID-19). Int J Surg. 2020;76:71–6.

Sokol R, Austin A, Chandler C, Byrum E, Bousquette J, Lancaster C, et al. Screening children for social determinants of health: a systematic review. Pediatrics. 2019;144(4):e20191622.

Somma D, Thomas BE, Karim F, Kemp J, Arias N, Auer C, et al. Gender and socio-cultural determinants of TB-related stigma in Bangladesh, India, Malawi and Colombia. Int J Tuberc Lung Dis. 2008;12(7):856–66.

Song S, Kucik JE. Trends in the utilization of recommended clinical preventive services, 2011-2019. Am J Prev Med. 2021;61:149–57.

Souch JM, Cossman JS. A commentary on rural-urban disparities in COVID-19 testing rates per 100,000 and risk factors. J Rural Health. 2021;37(1):188–90.

Srinivasan S, O'Fallon LR, Dearry A. Creating healthy communities, healthy homes, healthy people: initiating a research agenda on the built environment and public health. Am J Public Health. 2003;93(9):1446–50.

Stampfer MJ, Hu FB, Manson JE, Rimm EB, Willett WC. Primary prevention of coronary heart disease in women through diet and lifestyle. N Engl J Med. 2000;343(1):16–22.

Stokols D. Establishing and maintaining healthy environments: toward a social ecology of health promotion. Am Psychol. 1992;47(1):6–22.

Stokols D. Translating social ecological theory into guidelines for community health promotion. Am J Health Promot. 1996;10(4):282–98.

Sullivan PS, Satcher Johnson A, Pembleton ES, Stephenson R, Justice AC, Althoff KN, et al. Epidemiology of HIV in the USA: epidemic burden, inequities, contexts, and responses. Lancet. 2021;397(10279):1095–106.

Sutton S. Determinants of health-related behaviours: theoretical and methodological issues. The Sage handbook of health psychology. London: Sage; 2004.

Terrón-Pérez M, Molina-García J, Martínez-Bello VE, Queralt A. Relationship between the physical environment and physical activity levels in preschool children: a systematic review. Curr Environ Health Rep. 2021;8(2):177–95.

The Lancet Diabetes and Endocrinology. COVID-19: underlying metabolic health in the spotlight. Lancet Diabet Endocrinol. 2020;8:457.

Torres JM, Lawlor J, Colvin JD, Sills MR, Bettenhausen JL, Davidson A, et al. ICD social codes: an underutilized resource for tracking social needs. Med Care. 2017;55(9):810–6.

Van de Mortel TF. Faking it: social desirability response bias in self-report research. Aust J Adv Nur. 2008;25:40–8.

Wadhera RK, Wadhera P, Gaba P, Figueroa JF, Joynt Maddox KE, Yeh RW, et al. Variation in COVID-19 hospitalizations and deaths across new York City boroughs. JAMA. 2020;323(21):2192–5.

Webb Hooper M, Nápoles AM, Pérez-Stable EJ. COVID-19 and racial/ethnic disparities. JAMA. 2020;323(24):2466–7.

Wildeman C, Wang EA. Mass incarceration, public health, and widening inequality in the USA. Lancet. 2017;389(10077):1464–74.

Williams DR, Collins C. Racial residential segregation: a fundamental cause of racial disparities in health. Public Health Rep. 2001;116(5):404–16.

Wortham JM, Lee JT, Althomsons S, Latash J, Davidson A, Guerra K, et al. Characteristics of persons who died with COVID-19—United States, February 12-May 18, 2020. MMWR Morb Mortal Wkly Rep. 2020;69(28):923–9.

Yang J, Zheng Y, Gou X, Pu K, Chen Z, Guo Q, et al. Prevalence of comorbidities and its effects in patients infected with SARS-CoV-2: a systematic review and meta-analysis. Int J Infect Dis. 2020;94:91–5.

Zhang Y, Tzortzopoulos P, Kagioglou M. Healing built-environment effects on health outcomes: environment–occupant–health framework. Build Res Inform. 2018;47(6):1–20.

Part IV
Ethics, Bias, Privacy, and Fairness

Chapter 20
Personal Health Informatics Services and the Different Types of Value they Create

Thomas Wetter

Abstract Personal Health Informatics (PersHI) deals with ICT supported services for patients and citizens to safely enhance their health status. Internet search, online self support groups, or vital signs sensors connected to smart phones are examples. PersHI can create values for the individual or for society: *evidence, insight, mind set,* and *power*.

Evidence applies statistics like in phase III clinical trials. PersHI services are tested against classical treatments for significant superiority. Although such experiments do not epistemologically establish truth, they are deemed sufficient to approve a treatment. Examples of PersHI treaments with successful as well as failed demonstrations of evidence are iuxtaposed.

Compared to the stereotypical approach in evidence, *insight* is inductive and methodologically wide. Typical discoveries set out from lay language posts to social networks where ailments or cures are mentioned next to treatments. Machine Learning can "dig" for associations that are strong enough to suggest effects among terms harvested from posts. Typical discoveries are indication extensions of medications after off label uses or posts about adverse effects. Like an evidence, an insight is not a true fact either but depends on data quality and selected method. However, insight becomes available through data manipulation alone, without extra human subjects experimentation.

Access to information can change the *mindset* in the dimensions *knowledge, emotions, attitudes,* and *behaviors.* Patient education is central for Internet medicine and multiple effects have been shown. We see examples with effects in some dimension, some in isolation, some in combination with other dimensions. Paradoxically, we also see opposite effects in presumably coherent dimensions. Generally, effects tend to occur when the targeted population has a need *now*. Learning for a possible future need is not a common behavior.

T. Wetter (✉)
Institute for Medical Informatics, Heidelberg University Hospital, Heidelberg, Germany

Biomedical Informatics and Medical Education, University of Washington, Seattle, WA, USA
e-mail: thomas.wetter@urz.uni-hd.de

Online media can help citizens to achieve *power* for communities of patients suffering from similar medical conditions. For rare diseases nationwide coordination can lead to improved standards of care. For a debiliating headache we show how patient advocacy achieved access to a controlled substance and why this was ethical although in conflict with applicable law. We also see a patient initiative that stressed a health care system by insisting on vast public resources for a treatment without evidence.

PersHI achievements are ambivalent. The credibility of test theoretic evidence creation vs inductive identification of associations is a matter of debate. Design of trials needs a close eye on the subtleties of human behaviors. The relation between what patients know, feel, and do is sometimes irrational. Power gained through mobilized online crowds can let particulate interests overwhelm the common good. However, regarding the shortage of health care workforce, alternatives models of care delivery are a necessity. PersHI is such a model that draws on patients' active contribution.

Keywords Consumer health informatics · Personal health informatics · Internet Mobile applications · Internet-based intervention · Computer-assisted therapy Patient education · Health knowledge · Empowerment · Patient advocacy · Social determinants of health · Utility · Statistical data interpretation

Introduction

> The therapist is in, and automated to help
> (New York Times International June 10, 2021, about mental health apps)

With ever expanding Information and Communication Technology (ICT) based health related services for lay citizens the question needs to be asked what values—if any—such services create. Derived from the Latin word valere—to be worth—the first meaning of value is "the desirability or worth of a thing" (The International Webster's Comprehensive Dictionary of the English Language). This is the question of a broad evaluation of such health related services. By emphasizing the service character of Personal Health Informatics (PersHI) we follow a characterization as "information and communication technology based methods, services, and equipment that enable the lay citizen to safely play an active role in his health and preventive care" (Wetter 2016, p. 5).[1]

In this chapter we identify qualitatively different notions of "value" that PersHI services can achieve and aggregate studies where the creation—or loss—of such

---

[1] In (Wetter 2016) this definition was used for Consumer Health Informatics, at that time the common expression for patient centered services, which is meanwhile giving way to Personal Health Informatics,

values has been investigated. We consider the following four value dimensions: Evidence, Insight, Mindset, and Power.

Evidence in its general meaning is "that which makes evident or clear" (The International Webster's Comprehensive Dictionary of the English Language). In biomedical research, as in this text, the term is widely used in a specialized meaning of demonstrating superiority or sometimes non-inferiority of a new treatment in a planned experiment. Superiority, and analogously non-inferiority, can be concluded in application of a mathematical theory of statistical testing. In this theory such a conclusion necessarily comes with a likelihood p to err: to call the test outcome positive although it is not. By convention, a p value of <0.05 "indicates that the study evidence was good enough to support that hypothesis (of superiority) beyond reasonable doubt" (Kraemer 2019, p. E1). In this sense evidence is not necessarily truth. It is not less but also not more than a "negotiated social order (Marks 2000, p. 134) to accept an error likelihood of p to regard a successful intervention as unsuccesful. This is the prevailing paradigm of effectivenes research. Successfulness, though, is not clinical importance. "(P)articulary in studies with big data ... even trivial outcomes may have a p value of less than 0.05. "(Kraemer 2019, p. E1).

Insight is less clearly specified and more diverse. Therefore, the following examples may help. At a molecular level the identification of a membrane glycoprotein that a virus can dock to is such a discovery. At a population level we would call a treatment side effect coincidentially reported by many patients in health forums and discovered through text mining algorithms an insight.

Mindset is a combination of digital literacy, knowledge, judgmental capability, skills, emotions, and healthy behavioral patterns. A proper mindset in the sense of this definition allows a citizen to search and identify pertinent information or services, to understand what he finds, to distinguish scientifically sound from not so sound information, and subsequently to live up to what he learns.

Power is the capacity to hold or change affairs to one's will. Society wide, in open societies, power is distributed to different institutions, mainly legislation, administration, and jurisdiction. On the smallest scale of individual treatment decision power sharing between patient and physician is principally given through the autonomy maxim of medical ethics (Beauchamp and Childress 2013). Practically it has gained ground through the shared decision making (Charles et al. 1997) movement. Here we rather look at the middle scale between individual patient and society wide. We look at interest groups that drive agendas to gain or preserve assets for their followers. Citizen or patient associations take aim at processes in health care where decisions are routinely made over their minds. Decades ago this pertained to access to clinical trials for HIV medications. Patient self-help groups achieved that patients could opt to be included in trials rather than being identified and invited by their physicians (Kopelman 1994). HIV was a door opener for other patient self-help groups such that today patients can generally request to be included in trials where they meet the inclusion/exclusion criteria. We look at more recent examples where being organized through social media is instrumental to gaining new opportunities.

The values studied do not exist in isolation but overlap to some extent. The achievement of a value is not necessarily positive altogether. A gain of *power* for some may entail the loss of power of others. A Mindset may be fooled through conspiracy theories perfectly disguised in the coat of scientific evidence, insight, or utility.

While this four-value organization gives the chapter its shape and character, the following aspects that are also associated with Personal Health Informatics (PersHI) will play a marginal role at best. This is not a chapter about Electronic Health Records (EHRs) or patient-held EHRs, not about the methodology of evidence-based medicine, as in (Merlin et al. 2009), not about Medical Device regulation and safety, as in (Moshi et al. 2019). We rather look at end to end services and their value, where the devices and the software play a necessary but subordinate role. It is not about properties of scales, scores, questionnaires, repositories and other instruments that researchers use to acquire patient reported outcomes as in (Hensher et al. 2021) or (Broekhuis et al. 2019). We rather assume that researchers have used instruments that are meaningful to their ends and will ourselves proceed to how scales etc. were used to demonstrate the achievement of one of our values. This chapter does also not aim at promoting gender equity but rather to show the variability of study designs. If the best example known to the author to outline an approach to achieve a certain value is gender biased, we will mention this in the text but gender bias will not be a reason to not use that example.

In this chapter it will not be a reason to exclude an example because it failed. A lot can be learned from failures. Some success factors can best be demonstrated through their absence in failed projects. We will not hesitate to use such examples.

Writing this perspectives chapter mostly draws on established sources for scholarly writing such as pubmed (https://pubmed.ncbi.nlm.nih.gov) and the journals it lists and in a majority of cases offers free open access to. By "perspectives" we mean that, rather than mechanically retrieving and assessing all text that a systematic search brings forth, the author has actively searched for articles that best draw attention to the perspectives he wants to illustrate. Therefore, the claim that comes with this chapter cannot be to draw a true comprehensive picture of all there is qua being found through pubmed. The claim rather is to illustrate the chosen perspectives and how they influence the perception of health and health care delivery. For this end we take the liberty to use those article that best substantiate these perspectives.

The following, though, demonstrates that an attempt to systematically MeSH-search is prone to some misconceptions and biases and does not guarantee a systematic account. The reasons became visible when purposefully rather than systematically searching for this chapter. Once articles have been found work can proceed as we know it from systematic or scoping reviews. Finding, though, has to leave the preferred routes of identifying the MeSH keyword or keywords that characterize a topic and then to MeSH-search. Successful MesH search is based on two assumptions: That keywords exist for a chosen field and that new articles have been indexed. Neither is sufficiently satisfied for the fast advancing field of Personal Health Informatics. First initiatives began around 2000 (Kaplan and Brennan 2001).

The first reader (Nelson and Ball 2004) appeared in 2004, the first textbook (Wetter 2016) in 2016. An application of the author of this chapter for a MeSH keyword in 2012 was turned down because there was the marginally overlapping keyword Consumer Health Information. Not until 2018 was Consumer Health Informatics introduced in MeSH, at a time when the expression Consumer Health Informatics began to become disregarded because the word "consumer" is misleading about the roles and expectations of citizens in the medical arena. Therefore, to access the literature before 2018 he who searches has to invent terms that take him near, e.g. Internet (introduced in 1999), Mobile application (2014), Patient portal (2017), and most recently Internet-based intervention (2020). Which did not really help research for this chapter, because about 20 of all cited publications deal with Internet-based interventions and deserve the keyword, but 2/3 were published before 2020 and hence cannot have it. To summarize, creativity is required for spotting the sources to draw a picture like this chapter.

Values

Evidence

We concentrate on evidence as the demonstration that a therapeutic procedure is efficient. I.e. for the time being we argue within the paradigm of effectiveness research and disregard the critical remarks from (Kraemer 2019 and Marks 2000). For in order for a therapy to be FDA or respective authority outside the USA approved, proof of (superior) effectiveness is required and Randomized Controlled Trials (RCTs) together with statistical test theory are widely accepted as the decision theoretical model to establish effectiveness. This will be our reference point. We will look at variations on the theme of testing an experimental PersHI service against a standard therapy. We will outline different service designs which will address widely different health problems. In preparation of this text it appeared that among the health problems for which PersHi services are developed chronic somatic diseases and depression/anxiety type mental health problems are prevailing. A systematic review would, though, have to confirm that.

By design we primarily mean how and by what criteria subjects were recruited, what services were compared and how the comparison was organized, what primary and secondary outcomes were identified and how they could be recorded, knowing that the trustworthiness of subjects' perceptions may play a biasing role. Outcomes can be of different basic types, some of which are also touched upon in other parts of this chapter. They can, for example, be knowledge and literacy, attitudes and motivations, behaviours, or cures and mitigations of health problems. Since ultimately it only counts if we actually solve or reduce health problems, we mostly concentrate on the latter in this section: cures and mitigations. There are some exceptions, though. In the case of addiction including eating disorders, the changed behaviour comes close to being the cure. Therefore, we include in this section some trials about modifying addictive behaviours.

RCTs are no longer an oddity in the field of PersHI. As indication of maturity, we see primary outcomes clearly identified in most publications, find almost as many study designs published and registered as we find accomplished trials, and find trials that went through early termination because of obvious futility. But we will start with easy standard kind of designs with successful results.

(Wahlund et al. 2021) address the problem of COVID-19 dysfunctional worries and achieve a "brief digital and easily scalable self-guided psychological intervention (that) can significantly reduce … symptoms" (Wahlund et al. 2021, p. 1). In a randomized controlled design registered with ClinicalTrials.gov 670 Swedish adult citizens were randomized to either waiting list (WL) or the new online intervention. In the field of behavioural therapies WL is a standard control condition because it is the easiest to implement and it is realistic: Mostly therapists will not be available immediately for mental health problems and for patients it is a sad but normal experience that they have to wait. To be included in the study, besides some organizational facets, subjects had to have severe difficulty controlling COVID-19 worries and some consequences thereof, such as trouble sleeping or reduced work productivity. This was measured through the Coronavirus Health Impact Survey (CRISIS).[2] Severely depressive or suicidal citizens, according to the Montgomery Åsberg Depression Rating Scale Self-rated (MADRS-S), were excluded. Included patients in the experimental group received a specifically developed Internet based Cognitive Behavioral Intervention (CBI).[3] It consisted of extended texts, tasks to practice, and the opportunity to record progress in a work sheet. To assess and compare the effect of the intervention the primary outcome was the General Anxiety Disorder 7-items scale (GAD-7) in a version adapted to COVID-19 (https://osf.io/exh47/). There were several secondary outcomes regarding work (Work and Socal Adjustment Scale WSAS), sleep, depressive symptoms, tolerance of uncertainty, satisfaction with the intervention etc. GAD-7 and WSAS were taken at baseline and after 1, 2 and 3 weeks (end of the intervention) and 1 month later. At the 3-week endpoint there was a placebo effect, also called the Hawthorne effect in psychological experimentation: The untreated control arm improved on GAD-7, as did the intervention arm. However, the intervention arm was significantly better ($p < 0.001$) than the control arm in an intention to treat analysis. Regarding reduction of worries the intervention arm achieved 40%, and the control arm 17%. The intervention arm also

---

[2] Throughout this section numerous scales, scores, questionnaires etc. will play a role in recording baseline, progress, and cure of a disease. Providing references to all these secondary references would appear double the length of this chapter's bibliography without contributing to a better understanding of "Evidence". Therefore, we leave secondary references away, the more so since all primary references in this chapter point to "Free PMC Articles" in Pubmed. Therefore, the reader can follow up by himself at any time.

[3] The expressions Cognitive Behavioral Therapy (CBT) and Cognitive Behavioral Intervention (CBI) are both used for a widely applied therapy concept that sets out from helping the patient to understand and reflect his problem and then to equip him with solution or coping strategies.

improved on all secondary outcomes. Effects kept improving towards the 1-month follow up. Especially the latter is noteworthy because often effects fade fast after the end of an intervention. No serious adverse events were self-reported by the participants. Altogether this is a first example of a service that has shown that it is effective and safe and lends itself for deployment on a wide scale to citizens with COVID-19.

Another service from Sweden (Topooco et al. 2019) that added an interactive chat element to an unidirectional format like the above achieved even longer lasting healing for adolescents with depression. The article provides a rich overview about the value of interactive elements. The investigation described was made known through social media posts and through schools and youth centers. Of 162 who registered, 66 females and 4 males passed the inclusion/exclusion criteria checked through the Beck Depression Inventory II (BDI-II) and the standardized Mini-International Neuropsychiatric Interview (MINI) and were randomized to the intervention or to minimal control arm. The intervention consisted of eight Internet-delivered Cognitive Behavioral Therapy (ICBT) modules and eight individual 45-minute interactive chat sessions with a therapist over 8 weeks. At 8 weeks the intervention ended and primary outcome and various secondary outcomes were taken. At this time also the control arm patients were offered to transfer to the intervention treatment outside the trial. At 8 weeks 66 subjects responded and BDI-II showed significantly more improvement in the intervention arm than in the control arm (p < 0.001). At 12 months 29 of the 31 intervention arm patients who had answered at 8 weeks completed the measure again. They still had equally low BDI-II values, with larger variance, though. Without exception the secondary outcomes point in the positive direction. Scores for mood, quality of life, anxiety, social interaction, and self-efficacy had more improvement in the intervention than in the usual care arm. Two points of concern of an else very promising approach need to be mentioned. The distribution of males and females unintentionally is very skewed. A major reason certainly is the higher prevalence of depression among girls. Differences in help seeking behavior are also suspected such that campaigns to reach out to boys would have to be different. At this time, however, the investigation only allows conclusions about effectiveness for girls. For the second, this service does not scale up as easily as the former one because it requires human effort of 8 times 45 minutes plus documentary work per patient. A cost effectiveness study should investigate whether the remaining human workload is low enough to warrant the investment into the online offering. On the other hand, a service that combines a systematic impersonal online instruction with an empathetic human interaction may be the recipe for success and also bridge between personal and online medicine.

Cost effectiveness is investigated by (Paganini et al. 2019) in the context of an RCT for two Internet-based pain management therapies against waiting list. Patients with intensive pain other than cancer pain for more than 6 months and satisfying some organizational criteria were randomized to one of two ACT versions, ACTonPain$_{guided}$ and ACTonPain$_{unguided}$ or CG (waiting list Control Group). ACT stands for Acceptance and Commitment Therapy, a form of CBT. Here it consisted of seven modules, each meant for one week, which include information, metaphors, assignments, and mindfulness exercises. ACTonPain$_{guided}$ subjects were in addition contacted by human "eCoaches" weekly who provided feedback regarding the modules and typically spent 1.75 hours on one such activity. Statistically the investigation was powered for effectiveness. Descriptive economic analysis happened on top. The primary outcomes were percentage of subjects improved and quality of life according to the Assessment of Quality of Life 8D (AQoL-8D) instrument. While long-term effects at 6 months were all better for more elaborate treatments, the following test results, after Bonferroni correction for multiple testing, were also significant: For percentage positive treatment effect $ACTonPain_{guided} > ACTonPain_{unguided}$ and $ACTonPain_{guided} > CG$; for AQoL-8D $ACTonPain_{guided} > CG$. This may sound impressive but regarding absolute numbers it is still sad news about chronic pain: Even with the most effective $ACTonPain_{guided}$ only 45% of patients reported minimal or more improvement on pain level. Average quality of life was 0.28 on a scale from 0 to 1.

Nevertheless an exciting question remains whether the winner on effectiveness, $ACTonPain_{guided}$, is also the winner economically. After calculating the setup costs by treatment arm from their own expenses and figures from the software industry the authors have drawn on various public administration sources to collect values for running cost that would accumulate in 6 months. They aggregated direct medical (specialist visits, medication, etc.), direct non-medical (travel, domestic help, etc.) and indirect (mainly absenteism from work) costs. Together with setup the costs were 6945€ for $ACTonPain_{guided}$, 6560€ for $ACTonPain_{unguided}$, and 6908€ for CG. All these figures are mean values; standard deviations are also given and were used for the economic analysis. The underlying raw figures reflect the fact that the better the intervention, the lower the sick leave, medical treatment, and other costs are. So far it may nevertheless appear that all three are so close to each other that we cannot make a recommendation. But the farther reaching health economic question is how much cure we "buy" for the money we spend; in this case how much we pay per 1 patient cured and how much for a unit[4] of quality of life gained. We summarize a comprehensive modeling and simulation approach by (Paganini et al. 2019). From the gross figures the authors conclude that CG is more expensive than $ACTonPain_{unguided}$ although it achieves less, so there is no need to follow up on CG. $ACTonPain_{guided}$ consumes 45€ more than CG per additionally improved patient and 604€ more per improvement of quality of life by 1. Similarly, $ACTonPain_{guided}$ costs 2374 more than $ACTonPain_{unguided}$ per patient improved and 45,993 per quality of life improved by 1. In other words, for more healing we need to pay more and we have to ask the question of whether we are willing to pay more. Sensitivity analysis and stochastic simulation complement the point estimates and help to answer this question. Plotting simulation clouds of incremental costs (vertical axis) against incremental effects (patient cured or quality of life improved), with the origin of ordinates at zero effect and zero additional cost, $ACTonPain_{guided}$—$ACTonPain_{unguided}$ has a majority of points in the first quadrant, meaning that through paying more for

---

[4]This is a theoretical construct: increment of 1 unit of the chosen scale. Since quality of life only varies between 0 and 1 an increment of one can only be achieved in the extreme case from 0 to 1.

ACTonPain$_{guided}$ we achieve better numerical results. For ACTonPain$_{guided}$—CG, however, equally many points lie in the first and last quadrant, meaning that in the simulations it was equally likely to achieve better or worse numerical results for a price paid. Finally, the breakeven point to invest into ACTonPain$_{guided}$ to achieve a better cure was about 2000€ whereas to achieve an increment of 1 of quality of life required more than 40,000€. The underlying sophisticated model cannot work without making assumptions and all conclusions are as valid as modeling assumption and model structure truly map the reality of patients with pain. However, the simulation results clearly show that a moderate investment will likely help with pain and its dysfunctional aspect but quality of life will by far not improve equally. Citizens seeking cure from a program such as ACTonPain$_{guided}$ should, therefore, not nurture expectations that are unrealistic according to the presented modeling approach.

Paganini et al's paradigm was to show that a sophisticated experimental service achieves more medically and then to model how much more we would presumably have to pay for that service. We subsequently use one example to demonstrate a different economic perspective. The perspective is to first show that a new service it is non inferior to an existing one and then that it is less effort intensive, be it finance, workforce, or other. Of two examples, (Axelsson et al. 2020 and Maddison et al. 2019), we skip Axelsson's because it is about a health anxiety, as in (Wahlund et al. 2021). (Maddison et al. 2019) investigate cardiac rehabilitation (CR), either center-based (CBexCR) or as individualized exercise guidance through a dedicated telere-habilitation platform (REMOTE-CR). The study included patients with stable Coronary Heart Disease (CHD) identified through hospitals and outpatient units in Auckland and Tauranga (New Zealand). All had access to the rehab facilities of their health units. In a study of 12 weeks patients randomized to CBexCR received supervised exercise units in cardiac rehabilitation centers. Patients randomized to REMOTE-CR received a basic hardware—smartphone, wearable sensor—and access to web apps and a custom middleware. The whole package allowed concurrent exercise monitoring and retrospective analysis. Grounded in self-efficacy and self-determination theories and the Taxonomy of Behaviour and Change Techniques[5] it encouraged own goal setting, review of training data, behaviour change education and social support. During exercises specialists attended remotely to offer advice and feedback. At baseline, at the end of the intervention after 12 weeks, and after 24 weeks various parameters were recorded through the patient's equipment, cardiac rehabilitation center equipment, or through approved questionnaires. The primary outcome was VO$_2$max, an easy to measure indicator of exercise fitness and predictor of cardiovascular morbitiy and mortality. Metabolic parameters included blood lipids, glucose, and anthropometric values. Other parameters included self-efficacy, confidence, exercise adherence, quality of life, but also adverse events or subjectively experienced deterioration of health state. The recordings at the three checkpoints were taken by exercise physiologists who were blinded for the therapy arm of the patient. 82 (REMOTE-CR) and 80 (CBexCR) patients of mean ages 61

---

[5] For a basic treatment of self efficacy cf. (Bandura 1977)

and 61.5 years started. 69 and 70 were male. Cost data were captured by analyzing patient pathways and staff pathway and identifying costs along the way. For utilizsation of health care resources and medications data from the respective ministery were used. The assumptions were made that software was in a steady state and only costs maintenance and that no discounting was necessary for the short period of 24 weeks. Evaluation of the medical and behavioral value confirmed REMOTE-CR as a promising service. In a strict non-inferiority design the primary outcome VO_2max was not different between the two arms. At 12 weeks most parameters were in favor or REMOTE-CR or neutral, at 24 weeks all were in favor. Cost data lump sums for REMOTE-CR and CBexCR were 4920 vs 9535 New Zealand Dollars. To summarize (Maddison et al. 2019) provides a methodologically straight argument for a cardiac rehab service that can safely be managed through the distance and save about half the cost compared to the standard service. For the most part information and communication technology enable the patient to plan and monitor his effort and progress. Exercise physiologists secure the training sessions which one can do in parallel for several patients. The only downside is the overwhelming number of male subjects. This may reflect the proportions of citizens with CHD in the population but at this stage recommendations cannot be made for females.

(Bennell et al. 2020) also present an exercise program against a somatic disease. Knee osteoarthritis is a chronic disease that does not have a cure by itself and through its inclination for a sedentary life often entails other orthopedic, metabolic, and mental diseases. Motivating patients to exercise may prevent or delay the secondary ailments. Patients who had undergone a 12 week physiotherapist-supervised exercise program were encouraged to keep exercising and were randomized to either receiving regular motivating SMS (n = 56) or to untreated control (n = 54). After 24 more weeks various instruments were presented: self-reported home exercise adherence by Exercise Adherence Rating Scale (EARS) and number of days exercised in the past week as primary outcomes, plus many more about knee pain, physical function, quality of life, some about motivation, and some about anxieties regarding pain. The experimental group was significantly superior in the two primary outcomes but showed no effect in the secondary outcomes. Ironically this appears like a successful experiment with no effect. Designated primary outcomes improved but what makes up life: pain, function, quality of life, ... did not improve. There may be different explanations. For one, exercise might not really be good with knee osteoarthritis. This is unlikely, in light of several prior investigations. A more speculative explanation is the subject expectancy effect (Wetter 2016, p. 299 ff). It is known from psychological research and is also called demand characteristics. Subjects may unconsciously be stimulated to overreport what fulfills the express expectations of the experiment while truthfully reporting other observations. This explanation is speculative but supported through the following observation. The major longitudinal active agent of the intervention were SMSs focused and personalized on exercise behavior and attitude. It is exactly those variables where subjects reported improvement, while no improvement was reported for the variables pain, physical function, quality of life, anxieties ... which were not mentioned in the SMS, so lacking a stimulus to expect and to report changes. If this explanation is right (Bennell et al. 2020) seems to prove a positive adherence but actually it may as well show that answering behaviours can be manipulated through persistent SMS series of selective content.

We conclude "Evidence" with four noteworthy achievements and three suboptimal outcomes of investigations. The following are the noteworthy ones. (Bonnevie et al. 2020) show that most recent behavioral patterns in social media can be used to achieve health outcomes. (Kim and Utz 2019) overproportionally reach underserved population, (Corbett et al. 2015) reach a truly large sample with their intervention, and (Denis et al. 2019) save lives. We only mention (Bonnevie et al. 2020) here and deliver the details in section "Mindset" because the structure of the investigation is a literacy aware comparison between an experimental and a control arm on a large regional scale.

Attention to subjects' health literacy is also a distinguishing aspect in (Kim and Utz 2019)'s work to give diabetics better control of their condition. In an RCT they compared two health literacy sensitive intervention arms with control group and formed two strata by health literacy of subjects, so compared three times two arms. As literacy sensitive part patients outside the control group received an initial face-to-face education, easy-to-read material and the opportunity for action planning through either social media or phone calls, depending on which arm they were in. At baseline low literacy arm subjects' diabetes management was far inferior to high literacy subjects'. However, after 9 weeks the low literacy starters in the phone call arm had caught up with all high literacy starters. The intervention "was effective at mitigating the disadvantages faced by people with low literacy" (Kim and Utz 2019, p. 661), at the effort, though, of regular in-person synchronous contacts.

(Corbett et al. 2015) target age dependent cognitive decay. In an RCT with 6742 subjects older than 50 years they compared two fully automated interventions, General Cognitive Training (CT) and Reasoning Training (RT), to an untreated control group. The primary outcome was the IADL score—Instrumental Activities of Daily Living—among the subsample of subjects older than 60. This was purposefully selected because activities of daily living are pivotal to being able to live an independent life and the older subpopulatation is at higher risk at losing this capacity. In both, General and Reasoning Training, subjects improved significantly. Many other measures of cognitive function showed improvements. Since the "scale of benefit is comparable with in-person training (it indicates) potential as a public health intervention" (Corbett et al. 2015, p. 990).

In a multicenter RCT (Denis et al. 2019) demonstrated the lifesaving effects of giving patients after lung cancer treatment a permanently open web-based symptom monitoring form, for the patients to use whenever they felt a reason. This was compared to fixed schedule imaging follow-up (3 to 6 months laps times). Based on a sample of 121 patients the mean survival times estimated through Kaplan-Meier statistics were 19 months with the permanently open vs 12 months with the fixed schedule scheme. As a true highlight of Personal Health Informatics we see here that active attentive patients equipped with the right tool and service can achieve a lot for themselves.

Where there is light there is shadow. In the following we will try to learn from failed examples and what were the reasons for the failures. The failures are associated with high numbers of drop-outs, inappropriate statistical designs, and early termination of a trial after futile results of an intermediate evaluation.

(Walthouwer et al. 2015) attack the metabolic syndrome, one of the most addressed medical problems for which Personal Health Informatics services have been devised, see e.g. (Wetter 2016 Chap. 9). In industrialized countries and emerging markets overeating and lack of physical exercise pave the way for a diabetes pandemic. Many therapeutic concepts and technical and organizational implementations of weight control and reduction programs have been launched. In the present investigation two forms of intervention have been compared with untreated control. The interventions were 6 units of 15 minutes each, presented as videos in one or as material to read in the second arm. At a 6 month follow up 1015 of 1419 included subjects responded and provided data about their knowledge of diabetes control but also body mass index (BMI) and amount and type of energy uptake. Compared to control the video arm improved on all major variables and the material to read arm improved on energy uptake. Multiple imputation was applied to compensate for the drop-outs but its validity is questionable when almost one third of the values have to be invented. The drop-outs may also be a different less involved crowd for which those who stayed were not representative. Or, as (Lau et al. 2015, p. 9) comment in the discussion of an asthma intervention with an even more dramatic drop out rate: "Consumers must perceive the need … and must assign priority". This was apparently the case in (Denis et al. 2019, p. 3)' lung cancer intervention: "(n)o patients were lost to follow-up" while (Walthouwer et al. 2015)'s subjects did not feel an urgent need.

(Dear et al. 2015) address patients with generalized anxiety and comorbid disorders. In the investigation presented they tested two therapy concepts—Disorder Specific (DS) and Transdiagnostic (TD)—in the two settings Clinician Guided (CG) and Self Guided (SG). Patients were randomized to one of four combinations of concepts and settings. Therapy effects were studied for Generalized Anxiety Disorder (GAD), Major Depression Disorder (MDD), Social Anxiety Disorder (SAD), and Panic Disorder (PD). Many comparisons can be made. We look at CG vs SG because if Self Guided is not inferior, its automated scalable setting can take load off from human offered services. The developments of severity during the time span of the intervention (8 weeks, with 5 lessons to be studied) and up to 2 years were compared, among others, between CG and SG. No essential differences were found, just a somewhat different temporal development of severity among the MDD patients. The data look as if for all four diagnoses Clinician and Self Guided settings are equality good. Not more than "look as if" because the statistical design was to establish superiority of self guided, which failed. So equal effectiveness remains an impression, falling short of a statistically sound conclusion. It would have required a non-inferiority design as in (Maddison et al. 2019) to show equal effectiveness.

By contrast, (Heller et al. 2020) had a sound research design to test a guided Internet intervention for expecting mothers with moderate to severe signs of depression against care as usual. The intervention, MamaKits online, is a 5 week program that trains problem solving skills (PST). Starting before the 30th week of pregnancy women could enroll, had baseline assessments (T0, before randomization) in form of approved self fill questionnaires including Epidemiological Studies Depression Scale (CES-D) and Hospital Anxiety and Depression Scale—Anxiety subscale (HADS-A), and irrespective of treatment arm, additional assessments after the duration of the treatment (T1), at 36 weeks of pregnancy (T2) and 6 weeks post partum (T3). There were three primary outcomes: reduction of severity as of CES-D and HADS-A and child outcome, by gestational week, birth weight and need for emergency Cesarean. Based on sample size calculations, which included an attrition rate of 30%, 291 participants were targeted, to be included within 1 year.

Nothing of this worked as planned. After 3 years 159 women had been added to the study. Of these, 60% of the control and 43% (34/79) of the intervention arm were still available for T3. This is in accordance with only 37 women completing all five modules of PST, down to 9 who did not even complete one. No wonder that the situation after 3 years was not impressive. Within therapy arm and between Ts variances were high. In an intention to treat analysis no difference between control and intervention was significant. Only in the per protocol analysis, in disregard of the drop outs, some results suggested to be significant.

Regarding its original purpose that investigation cannot but be called a failure. But from a broader perspective it demonstrates the maturity of Personal Health Informatics as a sub discipline of therapy science. For the whole records of the investigation were not relegated to oblivion. Rather did the researchers seek approval for an interim analysis which was approved by the Medical Ethics Committee of the hosting academic institution. This led to the conclusion to terminate early based on futility of the available results. This process with its conclusion was submitted for scholarly publishing and was accepted by Journal of Medical Internet Research. The whole approach is fully documented such that future researchers in the field can study and try to learn lessons. They will know that enrollment and the risk of attrition will need special attention.

Insight

As opposed to Evidence, Insight applies inductive methodology. It proceeds from examples or instances to propositions. In radical inductionism instances may come to mind spontaneously, like some biological species seen in a place where it had not lived before or a so far unseen anatomic anomaly. Most insights of farther ranging value, though, do not come to mind spontaneously but need specific instrumentation and procedures.

Needless to say that in Medical Informatics and specifically in PersHI, instrumentation and procedures are data collection, storage, and algorithmic manipulation methods. Data in our case can be sensor data collected about him from the citizen's body or environment. In this case the citizen is the entity from which the collected data emerge but he does not actively contribute to their creation. Citizens may also be involved as "coders" of data. They read and upload values from measuring devices. This, however, does not differ fundamentally and will subsequently not be distinguished from data automatically uploaded from sensors, because the citizen only contributes mechanically, not qualitatively. He does contribute qualitatively when he subjectively evaluates his corporal, mental, emotional, nutritional, or other state and respective (new) observations and problems and shares them with providers or in general online media. From the patient's situation and perspective such sharing may equally well be hedonistic or altruistic: Wishing to showcase one's health and health problems or wishing to help others with similar problems. New insights may emerge from hedonistic and from altruistic activities. Whether a statement is meant to boast or to help may influence the veracity which researchers in this field should have on their minds.

Subsequently we will concentrate on data collected and stored as posts to social media. We will assume that they have been collected legally and their use for research purposes has in some way been approved. Examples worth studying go more than 10 years back.

In the early days of patientslikeme ®[6]when the platform had eleven condition related communities with 82,000 members altogether—it now has more than 2800 conditions and in the five communities analyzed here alone 250,000 members— (Frost et al. 2011) discovered a majority usage of neuroleptic drugs for other than their approved indications. For this purpose they found 1948 patient volunteered histories with modafinil mentions and 1394 with amitriptyline. While modafinil officially targets narkolepsie and amitriptyline targets depression, only 1% and 9% of the posts mentioned usage for these approved of conditions. Furthermore, off label users of amitriptyline were more satisfied than the regular users. Some users showed amazing creativity: While dry mouth is listed as adverse effect of using amitriptyline for depression, patients with amyotrophic lateral sclerosis reported successful use to control their symptom of excess saliva.

A more recent study (Nikfarjam et al. 2019b) reports similar insights from off label use of cancer medications found in www.inspire.com, a patient support platform that focuses on cancer, rare diseases and chronic conditions. Of 279 disease-drug co-occurences found in posts from 14 active support groups 96 were FDA approved, 9 were known off label uses and the majority of 174 were not known from a claims data base that was used to cross check. These 174 instances of disease-drug co-occurences found in posts concentrated on the following four disease-drug pairs: Temodar ™[7]/temozolomide, which is approved for brain tumors now showing for skin cancer; carboplatin discovered for prostate cancer, avastin ®[8] for breast cancer and paclitaxel for colorectal cancer. The relative novelty of temodar for skin cancer

---

[6] patientslikeme is a registered trademark of patientslikeme Inc.

[7] Temodar is a trademark of Merck Sharp & Dohme Corp

[8] Avastin is a registered trademark of Genentech, Inc.

can also be seen from the number of PubMed listed publications (on May 14, 2021): For skin cancer there are four, non of which is a clinical trial. By contrast, for brain tumors we find 299 articles, including 35 clinical trials. The authors mention two possible reasons for trying off label treatments. One is that physicians develop a deep understanding of drug targets and mutations that patients have and lets them conclude that a drug may be effective. The second and concerning reason is that "complexities of insurance coverage may lead to selection of off label alternatives" (Nikfarjam et al. 2019b, p. 304).

At about the same time as off label uses of modafinil and amitriptyline were discovered by (Frost et al. 2011) a study with breast cancer patients (Benton et al. 2011) pioneered the discovery of adverse drug reactions from social media. Respective self help platforms had already collected more than a million posts. The most active of eight platforms included in the investigation were breastcancer.org (70%), komen.org (16.5%) and csn.cancer.org (9.2%). Through sophisticated techniques of Natural Language Processing (NLP) and Medical Terminology mapping free texts were transformed into anonymized tokenized data sets that could be searched for cancer treatment regimes and adverse treatment effect encounters. Many posts were about adverse effects that were already listed in the medication labels or were about fear of rather than encounter of adverse effects. But some so far unknown adverse effects that patient actually suffered of, were discovered, including vaginal dryness with exemestane and letrozole, and as serious ones as high cholesterol with exemestane and fibromyalgia with anastrozole ®.[9] (Nikfarjam et al. 2019a) also contributed to this type of insight. With the same resource as above (www.inspire.com, cf. (Nikfarjam et al. 2019b)), they found mostly skin related and some other so far unknown adverse effects of two chemotherapy classes, erlotinib, and nivolumab resp. pembrozulizumab.

A very severe type of adverse drug reactions was addressed by (Golder et al. 2019): From Twitter ®[10] they identified mothers whose posts according to some preprosessing and human annotation could be classified as 'birth defect yes, unclear, or no'. Two groups were formed, one with 'yes' and one with 'no' and in these groups mentions of medications were sought. The list of the medications and their risk levels was taken from (www.tga.gov.au/prescribing-medicines-pregnancy-database). Besides presumed birth defects some suspected biographic factors for excess risk of birth defects were also recorded and tested in a multivariate logistic regression model. Among all factors associated with birth defects medication use stood out at an odds ration of 2.34 (1.24–4.44, p = 0.004). To summarize, the study creates real life data about impact of medications on fetuses. Such data could by no means be achieved from planned experiments for obvious ethical reasons.

A recent mini review of different pharmacovigilance methods and resources (Lavertu et al. 2021) puts such efforts into context. Published in Clinical

---

[9] Anastrozole is a registered trademark of AstraZeneca UK Limited
[10] Twitter is a registered trademark of Twitter, Inc.

Pharmacology and Therapeutics the review describes existing vigilance methods and resources such as Sentinel, PCORI, OHDSI and lists limitations such as insufficient capture of meaningful outcome measures and fragmentation across providers and focus. By contrast, social media profiles by and large are longitudinal, personal accounts of real life actions taken and experiences made by citizens. They have their own challenges: technical ones such as to transform lay plain language into medical terms and legal/ethical ones such as to protect privacy and to deal with withdrawn posts after they have been used in an analysis. "Ultimately, the combination of various data sources and expertise will result in safer and more effective pharmacovigilance …" (Lavertu et al. 2021, p. 1201).

Patient reported data not only reveal effects of medications, be they desired or adverse. In a new investigation (Oyebode et al. 2021) use a random selection from 47 million posts to Twitter, Facebook ®,[11] and YouTube to probe for sentiments that users of these platforms developed in response to the COVID-19 pandemic. The authors first cleansed the corpus. Among others they removed all web syntax expressions (hashtags, URLs, etc.) and special characters and converted online slang to English. Then they extracted key phrases which were matched against tokens in a lexicon that specializes on sentiment assignment (https://www.aaai.org/ocs/index.php/ICWSM/ICWSM14/paper/viewPaper/8109). Key phrases labeled as representing a positive or a negative sentiment were aggregated into categories or broader themes. 34 negative themes emerged of which 15 could be associated with the pandemic, including health related ones such as *struggling health system*, psychosocial ones such as *frustration due to life disruption*, or social ones such as *domestic violence* (Oyebode et al. 2021 p. 8). Positive themes were also found, fewer though, but encouraging as a diagnostic of population mental and social health: *public awareness, spiritual support.* Insights of both, positive and negative sentiments may help local health authorities to configure and deploy support programs and structures that meet the true physical and emotional needs and to make use of healing factors such as family connection and spiritual support.

Insights presented here draw on seeing the medical needle in the haystack of human texting in all its variations and messiness. It starts with misspelled pharmaceuticals, lay names for diseases or treatments, indications for affirmative vs negative, potential vs factual etc.. In the success case it ends with high fidelity classification of posts under categories studied. This requires large volumes of raw data, ethical consent to use them, large dictionaries and terminologies to compare against, and sophisticated algorithms to demonstrate the insights. The price is high but if the reward is new medical knowledge without need of experimentation with human subjects it should be worth the price.

---

[11] The registered trademark Facebook is owned by Facebook Inc.

Mindset

Mindset is in the first place understood as acquiring knowledge and skills, modifying attitudes and emotions that may induce behavior changes. Assistance in developing the mindset comes through ICT, mainly health apps and web sites, but also YouTube, Twitter, and other social media. The aspects of Mindset cannot be seen in isolation. *Aquired knowledge* can unleash other changes of the mindset. He who commands more knowledge may understand better what happens in him, around him, and to him. Concretely, as a patient he may better understand symptoms, how his environment reacts and what effects therapies are supposed to have. What was opaque and by that token terrifying becomes transparent and *emotions* such as anxiety may fade. Second, knowledge may also help to consciously develop *attitudes* towards medical institutions or procedures. All three, knowledge, emotions, and attitudes are drivers of *behaviours* which we will also study in this section. Ultimately the purpose of education in the field of biomedicine is healthy behaviors that lead to better healths *outcomes*. Outcome was mostly treated in section "Evidence", although there is considerable overlap.

Richards et al. (1998) already speculated about the "future role of the Internet in patient education". Written while the transition from static to animated and interactive contents was ongoing the authors imagined how this might help in future teaching, health assessment and decision support and that legislation and regulation were due. Meanwhile contents has far advanced but legislation and regulation faces ever new challenges.

Since Richards hundreds of articles have been written about using the Internet and mobile devices for health education. A clear majority addresses the following problems: How can we ascertain the correctness of published contents, be it as authors or in the role of a reviewer? And how can we present the material in such a way that our clients can comprehend and draw the right conclusions for themselves? The latter comes in different flavors: reading level classification of published material, health literacy/numeracy tests of the readers, variants for easier reading, animations etc.. We will not go deeper into these variations. We will rather take health related material as is, as it has been used in investigations that we study and will look closer at the questions, if, how, to what extent etc. the material has achieved Mindset changes, but also sometimes why not.

Knowledge

We will use five investigations to outline the impact of online material on knowledge. One of them, (Fraval et al. 2015), will appear again in its capacity to reduce anxiety. A key asset of this investigation is the patient's informed consent for surgery. To prepare the patient better the authors of the publication developed a web site http://www.orthoanswer.org/ (last viewed May 18, 2020). In a two arm RCT with 211 patients (42 were excluded due to insufficient reading skills) they compared standard conversation between patient and surgeon to standard conversation *plus* web site access. Besides satisfaction and anxiety, knowledge was the major outcome. It was measured through the Deaconess Informed Consent comprehension test, a validated questionnaire for knowledge of informed consent that was adapted to the orthopedic procedures. Correctness in the experimental arm was significantly higher: 69.25% vs 47.38% (p < 0.01); patients acquired significantly more knowledge.

Beerthuizen et al. (2020) investigate the effect of a sophisticated tailored self management support module to manage asthma. At the end of a 12 week high altitude treatment all patients received the standard discharge information. Patients in the experimental arm of the RCT additionally received PatientCoach, i.e. access to a whole set of tools. These included educational material such as understanding of asthma pathology, the purpose of their medications, the environmental influences, indicators for worsening breathing, and warning signs when to seek medical help, but also various bookkeeping, consumer electronics sensory, and self assessment instruments. These were tailored to the individual patient's severity and circumstances. At that time two major forms of asthma were known. For the study they were distinguished using the Asthma Control Questionnaire: *controlled asthma* with ACQ6 < 1.5. at therapy baseline, else *uncontrolled*. Patients were prompted to fill diverse questionnaires, including the ACQ6, at baseline and again at 3, 6, 9 and 12 months. With 91 missing of the due 310 questionnaires from 62 included patients a sophisticated data imputing regime was applied. Apart from this caveat about the quality of the data we see significantly better control knowledge in the PatientCoach arm throughout the follow up checkpoints. ACQ6 levels did gradually worsen over time in all subgroups. However, in the harder to treat *uncontrolled asthma* condition the control knowledge declined more slowly than in the *controlled asthma* condition which the authors characterize as "important and clinically relevant improvement". One might add that where the urge to control is clearly felt the motivation is there to preserve and apply the control knowledge.

The need may not be so clear in the following counterexample where Breastfeed4Ghana and @breastfeed4GH were rolled out through Facebook and Twitter to increase breastfeeding knowledge (Harding et al. 2020). 60 graphics with educational messages were created to convey basic knowledge and knowledge about breastfeeding in public and in the workplace. After an inaugural event with highranking officers the service was advertised within Facebook and Twitter plus through Whatsapp for 2 weeks and then the messages were deployed to registered citizens at a rate of three messages per day. Between week 15 and 22 the most visited messages were re-disseminated now also using influencers and paid ads. To note the performance of the campaign typical indicators such as likes, followers, etc. were recorded and clearly showed a substantial number of followers: 4096 in Facebook ® and 736 in Twitter. Surveys about the effect of the campaign were then filled by 451 subjects, about half of whom reported having been exposed to the campaign. Amazingly, 61% of the exposed could no longer remember what the campaign was about. Anyway, their knowledge was compared to the knowledge of non exposed subjects. A quiz with 7 questions, 4 multiple choice and 3 yes/no, was presented and correctness of answers was compared, with no significant difference between exposed and non exposed. Different, though, were the knowledge levels of those with child vs no child. A success factor that is prevailing among parents but only randomly present in the sample taken for the study is the pre-existing interest in the topic. Knowledge is gathered when there is a need; it is not taken on stock. Campaigns may go void when the target audiences do not see an actual purpose for the contents conveyed.

The next study demonstrates that knowledge can be conveyed and at the same time anxiety can be reduced. (Attai et al. 2015) report results from the Twitter support community #BCSM—Breast Cancer Social Media—where cancer patients can exchange knowledge and advice. In a very open Patient Reported Outcome Measure (PROM) setting the researchers asked 206 users of #BCSM, 191 of whom female, whether they believe that their knowlegde increased in different subdomains. Clear majorities affirmed to have gained general knowledge (80.9%), survivorship (85.7%), metastatic breast cancer (79,4%) and several more. Participants were also prompted about anxiety. Of 42 who reported "high" or "extreme" anxiety upfront, 29 reported "low" or "no" after membership in #BCSM; conversely, no participant moved the other way round. Since these were patient reported outcomes without any control, it cannot be excluded that some of the positive developments camouflage a subject expectancy effect (Wetter 2016, p. 299 ff); overreporting of results that presumably satisfy the researchers. But all percentages are so large that presumably there are true effects and emotion related effects go in line with knowledge related effects.

We now look an investigation from UK where anxiety stands in a complex relation to knowledge and sources of knowledge. Among the patients who receive secondary or tertiary care for Inflammatory Bowel Disease (IBD) through a hospital in Leeds a sample of 774 had already contributed to an earlier investigation. (Selinger et al. 2017) now invited them to reply about their disease state and various circumstances, including their resources to collect medical information and about their health related anxiety. Although this was not a truly old population official paper brochures still played the second largest role (used by 59,9%), after personal contacts with the hospital team (82,3%) and followed by official websites (53,5%). By contrast, alternative health websites were only used by 9%. Higher knowledge about the disease was among others significantly associated with level of formal education, membership with Crohn's and Colitis UK membership, and frequent use of official web sites. To the contrary frequent use of alternative health websites (homeopathy, nutritionist) and random web sites was significantly associated with higher anxiety. This is certainly hard to interpret. The authors concede that they cannot draw any conclusions on causality. The latter resources may spread information that induces anxiety but equally well may more anxious patients more likely be inclined to seek random sources. Whatsoever the reasons are, uncontrolled web sites deserve attention as to their effect on patient mindsets.

Attitude and Emotion

Our next direction of mindset is **attitude** and **emotion**. While emotions such as anxiety develop internally in response to external or internal stimuli an attitude rather is an outgoing positioning towards states or actions. One can be internally afraid of a vaccination in an emotional sense or have an attitude against vaccinations derived from knowledge or from following influencers etc. which makes one take— or avoid—actions.

The topic of vaccination is viral for the discussion about attitudes. We analyze dynamics of two pro vaccination and one anti vaccination campaign. The two pro campaigns were published in (Daley et al. 2018 and Bonnevie et al. 2020). Daley targets parents about childhood vaccinations, Bonnevie underserved adult communities about seasonal flu vaccinations. Daley used a conventional approach with two variants of a self developed dedicated web site while Bonnevie allowed herself the liberty to communicate her message to micro influencers and engaged them to give them the look and feel of their services.

In detail, Daley created three arms for an RCT: website with vaccine information plus social media components (VSM), website with vaccine information (VI), or usual care. 1093 expecting parents were recruited of whom 945 completed vaccine attitude surveys at enrollment (baseline), 3 to 5 and 12 to 15 months after birth (Timepoints 1 and 2). Among parents who were vaccine hesitant at baseline attitudes towards vaccination and its benefits improved significantly and almost equally at Timepoint 1 and improved more at Timepoint 2 with VSM showing the strongest increase. Participant who were already vaccination positive showed no change in attitude.

In detail, Bonnevie selected micro influencers with regional reach in a region where Kaiser Permanente had a large number of African American and Hispanic members. Results here were compared with results in a region that was not typically reached by the hired micro influencers and had similar proportions of African American and Hispanic citizens. Influencers were carefully selected to avoid engaging anti vaxers. Their followers were analyzed as to the proportion of African Americans and Hispanics. Selected influencers were instructed to let their messages be in accordance with the contents and aims of the campaign but were encouraged to give the posts their look and feel. Altogether 117 influencers where engaged most of whose post were on parenting (31%) or travel (10%), fashion or wellbeing, so a typical microcosmos, and 77,7% were female. Engagements such as likes or shares for posts happened both in English (49,471) and in Spanish (20,242). Representative samples from both regions were taken at baseline i.e. before the beginning of the 2018-19 flu seasons and after the season through a commercial opinion poll company. Various demographics were asked essentially demonstrating that the target populations were well matched. More than 50% of respondents were between 18 and 35, certainly an age cohort for whom subscribing to influencers is more typical than for retirement age.

Bonnevie's various results stand out in two aspects that may appear contradictory upfront. Experimental group i.e. in the targeted region versus control group i.e.

in a different region, asked at baseline and again after the campaign, voiced similar vaccination behavior percentages: "normally get vaccinated" (>50%), "some years" (25%), or "never" (~20%). Apparently there was no effect on actual behavior. By contrast "several measurements of specific knowledge and positive attitudes towards the flu vaccine were statistically significantly higher at follow up than at baseline" (Bonnevie et al. 2020, p. 7) in the exposed population. Significantly more subjects after the end of the season agreed that it is never too late for the vaccination, disagreed that healthy people do not need it, believed that government monitors safety, doubt that the vaccine is worse than the flu. Altogether, to affirm attitudes it proved successful to rely on the networks of trust between influencers and their followers and to conceal the top down character of the campaign but rather let it appear as bottom up. Whether this is ethical is a question in its own right. This notwithstanding the campaign effect is a cognitive underpinning for a basically positive attitude which may help to resist when tempted through challenging negative anti vaxer views.

Such cognitive intellectual reinforcement may be very necessary, because it can as well go the other way round, in the small and in the large. (Bradshaw et al. 2020) describe the sophistication and assertiveness of one anti vaccination campaign while (Wilson and Wiysonge 2020) analyze on a wide international level the use of social media to organize action and the level of negatively oriented discourse about vaccination.

Bradshaw's topic is "Vaccines Revealed" (https://www.vaccinesrevealed.com/about_us/), an outspoken anti vaccination URL and at the time of the investigation also the largest closed Facebook group on vaccination. It offers a documentary series to promote childhood vaccination exemptions and by that token is at odds with American Academy of Pediatrics guidelines. "Vaccines Revealed" impresses through three parents of vaccine injured children and a full slate of experts who in their entirety can apparently not be wrong. The MDs among the experts are notorious for their natural medicine preference for every condition. And there is a vaccine injury attorney and a CDC senior scientist. The ethics that drives the whole argument is a premise that is faulty upfront, howerver, in a way that lay citizens and even some scientists have hard times not to be fooled: "When it comes to vaccine risk, the only debate is the degree of risk that vaccines pose." This premise rightly paraphrases the medical ethics maxime "noli nocere"—above all prevent harm and then elaborates and substantiates through the witnesses and their rank and biography that vaccinations can cause harm—harm caused through action. Harm can, however, also be caused through non-action or omission. Not vaccinating a child may lethally harm the child when it contrives the disease and harm other citizens because he transmits the disease. Rationally, for all approved vaccines the risk of the action of vaccinating is by orders of magnitude lower than the risk of the omission, of refusing the vaccination. Emotionally, however, the risk of harming through action weighs by far higher than the risk through omission. This is over-expressed in the situation of childhood—minor—vaccinations where some parents are paralyzed through the fear to harm their loved ones through the "shot" (sic) while they disavow the risk of infection.

Bradshaw et al. (2020) have not investigated whether "Vaccines Revealed" actually caused vaccination exempts or refusals. Such is the aim of (Wilson and Wiysonge 2020). In contrast to Bradshaw, they investigate vaccinations in general, in disregard of the COVID-19 pandemic. Therefore, they are lacking some of the emotional and political aspects of making a decision as a legal guardian of a minor. Discussing their methods would go beyond the scope of this chapter. So we summarize their achievements from analyzing geocoded tweets world wide, opinion polls from 137 countries and WHO vaccination coverage data from 166 countries. In countries where Twitter is used intensely and by many to get organized, the belief that vaccines are unsafe is spread wide. Even more so, if misinformation spills across country borders vaccination coverage further declines in the inundated country. We have, therefore, to be aware that foreign social media intrusion does not only target elections or trade secrets but also public health in the affected countries.

Behavior

Finally we discuss one example where improved knowledge and attitude eventually transformed into action and one where it did not. Two related publications from Iran make the positive case using modest technology, SMS. The aim of (Mehran et al. 2012) was to improve the use of iodized salt for expecting mothers and young children in Tehran and by that token to foster normal brain development. In an RCT with 205 subjects control and experimental arm both received introductory information about the importance of iodized salt. The experimental "SMS" group additionally received one educational SMS per day for 6 weeks. At 8 weeks knowledge, awareness, iodine concentration in urine, and iodine concentration in salt samples from the households were checked. To the researchers' surprise differences were all but moderate at this endpoint. Knowledge and attitude did increase significantly more in the SMS arm, but both arms improved on all outcomes. However, in a follow up with the same housewives participating (Nazeri et al. 2015) the SMS group had sustained higher knowledge and awareness *and* higher measured iodine concentrations. Conversely, in the control group low awareness correlated with low urine concentrations. To conclude, the ultimate outcome improved sustainably under the more intense SMS intervention alone.

Rouf et al. (2020) addressed another nutrition issue. They tested in a three arm RCT with 211 students whether more intensive exposure to educational material about the developmental need of sufficient calcium intake increases intake. Their hypothesis that nutritional behavior can be improved was not supported through the results. While in the high intensitiy Facebook plus text messages therapy arm knowledge improved significantly, neither milk nor other calcium rich food uptake increased significantly and paradoxically increased more in the low intensity arms (Facebook without text messages, electronic leaflet). "Further research is needed" (Rouf et al. 2020, p. 2), as the authors conclude. Following observations by (Yu et al. 2014) a hypothesis to be tested would be to examine when enough is enough.

Busy individuals, in Yu's case hampered through a chronic disease, do not welcome additional intrusions into their lives unless they are obviously beneficial.

Personal Health Informatics efforts—be it top down from government, research, or public health institutions or be it bottom up through citizen driven social media campaigns—have educational aims of different kinds. We have seen examples where these could be achieved (Fraval et al. 2015; Beerthuizen et al. 2020; Attai et al. 2015; Mehran et al. 2012). We saw one failure ((Rouf et al. 2020) and some in between studies (Harding et al. 2020; Selinger et al. 2017; Bonnevie et al. 2020)). Two studies are ecological rather than interventional (Bradshaw et al. 2020; Wilson and Wiysonge 2020). They try to understand the effects of existing health related online media in populations. The diversity of results in this section clearly indicates that research should have a keen eye on effects on health related education emanating from a Pandora's box of originators.

Power

While in this chapter we often use the words citizen and client or subject—depending whether we refer to the day to day life situation or to experimental settings—the normal term for a person who needs help regarding his health is "patient". Patient derives from the Latin pateri which means to suffer. Besides conveying the need for help this also signals a passive role. The patient is treated, undergoes surgery, receives medication etc.. This section deals with changing roles. We will present stages of a more active and eventually powerful role of citizens facing health problems. The first association that the reader may have is "Shared Decision Making" (Charles et al. 1997) as a process between an individual patient and an individual physician or care team to agree about an individual treatment plan. This is *not*, what we will focus on. We will rather elaborate on situations where citizens or patients gather and aggregate their forces to build a pressure group and to achieve something on a general level that presumably helps the members of the pressure group. An example in recent history is the successful effort of HIV/AIDS patients in the 1990s to get access to new pharmaceuticals that were in clinical trials, both by giving them access to the trials or by giving them individually the right to use the substances. Patients overcame the so far prevailing paradigm that physicians take initiative and filter upfront who would be offered to enroll for a clinical trial (Kopelman 1994). This achievement was made in the early days of the Internet and social media did not yet play a helping role. The Treatment Action Group emerged from these activities and broadened the scope by actively searching for potential treatments. In the sequel we will concentrate on efforts where Internet and social media are widely available and see how they helped patients to push the borders of their activities. Some such movements have been initiated top down through researchers or authorities to instigate subsequent bottom up specification of requests to the health care system, e.g. (Dalton et al. 2018). Here we do *not* consider such originally top down activities but concentrate on genuinely bottom up ones.

Rare diseases seem to suggest themselves for bottom up engagement of affected patients or their parents. Actually, in the field of Dravet syndrome, a rare type of epilepsy, (Black and Baker 2011) report about the IDEA League, where IDEA League stands for International Dravet syndrome Epilepsy Action League. IDEA League pursued two goals. For families it offered advocacy and education. For the health care system an array of improvements were targeted. They included guidelines and standards of health care, support to coordinate and conduct research, develop policies for better funding, and achieve universal coverage of approved medications. The British branch has established a major fundraising institution, the Dean Henshall Memorial Fund, which is still active and today serves a broader range of purposes. A recent activity in support of Dravet syndrom patients (Brambilla et al. 2021) was an Internet conveyed survey conducted through employees of Dravet centers in several European countries to understand the impact of COVID-19 on Dravet syndrome patients.

Another interesting initiative where patients gained power and overthrew legal limitations is the therapy of cluster headache. (Kempner and Bailey 2019) investigate how the „Clusterbusters", a networked patient-led research initiative aggregated knowledge about therapy options for a so far untreatable debiliating disease. So debiliating that in the network suicide was a frequent topic and led to the somewhat sarcastic motto "Psychedelics or Suicide". According to (Kempner and Bailey 2019) the Clusterbusters have also exploited the opportunities of the Internet to allow the individual patient to make his treatment choices but to collectivize the reporting and interpreting of results. Here we concentrate on psychedelics, concretely, on mushrooms that contain Psilocybe. This substance was and still is only approved for industrial and research purposes and its private use is probihited. Clusterbusters nevertheless used it, reported about the effects and thereby helped therapy research. Through their act of civil disobedience they changed the rules and gained power and gained access to an otherwise restricted substance. This should not be taken as a recommendation for disobedience as the new virtue of patient behavior. But in this case we are facing a situation where legislation lags ethics (cf. Wetter 2016, p. 370f). According to (Beauchamp and Childress 2013) we find patient autonomy among four maximes of medical ethics. Autonomy, if seen in isolation, would permit psilocybe. Applicable law prohibits its use and in case of conflict applicable law outweighs ethics. So users of psilocybe violate applicable law. But do they act immorally? Applicable law is in accordance with another maxime, non-maleficence. It is known that Psilocybe may be lethal and prohibiting it avoids the harm of intoxications. Together, this poses a classical moral dilemma: autonomy and non-maleficence request different behaviors. Often, there is no solution to a dilemma. If, however, applicable law is not enforced, individual decisions and behaviors deviate from the normative ethics and rather give rise to a descriptive ethics: What is moral is not deduced from higher principles but emerges from undisputed behaviors.

Until this point using Psilocybe is a collection of individual behaviors. We could, though, go further for a society wide ethics that ratifies Psilocybe use, by drawing on the "Psychedelics or Suicide" "motto". If this is not meant sarcastic but reflects true sentiments, it means that not only allowing but also denying Psilocybe may cause harm. So we have the autonomy maxim in favor and the non-maleficience maxim in favor and in disfavor of Psylocybe permission. A utilitarian weighing of the maxims applied here—autonomy and non-maleficience in its two faces—could eventually lead to legislation that tolerates the substance use if requested by the citizen.

Polich (2012) provides a generic description of a bottom up patient initiated process to drive therapy research. Typically, enabled through the Internet and social media some pioneer patients volunteer anecdotes about accidential therapeutic effects or self initiated experiments and their outcomes. The range of therapies is much wider than in a typical two or sometimes three arm experimental trial. It is as wide as physicians or patients have ideas what off label uses of approved pharmaceuticals is worth giving a try. Outside the spheres of interest of academia and industry substances and modes of treatment including natural medicines which are otherwise stigmatized can be tried. This is usually a perfectly legal endeavour, as opposed to the claim to use Psilocybe, and may eventually even bring economic return for a pharmaceutical company if an indication extension of an approved pharmaceutical is discovered through the self experimentation of patients. Grassroots experiences made by the pioneers are then disseminated and may be commented and re-inforced by others. When a certain volume of observations has been shared and sighted, a stage is reached where (semi-)professional implementation in forms of data bases, systematic surveys etc. is required. Promising results at this stage may give rise to formal trials and sustainable funding. The more compelling the results from volunteered and aggregated date the more pressing is the question whether a trial is still due or whether the results be regarded as sufficient evidence. Along this way there are commonalities with and differences from professional led research. Since patient initiatives' common aims include to ultimately find their achievements published in professional media, they strive for systematic and reproducible action and observation/measurement in the veins of biostatistics or epidemiology. What they observe, however, reflects their intrinsic values. While professionals may "pursue academic, mechanistic questions … patients prioritize more pragmatic questions" (Polich 2012, p. 170). They study how their lives are affected and what unexpected and also what adverse effects may emerge. An example portal of a rare disease patient self support group can be found at https://www.anausa.org/index.php/.

Polich (2012) describes a research process initiated outside classical medicine and eventually entering the ranks of academic medicine. In the later years some patient driven initiatives have gained even more ground and have at some time become first tier resources, leaving the second tier for academia. (Whitsitt et al. 2015) describe this transition for dermatology. Starting point of their investigation ist Pinterest ®,[12] an Internet platform for the exchange of serious contents. Starting with five terms relevant in dermatology, e.g. *skin cancer awareness* and *sun*

---

[12] Pinterest is a registered trademark of Pinterest, Inc.

protection, they evaluated how and how often they were represented in pins—individual notices—and boards—ongoing threads of discussion. Findings in Pinterest could be expected as they were: mostly informative (49% of pins and 53% of boards), then advocacy (37% and 31%), then home remedies (14% and 16%). What amazed, even alarmed the authors: Only 24% of boards were created by M.D.s or advocacy groups. The ten top dermatology journals were nearly invisible and only one board was initiated by JAMA Dermatology. Dermatology has lost the place of primary information provider to an amourphous social media platform. "(D)ermatology organizations are relatively absent … This is a missed opportunity for targeted efforts to inform … on a multitude of skin related diseases." (Whitsitt et al. 2015, p. 3).

In the field of pediatric neurology the weight of Disease Advocacy Organizations (DAOs) is meanwhile even higher. As (Horrow et al. 2019) write, MDs in the field, according to a survey with 230, engage in four ways that speak a clear language with DAOs. They access or ***distribute*** DAO-produced materials; they consult DAOs; they collaborate in research; and they ***co-produce*** scholarly material with DAOs. It appears like the momentum is with the DAOs while doctors are junior partners. The authors discuss the observations very critically. Here are some quotes: "DAOs are expanding into clinical settings in many ways, …"—"The influence of DAOs may challenge the typical doctor-patient relationship."—"… close relationships with researchers can give DAOs increased influence over the research process and goals."—"… concerns … in the ethics literature … potential conflicts of interest with DAOs … industry funding." (Horrow et al. 2019, pp. 6 and 7). Whether a leading role of DAOs ultimately serves the purpose of ever improving services and outcomes for the affected patients is a different question. But in the field of pediatric neurology in these days the article finds a whole lot of power in the hands of the DAOs.

Also in neurology we find a recent similarly skeptical position taken by (Martini and Bragazzi 2021) about too much power in the hands of DAOs. Their concerns are mostly based on a view that neurological diseases need a highly complex and multidisciplinary approach and that there are many reasons to believe that patient held resources cannot deliver the necessary quality. They cite investigations about insufficient correctness and clarity of websites including misleading information about unapproved therapies and note possible conflicts of interest when industry funding for patient groups is involved. All these concerns are certainly right when applied to health resources on the Internet in their entirety. When applied to flagship advocacy organization the picture may be brighter because, like medical professional institutions, the DAOs depend on the trust of their members.

We have so far—with the exception of the "Clusterbusters"—made the silent assumption that when there is a will and sufficient reason to try an experimental treatment there is a way to get hold of the required substances. This is, however, anything but self evident. (Mackey and Schoenfeld 2016) have analyzed that in the USA it comes with a whole battery of mechanisms and a legal framework where the FDA deviates from various state legislations. This framework is in continuous motion and would deserve a book chapter in its own right. Because it is one important facet of patient striving for power through online media we will at least provide an introductory view. Only under the premise that pharmaceutical companies will make a substance available will the FDA check an application for "expanded access" or "compassionate use": use beyond approved indications. Pharmaceutical companies have their own agendas and are not obliged to comply. They may hope for indication extensions but also fear bad PR in case of an incident and approve or decline accordingly, for medical or for other reasons. At the same time states pass "Right to try" laws of which it is not sure whether they will be overridden through national legislation. This is a field for the general petition movement, where citizens can try to collect electronic support for philantropic, equal rights, or other purposes. Here, knowing what rhetoric makes a petition successful helps more than medical or clinical evidence expertise. Petitions can, therefore come from serious DAOs but equally well from ad-hoc crowds. In this sense they are not an indication of sustained power but of transient success. In a comment to (Mackey and Schoenfeld 2016; Hogan 2016, p. 4) argues that „only a disruptive force ... that addresses industry concerns ... will alter ... the expanded access campaigns as the method of choice for desperate patients ....".

Pullman, Zarzecny and Picard (Pullman et al. 2013), an ethicist, a public policy scholar, and an author, who closely followed the Canadian experience with the CCSVI movement, provide a more fundamental treatment of questions to be addressed and steps to be taken to give patient advocacy a sound basis beyond its present ad-hoc nature. CCSVI stands for Chronic Cerebrospinal Venous Insuffiency and some believe that it causes MS (Multiple Sclerosis) and that venoplasty is an effective therapy. Since its inception in the 2000s it has been among the most viral patient advocacy movements. For years it had positive public attention, fueled through its romantic flavor, a husband seeking a cure for his wife's untreatable disease. Petitions mushroomed and lawmakers could not but take action, although sound scientific proof was missing and warning of adverse events and some venular autopsy findings in the aftermath of vascular surgery were around. Federal money was invested into a registry and observational studies, while the provinces pursued different plans. Therefore, if judged by the confusion of the lawmakers this was a very successful disruptive campaign. An expert panel was convened which recommended a scientific process including a clinical trial. But a political process was put in place instead and evidence was ignored. Results from the regional trials came slower than the requests from politics for a plan, while a public opinion battle kept rolling. Politics and scientific medicine equally felt the pressure and blinded randomized controlled trials were considered but not approved. This all happened and burnt a lot of money while more promising MS therapies required funding for clinical trial and other frequent life threatening diseases such as cardiovasular or cancer required coverage. (Pullman et al. 2013) summarize their considerations with trenchant comments on the prospect and necessary limitations to patient advocacy. "Deliberate democracies cannot afford to be high-jacked by a cyber-mob. However, ... findings ... speculative or proven make their way into the public sphere ...." Academia may face a storm any time by an "interested, enthusiastic, and motivated public. Researchers and clinicians must learn to utilize these resources ...

". In the case of CCSVI no scientific evidence has meanwhile been found in its support. However, from the perspective of patients with so far untreatable diseases, new therapies and patient reports on their effects should still be taken seriously and not be discarded for the NIH-syndrome—Not Invented Here.

Discussion

The Roles of Personal Health Informatics in the Medical Industry

With some of its facets Personal Health Informatics (PersHI) is or is on the way to be a genuine part of the medical industry. Evidence for some Internet therapies is as conclusive as it is for other therapies. With other facets PersHI is totally at odds with the medical industry. Patients organize themselves to get access to prohibited substances, to funding, and to scholarly progress, sometimes bypassing professional organizations or public administration. Nevertheless, there is good reason to believe that PersHI is here to stay. For the first citizens will not let go of the opportunities of ubiquitous and equitable access to health information, services and structures. For the second PersHI has the potential to create values although not every technical achievement is also a value for the patient or the doctor. Finally regarding an imminent clinical workforce shortage (cf. Wetter 2016, Chap 2) aging societies need replacement for services that can equally well be delivered through technical means as through human beings. Therefore, we are challenged to identify the values that PersHI services create and to be alert to ambivalent or detrimental achievements.

In the field of clinical trials major challenges lie in the controversy between strictly enforced protocols in classical trials and the humble acknowledgment in PersHI trials that the therapy is what the patient understands and does and the result is what he reports. We have seen examples of knowledge and behavior mismatch in sections "Attitude and emotion" and "Behavior". Observation biases have been discussed in this chapter and are also a topic in other chapters of this volume. Still, Patient Reported Outcomes Measures (PROMs) are the most intimate traces of effects that treatments can have. They inform about perceived improvements or deteriorations that the patient truly senses and that no technical sensor may be able to map. Therefore, we need PROMs. To get the best of PROMS, as unbiased as possible reporting should be on the research agenda.

Drop outs have also been a problem. Here (Lau et al. 2015, p. 9)'s quote that "(C)onsumers must perceive the need … and must assign priority" points into the auspicious direction. Before we apply for funds, build something, let alone deploy and test it, we should have a clear picture whether it satisfies a pressing need of the patient and whether the burden imposed on him is small. Wishful thinking in this place leads to wasted effort. As long as numbers of drop-outs are moderate intention to treat analysis may cure the situation although we lose some statistical power.

In light of scarecity of human therapists and the opportunity it is often sufficient that a PersHI service is equally good. Or, as (Batterham et al. 2021, p. 1) summarizes in an article about a transdiagnostic Internet self-help intervention against depression: "… interventions can be beneficial … Despite low adherence and small effect size, the availability … is likely to fill a critical gap".

To demonstrate equal effectiveness biostatistics have developed non-inferiority designs and equivalence designs and statistical tests for the situation where the null hypothesis is that two treatments differ and where refutation of the difference is just what we want: evidence at a chosen p-value that two treatments are significantly **not** different. In light of this existing variant in statistical test theory it should become the standard that only when the goal is superiority of a treatment, superiority tests are applied. When, however, equal effectiveness is the goal only a successful equivalence test is accepted as proof, not a failed superiority test.

Assets beyond Insight

Insights make use of two environmental trends that develop independently: Citizens volunteer ever more data and observations about themselves in social media and computational power to find something in these observations still grows at unchecked speed. So, as long as it is legal and ethical to bring these trends together, it is more likely than unlikely that things are discovered that the eye cannot see and that could not be discovered 5 years ago. While the question of legal use is addressed in other chapters of this volume we will rather look at the assets that can be created and whether their values warrant their use.

Clear upside number one is that data map real lives of citizens who are not under the impression to be in an experiment when they post. So none of the biasing effects listed in the section "Evidence" should affect results. Second the data are there without extra cost and effort and the computational cost is neglegible. So, when out for medical discoveries we can choose to apply algorithms to existing data or dispose the data to oblivion and expose humans to experiments instead.

Assuming that we choose to use the data their exploitation runs in parallel or merges with other structures and processes in health care, mostly regarding the approval process of treatments. Overlapping with our discussion in section "Power" patients ad-hoc volunteer with substances or treatments where the pharmaceutical industry sets up a systematic phase II and partially phase I of a clinical trial. In PersHI patients develop an idea or trust some hearsay that something new cures their problem. They weigh their individual personal risks versus expected benefits, try and—if they survive—report. By isolated similar experiences a data set emerges that suggests the desired properties of a substance or treatment. "Suggests" because the procedure does not have the scrutiny of a planned experiment. So the ethical question is whether we can accept it despite concerns about the quality of the process and the data or whether we are compelled to let a planned experiment follow, i.e. to expose more citizens to the unknown risk.

At this stage, with promising volunteered outcomes which somewhat parallel a phase II, this is still at a moderate scale. Sound insights versus phase III trials, however, is the pivotal line of controversy. As of today, new treatments will only get approval after a Randomized Controlled Trial (RCT) has shown superior or equivalent effectiveness, depending on the research question and design. An undisputed necessity of this approach is to expose a large number of citizens—hundreds if not thousands—to one of two risks: to be denied an effected treatment in the control group or to be exposed to an unknown hazard in the intervention group. Now let us assume that an insight is so strong that noone can seriously deny that there is a desired effect. Among the investigations presented here (Frost et al. 2011) comes closest with more than 3300 patient reports about off label usages of neuroleptic pharmaceuticals. If these mentions withstand scrutinized proof of trustworthiness the Declaration of Helsinki about ethics of medical research (World Medical Association 2013, p. 2192) sets limits to further research: "… medical research involving human subjects may only be conducted if the importance of the objective outweighs the risks and burdens to the research subjects. When the risks are found to outweigh the potential benefits or *when there is conclusive proof of definitive outcomes, physicians must assess whether to continue, modify or immediately stop the study*." This was implicitly applied—although whe did not mention it—in the negative sense in (Heller et al. 2020), where there was no more prospect for a proof of effectiveness and consequently the trial was stopped. Here it must be considered in the positive sense: is it ethical to expose thousands of subjects to an experiment of which we kind of know the positive outcome? Or would it not be more ethical to apply the best possible diligence to assure the quality of the available data rather than planning, getting approval, running, and evaluating an experiment to get new data? Let alone the time lost for patients to have the effective treatment right when the insight is there?

While phase III RCTs are in sharp contrast to insights methodologically and philosophically, phase IV is on a clear path of convergence with insights which have already been "welcomed" as a complementary method of pharmacovigilance (Lavertu et al. 2021).

Mindset

In an earlier version the section was called "Education". This, however, turned, out too narrow and too unidirectional. Of course can it be the aim of a service to educate patients or citizens. But what does that actually mean? And who learns from whom? We have discerned three directions of mindset, knowing that in psychology distinctions are by far more subtle. However, for the purpose of this volume we try to distinguish what people know from how they feel and how they behave. We do it with a warning voice, briefly reviewing examples to demonstrate that knowing, feeling, and doing are not necessarily in sync. Knowledge and feelings can correlate positively (Fraval et al. 2015; Attai et al. 2015) or the absence of a positive feeling can make cognitive training useless (Harding et al. 2020). Knowledge from different sources can influence feelings positively or negatively (Selinger et al. 2017). Knowledge can increase and behavior can change (Mehran et al. 2012; Nazeri et al. 2015) or does not change accordingly (Bonnevie et al. 2020; Rouf et al. 2020). And last but not least: self declared healers (e.g. https://cancer.mercola.com/) and conspiracy theorists (example in (Bradshaw et al. 2020)) are also spreading their wisdoms and target the mindset like serious providers do. It must be concluded that there are no easy and straight answers. Gaining in one dimension of Mindset does not warrant that the other dimensions follow suit.

Power and the Whole Picture

Historically (e.g. (Kopelman 1994)), patient power has emerged from a shared medical problem for which affected patients and their kin pushed for being granted opportunities to try a new solution for the problem.

This has happened more or less in accordance and mutual support or in competition between the medical "establishment" and the "newbies". The Dravet syndrom initiative (Black and Baker 2011) aimed to make the "establishment" aware of a rare disease. Achievements were sought through the means of existing structures while scientific progress from within the Dravet self support group was published through the same channels that professionals use. (Polich 2012) provides a review how such symbiosis can form naturally, by letting the best qualified party for each step contribute and by seeking synergy. (Kempner and Bailey 2019) report about controlled substance use against cluster headache is an off all limits endeavour. It happens mostly outside structures of medical care and in disregard of public legislation. It could be regarded as an innocent anomaly on the margins if it were not a precedence for tolerating an illegal act. The public answer in the US to such points of controversy is all but clear. Different states have different "expanded use" legislation—legislation when to grant patients access to pharmaceuticals outside their approved indications—and the industry can decide by itself whether to deliver (Mackey and Schoenfeld 2016).

Other initiatives collide with existing structures diametrally. The dermatology and pediatric neurology initiatives (Whitsitt et al. 2015; Horrow et al. 2019) establish research structures of their own, skeptically but not constructively eyed by the professional organizations. Duplicate or wasted effort and disorientation on the part of patients about authoritative sources are likely consequences.

Among patients who suffer from the same medical problem or see the same solution and are enabled to communicate, groupthink patterns may over time develop (Howard and Howard 2019, pp. 29–30). These include mechanisms to reinforce the group's beliefs and to devaluate, rationally and morally, positions and individuals that are in contrast with the group's beliefs. In the case of disease or treatment self support and advocacy groups this means that group members truly believe that their position is correct and that this gives them the right to push. (Pullman et al. 2013) have shown that such egomaniacal behaviors, as comprehensible as they may be, can take a health care system to the brink. The health care related administration and structures of Canada were not prepared to arbitrate between the aggressive advocacy for CCSVI versus many other and partially more promising requests for research or coverage. On a wider scale we may have to acknowledge that technology has moved faster than ethics, or, as (Goodman 2015, p. 71) writes: "... time and again in the history of technology: The development and use of an exciting new tool has utterly outstripped the ethical and legal resources required to ensure its appropriate use."

All this is happening while we speak and will not likely go away. There is definitely value of different sorts in many Personal Health Informatics services. We are responsible to identify where there are true values to let them bear fruit while preserving approved health care processes and structures. So hopefully the answer to the following question becomes more and more "yes":

The therapist is in 24/7. But will it be able to help YOU?

Learning Objectives

Readers shall become aware that Personal Health Informatics services create values of different types.

Readers shall become aware that evidence of effectiveness is one such value.

Readers shall be able to outline the character of different values through examples.

Readers shall become aware that values can be ambivalent and positive achievements may have a "price" to pay.

Review Questions

Q: Which values are distinguished in this chapter?

A: evidence, insight, mindset, power

Q: To establish two of the four values draws heavily on formal methods such as statistics or algorithms? Which ones?

A: evidence, through statistical test theory; insight, through data and text mining algorithms

Q: How are the other two values established?

A: **mindset** (There is not the one and only answer here; the following gives orientation about the type of the answer) Through diverse informative and motivational service offerings—simple sequences of SMSs to sophisticated influencer mediated campaigns—that were built with some knowledge, attitude, or behavior goal in mind.

power (There is not the one and only answer here; the following gives orientation about the type of the answer) Through online communities which act as pressure groups, somewhat like petition campaigns. They circulate observations from or encouragements to members to get more options to act than the health care system in the present form assigns them

Q: Name and outline a service that you would call a (near) perfect success.

A: Several answers are possible. Here come some article references and keywords in what respect they stand out.

(Corbett et al. 2015) size and convincing results

(Wahlund et al. 2021) long lasting effect

(Denis et al. 2019) save lives

(Golder et al. 2019) make severe risks known

Q: Name and outline a service that you would call a (near) complete failure.

A: Several answers are possible. Here come some article references and keywords in what respect they stand out negatively.

(Heller et al. 2020) trial terminated prematurely

(Rouf et al. 2020) planned result not achieved, paradoxical observations

(Dear et al. 2015) wrong research design

Clinical Pearls

Personal Health Informatics services can save lives.

Fully automated Personal Health informatics services can be efficient and safe.

Many Personal Health Informatics services are available 24/7.

References

Attai DJ, Cowher MS, Al-Hamadani M, Schoger JM, Staley AC, Landercasper J. Twitter social media is an effective tool for breast cancer patient education and support: patient-reported outcomes by survey. J Med Internet Res. 2015;17(7):e188. https://doi.org/10.2196/jmir.4721.

Axelsson E, Andersson E, Ljótsson B, Björkander D, Hedman-Lagerlöf M, Hedman-Lagerlöf E. Effect of internet vs face-to-face cognitive behavior therapy for health anxiety: a randomized noninferiority clinical trial. JAMA Psychiat. 2020;77(9):915–24. https://doi.org/10.1001/jamapsychiatry.2020.0940.

Bandura A. Self-efficacy: toward a unifying theory of behavioral change. Psychol Rev. 1977;84(2):191–215. https://doi.org/10.1037/0033-295X.84.2.191.

Batterham PJ, Calear AL, Farrer L, Gulliver A, Kurz E. Efficacy of a Transdiagnostic self-help internet intervention for reducing depression, anxiety, and suicidal ideation in adults: randomized controlled trial. J Med Internet Res. 2021;23(1):e22698. https://doi.org/10.2196/22698.

Beauchamp TL, Childress JF. Principles of biomedical ethics. 7th ed. Oxford University Press; 2013.

Beerthuizen T, Rijssenbeek-Nouwens LH, van Koppen SM, Khusial RJ, Snoeck-Stroband JB, Sont JK. Internet-based self-management support after high-altitude climate treatment for severe asthma: randomized controlled trial. J Med Internet Res. 2020;22(7):e13145. https://doi.org/10.2196/13145.

Bennell K, Nelligan RK, Schwartz S, Kasza J, Kimp A, Crofts SJ, Hinman RS. Behavior change text messages for home exercise adherence in knee osteoarthritis: randomized trial. J Med Internet Res. 2020;22(9):e21749. https://doi.org/10.2196/21749.

Benton A, Ungar L, Hill S, Hennessy S, Mao J, Chung A, Leonard CE, Holmes JH. Identifying potential adverse effects using the web: a new approach to medical hypothesis generation. J Biomed Inform. 2011;44(6):989–96. https://doi.org/10.1016/j.jbi.2011.07.005.

Black AP, Baker M. The impact of parent advocacy groups, the internet, and social networking on rare diseases: the IDEA league and IDEA league United Kingdom example. Epilepsia. 2011;52(Suppl 2):102–4. https://doi.org/10.1111/j.1528-1167.2011.03013.x.

Bonnevie E, Rosenberg SD, Kummeth C, Goldbarg J, Wartella E, Smyser J. Using social media influencers to increase knowledge and positive attitudes toward the flu vaccine. PLoS One. 2020;15(10):e0240828. https://doi.org/10.1371/journal.pone.0240828.

Bradshaw AS, Treise D, Shelton SS, Cretul M, Raisa A, Bajalia A, Peek D. Propagandizing anti-vaccination: analysis of vaccines revealed documentary series. Vaccine. 2020;38(8):2058–69. https://doi.org/10.1016/j.vaccine.2019.12.027.

Brambilla I, Aibar JÁ, Hallet AS, Bibic I, Cardenal-Muñoz E, Prpic I, Darra F, Specchio N, Nabbout R. Impact of the COVID-19 lockdown on patients and families with Dravet syndrome. Epilepsia Open. 2021;6(1):216–24. https://doi.org/10.1002/epi4.12464.

Broekhuis M, van Velsen L, Hermens H. Assessing usability of eHealth technology: a comparison of usability benchmarking instruments. Int J Med Inform. 2019;128:24–31. https://doi.org/10.1016/j.ijmedinf.2019.05.001.

Charles C, Gafni A, Whelan T. Shared decision-making in the medical encounter: what does it mean? (or it takes at least two to tango). Soc Sci Med. 1997;44(5):681–92. https://doi.org/10.1016/s0277-9536(96)00221-3.

Corbett A, Owen A, Hampshire A, Grahn J, Stenton R, Dajani S, Burns A, Howard R, Williams N, Williams G, Ballard C. The effect of an online cognitive training package in healthy older adults: an online randomized controlled trial. J Am Med Dir Assoc. 2015;16(11):990–7. https://doi.org/10.1016/j.jamda.2015.06.014.

Daley MF, Narwaney KJ, Shoup JA, Wagner NM, Glanz JM. Addressing parents' vaccine concerns: a randomized trial of a social media intervention. Am J Prev Med. 2018;55(1):44–54. https://doi.org/10.1016/j.amepre.2018.04.010.

Dalton JA, Rodger D, Wilmore M, Humphreys S, Skuse A, Roberts CT, Clifton VL. The health-e babies app for antenatal education: feasibility for socially disadvantaged women. PLoS One. 2018;13(5):e0194337. https://doi.org/10.1371/journal.pone.0194337.

Dear BF, Staples LG, Terides MD, Karin E, Zou J, Johnston L, Gandy M, Fogliati VJ, Wootton BM, McEvoy PM, Titov N. Transdiagnostic versus disorder-specific and clinician-guided versus self-guided internet-delivered treatment for generalized anxiety disorder and comorbid disorders: a randomized controlled trial. J Anxiety Disord. 2015;36:63–77. https://doi.org/10.1016/j.janxdis.2015.09.003.

Denis F, Basch E, Septans A-L, Bennouna J, Urban T, Dueck AC, Letellier C. Two-year survival comparing web-based symptom monitoring vs routine surveillance following treatment for lung cancer. JAMA. 2019;321(3):306–7. https://doi.org/10.1001/jama.2018.18085.

Fraval A, Chandrananth J, Chong YM, Coventry LS, Tran P. Internet based patient education improves informed consent for elective orthopaedic surgery: a randomized controlled trial. BMC Musculoskelet Disord. 2015;16:14. https://doi.org/10.1186/s12891-015-0466-9.

Frost J, Okun S, Vaughan T, Heywood J, Wicks P. Patient-reported outcomes as a source of evidence in off-label prescribing: analysis of data from PatientsLikeMe. J Med Internet Res. 2011;13(1):e6. https://doi.org/10.2196/jmir.1643.

Golder S, Chiuve S, Weissenbacher D, Klein A, O'Connor K, Bland M, Malin M, Bhattacharya M, Scarazzini LJ, Gonzalez-Hernandez G. Pharmacoepidemiologic evaluation of birth defects from health-related postings in social media during pregnancy. Drug Saf. 2019;42(3):389–400. https://doi.org/10.1007/s40264-018-0731-6.

Goodman KW. Ethics, medicine, and information technology: intelligent machines and the transformation of health care. Cambridge University Press; 2015.

Harding K, Aryeetey R, Carroll G, Lasisi O, Pérez-Escamilla R, Young M. Breastfeed4Ghana: design and evaluation of an innovative social media campaign. Matern Child Nutr. 2020;16(2):e12909. https://doi.org/10.1111/mcn.12909.

Heller HM, Hoogendoorn AW, Honig A, Broekman BFP, van Straten A. The effectiveness of a guided internet-based tool for the treatment of depression and anxiety in pregnancy (MamaKits online): randomized controlled trial. J Med Internet Res. 2020;22(3):e15172. https://doi.org/10.2196/15172.

Hensher M, Cooper P, Dona SWA, Angeles MR, Nguyen D, Heynsbergh N, Chatterton ML, Peeters A. Scoping review: development and assessment of evaluation frameworks of mobile health apps for recommendations to consumers. Journal of the American Medical Informatics Association: JAMIA. 2021; https://doi.org/10.1093/jamia/ocab041.

Hogan M. (R)evolution: toward a new paradigm of policy and patient advocacy for expanded access to experimental treatments. BMC Med. 2016;14:39. https://doi.org/10.1186/s12916-016-0586-6.

Horrow C, Pacyna JE, Cosenza C, Sharp RR. Examining physician interactions with disease advocacy organizations. AJOB Empirical Bioethics. 2019;10(4):222–30. https://doi.org/10.1080/23294515.2019.1652213.

Howard S, Howard J. Cognitive errors and diagnostic mistakes. Springer International Publishing; 2019. https://link.springer.com/book/10.1007%2F978-3-319-93224-8.

Kaplan B, Brennan PF. Consumer informatics supporting patients as co-producers of quality. Journal of the American Medical Informatics Association: JAMIA. 2001;8(4):309–16. https://doi.org/10.1136/jamia.2001.0080309.

Kempner J, Bailey J. Collective self-experimentation in patient-led research: how online health communities foster innovation. Soc Sci Med. 2019;(1982, 238):112366. https://doi.org/10.1016/j.socscimed.2019.112366.

Kim SH, Utz S. Effectiveness of a social media based, health literacy sensitive diabetes self-management intervention: a randomized controlled trial. Journal of Nursing Scholarship: An Official Publication of Sigma Theta Tau International Honor Society of Nursing. 2019;51(6):661–9. https://doi.org/10.1111/jnu.12521.

Kopelman LM. How AIDS activists are changing research. In: Monagle J, Thomasma DC, editors. Health care ethics: critical issues. Aspen; 1994.

Kraemer HC. Is it time to ban the P value? JAMA Psychiat. 2019;76(12):1219–20. https://doi.org/10.1001/jamapsychiatry.2019.1965.

Lau AYS, Arguel A, Dennis S, Liaw S-T, Coiera E. "Why Didn't it work?" lessons from a randomized controlled trial of a web-based personally controlled health management system for adults with asthma. J Med Internet Res. 2015;17(12):e283. https://doi.org/10.2196/jmir.4734.

Lavertu A, Vora B, Giacomini KM, Altman R, Rensi S. A new era in pharmacovigilance: toward real-world data and digital monitoring. Clin Pharmacol Ther. 2021;109(5):1197–202. https://doi.org/10.1002/cpt.2172.

Mackey TK, Schoenfeld VJ. Going "social" to access experimental and potentially life-saving treatment: an assessment of the policy and online patient advocacy environment for expanded access. BMC Med. 2016;14:17. https://doi.org/10.1186/s12916-016-0568-8.

Maddison R, Rawstorn JC, Stewart RAH, Benatar J, Whittaker R, Rolleston A, Jiang Y, Gao L, Moodie M, Warren I, Meads A, Gant N. Effects and costs of real-time cardiac telerehabilitation: randomised controlled non-inferiority trial. Heart. 2019;105(2):122–9. https://doi.org/10.1136/heartjnl-2018-313189.

Marks HM. The progress of experiment: science and therapeutic reform in the United States, 1900-1990. Cambridge Univ. Press; 2000.

Martini M, Bragazzi NL. Googling for neurological disorders: from seeking health-related information to patient empowerment, advocacy, and open, public self-disclosure in the neurology 2.0 era. J Med Internet Res. 2021;23(3):e13999. https://doi.org/10.2196/13999.

Mehran L, Nazeri P, Delshad H, Mirmiran P, Mehrabi Y, Azizi F. Does a text messaging inter-
    vention improve knowledge, attitudes and practice regarding iodine deficiency and iodized
    salt consumption? Public Health Nutr. 2012;15(12):2320–5. https://doi.org/10.1017/
    S1368980012000869.
Merlin T, Weston A, Tooher R. Extending an evidence hierarchy to include topics other than treat-
    ment: Revising the Australian "levels of evidence.". BMC Med Res Methodol. 2009;9:34.
    https://doi.org/10.1186/1471-2288-9-34.
Moshi MR, Parsons J, Tooher R, Merlin T. Evaluation of Mobile health applications: is regulatory
    policy up to the challenge? Int J Technol Assess Health Care. 2019;35(4):351–60. https://doi.
    org/10.1017/S0266462319000461.
Nazeri P, Mirmiran P, Asghari G, Shiva N, Mehrabi Y, Azizi F. Mothers' behaviour contributes to
    suboptimal iodine status of family members: findings from an iodine-sufficient area. Public
    Health Nutr. 2015;18(4):686–94. https://doi.org/10.1017/S1368980014000743.
Nelson R, Ball MJ, editors. Consumer informatics: applications and strategies in cyber health care.
    Springer; 2004.
Nikfarjam A, Ransohoff JD, Callahan A, Jones E, Loew B, Kwong BY, Sarin KY, Shah NH. Early
    detection of adverse drug reactions in social health networks: a natural language processing
    pipeline for signal detection. JMIR Public Health Surveill. 2019a;5(2):e11264. https://doi.
    org/10.2196/11264.
Nikfarjam A, Ransohoff JD, Callahan A, Polony V, Shah NH. Profiling off-label prescriptions in
    cancer treatment using social health networks. JAMIA Open. 2019b;2(3):301–5. https://doi.
    org/10.1093/jamiaopen/ooz025.
Oyebode O, Ndulue C, Adib A, Mulchandani D, Suruliraj B, Orji FA, Chambers CT, Meier S, Orji
    R. Health, psychosocial, and social issues emanating from the COVID-19 pandemic based
    on social media comments: text mining and thematic analysis approach. JMIR Med Inform.
    2021;9(4):e22734. https://doi.org/10.2196/22734.
Paganini S, Lin J, Kählke F, Buntrock C, Leiding D, Ebert DD, Baumeister H. A guided and
    unguided internet- and mobile-based intervention for chronic pain: health economic evalu-
    ation alongside a randomised controlled trial. BMJ Open. 2019;9(4):e023390. https://doi.
    org/10.1136/bmjopen-2018-023390.
Polich GR. Rare disease patient groups as clinical researchers. Drug Discov Today.
    2012;17(3–4):167–72. https://doi.org/10.1016/j.drudis.2011.09.020.
Pullman D, Zarzeczny A, Picard A. Media, politics and science policy: MS and evidence from the
    CCSVI trenches. BMC Med Ethics. 2013;14:6. https://doi.org/10.1186/1472-6939-14-6.
Richards B, Colman AW, Hollingsworth RA. The current and future role of the internet
    in patient education. Int J Med Inform. 1998;50(1–3):279–85. https://doi.org/10.1016/
    s1386-5056(98)00083-5.
Rouf A, Nour M, Allman-Farinelli M. Improving calcium knowledge and intake in Young adults
    via social media and text messages: randomized controlled trial. JMIR Mhealth Uhealth.
    2020;8(2):e16499. https://doi.org/10.2196/16499.
Selinger CP, Carbery I, Warren V, Rehman AF, Williams CJ, Mumtaz S, Bholah H, Sood R, Gracie
    DJ, Hamlin PJ, Ford AC. The relationship between different information sources and disease-
    related patient knowledge and anxiety in patients with inflammatory bowel disease. Aliment
    Pharmacol Ther. 2017;45(1):63–74. https://doi.org/10.1111/apt.13831.
Topooco N, Byléhn S, Dahlström Nysäter E, Holmlund J, Lindegaard J, Johansson S, Åberg
    L, Bergman Nordgren L, Zetterqvist M, Andersson G. Evaluating the efficacy of internet-
    delivered cognitive behavioral therapy blended with synchronous chat sessions to treat adoles-
    cent depression: randomized controlled trial. J Med Internet Res. 2019;21(11):e13393. https://
    doi.org/10.2196/13393.
Wahlund T, Mataix-Cols D, Olofsdotter Lauri K, de Schipper E, Ljótsson B, Aspvall K, Andersson
    E. Brief online cognitive Behavioural intervention for dysfunctional worry related to the
    COVID-19 pandemic: a randomised controlled trial. Psychother Psychosom. 2021;90(3):191–9.
    https://doi.org/10.1159/000512843.

Walthouwer MJL, Oenema A, Lechner L, de Vries H. Comparing a video and text version of a web-based computer-tailored intervention for obesity prevention: a randomized controlled trial. J Med Internet Res. 2015;17(10):e236. https://doi.org/10.2196/jmir.4083.

Wetter T. Consumer health informatics. Springer International Publishing. 2016; https://doi.org/10.1007/978-3-319-19590-2.

Whitsitt J, Mattis D, Hernandez M, Kollipara R, Dellavalle RP. Dermatology on pinterest. Dermatol Online J. 2015;21(1)

Wilson SL, Wiysonge C. Social media and vaccine hesitancy. *BMJ*. Glob Health. 2020;5(10) https://doi.org/10.1136/bmjgh-2020-004206.

World Medical Association. World medical association declaration of Helsinki: ethical principles for medical research involving human subjects. JAMA. 2013;310(20):2191–4. https://doi.org/10.1001/jama.2013.281053.

Yu CH, Parsons JA, Mamdani M, Lebovic G, Hall S, Newton D, Shah BR, Bhattacharyya O, Laupacis A, Straus SE. A web-based intervention to support self-management of patients with type 2 diabetes mellitus: effect on self-efficacy, self-care and diabetes distress. BMC Med Inform Decis Mak. 2014;14:117. https://doi.org/10.1186/s12911-014-0117-3.

Chapter 21
Electronic Health Records: Ethical Considerations Touching Health Informatics Professionals

Eike-Henner W. Kluge

Abstract Health informatics professionals (HIPs) are responsible for the technical aspects of the construction, storage, maintenance and communication of electronic health records (EHRs). They therefore function as the technical interface between patients on the one hand and health care professionals as well as institutions on the other when these, directly or indirectly, are engaged in the delivery of health care. EHRs, in turn, function as patient analogues in such a context. HIPs, therefore, stand in a fiduciary relationship to the subjects of EHRs. This means that while there is an overlap with some of the technical aspects of informatics in other areas of electronic record keeping—issues such as privacy, security and accessibility are implicated—the role of HIPs in health care is subject to special ethical considerations. Precision medicine, being genetically focused, adds another special parameter, as does the increased mobility of patients and the fact that modern health care frequently crosses jurisdictional boundaries where distinct legal informatic provisions are operative and different ethical considerations may be followed. Moreover, the fact that EHRs tend to be stored in different ways, varying from proprietary servers to the cloud, adds further ethical complications for HIPs, as does the fact that the data that are contained in EHRs are potentially valuable items. This chapter outlines some of the ethically relevant features that are involved in all of this and sketches some considerations that may guide the behaviour of HIPs in a global setting.

Keywords Patient analogue · Electronic health records · Ethics · Fiduciary relationship · Precision medicine · Privacy · Security · Accessibility · Confidentiality

E.-H. W. Kluge (✉)
Department of Philosophy, University of Victoria, Victoria, BC, Canada
e-mail: ekluge@uvic.ca

P.-Y. S. Hsueh et al. (eds.), *Personal Health Informatics*, Cognitive Informatics in Biomedicine and Healthcare, https://doi.org/10.1007/978-3-031-07696-1_21

Learning Objectives
1. Ability to identify ethically relevant differences between EHRs as patient analogues and other types of person-oriented electronic records.
2. Ability to identify and address ethical issues that arise for HIPs in view of their fiduciary relationship to patients in connection with health care professionals and health care institutions.
3. Ability to incorporate appropriate ethical as opposed to legal considerations into the construction, maintenance, communication and storage of EHRs.
4. Ability to address and deal with ethical issues that arise for HIPs relative to EHRs in the context of personalized medicine.

Introduction

Medical record keeping has changed in many important ways since such records first began to be kept, both with respect to the media in which they are kept as well as with respect to their content and the reasons for keeping them. The traditional way of outlining what happened is that they were first kept in stone, clay and string (quipus) and sometimes even wax (Brosius 2003; Nesbit 1914; Ascher and Ascher 1981), but that this was ultimately superseded by paper-based recordkeeping, and that by the second half of the twentieth century even this began to be replaced by electronic[1] methods of recording and storage—a process that is still ongoing.

This way of presenting the evolution medical record keeping, however, is somewhat limited in scope. It not only ignores the fact that the reason why they were kept as well as that their content changed in significant ways and what they came to be used for, it also ignores who is involved in their construction and their handling in this new electronic form, as well as the fundamental changes that they underwent in their ethical nature.

Thus, originally medical records were essentially no more than *aides-mémoires* and as such were kept only by health care professionals and only for their own diagnostic, treatment and teaching purposes. Moreover, they only contained what the professionals considered medically relevant data about their particular patients. With the advent of organized health care institutions such as modern hospitals and clinics, however, they came to include data about next-of-kin, patient-specific socio-economic data such as a patient's particular profession and the manner of reimbursement for their health care expenses, etc., and with the advent of personalized medicine even genetic data came to be included. In other words, they became health records in the general sense of that term. Further, in their electronic form they came to function as the technical interface between patients on the one hand and health care professionals and institutions on the other, and became involved in the various

---

[1] The term 'electronic' is intended to cover both electronic and photonic methods of recording and storing.

kinds of decisions that were made about patients in the overall health care context. With this, they came to function as patient analogues in information and decision-space.

As yet, this development is still ongoing because the structure of these electronic health records (EHRs) is still evolving, as is their relationship to new electronic methods of analysing and evaluating the data that are contained in them by means of expert systems and so-called artificial intelligence. Nor have they yet been fully integrated into all aspects of health care delivery and planning in all jurisdictions. Nevertheless, the process is well under way.

All of this has important ethical implications. However, these implications are not confined to the health care professionals and institutions who actually use them in their planning and in their delivery of health care, because the technical aspects of the construction, storage, maintenance, communication and handling of EHRs has given rise to a new kind of professional: namely, the health informatics professional (HIP). And while there is an overlap in some of the technical aspects of their role with what is performed by informatics professionals in other areas of electronic record keeping—for instance, issues such as privacy, security and accessibility constitute common areas of concern—the ethical implications for HIPs are different because these implications straddle two distinct realms: the realm of patient-relevant considerations that are grounded in the role of EHRs as patient analogues on the one hand, and the realm of health care professional- and institution-relevant considerations that are grounded in the latter's role as deliverers of health care on the other.

At this juncture, and before proceeding any further, it may be appropriate to explain in what sense EHRs are patient analogues, and how the concept of patient analogue will be understood in what follows. An analogue is something that performs a similar function to, or that can be substituted for, that of which it is the analogue. It is in this sense that EHRs as originated by health care professionals should be understood as being patient analogues. As originated by health care professionals, they form the basis of the patient profiles that are developed by the latter and that function as the basis of health care decision-making about patients, whether that be at the hands-on or the administrative level. They may not be entirely accurate or even complete. For instance, the data that they contain may be situation- and context-dependent, and they may fail to contain information that would be relevant about their subjects but that would not be available in the purely professional setting. That, however, does not detract from the role they play in the delivery of professional health care, and it is this role that stamps them as patient analogues (Kluge 2020a).

Ethics Preamble

Continuing, then, and as a procedural preamble before outlining the nature of the ethical implications that surround the development, storage, use and communication of EHRs as patient analogues in this sense of the term, it may be useful to clarify what is meant by saying that the implications are ethical in nature.

Ethical considerations differ from legal and administrative considerations in that they are not grounded in rules or laws that have been passed by a duly established authority or that are the result of decisions that have been made by administrators. They are grounded in fundamental ethical principles that apply to actions that affect persons insofar as they are persons.

This, in turn, may also benefit from some clarification because how the notion of person is understood also has implications for whether the strictures that apply to the relationship between HIPs and health care institutions are purely administrative, contractual or legal in nature or whether they are also have ethical parameters.

Thus, the notion of a person may be understood in two distinct senses: once as referring to a so-called natural person—i.e., a living member of the species *homo sapiens* who has the capacity for sentient cognitive awareness and volition—and once as referring to what is generally called a constructive person, such as a corporation. Patients are persons in the first sense of the term, as are health care professionals, HIPs and administrators. However, groups of individuals may function in a unified fashion as an individual, and as such may be aware of certain facts, have certain values and aims, and may make decisions on that basis. This is formally acknowledged in the concept of a corporate or constructive person (Kluge 2020a; List and Pettit 2011). Health care institutions, therefore, are persons in this second sense of the term. Both types of persons, however, are subject to ethical considerations because both have the capacity to apprehend facts and of voluntary decision-making. All of this has important implications for HIPs, because it means that not only are their interactions with health care professionals and patients subject to ethical constraints, but also their interactions with health care institutions.

Ethical considerations, in turn, are different from considerations that are grounded in ethos, custom or law. While these latter derive their applicability—and, indeed, their validity—from the traditions that have established them or by having been promulgated by a duly established authority, ethical considerations are independent of such derivation. They derive their validity from the fundamental principle of ethics, which in turn are grounded in what it is to be a person. These principles are echoed by the *Universal Declaration of Human Rights* (United Nations 1948) and hence are recognized as being universally valid. Therefore the ethical acceptability of a given action, behaviour, stance or situation that involves persons in either sense of that term is subject to their constraints.

The fundamental principles of ethics include the *Principle of Autonomy* (Every person has the right to self-determination, subject only to the equal and competing rights of others.), the *Principle of Equality* (All persons, insofar as they are persons, are equal and have the right to be treated accordingly.), the *Principle of Beneficence* (Everyone has the duty to advance the good of others in keeping with the competent values of the other person if it is possible to do so without undue harm to oneself.), and the *Principle of Nonmaleficence* (Everyone has the duty to prevent harm to others in keeping with the competent values of the other person if it is possible to do so without undue harm to oneself.) (Kluge 2020a). The *Principle of Impossibility* (All rights and duties hold subject to the condition that it is possible to fulfil them under the circumstances that obtain.), while not strictly an ethical principle, functions like a n ethical principle in that it conditions all rights and duties that derive from the fundamental principles of ethics. It therefore also plays a role in determining whether a given action is ethically appropriate. Moreover, these principles apply to actions as well as inactions. In other words, the failure to engage in an action when there is a duty to do so would count as an ethical failing.

These principles, then, structure the framework of what counts as ethically appropriate treatment of persons in both senses of the term "person", and they entail both rights and duties. Rights define how the right-holders themselves should be treated by other persons, whereas duties impose obligations on individuals with respect to how they should treat other persons. Rights and duties, therefore, are correlatives, which means that for every right there is a corresponding duty or obligation, and for every duty or obligation there is a corresponding right. At the same time, whereas a right may be exercised at the discretion of the right-holder, a duty obligates the individual who has that duty and, unless the Principle of Impossibility applies, discretion on part of the duty-holder is not an ethically acceptable option.

It should be clear from the preceding that while ethical considerations apply to the conduct of HIPs as well as patients, health care professionals and health care institutions, they do not apply—at least not directly—to such things as expert systems or to systems that are frequently referred to by the term "artificial intelligence" simply because these are not persons. Ethical considerations apply to them only indirectly in that they apply to their construction and usage, and it is those who construct, contract for or use them to whom the ethical considerations apply directly.

It should also be clear that ethical considerations do not apply directly to EHRs because these are only patient analogues and therefore are not persons in their own right. However, ethical considerations do apply to them derivatively precisely because they are person analogues, and they apply derivatively insofar as they are related to persons. So, for instance, ethically grounded privacy considerations apply derivatively to EHRs because they reflect the right to privacy that belongs to their subjects.

Finally, it should be clear that ethical considerations do not directly apply to the databases in which EHRs are stored; and that while it may be appropriate to say that certain types of such databases are unethical, this is correct only in a manner of speaking. It is really an abbreviated way of saying that how they are established and maintained, how their content is determined and how they are used redounds to those who actually establish, maintain or use them.

Ethical Considerations for HIPs

The fact that HIPs are centrally involved as technical facilitators in the establishment and use of EHRs and the fact that EHRS function as patient analogues entails that HIPs have ethical obligations towards both the patients themselves and towards the health care professionals and the institutions that use them. At the same time, however, it is important to note that considerations that affect how HIPs function on the basis of social, cultural or educational considerations do not necessarily have ethical relevance and may not even be ethically appropriate, because these considerations are ultimately grounded in historical parameters that may not themselves be ethically valid. A good example of this would be the social, cultural and educational parameters that condition the behaviour of HIPs in totalitarian or religious societies whose standards are at variance with the fundamental ethical principles that ground the *Universal Declaration of Human Rights*.

Patients

The ethical obligations that HIPs have towards patients derive from the Principles of Autonomy, Equality and Nonmaleficence. Thus, the Principle of Autonomy, which is to the effect that every person has the right to self-determination, entails that patients not only have the right to control access to their physical persons but also to the EHRs that are their analogues (where the notion of analogue is understood as was indicated a few paragraphs ago). Consequently HIPs, as facilitators of the construction and use of EHRs, have an obligation design them in such a way that the privacy rights that belong to the patient-subjects of EHRs are integrated into the structure, access controls and similar aspects of EHRs.

At the same time, individual patients may consider the provision of health care to be more important than privacy or related issues. By the Principle of Autonomy, this would be entirely within their right. Consequently HIPs would be ethically obligated to structure EHRs in a way that takes this into account so that the subjects of EHRs have the chance to decide whether to exercise their right to privacy even if this means possibly foregoing relevant health care services.

However, as was mentioned before, the Principle of Autonomy has a qualifying clause: namely, "subject to the equal and competing rights of others." Therefore it does not give patients an absolute right to control the privacy of their records. Thus, there may be circumstances—for instance, when a patient's health condition may reasonably be presumed to pose a threat to the welfare of other members of society—when the Principle of Nonmaleficence overrules what would otherwise be the patient's right to privacy, and when access to their records would be ethically appropriate even against a patient's wish and without their consent. Consequently a patient's right to privacy is conditional, and HIPs have an obligation to structure the protocols that surrounded access to patient records accordingly. At the same time, however, it is also ethically appropriate that HIPs take measures to ensure patients are made aware of this limitation.

As to the Principle of Equality, given that all persons insofar as they are persons are equal and should be treated the same, HIPs have an obligation to do their best to ensure that the same security, privacy and other informatic considerations apply to all EHRs unless there are ethically relevant differences between the persons themselves. Any such exceptions, however, should be justified and should be made known to the subjects of the EHRs themselves.

The Principle of Nonmaleficence, in turn, entails that because the EHRs are essential to the delivery of health care for the patients whose analogues they are, HIPs have an obligation to structure EHRs and their disposition as best as possible so as to ensure their security, accessibility, availability and integrity in order to minimize the possibility of technology-based harm to the patients whose analogues the EHRs are. This may present challenges in light of the increased mobility of modern patients and in light of the fact that contemporary health care consults sometimes cross jurisdictional boundaries where distinct legal informatic provisions are operative and different ethical considerations may be followed. The ethical obligations that HIPs have towards patients, however, entail that ethical considerations that are grounded in the *Universal Declaration of Human Rights* take priority over any legal provisions and over rules that are based on purely culturally based considerations. HIPs should therefore structure the EHRs and the access to them accordingly and should ensure that, with the exceptions noted above, patient consent for their usage and disposition is ethically mandated. Such consent may take several forms. In this connection, however, HIPs should always remember that a patient's signature does not in itself indicate that the patient has given consent. It may simply be indicative of a patient's automatic reaction to a protocol that requires a signature. Therefore— insofar as this lies within their power—HIPs should also take appropriate steps to ensure that the signature protocol itself warrants that patients understand the nature and significance of what a signature entails, and when it is ethically valid.

Health Care Professionals and Institutions

As to the ethical obligations that HIPs have towards health care professionals and institutions, these derive from the fact that the professionals and institutions rely on the data that are contained in the EHRs when making decisions about patients and when developing the institutional framework in which health care is delivered. Security, accessibility and availability are here implicated and once more are grounded in Equality, Beneficence and Nonmaleficence. This is particularly important in the case of health care professionals who, ever since the time of Hippocrates, have an ethical obligation to always act in the best interest of their patients (Edelstein 1943). In the modern setting, health care professionals cannot fulfil this obligation unless they can be certain that what is contained in the EHRs of their patients is secure from alterations or modifications that do not originate in their own professional actions. In other words, the security of EHRs becomes a central feature of HIPs' obligations towards health care professionals. With due alteration of detail, the accessibility and technical usability of EHRs are also implicated, because health care professionals cannot fulfil their patient-oriented duties unless they have access to the patients' EHRs.

Similarly, health care institutions cannot structure the frameworks in which professional health care is delivered unless the institutions have access to data about the appropriateness and effectiveness of the procedural provisions that they put in place,and with respect to the tools and devices with which they supply the professionals who work in their particular setting. This is possible only if HIPs construct and operationalize the institutions' technical frameworks appropriately. While this obligation may find legal reflection in the contracts that bind HIPs and health care institutions, it is ultimately grounded in the Principles of Beneficence and Nonmaleficence, and it extends beyond what may be—and, indeed, beyond what can be—stated in purely contractual terms. Further, this obligation includes such things as the duty to ensure that the formatting of the EHRs is consistent with the requirements of the relevant parties who need access them, and that the necessary means for accessing them are available so that the EHRs can in fact be accessed as and when this is needed. Along similar lines, it also includes an obligation to ensure that so-called legacy systems—technology and computer programs that are outdated and no longer generally in use—are replaced in due time and in a technically appropriate manner; and it includes the obligation to ensure—all other things being equal—that the EHRs are protected by appropriate back-up measures.

However—and this explains the qualifier "all other things being equal"—HIPs can fulfil these obligations only if they have appropriate and sufficient resources to fulfil these tasks. The Principle of Impossibility is here engaged. If these resources are insufficient, the obligation loses its force and is replaced by the obligation to take appropriate steps to ensure that both the health care professionals and the health care institutions with whom they are affiliated are aware of this shortcoming, understand it implications and do their best to remedy any such situation.

Implications of Modern Health Care

The changes in health record keeping are not, however, confined to the development of EHRs. They also include their storage, communication and content, all of which have corresponding ethical implications for HIPs.

Beginning with storage, traditional paper-based patient health records were stored in material places and their security could be assured by suitable material measures. Moreover, access to them—and hence their privacy and security—could be safeguarded by instituting appropriate identification procedures that would distinguish between those who could legitimately have access to them and those who did not, and under what conditions. While essentially the same security and privacy requirements exist for EHRs, the fact that they are electronic in nature calls for fundamentally distinct solutions: not simply in technical but also in functional terms.

For instance, to consider only three examples, EHRs can be stored either in machines that belong to health care professionals who are not members of a health care institution, in servers that are part of a health care institution, or they can be stored in the cloud: i.e., in servers that do not belong either to health professionals or to health care institutions but to corporations with whom these have contractual arrangements. In each case, however, the possibility exists that these storage facilities may be hacked and, as recent experience has shown, it is almost impossible to prevent this unless the facilities are freestanding and unreachable by external electronic means—which of course would make them of limited use except in the setting of the storage facilities themselves.

Likewise, the fact that there can be multiple entry points for accessing EHRs as well as the fact that it is possible to control access to specific parts of the record in keeping with the qualifications of those who seek such access and the role that they play in health care delivery provides HIPs with challenges for the ethically appropriate construction and embedding of EHRs. While these challenges also existed for paper-based records, they assume different proportions in the case of EHRs. Similar considerations apply with respect to the ease with which EHRs may be copied or transferred. Therefore modern health care, which increasingly relies on electronic record keeping and methods of communication, presents these traditional challenges to HIPs in a new—and sometimes difficult—form.

Privacy Considerations

All of this presents a particular challenge for HIPs in an institutional setting. To put this into context, it may be useful to outline what is here at issue. Purely logically speaking, every kind of health care professional is associated with a particular domain of data that satisfies the data needs that are associated with their professional activities: i.e., with what may be called their characteristic data-need domain. Such data-need domains may overlap, as for instance the data-need domain of a cardiac surgeon will overlap with that of an anaesthesiologist, that of a psychiatrist with that of a hospitalist, and all of these may overlap with the data-need domains of the clinical nurses who take care of individual patients. Nevertheless, they will not be exactly coextensive, and each kind of professional will have a central data domain that is unique to their particular professional specialty.

However, if HIPs construed their ethical obligation to ensure the privacy and security of EHRs in the institutional setting by putting in place electronic safeguards that would absolutely prevent their being accessed by individuals whose data demands did not match their characteristic data-need domains, this would be too extreme. It would mean that the professionals would not be able develop innovative approaches for dealing with health issues, could not improve on established methods of providing care or simply develop more effective ways of delivering the type of care that was characteristic of their profession. Consequently, the privacy safeguards that HIPs build into EHRs and into the informatic structures of health care institutions should take this into account, both because of the ethical obligations that HIPs have towards the patients who are the subjects of such records as well as the obligations that they have towards the health care professionals and health care institutions.

One way of doing so would be to structure the privacy shield that surrounds EHRs by not only requiring the identification of whoever seeks such access as a health care professional who was actively involved in care of the particular patient whose EHR they are trying to access—where failure to meet this requirement would trip an automatic blockage—but also by diverting such an attempt to an appropriately positioned institutional administrative security authority, so that whoever made such an attempt could justify their action. That authority would then have the option of lifting the blockage that the HIPs had put in place.

However, despite the best measures that HIPs can put in place to guard against it, inappropriate access by unauthorized individuals to the servers in which EHRs are stored—and thus to the EHRs themselves— is possible. This is commonly referred to as hacking, and it can occur irrespective of whether the EHRs are stored in proprietary servers of health care professionals, in the servers of health care institutions, or in the cloud. The only way to protect the privacy of the subjects of EHRs in this regard is for HIPs to design the informatic structures of the EHRs themselves—as well as their content—in a way that would minimize the possibility of a privacy breach even if an inappropriate access to the EHRs did occur.

A way of doing this would be integrate the logical aspects of the privacy rights that belong to the patient-subjects of EHRs into the format in which data are entered into the EHRs themselves. That is to say, patient data come in various forms. There are identified data—i.e., data that are specific to a particular patient and that carry an explicit patient identifier which, simply by becoming known, would directly allow the identification of that patient. Then there are deidentified data—i.e., data where the identifiers that would allow the direct identification of the patient have been deleted. There are also pseudonymized patient data—i.e., data that have been supplied with a fictitious identifier and which, consequently, cannot be attributed to the specific individual about whom they are unless the pseudonym is somehow connected with the true identity of the patient. Finally, there are anonymized data, which are data that have been stripped of all identifying features including pseudonyms, so that the patients about whom the data are remain anonymous even when the data themselves become known.

Since the obligation of HIPs to protect patient privacy extends beyond simply protecting EHRs from unauthorized access but includes protecting the privacy of their subjects as much as possible even when unauthorized access does occur, this means that HIPs have an ethical obligation to take the data-parameters that were just mentioned into account when structuring the formats of EHRs.

One way of doing this would be for HIPs to design EHRs in such a way that the patient-data that are entered into them would automatically be pseudonymized or de-identified. However, as past experience has shown, neither pseudonymization nor de-identification would necessarily be successful in protecting patient privacy. Anonymization at entry would therefore seem to be the appropriate alternative for HIPs to adopt in their design of EHRs. However, some authorities have argued that not even this would inevitably be successful. They have pointed out that even when patient data in an EHR are anonymized, re-identification is possible given access to three distinct data in the EHR when these data are linked to prescription records and some other medical data (Emam et al. 2009; Porter 2008; Richardson et al. 2015). If that is correct, then HIPs can be sure of fulfilling their patient-oriented privacy obligation only by structuring EHRs in such a way that the EHRs themselves and everything in them is encrypted. Therefore it would follow that if HIPs wanted to be sure of fulfilling their privacy obligations towards the subjects of EHRs, then they would be obliged to inform whoever employs their services of these facts, and to request that they be authorized to structure the development and storage of EHRs along the relevant lines.

Consequently, it would seem that HIPs would have fulfilled their ethical obligation towards the subjects of EHRs and that they would be absolved of ethical responsibility if such authorization was not forthcoming and a privacy violation did occur. However, that is not entirely clear. For, it would remain a distinct question whether HIPs would be acting ethically as professionals if they accepted employment under such conditions in the first place.

Precision Medicine

Another matter that has ethical significance for HIPs with respect to EHRs is that modern medical practice has evolved to include precision medicine.

That is to say, the traditional model of health care intervention considers the particular physiological and psychological characteristics of a patient as well as their lifestyle and environmental embedding and then—in order to shape their diagnosis, prognosis and proposed intervention—applies to this the results of the controlled health care research that results in statistically valid conclusions. In other words, the traditional model of health care delivery essentially relies on health-related information that has been derived in a controlled fashion.

However, given the controlled nature of this research, the conclusions that are reached in this sort of research essentially constitute a "one-size-fits-all" model. By contrast, personalized medicine is based on the thesis that the success profile of a given intervention cannot be meaningfully determined solely on the basis of traditional and standard research protocols: that it should also take into account how the statistically valid results of such research actually perform when they are used in the uncontrolled health care setting of actual hands-on practice. Moreover, and indeed above all, it is based on the realization that the genetic endowment of an individual determines how the individual reacts to a particular intervention—in particular, to a pharmaceutical—and how the individual reacts to such an intervention in their particular socio-economic setting.

The reason this move to personalized medicine has ethical implications with respect to EHRs and HIPs is that the research that is involved in establishing the parameters of personalized medicine is importantly different from standard research because it predominantly involves the use of EHRs.

More specifically, there are two fundamentally distinct methods of conducting health research: There is hands-on research, which involves direct interactions between researchers and controlled groups of patients in controlled settings on the basis of research protocols that have been approved by a duly established authority. If scientifically successful, this research leads to the formal approval of the intervention in question. Then there is health care research that is essentially data-based, and that looks at the relationship between various types of health data that are contained in patient records and tries to establish correlations.

However, health care as it is practiced in real life does not deal with controlled groups of patients in controlled settings. Not only do variations in the environmental and lifestyle factors of individual patients play an important role in the success or failure of an intervention in hands-on health care, so does the genetic endowment of the individual patients. Modern health care professionals, therefore, realized that if they were to follow the ethical injunction that they should always act in the best interest of their patients (Edelstein 1943), these factors should also be taken into account when deciding whether a given intervention would be appropriate on a given occasion.

Precision medicine does just that. As was said, it is based on the realisation that a patient's genetic endowment plays a critical role in whether—and in how well—a particular intervention works for the individual patient, since it is the individual's genetic endowment that ultimately determines how the patient will react to any intervention. This, however, cannot be determined even by taking into account the data from Phase IV trials, which are sometimes called post-marketing surveillance studies. These are reports that have been filed about an intervention's performance in actual practice. The point is that these reports are not statistically valid because they essentially deal only with the adverse side-effects of an intervention, and reporting this is often voluntary in nature. Moreover, except under very unusual circumstances, they do not include the genetic factors that may be involved in the performance of the intervention in question. Therefore they do not offer a firm scientific basis for evaluating the actual success-profile of a given intervention (McNeil et al. 2010).

At the same time, like all other forms of medicine, precision medicine cannot simply be based on observations that have been made in individual cases. To be scientifically valid, it has to be based on properly controlled research. Since hands-on genetic research would involve experimenting on human beings through genetic manipulation and this, as opposed to purely scientific experimenting on tissues that do not leave the laboratory, is considered to be ethically highly questionable, research for precision medicine looks at the data that are in EHRs inclusive of the genetic profiles of their subjects as well as the environmental and lifestyle factors, and it pays particular attention to the relationship between the genetic profiles of the subjects and the interventions in question. The outcomes of such studies are then used to refine the statistical profiles of the interventions as these are developed on the basis of standard hands-on research. Consequently, an essential component of precision medicine research involves data mining.

This means that it is crucial for the development of precision medicine that its researchers have access to EHRs even though they may not currently be involved in therapeutic interactions with the relevant patients. However, as the preceding discussion has pointed out, EHRs are surrounded by a sphere of privacy that is ethically grounded in the privacy rights of the subjects of the EHRs. Consequently, this means that if precision medicine research is to succeed, the access controls for EHRs that were mentioned above have to be modified in important ways.

More specifically, the HIPs who technically establish the EHRs should structure the access controls in such a way that researchers who are engaged in precision medicine protocols that have been approved as scientifically and ethically valid by a duly constituted research authority will not be excluded from having access to the EHRs despite the fact that they are not engaged with the subjects of the EHRs in a therapeutic manner.

However, since the identity of the patients whose EHRs would be accessed in such research would essentially be irrelevant for establishing the influence of genetic determinants on the success of a given intervention, this means that HIPs are ethically obligated to structure the technical format of EHRs in such a way that, unless it was absolutely impossible to do so, the data-identifiers in the EHRs are separated from the data themselves, and that the researchers have access only to the pure data. It also means that, in keeping with what was previously said about data-need domains, the researchers should only be allowed to access to the data domains that are in keeping with the domains that are indicated in the approved precision medicine research projects. Finally, it means that if HIPs have encrypted the EHRs—as was also suggested as being ethically appropriate—the encryption keys be supplied to the precision medicine researchers by whoever is administratively responsible for the security and privacy of the EHRs.

Expert Systems and Artificial Intelligence

As was indicted a moment ago, precision medicine research involves a lot of data mining. In the contemporary context, this is not generally carried out by the researchers themselves in a hands-on fashion and on a step-by-step basis by looking at and correlating the data that are contained in the various records. It is generally done by expert systems, and by what is sometimes referred to as artificial intelligence. Moreover, it is not only precision medicine research that makes use of these tools. Modern health care is increasingly taking advantage of expert systems and artificial intelligence, and not only with respect to data mining but also in the context of health care delivery itself—for instance, in telemedicine, where this may involve diagnostic as well as treatment modalities. HIPs, again, are instrumentally involved both with respect to the design and the functioning of these tools. The question, therefore, arises whether this poses ethical issues for HIPs and for EHRs that are distinct from those that have been considered so far.

In short, the answer is a qualified NO. However, to explain this answer, it may be useful to begin by briefly clarifying the notion of an expert system and that of an artificial intelligence.

Expert systems are computer programmes that emulate the decision-making ability of human experts in a particular field. Some are specifically designed to computationally scan huge data sets that include not only medical data but also such things as social, economic and behavioural data in order to identify patterns, trends and to make associations. These are especially useful in precision medicine, in hands-on health care, in research contexts, as well as in health care planning. In the context of hands-on health care and precision medicine expert systems are used to scan the relevant data in EHRs, reach a diagnosis, make a prognosis, and suggest possible treatment options that the attending health care professionals may then present to their patients for consent. These systems tend to do so on the basis of probability calculations whose nature has been programmed into them, and they may follow neural network models (Hinton et al. 2012; Krizhevsky et al. 2012). Once employed, they function without direct human input, and when they are properly designed they can even refine their interpretational subroutines to reach ever more accurate conclusions as more data become available to them. In short, they then are self-modifying learning systems. Moreover, when they are integrated into a medical equipment structure, they can even perform medical interventions such as surgery, both directly as well as remotely when the patients are in different locations from their attending health care professionals (Eadie et al. 2003; Hung et al. 2018). The ethically important point is that such expert systems do not function independently of the health care professionals who employ them on specific occasions and for the specific tasks for which they are designed.

By contrast, artificial intelligence systems—i.e. artificial intelligence (AI) systems in strict or strong sense of that term—are different from expert systems in that they can perform all of the functions that expert systems can perform inclusive of medical interventions such as surgery, except that they can do so independently of the instigation and supervision of health care professionals. Moreover, they can not only learn from their mistakes and improve their performance by incorporating the data from the outcomes of their interventions into their subroutines, they can even change their valuational frameworks either on the basis of these outcomes or as based on the values of the patients themselves. In other words, AIs in this full-blooded sense of the term are computer systems that could completely take over the function of health care professionals and could substitute for them in all ways. They could even be employed on a consultative basis when expert advice that exceeded the qualifications of a general practitioner was called for, or substitute for human medical practitioners in eHealth and telemedicine.

At present, there are no AIs of this kind. There only are expert systems in the preceding sense of that term (Kluge 2020b). Therefore, an analysis of the ethical challenges that full AIs would present transcends the limits of the present discussion and therefore will be put off to another occasion.

Returning, then, to the question whether expert systems in the standard sense of the term pose ethical issues for HIPs and EHRs that are distinct from those that have been considered so far, it should be clear why the question was answered by a qualified negative. HIPs construct expert systems only on the basis of the parameters that they have been given by health care professionals and, as was said, the expert systems are only employed by health care professionals as tools that complement their own professional actions. Therefore ethical concerns would rise for HIPs only with respect to the ethical acceptability of the instructions that they receive, and with respect to how the expert systems are used to perform what would otherwise be performed by the professionals themselves, such as surgery.

As to the first, the instructions for constructing expert systems stipulate what data in the EHRs should be selected, how they should be correlated and what conclusions should be drawn from them. At first glance, these are purely medical matters and therefore are ethically neutral. However, to argue thus would be to ignore the fact that these instructions are themselves embedded in a valuational framework that identifies what types of data the expert system should treat as relevant, and what degree of significance it should assign to the data. However, the values that structure this framework may not be objectively medical in orientation. For instance, they may be racially (Hall et al. 2015) or sexually biased (Brezinka 1995) and therefore the systems that are based on them may not select certain data that would be factually relevant. Alternatively, the subroutines may select the medically appropriate data but accord them degrees of significance that would be in accordance with the value perspective of the professional who gave the instructions for the construction of the expert systems, where this perspective may be biased in a cultural, social or even religious, etc. sense. Ethically that would be problematic, for the values that frame the instructions that the HIPs are given for constructing expert systems should be consistent with the fundamental principles of ethics that were outlined above. Therefore, HIPs should be aware of such matters and would be ethically obliged to refuse to devise such an expert system. Unfortunately, however, it remains a conundrum how HIPs could determine whether such a bias was in fact the case.

As to the usage of expert systems, an ethical consideration that arises concerns expert systems that are integrated into medical equipment structures and that perform medical interventions such as surgery, whether that be directly or remotely when patients and health care professionals are in different locations. Such expert systems are not like other expert systems because, once put into operation, they take the place of the professionals themselves. Arguably, therefore, just as a health care professional require patient consent in order for another professional to step into their place and perform the surgery that is indicated, these systems should be designed in such a way that they would remain inoperative unless, in accordance with the Principle of Autonomy, the consent for their usage was entered into their subroutines by the patients themselves or by the latter's duly empowered substitute decision-makers. HIPs therefore have an ethical obligation to ensure that these considerations are built into the employment of such expert systems.

Conclusion

Contemporary health care has evolved in the direction of replacing paper-based patient records with electronic patient records, and has expanded the ambit of these records to include all patient-based parameters that are considered relevant to delivering health care to patients on an individual basis. They therefore tend to include not only individual physiological and psychological patient-based data but also genetic information, environmental data insofar as these are considered medically relevant, social parameters insofar as these affect the health status of individuals, and in some cases even employment and financial information. In short, paper-based patient records have evolved into EHRs. This, in turn, raises ethically based privacy and security issues that are different from, and that transcend the scope of, the issues that exist for paper-based patient records. Moreover, they require the involvement of health informatic professionals as interfaces between the patients, the health care professionals and the institutions in which health care is delivered. The preceding discussion has outlined some of these issues. By way of conclusion, however, it should always be kept in mind that EHRs are patient analogues in the sense that was outlined in the begining, and that their construction and usage is subject to the fundamental Principles of Ethics that govern the framework in which health care is delivered. This, however, means that the ability of HIPs to meet the requirements of ethically appropriate action is always subject to the Principle of Impossibility: i.e., subject to the fact that one cannot have an obligation to do what is impossible. Therefore the funding and working conditions for HIPs who are involved in the construction and use of EHRs should always be appropriate.

Review Questions

1. How do ethical considerations differ from considerations that are based on ethos, tradition or law?
2. What is the difference between paper-based patient records and electronic health records (EHRs) and why are EHRs patient analogues?
3. Why (and how) do ethical considerations apply to EHRs?
4. Why are the ethical considerations relevant when considering the role of HIPs, and what are some of these ethical considerations?
5. What is special about personalised medicine with respect to EHRs?
6. What are the ethical implications of expert systems (and artificial intelligence) for HIPs?

Answers

1. Ethical considerations are based on universally accepted fundamental ethical principles (Autonomy, Equality, Beneficence and Nonmaleficence) as these are reflected in the *Universal Declaration of Human Rights*, and the rights and duties that derive from them are only subject to the Principle of Impossibility. By contrast, considerations that are based on ethos, tradition or law are not necessarily consistent with these ethical principles because they are based on what a given society finds (or has found) appropriate.

2. Paper-based patient records differ from EHRs not merely in that they are purely material in nature but also in that they are not patient analogues, nor can they function as the interface between the material patients and health care professionals and institutions in distanced interactions. Moreover, they cannot be incorporated into modern health care delivery systems such as tele-surgery.

3. Ethical considerations apply to EHRs because they are patient analogues. However, they do not apply directly but derivatively in that the ethical considerations that apply to EHRs are grounded in the ethical considerations that apply to the patients whose analogues they are.

4. The ethical implications of EHRs for HIPs are grounded in the fact that it is the HIPs who construct and maintain EHRs, and that they are responsible for the technical aspects of their privacy, security, accessibility and availability. They therefore are responsible for the technical aspects of the interaction between patients and health care professionals and institutions.

5. Personalised medicine attempts to adjust the delivery of health care to individual patients by taking into account how the genetic endowment of individual patients affects the success-profiles of standardly approved health care interventions, and in particular with respect to pharmaceuticals. It therefore is the closest that health care professionals can come to following the Hippocratic injunction to always act in the best interest of their patients. EHRs are centrally involved in this because the research that establishes the relevant parameters involves the data mining of EHRs.

6. HIPs construct expert systems according to the instructions that they receive from health care professionals. It is therefore ethically obligatory for HIPs to make sure that these instructions are based solely on medical factors and are in accordance with fundamental ethical principles and free of professionally-based value biases.

References

Ascher M, Ascher R. Code of the quipu: a study in media, mathematics, and culture. Ann Arbor: University of Michigan Press; 1981.

Brezinka V. Ungleichheiten bei Diagnostik und Behandlung von Frauen mit koronarer Herzkrankheit. Eine Ubersicht [Gender bias in diagnosis and treatment of women with coronary heart disease. A review]. Z Kardiol. 1995;84(2):99–104.

Brosius M, editor. Ancient archives and archival traditions: concepts of record-keeping in the ancient world. Oxford: Oxford University Press; 2003.

Eadie LH, Seifalian AM, Davidson BR. Telemedicine in surgery. Br J Surg. 2003;90(6):647–58.

Edelstein L. The Hippocratic oath, text, translation and interpretation. Baltimore: The Johns Hopkins Press; 1943.

Emam KE, Dankar FK, Vaillancourt R, Roffey T, Lysyk M. Evaluating the risk of re-identification of patients from hospital prescription records. Can J Hosp Pharm. 2009;62(4):307–19.

Hall WJ, Chapman MV, Lee KM, Merino YM, Thomas TW, Payne BK, Eng E, Day SH, Coyne-Beasley T. Implicit racial/ethnic bias among health care professionals and its influence on health care outcomes: a systematic review. Am J Public Health. 2015;105(12):e60–76.

Hinton GE, Srivastava N, Krizhevsky A, Sutskever I, Salakhutdinov RR. Improving neural networks by preventing co-adaptation of feature detectors. arXiv. 2012;arXiv:12070580.

Hung AJ, Chen J, Shah A, Gill IS. Telementoring and telesurgery for minimally invasive procedures. J Urol. 2018;199(2):355–69.

Kluge E-H. The electronic health record: ethical considerations. Cambridge, MA: Academic; 2020a.

Kluge EW. Artificial intelligence in healthcare: ethical considerations. Healthc Manage Forum. 2020b;33(1):47–9.

Krizhevsky A, Sutskever I, Hinton G. ImageNet classification with deep convolutional neural networks. Adv Neural Inf Process Syst. 2012;25:1097–105.

List C, Pettit P. Group agency: the possibility, design, and status of corporate agents. New York: Oxford University Press; 2011.

McNeil JJ, Piccenna L, Ronaldson K, et al. The value of patient-centred registries in phase IV drug surveillance. Pharm Med. 2010;24(5):281–8.

Nesbit WM. Sumerian records from Drehem. New York: AMS Press; 1914.

Porter CC. De-identified data and third party data mining: the risk of re-identification of personal information. Washington J Law Technol Arts. 2008;5(1):1–8.

Richardson V, Milam S, Chrysler D. Is sharing de-identified data legal? The state of public health confidentiality laws and their interplay with statistical disclosure limitation techniques. J Law Med Ethics. 2015;43(1_suppl):83–86.11.

United Nations. (1948). Universal declaration of human rights. https://www.un.org/en/about-us/universal-declaration-of-human-rights

Chapter 22
Healthcare Organizations as Health Data Fiduciaries: An International Analysis

Paul R. DeMuro and Henry E. Norwood

Abstract The healthcare marketplace is in an evolutionary race with electronic health data as the ultimate prize. The global movement towards digitalization of health data has increased providers' abilities to share, accumulate, and analyze data, focused on benefitting healthcare consumers and treatment. Third party actors beyond the provider and consumer have also shown a willingness to pay for access to this data, driving up the value of health data and monetizing the value of such data. The growing ability of actors beyond the patients and providers to access, use and profit from health data has placed patients' sensitive health data in a place of vulnerability. Healthcare providers and larger healthcare organizations have legislatively imposed legal requirements to ensure health data is maintained and protected from unauthorized use or disclosure. Jurisdictions all over the world have imposed specific duties on organizations who act as "health data fiduciaries" related to this information. The more recent recognition of the fiduciary concept to health data recognizes a higher standard of care on those in possession of health data than many statutes have specifically recognized in the past. This chapter introduces the idea of the health data fiduciary and specifically describes the application of this term to the duties owed by healthcare providers and organizations to the patients they serve. The chapter begins with an overview of the major changes in the healthcare landscape that necessitated the recognition of the health data fiduciary relationship. The chapter then briefly discusses fiduciary relationships, generally, and describes the nature of fiduciary relationships between healthcare providers and healthcare organizations and their patients, along with showing how these relationships work to establish the health data fiduciary relationship. The chapter goes on to provide an illustrative survey describing the data privacy acts from various jurisdictions,

P. R. DeMuro
Nossaman LLP, Austin, TX, USA
e-mail: pdemuro@nossaman.com

H. E. Norwood (✉)
Herman Law Firm, Brookline, MA, USA

© The Author(s), under exclusive license to Springer Nature
Switzerland AG 2022
P.-Y. S. Hsueh et al. (eds.), *Personal Health Informatics*, Cognitive Informatics
in Biomedicine and Healthcare, https://doi.org/10.1007/978-3-031-07696-1_22

including internationally, to describe how various jurisdictions have addressed the emergence of the health data fiduciary relationship. The chapter concludes with recommendations for future legislation governing and addressing health data fiduciaries.

Keywords Data · Healthcare · Fiduciary · International · Privacy

Introduction

Conducting business in today's technologically driven world has led to many new questions regarding the concept of trust between organization and client. Organizations, particularly those operating in the healthcare industry, maintain an ever-increasing amount of patient **protected health information** (PHI), that is, information relating to an individual's physical or mental health condition, the healthcare provided or recommended for that individual, or the payment information regarding the provision of healthcare to the individual, which either identifies a specific person or which can reasonably identify that person. **Personal health records** (PHRs) are records in the possession of healthcare providers containing sensitive, health-related information regarding a patient, often including a patient's name, phone number, address, financial information, insurance information, and health history. This leads to a number of concerns from patients regarding their information privacy. **Privacy** is the right of individuals to control access to their person (body privacy) or information about themselves (information privacy). Further, the sensitive and valuable nature of the information contained within health records make them valuable for both legitimate and illegitimate purposes. Given the high value and sensitive nature of a patient's health records, along with the growing occurrence of healthcare data breaches, the question arises as to whether healthcare organizations in control of protected health information should owe a fiduciary duty to patients.

Monetization of Health Data

In today's world, data has great value. Health data, specifically, has value to specific marketplace actors (Shah and Patel 2021). The monetization of health data is a major industry in and of itself and it is expanding as more health data is being shared (Shah and Patel 2021).

Healthcare providers possess vast amounts of health data, but third-party vendors have traditionally profited off patient data (Shah and Patel 2021). Third-party vendors, typically electronic health record (EHR) vendors, obtain patient health data and, in turn, sell it to buyers attempting to gain insightful market information from the data (Shah and Patel 2021). The third-party vendors de-identify the patient information before selling it for privacy and legal compliance purposes (Shah and Patel 2021). The purchasers of de-identified health data include research organizations, pharmaceutical companies and investment firms among others (Shah and Patel 2021). Monetization of health data can generally be categorized under two methods of monetization: (1) indirect monetization and (2) direct monetization (Shah and Patel 2021).

Indirect monetization occurs where a healthcare provider organization profits off health data that remains in its possession (Shah and Patel 2021). This is most often accomplished where the provider organization utilizes the data it collects directly from its patients to improve the organization's internal operations (Shah and Patel 2021). Indirect monetization can also occur where providers utilize their patient data to perform medical research via case studies to improve the provision of care (Shah and Patel 2021). Indirect monetization is also performed in the financial departments of healthcare organizations where departments utilize patient health, health device, and insurance data to streamline patient payments, execute more advantageous supply contracts, and to eliminate unnecessary expenditures of resources (Shah and Patel 2021).

Direct monetization occurs where health data is sold to parties outside of the provider organization for monetary gain (Shah and Patel 2021). Direct monetization can also occur where providers exchange access to health data with a third-party in exchange for data processing and analytic services, whereby the third-party will receive access to the de-identified data and, in return, will analyze the data and provide the provider organization with useful insights (Shah and Patel 2021).

While direct monetization has been the traditional form of health data monetization, this may be shifting. A new organization called Truveta Inc., is made up of several of the largest healthcare provider organizations in the U.S. (Millard 2021). Truveta is committed to retaining control over how their patients' de-identified data is shared and for what purposes it is used (Millard 2021). It is estimated Truveta will have access to nearly 13% of all patient data in the U.S. (Shah and Patel 2021). Truveta strives to improve patient care by using the data in its possession to advance treatment, as opposed to selling the data to outside parties (Millard 2021). Here we see indirect monetization being prioritized over direct monetization allegedly for the benefit of the patient.

As data is being shared with and monetized by an increasing number of organizations, health data is at an increasing risk of being compromised, either through improper disclosure from an entity properly in possession of the data or through a cyber breach initiated by a bad actor (Snell 2017). While de-identification of health data reduces the risks associated with improper disclosures or data breaches, it is possible to overcome de-identification methods and establish the identities of patients (Hern 2019).

The increase in health data monetization necessitates health organizations review their methods of maintaining health data, the emerging technologies involved in processing and sharing health data, the risks to health data from outside parties, and the legal landscape regarding a heightened duty to safeguard health data.

How Health Data Is Maintained by Healthcare Organizations

Healthcare organizations are storing larger and larger amounts of health data. Aside from the typical practice of converting provider notes and patient intake documents into digital form, healthcare organizations and their patients are now also syncing their smart devices to a shared storage area, dramatically increasing the data held in the possession of healthcare organizations (O'Dowd 2017). The need to store and manage this data effectively is critical to the organization's success and to patients' safety.

The traditional method used by healthcare organizations to maintain health information is on-site data storage (O'Dowd 2017). Prior to the digital revolution, on-site storage of health information involved storing physical, paper patient files into a physical filing system. Some healthcare organizations continue to use this approach and some use a hybrid approach of maintaining certain physical files for a length of time while also converting the files to a digital format. The benefits of physical or paper maintenance of health information is that the information is protected from any form of hacking attempt, the information is more difficult to alter, and sharing the information requires a more intentional process of physically handing or sending the information to a party, which may reduce the likelihood of an unauthorized disclosure. The drawbacks of the physical storage method are the expenditure of resources creating paper files, the necessity of space to store physical files, less-efficient access to information when compared to digital files, which can be searched automatically, and the threat of physical theft or unauthorized physical access. Most healthcare organizations are moving away from this method, in whole or in part, and digitalization of health information is becoming the norm.

On-site digital data storage involves the healthcare organization maintaining its own data on its own servers, without connecting to an outside digital space (O'Dowd 2017). This method brings with it the advantage of greater control over the data as well as ease of access since the data is readily available to the organization (O'Dowd 2017). Further, because on-site storage only requires a connection to a local network, it is arguably the safest option when considering the threat of an external threat (O'Dowd 2017). The downsides of on-site data storage include limited physical space to house servers which becomes necessary as the volume of stored data increases, the need for continuous power supply and cooling mechanisms, the need for regular IT support, and lesser adaptability to software or storage updates (O'Dowd 2017).

Some health organizations opt to store their health information off-site from their normal area of operations in a separate location maintained by the organization (Bednar 2020). This brings the benefit of space and retention of control by the organization (Bednar 2020). Further, off-site storage insulates stored data from crises that may occur at the organization itself (Bednar 2020). On the downside, the organization is responsible for ensuring a continuous energy supply, IT maintenance, and personnel at the off-site location (Bednar 2020).

Health information may also be stored by a third-party vendor, either a healthcare clearinghouse or a health information data processing center. The former converts health information received from the provider organization into coded billing information for transmission to health insurers (Compliancy Group 2021). The latter stores the health information from several healthcare organizations as a professional service (Assoc. of Healthcare Internal Auditors 2013). The benefit of the third-party vendor method of data storage is largely that of convenience—the vendor undertakes the burdens involved with maintaining the data and housing the necessary servers, as well as any needed IT services (Assoc. of Healthcare Internal Auditors 2013). The downsides of the third-party vendor option include the lesser degree of access and control of the stored data by the provider organization as well as the centralization of health data from multiple organizations into one location (Davis 2019). Cybercriminals have targeted third-party heath information vendors and, given the volume of information stored by these institutions, they will likely remain an attractive target to cybercriminals (Davis 2019).

Cloud storage is the latest frontier in data storage. Cloud data storage enables what is perhaps the greatest ease of access for the provider organization and the patient alike (Siddhartha 2020). The problem of physical space is removed and operating costs for IT services are greatly diminished (Siddhartha 2020). The cloud storage method is also ideal for the constant changes in the data storage field, as updates to a cloud storage system are generally accomplished with ease (Siddhartha 2020).

The EU has created "eHealth," an electronic records database operated by EU Commission. The eHealth database provides Europeans with access to their medical records while providing for the maintenance and security of their health data (European Commission 2021). Health providers throughout the EU may access an individual's health data through eHealth upon obtaining the individual's informed consent (European Commission 2021). Storage on the eHealth system has many benefits, including accessibility across national borders and between health providers, limited cost to organizations to access patient data, and the provision of security by an international agency (European Commission 2021). On the other hand, such large-scale centralization of health data poses security risks and may make the eHealth system an attractive target to cybercriminals (European Commission 2021).

The Expansion of Healthcare Technology

As healthcare continues moving in the direction of digital information, healthcare organizations must evolve their practices to uphold their responsibilities to their patients, ensure compliance with laws and regulations, and maintain the trust of patients when it comes to privacy. In order for the benefits of digitized health services to be realized, companies need to ensure the safety of their patients' data. **Security** of protected health information refers to ensuring the protection of information and information systems from unauthorized access, use, disclosure, disruption, modification, or destruction in order to provide confidentiality, integrity, and availability. In addition to security, healthcare organizations that also serve as providers of health services must also maintain the confidentiality and privacy of patient data. **Confidentiality** refers to the obligation to ensure health information is not disclosed to unauthorized recipients or exposed to threats of unauthorized access. **Integrity** refers to ensuring that data or information has not been altered or destroyed in an unauthorized manner. Newer health information technologies will result in more health information being accumulated by organizations, requiring more trust in these organizations by patients.

Big Data, a field dedicated to finding solutions to analyze data sets that are too large or complex to be analyzed using traditional data-processing application software, and the **Internet of Things** (IoT), referring to physical objects implanted with software that connects and exchanges data with other systems via networks, have expanded the categories of and the extent to which health information is collected (Licea 2019). Wearable technology, such as watches, bracelets, rings, and phone applications, can detect a wearer's heart rate, activity, location, blood pressure, heart rate, oxygen levels, glucose levels, and fertility, among other statistics (Licea 2019). Constant monitoring of vital statistics allow healthcare organizations to provide more accurate, efficient treatment plans and give providers a more detailed picture of their patients' health (Licea 2019). Increasing the efficiency of care through increased data from wearable technology can save healthcare organizations time and money, which is likely why this technology is backed by the healthcare and insurance industries (Licea 2019). Of particular relevance, the new technology advanced through Big Data and the IoT will result in larger quantities of patient data in the hands of healthcare organizations (Licea 2019).

The use of **Artificial Intelligence** (AI), intelligence, such as reasoning ability, demonstrated by machines, is expanding the rate at which healthcare organizations are able to access health information in furtherance of providing patient care (Davenport and Kalakota 2019). Many AI technologies are capable of sifting through vast amounts of patient data and health research to determine solutions to health problems and, to a certain extent, render predictive models regarding patient outcomes when treated using a proposed method (Davenport and Kalakota 2019). AI in healthcare could greatly improve patient outcomes and efficiency of care, but it is entirely reliant on the availability of patient health data of which to make use in rendering predictive models.

Telehealth, the provision of healthcare services via electronic information and telecommunication technologies, has become more prevalent over the past year, particularly due to the COVID-19 pandemic (Pennic 2020). The shift to telehealth demonstrated the capability in the healthcare field to move toward remote care (Pennic 2020). As the pandemic abates, telehealth care may recede as well, but it is unlikely to return to pre-pandemic levels as both providers and patients have enjoyed its convenience (Pennic 2020). Telehealth relies on the transmission of health information digitally, either through a webcam or though uploads to a cloud space or server used by the organization, requiring a level of trust on the part of the patient that the organization will maintain the privacy and security of that information (Pennic 2020).

The common denominator of most advances in healthcare technology is the prevalence of electronic data sharing between patient and provider. The corresponding responsibility on the part of healthcare organizations to care for this information will increase accordingly.

The Right to Be Forgotten

An individual's right to restrict or eliminate their personal information on the internet is currently the subject of much debate (Singleton 2015). The "**right to be forgotten**" as this right is referred to, has become popularized in the EU and is inspiring support among policymakers in other countries as well. While a right to be forgotten had already been established to certain degrees, it received judicial recognition in *Google Spain SL v. Agencia Espanola de Proteccion de Datos*. In *Google Spain*, a case heard in Spain, the Court of Justice of the European Union held that the right to be forgotten on the internet is a right held by all members of the EU (Case C-131/12 2014). This right, however, must be balanced against the public right to freedom of information (Leiser 2020). For matters which are more private in nature (e.g., information regarding an individual's health), the information should be deleted by the data controller pursuant to the right to be forgotten (Brougher 2016). The right to be forgotten would also be codified into the EU's overarching data protection law, discussed later in this chapter. The decision in *Google Spain* focused on internet search engines, such as Google, but the decision has ramifications for other data controllers as well, including health data controllers.

Health data sharing has expanded in modern times and it is no longer the case that an individual will only share their personal health information with a medical provider in furtherance of receiving medical treatment (Licea 2019). Patients themselves are inputting their health information to health apps and electronic programs, which are operated by organizations collecting their health data (Licea 2019). If these organizations are collecting health data from members of the EU, then once these organizations receive an individual's data, they become data controllers under the EU's right to be forgotten (GDPR.EU 2021). EU members have the right to demand health data controllers delete the health information in the possession of an organization, assuming the organization held the information subject to the individual's consent or that the purpose for which the organization held the individual's health information is no longer necessary (GDPR.EU 2021).

The right to be forgotten is an emerging area of law and has not yet gained global acceptance. The U.S., where many of the larger internet search providers are based, has not yet formally accepted the right to be forgotten. The major implications of the right to be forgotten on the healthcare industry remain to be seen.

The Threat of Cybercrime

Because health information is predominantly stored in electronic form, it can be compromised by cybercriminals. Cybercrime involving protected health information threatens to undermine the level of trust between patients and the health organizations maintaining their information. The growing market for health data ensures health data will be shared with an increasing number of parties, spanning far from the original party with whom the individual's health information was shared – likely, the individual's healthcare provider (Davis 2019). This increased sharing leads to a larger threat that the shared data will be compromised through a cyberattack as cybersecurity safeguards and measures will likely not be uniformly stringent among the multiple actors possessing valuable health data (Davis 2019). **Safeguards** refer to protective measures prescribed to meet the security requirements (i.e., confidentiality, integrity, and availability) specified for an information system. A brief overview of the various threats cybercriminals employ demonstrates the varied threat posed by cybercrime to the safety of health information.

Phishing is a method of cyber hacking involving emails sent to a member of an organization or to several members of an organization that appear to be sent from a credible source (Ingalls 2021). The hacker who sent the email attempts to induce the recipient to disclose sensitive information regarding the organization, such as login or password information (Ingalls 2021). The hacker may also attempt to lure the member into opening a fraudulent webpage, resulting in the installation of malware onto the organization's computer (Ingalls 2021). *Spear phishing* is a specific form of phishing in which a message is targeted to a specific employee of an organization (Ingalls 2021).

Keylogging refers to the activity of covertly logging a computer user's keystrokes on the computer's keyboard by infecting the target computer (Ingalls 2021). The user is generally unaware their keystrokes are being logged and, therefore, may unwillingly be transmitting sensitive information to the hacker (Ingalls 2021).

Ransomware is a type of computer malware designed to extort ransom payments from its targets (DeMuro 2017). Ransomware acts by infecting a computer, disabling the entire computer or disabling specific functions of the computer, and presenting a message on the computer screen demanding a ransom payment in exchange for regaining the computer's functionality (DeMuro 2017). Ransomware has taken on many different forms and continues to evolve since its creation many years ago (DeMuro 2017). All healthcare organizations need to be prepared to prevent, protect against, and manage a ransomware attack to ensure the privacy of their patients and others who have entrusted the organization with their data.

Denial-of-Service (DoS) attacks occur when hackers disrupt an organization's computer systems by flooding them with multiple, unnecessary requests, over-whelming the system (Ingalls 2021). DoS hackers often make use of several, internet-connected devices to send the target system unnecessary requests in a coor-dinated manner (Ingalls 2021). The use of a network of devices in this manner is often referred to as a "botnet." (Ingalls 2021).

Malware is a general term referring to software designed to cause damage to a computer system (Ingalls 2021). *Adware* is a specific form of malware designed to automatically generate advertisements for specific companies onto the infected computer (Ingalls 2021). S*pyware* is a form of malware that tracks the information stored onto a computer as well as the computer's activity and transmits the informa-tion to an outside source (Ingalls 2021).

The techniques hackers use to compromise sensitive data, including health data, are constantly evolving. A strong cybersecurity framework and consistent anti-hacking practices can reduce the risk of cybercrime, but even unsuccessful attempted cybercrimes can erode patient trust in the security of their information. The threats posed to health information, as well as its value, call into question the level of duty healthcare organizations owe to their clients to keep their information safe.

Fiduciary Relationships in the Field of Healthcare

Fiduciary relationships describe a variety of interactions between health care pro-viders and patients, in which patients rely upon individuals and organizations with greater knowledge, skills, and power than themselves to promote their best interests regarding their health (Furrow 2009). Generally speaking, the legal concept of a **fiduciary** requires those with greater power and knowledge to exercise the skill, judgment, integrity, and discretion necessary to protect the individual with less power who is generally dependent on the stronger party (Furrow 2009).

Judiciaries have recognized many different types of fiduciary relationships, including the relationships between: attorney and client, corporate management and shareholder, guardian and ward, trustee and beneficiary, bank and customer, agent and principal, as well as doctor and patient (Furrow 2009). A fiduciary relationship generally involves: (1) a party providing a service or good requiring a level of knowledge and expertise beyond that possessed by the general public; (2) a second-party, without the requisite knowledge and expertise of the first, availing itself of the service or good offered by the first-party; (3) reliance by the second-party on the first-party regarding the rendering of the service or good (Furrow 2009). These elements generally create a **fiduciary duty**, that is, a legal duty on the part of the fiduciary holder to act with a degree of care, honesty, integrity, discretion, judgment, knowledge, and skill, which is greater than the degree of care owed by a person not acting as a fiduciary (Furrow 2009). Fiduciary duties are generally separate from the ordinary duties owed under tort law to conform to some standard of reasonable care (Furrow 2009). Breach of a fiduciary duty can expose the fiduciary holder to liability from those dependent upon them (Furrow 2009).

The Fiduciary Relationship Between Medical Provider and Patient

Some jurisdictions have long recognized the existence of a fiduciary relationship between a medical provider and their patients. Arguably, the Hippocratic Oath, established by early Greek physicians, sought to impose a heightened standard of care on physicians regarding their patients, which could be viewed as a fiduciary duty (Hajar 2017). The physician-patient fiduciary duty is generally viewed as an equitable or moral doctrine (Furrow 2009).

The parameters of the physician-patient fiduciary vary by jurisdiction. Generally, the physician-patient relationship requires physicians to prescribe and apply treatment with the competence, knowledge, care, discretion, and judgment in the best interests of the patient (Furrow 2009). Physicians are generally prohibited from willfully failing to disclose pertinent information regarding the patient's health or possible treatment options (Murray 2012). There are generally exceptions to this prohibition, involving the incapacity of the patient, such that the patient would be unable to comprehend the information communicated to them and also where the potential harm caused by delivering the information would likely outweigh the benefits (Murray 2012). Physicians are generally prohibited from disclosing the patient's health status to unauthorized individuals or organizations (Furrow 2009). Physicians are further prohibited from exerting influence over a patient for their own personal gain. While this type of personal gain can take many different forms, it often takes the form of financial gain.

The concept of the medical provider as a holder of a fiduciary duty carrying the responsibility to safeguard patients creates a special relationship between provider and patient (Furrow 2009). The provider is in a unique position of power, given their education, training, and skill, which are not available to the general public and given the particular vulnerabilities of their patients (Furrow 2009). At its core, the fiduciary duty owed by individual provider to patient, is grounded in the personal nature of the relationship between the two (Furrow 2009). Such a relationship is generally not present in the relationship between patient and health organization.

The Fiduciary Relationship Between Healthcare Organizations and Patients

Unlike individual providers of healthcare, healthcare organizations, including hospitals, medical offices, nursing homes, pharmacies, etc., are businesses (Furrow 2009). The relationship between the healthcare organization and the patient is more distant than the relationship between healthcare provider and patient (Furrow 2009). Often, this distance gives the patient the impression that their relationship and the duty owed to them emanates from the provider, as opposed to the organization. However, the unique vulnerabilities of healthcare patients dependent on, not merely the provider, but also the system governing the provider and, to a certain extent, governing the care provided to the patient (Furrow 2009).

Healthcare organizations have been found to owe a fiduciary duty to their patients in certain jurisdictions (Furrow 2009). As examples, hospitals, nursing homes, health insurance providers, and pharmaceutical organizations have, to some degree, all been held to a higher degree of care in regard to their clients than a non-healthcare organization, suggesting the existence of a fiduciary duty (Furrow 2009). However, the parameters of this duty are not established to the degree of the fiduciary duty imposed on physicians, which has existed long before any fiduciary duty imposed on a healthcare organization.

Legal scholars have argued that the current state of fiduciary law as it pertains to the healthcare field, fails to adequately protect patients due to the increased complexity regarding how care is provided and how payment is received (Miller 1983). Healthcare in some jurisdictions, such as the United States, has shifted toward an institutional model, whereby care is rendered by one or more providers, but payment is subject to a separate process, often with an intermediary, a health insurance company, present in the relationship (Tikkanen et al. 2020). Health insurance in these jurisdictions has become more prevalent nationwide and has assumed an increasing amount of the financial burden regarding the provision of care. Often, the cost to the patient of the care they are receiving is unknown until the patient's insurance company weighs in pursuant to the contract between the patient and their insurer (Tikkanen et al. 2020).

On the other hand, many countries in the EU have shifted toward a universal health model of medicine, whereby the cost and quality of care are regulated by national government entities (Janus and Minvielle 2017). Citizens are required to pay into this system, generally through taxation (Janus and Minvielle 2017). After a citizen has paid in to the system, they are generally free to obtain care from any healthcare provider of their choosing, while the national government provides for the cost of care (Janus and Minvielle 2017).

These systems call into question which parties hold fiduciary duties and to what extent? In institutional models, health insurers often wade into the provider's role regarding the necessity of care rendered to the patient and will generally only cover services allowed under the contract between insurer and insured that are reasonably necessary to treat an insured's medical condition. Of course, prescribing treatment that is necessary to treat a patient's medical condition has traditionally been at the core of the fiduciary duty owed by the provider. In universal health models, national governments generally provide for the payment of health services, through taxation, but the governments also ensure the quality of care provided and, in certain EU countries, healthcare providers are considered employees of the national government. The abilities of insurers or governments to weigh in on the quality of care and the payment of care decisions clouds the nature of the fiduciary duty owed by the provider, the insurer, or the government.

Furthermore, patients worldwide no longer receive care exclusively from a single point of service, as was more common historically (Arora et al. 2015). The field of medicine has become more specialized and providers will generally refer a patient to a number of different providers in order to address a patient's diverse health needs (Arora et al. 2015). As the healthcare field has also grown in complexity, providers have moved toward outsourcing the financial and management aspects of healthcare to separate departments or, in some circumstances, to separate organizations altogether (Arora et al. 2015). This results in a multitude of relationships involving the patient, which may or may not involve fiduciary duties.

The assumed roles of healthcare organizations, health insurers, and national governments, regarding the payment and quality of a patient's care represent a blending of roles traditionally held exclusively by the healthcare provider necessitates that the patient's health data will be shared among members of at least two of these institutions. When the patient's health data was merely in the possession of the healthcare provider, it was clear that the duty to maintain the patient's health data rested with the provider. However, the intermingling of responsibilities among providers, insurers, and governments, makes it less clear which actors hold the responsibility to maintain and safeguard a patient's information.

The Fiduciary Duty of a Healthcare Organization to Maintain Health Data

The threat of losing clients is not sufficient to encourage those in possession of health data to protect their client's privacy interests (Dobkin 2018). A person who relinquishes their health data generally is not fully aware how their data will be used or who will ultimately possess their data (Dobkin 2018). The increases in the monetary value of health data and health data sharing, as well as the constant, often high-profile, threat of cyberattacks targeting health data, has led to heightened duties of care being imposed on organizations regarding their maintenance of individual health data (Dobkin 2018).

Physicians and other healthcare providers generally owe a duty to their patients to maintain the confidentiality of communications regarding the patient's health (Furrow 2009). This duty falls under the fiduciary duty owed by physicians (Furrow 2009). This same duty is generally extended to healthcare organizations which are often provided information as either providers of care themselves or pursuant to an agreement between the organization and the physician to maintain the confidentiality of a patient's health information (Furrow 2009).

The digital age, while vastly improving the quantity and quality of health information available to healthcare providers, has complicated the nature of the duty providers and health organizations owe to patients regarding patient health information. The shift toward electronic information necessitates the assistance of non-health professionals to maintain the integrity and security of patient information. Further, the threat of cybercriminals attempting to access health information poses challenges health providers in the pre-digital age could not have fathomed.

Complicating the nature of a fiduciary duty owed by healthcare organizations to the individuals whose data is in the possession of the organizations, are the increasing number of organizations in the business of health, but not as direct providers of care. Organizations focused on health technology, such as exercise, diet, or lifestyle applications, but not actually providing healthcare to a patient, operate in the health market and often possess health data (Licea 2019). Unlike the relationship between a healthcare provider and patient in which a patient discloses their health information in a collaborative effort to ensure they receive the highest quality and most accurate care from the provider, the relationship between a health application and user is quite different in that the user inputs their health data to the device in their efforts to obtain the greatest use from the device (Licea 2019). Viewing the health app device as merely a tool, can lead users to fail to consider that their health data may be accessed from the device by the owners of the app and, potentially, by third parties (Licea 2019).

These rapid changes in the health information landscape brings forth yet another issue regarding the fiduciary duties owed to individuals by healthcare organizations: whether a fiduciary duty is owed by a healthcare organization to maintain a patient's electronic health information. When viewed in a more basic context – whether an individual healthcare provider owes a fiduciary duty to maintain a patient's health information – answering this issue in the affirmative seems simple. However, as discussed previously, the model of healthcare has become more complex globally. Can this issue be answered as easily when, instead of a health provider, an organization which does not directly provide care is maintaining the patient's information? Should health insurers be held to this same duty? What duty is owed by organizations tasked solely with housing healthcare information? Should developers of "smart" products and "smart" electronic applications, such as fitness appliances, which track a user's health information, be held to the same fiduciary duty to maintain the user's health information? These are the issues facing lawmakers, courts, healthcare providers, health organizations, developers of health-related products, patients, and consumers. These issues have lead some to call for the creation of fiduciary duties being placed on individuals in possession of health data, referred to as **health data fiduciaries**, which are individuals or organizations which determine the purpose and means by which personal information will be processed and are, as a result of the valuable and sensitive information they possess, held to comply with higher standards of care than individuals or organizations that are not in possession of protected health information.

Definitive answers to these questions are rare given the constant expansion of healthcare and health technology, outpacing international legal and legislative systems. As such, the concept of a health data fiduciary remains poorly developed. However, many jurisdictions have made efforts to establish legal frameworks governing the maintenance, sharing, and security of health information with some jurisdictions imposing the equivalent of a fiduciary duty on the part of organizations in regard to health data. These frameworks vary by country and, in some instances, by regional divisions within countries. Some countries have addressed health information within laws separate from other forms of sensitive information, while other countries have addressed health information within the same laws as other forms of information. A review of a selection of these legal frameworks from across the globe demonstrates that lawmakers in each country will often incorporate aspects of another country's framework into their own laws. This review is helpful to understand the means by which health information is being protected across many jurisdictions but is also helpful to predict how other countries may form their own health information laws in the future by using the existing laws as models.

National Health Data Privacy & Security Laws

Data privacy laws currently exist in a majority of nations worldwide (iSight 2021). This section provides an illustrative scan of data privacy laws in nations on each continent. The select nations were chosen as a representative sample of those nations which have passed health data privacy and security legislation intended to apply nationwide. The privacy laws discussed represent attempts to structure the duties owed by healthcare organizations and third parties over patient health data in their possession.

The United States of America

In the United States, fiduciary duties have been held to apply to trustees, bankers, corporate board members, guardians, lawyers, and medical providers. There is no consensus among United States' courts to extend fiduciary duties to all entities in possession of private health information aside from the direct provider of care. This issue is dealt with more specifically by the United States' signature health information privacy law.

In 1996, the United States passed the Health Insurance Portability and Accountability Act (HIPAA), addressing the privacy of patient health information. HIPAA establishes patient rights to access their private health information, trust that their information is being held securely and only being used for purposes consistent with their well-being and amend or correct their information for accuracy (Health Insurance Portability and Accountability Act (1936)). Informed consent is necessary for the initial collection of personal health information and for uses of personal health information outside of the scope of medical treatment. HIPAA can be divided, for purposes of simplicity, into three broad categories of rules, each designating a primary goal of HIPAA: (1) Privacy Rule; (2) Security Rule; and (3) Breach Notification Rule.

The HIPAA Privacy Rule creates standards applicable across the entire United States designed to protect private health information. The Privacy Rule applies to a certain type of information, known as "protected health information." Protected health information, also referred to as "individually identifiable health information," is information relating to: *"[T]he individual's past, present, or future physical or mental health or condition; the provision of health care to the individual; or the past, present, or future payment for the provision of health care to the individual,"* which either identifies a specific person or which can reasonably identify that person.

Individually identifiable health information cannot be used by entities covered by HIPAA for any reason other than the treatment-related reasons allowed in the Privacy Rule or if the individual, whose information is at issue authorizes, in writing, the information to be used for specific purposes. The information cannot be disclosed by covered entities unless it is disclosed to the individuals themselves, upon request, or to certain government agencies if there is an ongoing investigation. Covered entities also may use or disclose this information for the organization to treat, pay, and conduct other healthcare activities.

The HIPAA Security Rule requires that entities covered by the Act implement measures that can lower an entity's risk of a cyberattack. The Security Rule applies to a specific type of protected health information, referred to as "electronic protected health information." Electronic protected health information is protected health information transmitted by the organization using some electronic means.

The Security Rule requires organizations to conduct regular risk analyses to detect potential vulnerabilities to the electronic protected health information being stored by the organization. The organization then must work to minimize these vulnerabilities. Organizations must have protocols in place to detect and prevent malicious software from infecting their computer systems. Users of healthcare organizations' computer systems must be trained on how to protect their systems against malicious software and report any suspicions that malicious software has infected one of the organization's systems.

The Security Rule further requires healthcare organizations to use access controls, allowing only necessary users to have access to electronic protected health information. The Security Rule requires organizations to conduct risk analyses of all threats to any electronic protected health information generated by the organization or its affiliates to determine if any electronic protected health information is in jeopardy of theft, exposure, or loss. Covered entities must also demonstrate that their entire workforce is in compliance with the Security Rule.

To put individuals who have been negatively affected by a breach of personal health information on alert, HIPAA provides for a number of rules requiring healthcare organizations to notify different parties in the case of a breach. These provisions are in HIPAA's Breach Notification Rule. The Breach Notification Rule applies to all protected health information, not only electronic protected health information.

Under title 45, section 164.402 of the U.S. Code of Federal Regulations, a breach is defined as: *"[T]he acquisition, access, use, or disclosure of protected health information in a manner not permitted,. .. which compromises the security or privacy of the protected health information"* (45 C.F.R. § 164.402). Any impermissible use of protected health information is presumptively a breach requiring notification, unless the covered entity is able to demonstrate that there is a low likelihood that the protected health information was actually compromised. If a covered entity commits a breach that involves unsecured protected health information, the entity is required to make disclosures to the U.S. Department of Health and Human Services, any individuals who may be affected by the breach, and, depending on the circumstances, to the public through the media.

HIPAA permits an organization to share health information with a third-party organization, upon the execution of a third-party vendor agreement. If the organization initially hosting the health information shares the information with a third-party vendor, the initial organization retains responsibility over the information and must still ensure its use and security is compliant with HIPAA.

There are some forms of health information that are not covered by HIPAA and are dealt with more specifically by other U.S. laws, such as genetic information, which is addressed by the Genetic Information Nondiscrimination Act of 2008 (GINA) (United States of America, Genetic Information Nondiscrimination Act (2009)). The primary purpose of GINA is to prohibit discrimination based genetic information. GINA has separate parts dealing with discrimination regarding health insurance and discrimination regarding employment. Federal legislation creating the Substance Abuse and Mental Health Services Administration (SAMHSA) also created regulations regarding the privacy and authorized disclosures of patient substance abuse records (Confidentiality of Substance Use Disorder Patient Records (2017)). The Privacy Act of 1974 provides for the regulation of personal information held by U.S. government agencies (Privacy Act of 1974 (1974)). These federal statutes pertain less to personal health information, so they are only briefly mentioned here. Many individual states within the United States also have their own health information privacy laws applicable to individuals and organizations operating within the confines of the state's borders, including biometric information privacy laws, which are growing in prevalence in the United States.

The European Union

The General Data Privacy Regulation (GDPR) is a regulation passed by the European Union (EU) in 2016 (EU General Data Protection Regulation: Regulation (2016)). More than any other national data privacy law, the GDPR has served as a model data privacy law for other nations. The GDPR applies to all EU member states and many EU member states have passed their own data privacy laws implementing the GDPR.

Under the GDPR, organizations maintaining personal health information must inform patients of the organizations use of the patient's information and may only use such information for a legitimate purpose. Organizations may only retain health information until its purpose is completed and may only use the health information necessary to complete its purpose.

Patients have the right to know what information is being used and the purpose for the use, as well as to amend incorrect information. Informed consent from the patient is required if their health information will be used by the organization outside of its original purpose.

The GDPR also contains several information security provisions. Organizations must establish minimum, documented procedures to safeguard the health information in its possession. Information security trainings are also required to be conducted by the organization for any employees maintaining the information. It is recommended, under the GDPR, that organizations assign a data protection officer, whose role it is to oversee the organization's compliance with the GDPR and to ensure the security of the stored information. The GDPR also features breach notification provisions, requiring an organization to notify those negatively impacted by an information security breach within seventy-two hours.

Information-sharing by the organization with third-parties is permitted under the GDPR, however, the sharing organization retains responsibility for any compromise of the shared information and is further responsible for ensuring the third-party complies with the GDPR in relation to the shared information.

The "right to be forgotten" is featured in Article 17 of the GDPR and provides that health organizations must erase any health information in its possession upon the individual's request if the purpose for which the organization held the information has been accomplished, the organization only used the information for marketing purposes, or if the organization only used the individual's information subject to the individual's consent and that consent has now been revoked.

In addition to the GDPR, another important health data protection law in the EU is the establishment of the Working Party on the Protection of Individuals with regard to the Processing of Personal Data (Article 29 of Directive 95/46/EC (2007)). Article 29 addressed the EU health care industry directly. Article 29 provides requirements for health information collected by healthcare organizations in electronic form. The collection of health information must be for the purpose of providing healthcare services.

Canada

In Canada, the Personal Information Protection and Electronic Documents Act (PIPEDA) is the primary health data protection law applying to Canada (Canada, Personal Information (2000)). PIPEDA applies to Canadian organizations maintaining, collecting, and using personal information, including personal health information.

The provinces of Alberta, British Columbia, Labrador, New Brunswick, Newfoundland, Nova Scotia, and Quebec have their own privacy laws as well, which are substantially similar to PIPEDA. Organizations with substantially similar privacy laws are exempt from PIPEDA regarding the maintenance, storage, and use of health information within the particular province.

PIPEDA generally requires organizations in possession of patients' health information to abide by ten equitable principles in regard to the organization's handling of the health information.

1. The principle of Accountability requires organizations to appoint an information privacy official responsible for the organization's compliance with PIPEDA and for the maintenance. The organization must, further, maintain the health information in its possession and implement reasonable measures to protect the information in its possession.

2. The principle of Identifying Purposes requires organizations to identify the purposes for the organization's collection and use of a patient's personal health information. In the event the organization seeks to fulfill a new purpose, it is required to obtain the patient's consent to the new purpose.

3. The principle of Consent requires the organization obtain informed consent from the patient upon collecting, using, and disclosing the patient's personal health information. Consent can be withdrawn by the patient at any point in time. There is not a strict rule under PIPEDA regarding the form of consent, but instead the form of consent should be commensurate with the sensitivity of the information or transaction involved.

4. The principle of Limiting Collection requires organizations to only collect the amount of patient health information that is necessary for the organization to fulfill its consented-to purpose. It is further required that organizations only collect information using legitimate, lawful methods.

5. Similar to the previous principle, the principle of Limiting Use, Disclosure, and Retention requires organizations to limit the information used, disclosed, and retained only to the extent necessary to fulfill its stated purpose. The organization must also be capable of explaining the reasoning behind its use, disclosure, and retention of health information.

6. The principle of Accuracy requires organizations to make reasonable efforts to ensure the patient health information in its information is accurate and current. The organization is recommended to implement policies regarding regularly updating certain categories of information.

7. The principle of Safeguards requires organizations to put into practice security policies designed to protect patient health information. These policies are required to be regularly reviewed and updated. Employees handling health information must be trained and made aware of the organization's safeguard policies. The level of protection offered by an organization's safeguards should be commensurate with the value, sensitivity, and risk posed to the information in the organization's possession.

8. The next principle, Openness, requires organizations to make their information management and privacy policies available to the general public, clear, and reasonably understandable.
9. The principle of Individual Access grants individuals the right to access their health information in the possession of an organization. The organization must respond to patient requests to access their information within 30 days upon receipt of the patient's request. This 30-day limit may only be extended in circumstances under which it would be unreasonable for the organization to respond within 30 days. In addition to patient information itself, the organization must also disclose how a patient's information has been used by the organization. This principle also gives patients the right to have their information amended for accuracy.
10. The final principle, that of Challenging Compliance, gives individuals the right to challenge an organization's compliance with PIPEDA. A successful challenge alleging an organization has failed to comply with the PIPEDA principles will require the organization to come into PIPEDA compliance. Organizations must have procedures regarding the handling of PIPEDA compliance challenges.

Mexico

Mexico recognizes the privacy of personal data as a constitutional, fundamental right. Mexico then passed the Federal Law on Protection of Personal Data Held by Private Parties in 2010 (United Mexican States (2010)). In 2013, the National Institute for Access to Information and Protection of Personal Data (INAI), issued the Guidelines on Privacy Notices, establishing the primary information privacy framework applicable to health information in Mexico (National Institute for Access to Information and Protection of Personal Data (2013)).

Under the guidelines, an organization must obtain a patient's written, informed consent before possessing their health information. Certain exceptions apply to the consent rule, such as in situations where consent cannot be given due to the health condition of the patient and medical care is necessary to prevent additional harm.

Generally, an organization is bound by the principles of legality, consent, quality, loyalty, proportionality, and accountability in its obligations to maintain a patient's personal health information. Organizations are required to implement security measures intended to safeguard personal health information from loss, unauthorized use, or unauthorized access. Further, organizations must only use health information in accordance with the purpose stipulated by the patient and the information may be altered or destroyed at the direction of the patient. Patient health information may only be possessed by an organization for as long as necessary to fulfill its stated purpose.

The guidelines permit transfers of health information to third-parties. Transfers of health information require the execution of data transfer agreements. Further, the informed consent of the patient must be granted as well.

Organizations maintaining health information are required to appoint a data protection officer. The data protection officer is tasked with ensuring the organization's compliance with the guidelines, ensuring the protection of health information, and responding to patient inquiries regarding their information.

The guidelines provide for a breach notification requirement. Organizations maintaining health information are required to disclose, immediately, the existence of any breach, unauthorized disclosure, or unauthorized use of a patient's health information to the patient. The nature of the incident, the information at risk, recommendations, remedial actions, and a method of obtaining additional information must, at a minimum, be included in the organization's disclosure.

Brazil

On August 14, 2018, Brazil passed its signature legislation providing for the protection of individual data, including health data (Federative Republic of Brazil (2018)). The Lei Geral de Protecao de Dados (LGPD) was modeled after the GDPR and defines personal data to include health, genetic, and biometric data.

The LGPD provides ten bases for which and organization may collect health data, which includes collecting data with the consent of the individual. Consent to the collection of an individual's health data must be informed and provided in writing. An individual's consent to the collection and use of their health data must provide for the purpose of the collection and the permitted uses of the individual's health data. The organization must remain within the permitted purpose and permitted use to which the individual gave their consent. The individual has the right to revoke their consent at any point in time.

The individual has the right to access their health information upon request and may also request to the organization cease to use their health information even if the organization remains within the permitted use of the information.

The LGPD also provides requirements for the security of health information in the possession of organizations. Organizations are required to adopt reasonable security measures to protect an individual's personal health information. Further, organizations are required to notify an individual if their health information has been compromised. Organizations must also notify the regulatory agency tasked with enforcing the LGPD of any comprise of personal health information.

Argentina

The Argentina Protection of Personal Information Act (POPIA) was passed in the year 2000 (Argentine Republic (2000)). A new personal data protection bill has been proposed in Argentina with similarities to the GDPR, but has yet to be passed. POPIA remains the primary legal authority in Argentina regarding personal data, including health data, privacy.

According to POPIA, personal health data may only be collected and used by an organization upon receiving written, informed consent from the individual. However, if the personal health data has been anonymized, it ceases to be considered *personal* health data under POIA and no consent is necessary to collect and use the anonymized data.

Personal health data may only be collected for legal, relevant purposes and may not be used beyond the scope of the intended purpose. Individuals have the right to request a full accounting of their personal health data, including copies of the data in the organization's possession, the purpose for the collection, and any use of the data. Transfer of an individual's personal health information is impermissible without the individual's informed, written consent.

POPIA uses the term "data controllers," but does not define the term. A data controller under POPIA seems to function similarly to a data control officer, which is provided for in other national personal data privacy laws. Data controllers, under POPIA, must be designated by organizations in possession of personal health data. The controllers must implement technical security measures to protect personal information in the organization's possession. Data controllers must also ensure health information remains private and secure in the organization's care.

South Africa

South Africa passed its Protection of Personal Information Act (POPIA) on November 19, 2013 (Republic of South Africa (2013)). Under POPIA, "special personal information" is protected and this term specifically includes personal health information. POPIA features eight conditions by which organizations in possession of special personal information must abide.

1. **Accountability**: This Condition requires organizations to ensure the remaining conditions are complied with before collecting or using personal health information. The Condition also requires continued compliance with POIPA throughout the organization's use of the information.
2. **Processing Limitation**: This Condition requires organizations to use personal health information only in a manner that does not risk the individual's privacy. Organizations must only use the amount of data and only the data relevant to fulfill its stated purpose to which the individual has consented. Consent must also be granted by the individual prior to the organization's collection or use of their health information and the individual may withdraw their consent at any time. The organization may only collect health information from the individual to whom the information is regarding unless the information is available in a public record or the individual consents to collecting their information from another source.
3. **Purpose Specification**: This Condition requires an organization to only collect or use health information for a specific purpose, which is defined, of which the individual is aware, and to which the individual has consented. The purpose must

be lawful. Once this purpose has been completed, the organization must destroy or de-identify the health information in its possession.

4. **Further Processing Limitation**: This Condition, similar to Condition 3, requires organizations to cease using health information once its purpose for using the information is complete unless the individual has given their consent to continue using the information, the health information is available in a public record, or if the information is necessary to comply with South African law.

5. **Information Quality**: This Condition requires organizations to ensure the health information it collects and uses is complete and accurate. Individuals have the right to amend or supplement the health information in an organization's possession if doing so would render the information more complete or accurate.

6. **Openness from the organization**: This Condition requires organizations using health information to document the information in its possession as well as to document the uses of the information. Individuals are entitled to know under POPIA how their information is collected, what information has been collected, the purpose of the collection, the organization's contact information, intentions to transfer the information to a third-party, and the legal requirements regarding the collection and use of their information.

7. **Security Safeguards**: Under this Condition, organizations must provide for the security of health information in their possession. The Condition requires the implementation of technical safeguards, employee awareness and security training, risk assessments, and threat analyses. Breach notification requirements are also provided for under Condition 7, requiring organizations to make individuals affected by a breach of their information aware of the breach and the extent to which their information may have been compromised. Third-party sharing of information is permitted under this Condition, but only with the individual's consent and upon execution of a third-party agreement, by which the third-party accepts its compliance obligations under POPIA.

8. **Data Subject Participation**: The rights of individuals regarding the collection and use of their health information are provided for in this Condition. Individuals have the right to access their information within a reasonable time. Individuals have the right to be made aware of uses of their information, the information collected, and the purposes behind the uses and collection. Further, individuals have the rights to amend or supplement their information.

Uganda

In February 2019, Uganda passed its Data Protection and Privacy Act (DPPA), which seeks to protect its citizens' expectations of privacy regarding the collection and use of their personal information, including health information (Republic of Uganda (2019)). The Act broadly prohibits organizations from collecting, holding, and using personal information which invades the privacy of an individual.

The Act requires organizations to be accountable for the health information in their possession. Organizations may only collect and use information for lawful purposes.

Only the minimal amount of information may be collected and used to fulfill the lawful purpose. The information may only be retained by the organization for the amount of time needed to fulfill its purpose. The information in the organization's possession must be complete and accurate and individuals have the right to amend their information. Further, informed consent on the part of the individual is required before their health information may be collected or used by an organization.

Transparency is required in an organization's relations with the individual whose health information is in its possession. Individuals have the right to access their health information. The Act further gives individuals the rights to amend or supplement their health information and to demand an organization cease its use of their health information.

Security safeguards must be implemented to protect personal health data. Safeguards should include risk assessment, threat analyses, and training of employees. Complaints may be made to government authorities for an organization's failure to comply with DPPA.

Japan

Japan passed one of the earliest privacy laws in Asia. Passed in 2003, the Act on the Protection of Personal Information (APPI), is Japan's primary personal health data privacy law. It has been amended and enhanced in recent years to keep pace with technological developments (Japan (2003)). The recent changes make the APPI more similar to the GDPR.

Like the GDPR, the APPI requires the individual's informed consent prior to the collection and use of personal health information. Personal health information may only be transferred to third parties upon the organization's obtaining written, informed consent from the individual. As with most data privacy laws, the organization is only permitted to obtain a reasonable amount of information to further the organization's proper purpose and the individual has the right to access, amend, or supplement its data.

The APPI established a Personal Information Protection Commission (PPC), the governing authority regarding data protection in Japan. The APPI contains breach notification provisions, under which an organization in possession of personal health information must notify the PPC and the individual involved, in the event of a compromise or breach of personal health information.

Organizations are required to maintain the security of personal health information. The APPI requires reasonable steps be taken to ensure the accuracy, security, privacy, and supervision of personal health information. Unlike other data privacy laws, the APPI does not require the appointment of a data protection officer. Organizations are tasked with ensuring their own compliance with the APPI and for maintaining the security and privacy of the health data in their possession and, despite the fact that the APPI does not require the appointment of a data protection officer per se, the APPI does require organizations to name an individual who will control the personal health information in the possession of the organization.

Importantly, the more recent amendments to the APPI allow organizations to avoid many of the individual rights provisions of the APPI if the organizations anonymize the health data in their possession to the extent the data cannot reasonably be traced to the individual. This provision was not featured in the original APPI.

South Korea

Enacted in 2011, South Korea's Personal Information Protection Act (PIPA) is among Asia's most stringent personal data protection laws (Republic of Korea (2011)). PIPA's definition of personal data includes health data and biological data.

Organizations in possession of personal health data are required by PIPA to make their data privacy and protection policies public. Individuals are entitled to access their personal health information within 10 days of requesting said information and an individual's information cannot be obtained or used without the individual's informed consent. The purpose for which organizations collect and use personal health data must be legitimate and organizations must operate within that purpose.

Under PIPA, organizations are required to maintain and secure the personal health information in its possession. Organizations are required to ensure the information in its possession is complete and accurate and individuals maintain the rights to amend and to order the destruction of their personal health data.

Philippines

In 2012 the Philippines passed its Data Privacy Act, the comprehensive personal data privacy law for the country (Republic of the Philippines (2011)). The law is applicable to all individuals or organizations that possess and use personal data, including health data. The Data Privacy Act also created a National Privacy Commission designated as the government enforcement agency of the Act. The final rules and regulations regarding the Data Privacy Act were applied in 2016.

As with the personal data laws in other nations, the Data Privacy Act in the Philippines requires organizations to designate a legitimate, legal purpose for its collection and use of personal health information. The individual's consent is required prior to the organization's collection and use of that individual's health data and the organization may only use an individual's health data within the purpose to which the individual consented.

Third-party sharing of personal health information is permitted by the Data Privacy Act. Organizations must, however, enter into agreements with the third parties who will possess and use the personal health data, subjecting the Third-party to the same obligations under the Data Privacy Act as the original organization.

The Data Privacy Act features a security framework, providing for the protection of personal health data. Organizations are required to maintain the reasonable expectations of privacy that individuals have in regard to their health information.

An organization's compliance, or lack thereof, with the Data Privacy Act, is reviewable by the National Privacy Commission. Technical safeguards, employee training, risk and threat analyses are all encompassed under the Data Privacy Act.

The law further provides for notification of affected individuals in the event of a data breach. Where personal health information has been compromised or disclosed without authorization, the organization originally holding the information must disclose the breach to the individual if: (1) the information breached is sensitive in nature; (2) the organization holds a reasonable belief that the health information has been acquired by an unauthorized party; (3) there is a risk to the individual; and (4) the potential harm to the individual is serious in nature.

Russia

The primary national law in Russia in the area of data protection is the Personal Data Law (Russian Federation (2006)). The Personal Data Law protects all personal data, including data pertaining to special categories of privacy, such as race, nationality, political opinions, religious beliefs, biometrics, and health.

A data operator can delegate the processing to a Third-party, subject to the data subject's consent, who will be acting under the data operator's authorization based on a processing agreement, or by operation of a special state or municipal act (Article 6(3), Personal Data Law).

Organizations may only collect health information lawfully and pursuant to fairness considerations. Only the amount of health information necessary to fulfill the organization's purpose may be collected and the information may only be possessed for the length of time necessary to fulfill the organization's purpose. The organization may only use the information to fulfill its stated purpose.

An organization is under the obligation to maintain the security and privacy of the health information in its possession pursuant to the Personal Data Law. The Law requires organizations to designate a data protection officer who is tasked with ensuring the information in the possession of the organization is secure and that the organization is compliant with the Personal Data Law. Impact assessments and threat analyses must be performed regularly by the data protection officer and employees handling personal information must be trained to comply with the organization's information security policies.

Patients are granted certain rights in regard to their information under the Personal Data Law. Patients have the right to access their information upon request and the organization must respond to a patient's request within 30 days of receipt. Patients have the right to amend their health information if it is inaccurate or incomplete. The organization must inform patients if information regarding them has been obtained from another source. Informed consent from the patient is required before any use or collection of their information.

The Personal Data Law does permit organization's to share health information with third-parties, but only upon obtaining the informed consent of the patient and only when, and to the extent, necessary to fulfill the organization's stated purpose for using the information.

People's Republic of China

On November 6, 2016, the People's Republic of China (PRC) passed its Cybersecurity Law of the People's Republic of China, which became effective in June, 2017 (People's Republic of China (2016)). The Cybersecurity Law is broad in scope, applying to personal information, information regarding the country's critical infrastructure, and the cross-border transfer of information.

Organizations maintaining personal information are prohibited from disclosing, altering, or destroying personal information in its possession without the authorization of the individual whose personal information has been collected. Individuals have the right to request their information be amended, deleted, or released to them. An individual's informed consent is needed to allow an organization to disclose the individual's information to a Third-party. It should be noted however, that these privacy and consent provisions do not apply where the organization has de-identified the individual's personal information. The PRC Cybersecurity Law establishes a breach notification requirement where personal information has been improperly disclosed or improperly accessed by an unauthorized Third-party.

The Cybersecurity Law further establishes a penalty structure for noncompliant organizations. Penalties are assessed by regulatory agencies and range from monetary penalties, to licensure suspension.

On August 20, 2021, the PRC passed a new information privacy and security law, the Personal Information Protection Law (PIPL). The text of the PIPL has not been released at the time of this writing, but is scheduled to become effective on November 1, 2021. Organizations will need to be in compliance with PIPL by the date of its effect to avoid penalties. While the full text of the PIPL remains to be seen, the law is intended to serve as the primary data protection law in the PRC.

India

India has proposed its Personal Data Protection Bill (PDPB) in 2019, but at the time of this writing, the Bill has yet to become law (Republic of India (2019)). Many expect the Personal Data Protection Bill to be signed into law in 2021. The Personal Data Protection Bill draws heavily from the EU's GDPR. The Bill imposes compliance requirements for all personal data, including health data.

The Bill specifically proposes the term "data fiduciary," which is an individual or organization which determines the purpose and means by which personal information will be processed. While the requirements the Bill would impose on a data fiduciary are similar to the requirements other national data protection laws impose on organizations collecting personal health information, the Bill is unique in its designation of all entities processing personal information as "fiduciaries."

Under the Bill, organizations are required to obtain an individual's informed consent before collecting or using their personal health information. Health information may only be used for the purposes to which a patient has given their informed consent. Informed consent is also required before making any disclosure of a patient's health information to a third-party.

The Bill requires organizations to provide for the security of health information. Organizations must implement security safeguards and provide training to its employees regarding the handling and safety of health information. Where several other national data protection laws require the selection of a data protection officer, The Personal Data Protection Bill would require organizations to select "significant data fiduciaries." Similar to the data protection officers featured in other national data protection laws, significant data fiduciaries will be tasked with ensuring the organization's compliance with the Bill, conducting information security analyses and audits, and ensuring the security of the information in the possession of the organization.

Australia

The Australia Privacy Principles (APPs) contained within Australia's Privacy Act 1988, constitute the primary, national health information protection laws in the country (Commonwealth of Australia (1988)). Regulations within Australian state and territories also regulate health information privacy. The APPs are divided into 13 categories of privacy protection.

The Principles require open and transparent management of personal information. This Principle requires organizations maintaining health information to have a current, express APP privacy policy. Organizations must make reasonable efforts to implement procedures to ensure compliance with the APPs.

Under the anonymity and pseudonymity Principles, organizations maintaining health information must offer patients the option of anonymity or pseudonymity with regard to their health records, with limited exceptions applying if Australian law otherwise requires the disclosure of the patient's identity or if it would not be reasonably practicable for the organization to maintain the patient's anonymity or pseudonymity.

The collection of solicited personal information Principle, details when an organization is permitted to collect solicited personal information. An organization is only permitted to solicit and collect personal information that is reasonably necessary for or directly related to a proper purpose. Informed consent from the patient is necessary for an organization to collect solicited health information and the organization may only collect this information from the patient themselves.

The collection of unsolicited personal information Principle pertains to health information collected by an organization that has not been requested by the organization. If the organization collects health information it has not specifically requested and that it could not obtain from a pubic source, the organization must destroy or deidentify the health information. If the information is obtainable from a public source, the organization need not destroy or deidentify the information.

The Principle regarding notification of the collection of personal information pertains to the circumstances where an organization maintaining health information must make disclosures to the patient. If a third-party comes into possession of the patient's health information, either intentionally or unintentionally, the organization must take reasonable steps to notify the patient.

The Principle pertaining to the use or disclosure of health information details where an organization may use or disclose health information in its possession. An organization may only disclose health information with the informed consent of the patient or, if no informed consent is granted, then only for the original use the information was entrusted to the organization.

Two Principles pertain to cross-border disclosures of personal health information and the use of government-related identifiers respectively.

The Principle regarding the quality of the health information in the possession of the organization, requires organizations to take reasonable measures to ensure the accuracy of the health information in its possession and to ensure the information is current. The organization must provide for the same requirements with regard to information it permissibly discloses to third parties.

The security of health information is detailed in a separate Principle. Organizations are required to take reasonable measures to ensure the protection of the health information in its possession from theft, misuse, loss, improper disclosure, and loss. This same Principle requires organizations to destroy records it no longer requires for its permitted use unless the records are publicly available.

Access to health information is encompassed in another Principle. This Principle requires an organization to provide a patient their health information upon request. Few exceptions apply to this Principle permitting the organization to refuse a patient's right to access their information.

The final Principle grants patients the right to correct the health information in the possession of the organization. The organization is required to affirmatively take reasonable measures to ensure the accuracy of the information it possesses.

A Closing Look at International Health Data Legal Frameworks

This survey demonstrates many of the legal efforts made by nations to address the lack of clarity regarding a health data fiduciary role applicable to healthcare organizations. Many nations have taken steps toward creating a clear health data fiduciary duty. India, in particular, in its pending data privacy legislation, explicitly uses the term "data fiduciary." This term is important as it leaves less doubt as to the nature of the relationship between individuals and health data holders. The explicit use of the term may also aid judiciaries in interpreting national data privacy acts to determine novel legal issues in this area. Furthermore, future health data privacy legislation should place heavier consideration on the issue of health data monetization and whether, as a matter of policy, nations wish to regulate whether and the extent to which personal health data is permitted to be sold for profit (Tables 22.1 and 22.2).

Table 22.1 Distinctions among terms

Terms	Definitions
Artificial intelligence	Intelligence, such as reasoning ability, demonstrated by machines.
Big data	A field dedicated to finding solutions to analyze data sets that are too large or complex to be analyzed using traditional data-processing application software.
Confidentiality	Data or information is not made available or disclosed to unauthorized persons or processes.
Fiduciary	A legal concept in which a heightened duty is owed by an individual with greater power and knowledge than another, to exercise the skill, judgment, integrity, and discretion necessary to protect the individual with less power who is generally dependent on the stronger party
Fiduciary duty	A legal duty on the party of a party to act with a degree of care, honesty, integrity, discretion, judgment, knowledge, and skill, which is greater than the degree of care owed by a person not acting as a fiduciary.
Health data fiduciary	Individuals or organizations which determine the purpose and means by which personal information will be processed and are, as a result of the valuable and sensitive information they possess, held to comply with higher standards of care than individuals or organizations that are not in possession of protected health information.
Integrity	Data or information have not been altered or destroyed in an unauthorized manner.
Internet of things (IOT)	Physical objects implanted with software that connects and exchanges data with other systems via networks.
Personal health records (PHR)	Records in the possession of healthcare providers containing sensitive, health-related information regarding a patient, often including a patient's name, phone number, address, financial information, insurance information, and health history.
Privacy	The practice of maintaining the confidentiality and security of protected health information.
Protected health information (PHI)	Information relating to an individual's physical or mental health condition, the healthcare provided or recommended for that individual, or the payment information regarding the provision of healthcare to the individual, which either identifies a specific person or which can reasonably identify that person.
Right to be forgotten	An individual's right to restrict or eliminate their personal information on the internet.
Safeguards	Protective measures prescribed to meet the security requirements (i.e., confidentiality, integrity, and availability) specified for an information system. Safeguards may include security features, management constraints, personnel security, and security of physical structures, areas, and devices. Synonymous with security controls and countermeasures.
Security	Protecting information and information systems from unauthorized access, use, disclosure, disruption, modification, or destruction in order to provide confidentiality, integrity, and availability.
Telehealth	The provision of healthcare services via electronic information and telecommunication technologies

Table 22.2 International health information privacy & security legislation survey

Nation	Signature health information privacy & security legislation	Year of effect
United States of America	Health insurance portability and accountability act (HIPAA)	1996
The European Union	The general data privacy regulation (GDPR)	2016
Canada	Personal information protection and electronic documents act (PIPEDA)	2000
Mexico	Federal Law on protection of personal data held by private parties	2010
Brazil	Lei Geral de Protecao de dados (LGPD)	2018
Argentina	Argentina protection of personal information act (POPIA)	2000
South Africa	Protection of personal information act (POPIA)	2013
Uganda	Data protection and privacy act (DPPA)	2019
Japan	Act on the protection of personal information (APPI)	2003
South Korea	Personal information protection act (PIPA)	2011
Philippines	Data privacy act	2012
People's Republic of China	Cybersecurity Law of the People's Republic of China	2016
	Personal information protection Law (PIPL)	2021
India	Personal data protection bill (PDPB)	2019
Russia	Personal data Law	2006
Australia	Australia privacy principles (APPs)	1988

Conclusion

The concept of healthcare organizations acting as health data fiduciaries is becoming an accepted legal norm globally. Regardless of whether the term "fiduciary" is used in health data privacy laws, the heightened duties and expertise of a fiduciary are being imposed on designated individuals within healthcare organizations. As healthcare continues to expand in its complexity and more actors join the healthcare framework, courts and legislators will have additional opportunities to weigh in on this issue, which will provide a more robust body of jurisprudence regarding organizational health data fiduciaries.

Discussion Questions
1. What is the value of protected health information considering the various parties involved in the creation, collection, and storage of protected health information?
   Health information has value to specific marketplace actors. Healthcare providers use health information in the course of providing health services to patients and to perform research in furtherance of the provision of health services. Health information has value to health insurers in that the information can provide insights regarding coverage decisions, risk, and possible coverage options. Health information has value to non-healthcare marketplace actors seeking to utilize the information in the furtherance of selling their products or procuring new clients/customers. Health information has value to bad faith

actors seeking to leverage privacy and sensitivity of health information in exchange for profit. Health information also has value, typically non-monetary value, to the individual whose health information is at issue due to the privacy and confidentiality concerns of the individual.

2. How is protected health information stored and what are the various considerations that come into play when deciding on various methods of information storage?

Health information can be stored using a variety of methods. On-site physical storage involves the storage of health information in a physical format within the storing organization's property. The benefits of this form of storage include protection from cybercrime and ready availability of the information. The drawbacks of this form of storage include the lack of efficiency and lack of navigation ease when storing large amounts of information in a physical form, as well as the limitations placed by the physical space available to store the information. On-site digital storage of health information involves organizations storing health information in a digital format on its own servers. This method of storage features the drawbacks of cyber hacking and the requirement that the organization maintain its digital network, while providing the benefits of ease of access, navigation, and greater storage capacity when compared with physical storage. Off-site digital storage involves the storage of health information by a contracted third-party. This method features the benefits of storage capacity and professional data management services, while featuring the drawbacks of third-party involvement and cyber hacking. Cloud storage of health information involves storing health information on a cloud network. This method features the benefits of storage capacity, accessibility, ease of navigation, and low maintenance requirements, while featuring the drawbacks of cyber hacking.

3. What are the basic elements that generally establish a fiduciary duty and do these elements apply to an individual or organization in possession of protected health information?

A fiduciary relationship generally involves: (1) a party providing a service or good requiring a level of knowledge and expertise beyond that possessed by the general public; (2) a second-party, without the requisite knowledge and expertise of the first, availing itself of the service or good offered by the first-party; (3) reliance by the second-party on the first-party regarding the rendering of the service or good. An individual or organization in possession of protected health information generally must possess at least the knowledge required to store and maintain the information in accordance with the applicable data privacy and security law. This level of knowledge is generally greater than that possessed by the relying party (often a patient), particularly when the health information is being stored in a digital format, as is common, because this raises additional concerns regarding cybersecurity. The first element of the fiduciary relationship test would be satisfied. The relying party in the healthcare context is seeking to avail itself of the services or products of the healthcare provider. The second element of the analysis would also be satisfied. The provider will normally request a patient's health information in furtherance of the provision of care and the patient generally has little control regarding the methods by which their information will be stored, maintained, or secured. The third element of this analysis would also be satisfied. Because the three elements of the fiduciary relationship are satisfied when viewed in light of a party in possession of protected health information, it stands to reason that a party in possession of protected health information should be held to the heightened standard of a fiduciary.

References

45 C.F.R. § 164.402.

Argentine Republic. Protection of personal information act; 2000.

Arora V, Moriates C, Shah N. The challenge of understanding health care costs and charges. AMA J Ethics. 2015;17(11):1046–52. available at: https://journalofethics.ama-assn.org/article/challenge-understanding-health-care-costs-and-charges/2015-11

Article 29 of Directive 95/46/EC, Working Document on the Processing of Personal Data Relating to Health in Electronic Health Records (EHR), 2007 O.J. (WP 131), available at http://ec.europa.eu/justice/policies/privacy/docs/wpdocs/2007/wp131_en.pdf [http://perma.cc/E6SY-95PA] [hereinafter Article 29].

Assoc. of Healthcare Internal Auditors, Third-Party Relationships and your Confidential Data: Assessing Risk and Management Oversight Processes, *2–3, (2013). available at: https://ahia.org/assets/Uploads/pdfUpload/Whitepaper.pdf.

Bednar L. The need for an offsite backup for electronic health records (EHR). Secure Drive; (Jan. 15, 2020), available at: https://www.securedrive.com/blog/need-for-offsite-backup-for-ehr.

Brougher JD. The right to be forgotten: applying European privacy Law to American electronic health records. Ind Health L Rev. 2016;13:510.

Canada, Personal Information Protection and electronic documents act, SC 2000, c 5. https://canlii.ca/t/541b8. Retrieved on 2021 April 01.

Case C-131/12, Google Spain SL, Google Inc. v. Agencia Espan ola de Proteccion de Datos (AEDP), Mario Costeja Gonzalez, 2014 ECLI:EU:C:2014:317, 100(3) (May 13, 2014), http://curia.europa.eu/juris/document/document.jsf?text= & docid=152065 & pageIndex=0 & doclang=en & mode=1st & dir= & occ=first & part=1 & cid=356089.

Commonwealth of Australia. Privacy Act 1988 (Cth) https://www.legislation.gov.au/Details/C2018C00292.

Compliancy Group, Healthcare Clearinghouses HIPAA Privacy Rule, (last visited: 4/4/2021). available at: https://compliancy-group.com/healthcare-clearinghouses-hipaa/.

Confidentiality of Substance Use Disorder Patient Records, 82 Fed. Reg. 11, 4162–20 (01/18/2017); U.S. Department of Health & Human Services, Substance Abuse Confidentiality Regulations: Fact Sheets regarding the Substance Abuse Confidentiality Regulations (3/30/2021), available at: https://www.samhsa.gov/about-us/who-we-are/laws-regulations/confidentiality-regulations-faqs.

Davenport T, Kalakota R. The potential for artificial intelligence in healthcare. R College Phys Future Healthc J. (June, 2019), available at: https://www.ncbi.nlm.nih.gov/pmc/articles/PMC6616181/.

Davis J. Third-party vendors behind 20% of healthcare data breaches in 2018, Health IT Security; (April 15, 2019), available at: https://healthitsecurity.com/news/third-party-vendors-behind-20-of-healthcare-data-breaches-in-2018.

DeMuro PR. Keeping internet pirates at bay: ransomware negotiation in the healthcare industry. Nova L Rev. 2017;41:347, 352–5.

Dobkin A. Information fiduciaries in practice: data privacy and user expectations. Berkely Tech. LJ. 2018;33(1):1–52.

EU General Data Protection Regulation (GDPR): *Regulation (EU)* 2016/679 of the European Parliament and of the Council of 27 April 2016 on the protection of natural persons with regard to the processing of personal data and on the free movement of such data, and repealing Directive 95/46/EC (General Data Protection Regulation), OJ 2016 L 119/1.

European Commission. eHealth: Digital Health and Care, (last visited: 4/4/2021), available at: https://ec.europa.eu/health/ehealth/home_en.

Federative Republic of Brazil. Lei Geral de Protecao de Dados; 2018

Furrow BR. Patient safety and the fiduciary hospital: sharpening judicial remedies. Drexel L Rev. 2009;1:439.

GDPR.EU. Everything you need to know about the "right to be forgotten"; 2021., available at: https://gdpr.eu/right-to-be-forgotten/.

Hajar R. The Physician's oath: historical perspectives. Heart Views; 2017. available at: https://www.ncbi.nlm.nih.gov/pmc/articles/PMC5755201/

Health Insurance Portability and Accountability Act. Pub. L. No. 104–191, § 264, 110 Stat.1936.

Hern A. 'Anonymised' data can never be totally anonymous, says study. The Guardian;s (July 23, 2019), available at: https://www.theguardian.com/technology/2019/jul/23/anonymised-data-never-be-anonymous-enough-study-finds.

Ingalls S. Types of malware & best malware protection practices. ESecurity Planet; (Feb. 16, 2021), available at: https://www.esecurityplanet.com/threats/malware-types/#phishing.

iSight, A practical guide to data privacy laws by Country [2021], (March 5, 2021), available at: https://i-sight.com/resources/a-practical-guide-to-data-privacy-laws-by-country/.

Janus K, Minvielle E. Rethinking health care delivery: what European and United States health care systems can learn from one another. Health Aff. 2017; available at: https://www.healthaffairs.org/do/10.1377/hblog20171214.835155/full/

Japan, The act on the protection of personal information, 2003. available at: https://www.cas.go.jp/jp/seisaku/hourei/data/APPI.pdf..

Leiser MR. 'Private jurisprudence' and the right to be forgotten balancing test. Comput Law Sec Rev. 2020;39:105458

Licea M. All the scary ways health apps are using your data. New York Post; (Nov 11, 2019), available at: https://nypost.com/2019/11/11/all-the-scary-ways-health-apps-are-using-your-data/.

Millard M, Truveta, Formed wit Big-Name Health Systems, Aims for AI-Powered Data Advances. Healthcare IT News; (Feb. 11, 2021), available at: https://www.healthcareitnews.com/news/truveta-formed-big-name-health-systems-aims-ai-powered-data-advances.

Miller FH. Secondary income from recommended treatment: should fiduciary principles constrain physician behavior? In: Gray BH, editor. New health care for profit: doctors and hospitals in a competitive environment; 1983.

Murray L. Informed consent: what must a physician disclose to a patient? AMA J Ethics. 2012; available at: https://journalofethics.ama-assn.org/article/informed-consent-what-must-physician-disclose-patient/2012-07#:~:text=If%20disclosure%20is%20likely%20to,to%20refuse%20a%20specific%20treatment

National Institute for Access to Information and Protection of Personal Data. Guidelines on privacy notices. National Institute for Access to Information and Protection of Personal Data ('INAI'); 2013.

O'Dowd E. Healthcare data storage options: on-premise. In: Cloud and hybrid data storage. HIT Infrastructure; (Mar. 4, 2017), available at: https://hitinfrastructure.com/features/healthcare-data-storage-options-on-premise-cloud-and-hybrid-data-storage.

Pennic J. Telehealth and cybersecurity: what you should know. HIT Consultant; (7/22/2020), available at: https://hitconsultant.net/2020/07/22/telehealth-cybersecurity-what-you-should-know/#.YHL9t-hKhPY.

People's Republic of China. Cybersecurity Law of the People's Republic of China; 2016.

Privacy Act of 1974, 5 U.S.C. §552a (1974).

Republic of India. Personal Data Protection Bill, 2019., retrieved from: http://164.100.47.4/BillsTexts/LSBillTexts/Asintroduced/373_2019_LS_Eng.pdf.

Republic of Korea. Personal Information Protection Act (PIPA); 2011.
Republic of South Africa. Protection of personal information act. Government Gazette, 26
    November 2013., Retrieved from: https://www.gov.za/sites/default/files/gcis_document/20140
    9/3706726-11act4of2013protectionofpersonalinforcorrect.pdf
Republic of the Philippines. Data Privacy Act; 2011.
Russian Federation. Federal Law of 27 July 2006 N 152-FZ on Personal Data, 2006., available at:
    https://pd.rkn.gov.ru/authority/p146/p164/.
Shah AB, Patel NB, Contributed: unlocking value in health data: Truveta's data monetization strat-
    egy carries big risks and responsibilities. Mobi Health News; (March 5, 2021), available at:
    https://www.mobihealthnews.com/news/contributed-unlocking-value-health-data-truveta-s-
    data-monetization-strategy-carries-big-risks
Siddhartha, The data storage challenges of the healthcare industry, SD Global; (Jan. 22, 2020), available
    at: https://www.sdglobaltech.com/blog/the-data-storage-challenges-of-the-healthcare-industry.
Singleton S. Balancing a right to be forgotten with a right to freedom of expression in the wake of
    Google Spain v. AEPD. Ga. J. Int'l & Comp. L. 2015;44:165.
Snell E. Benefits. In: Challenges of secure healthcare data sharing. Health IT
    Security; (Oct. 20, 2017), available at: https://healthitsecurity.com/features/
    benefits-challenges-of-secure-healthcare-data-sharing.
The Republic of Uganda. The Data Protection and Privacy Act; 2019.
Tikkanen R, Osborn R, Mossialos E, Djorjevic A, Wharton GA. International health care systems
    profiles: United States, The Commonwealth Fund; June 5, 2020., available at: https://www.
    commonwealthfund.org/international-health-policy-center/countries/united-states
United Mexican States. Federal Law on Protection of Personal Data Held by Individuals
    (LFPDPPP); 2010.
United States. The genetic information nondiscrimination act of 2008 (GINA). Washington, D.C.:
    U.S. Dept. of Labor, Employee Benefits Security Administration; 2009.

Chapter 23
Ethical, Legal, and Social Issues Pertaining to Virtual and Digital Representations of Patients

Bonnie Kaplan

Abstract As precision and personalized medicine prove their worth, care shifts more towards treating representations of patients rather than patients' persons and bodies. Something is gained and something is lost by virtualizing patients and mediating care through technology. Because benefits are clear, the chapter highlights ethical, legal, and social issues surrounding quality of care, privacy, bias, and fairness to consider what could be lost.

I argue that virtualization reduces distinctions between individuals and reduces knowledge of each patient and patient's body. That changes relationships between patients and clinicians and shifts the locus of care away from the patient. It also decontextualizes data on which treatment and algorithmic recommendations are based. The data and algorithms all lack transparency, yet their predictions influence care. Not only can care be compromised, but both patients' and clinicians' personhood and autonomy are threatened.

Privacy, too, is endangered by the push to generate, collect, and aggregate data as all data become health data, used repeatedly and combined into multiple datasets. It is impossible to predict what those datasets will be, how data will be used, and what they will yield. Anonymity and consent both lose meaning. Privacy concerns can undermine confidentiality, which, in turn, can undermine trust, and therefore, can compromise care.

Algorithmic predictions based on sorting patients into algorithmically derived groups can harm group members. Care influenced by algorithmic recommendations may not be appropriate for all patients in the group, and predictions may stem from, or result in, bias, stigmatization, negative profiling, or disparate services.

The chapter concludes with a framework for analyzing ethical, legal, and social issues. It expands the scope of bioethics to more generally include information technologies in healthcare. To realize the promise of personalized medicine in ethical ways, individuals and their bodies should be central and personalization personal.

B. Kaplan (✉)
Yale University, New Haven, CT, USA
e-mail: Bonnie.Kaplan@yale.edu

P.-Y. S. Hsueh et al. (eds.), *Personal Health Informatics*, Cognitive Informatics
in Biomedicine and Healthcare, https://doi.org/10.1007/978-3-031-07696-1_23

Keywords Personalized medicine · Precision medicine · Virtualized patients
Representations of patients · Algorithms · Big data · Ethical issues · Quality of
care · Privacy · Bias · Ethics framework · ELSI

Learning Objectives
- To be able to analyze current and emerging ethical, legal, and social issues
  related to virtual healthcare and to personalized medicine and quality of
  care, privacy, bias, and fairness
- To recognize both benefits and limitations of mediating care through information technologies, virtualizing patients, and informing care with data
  representations of patients and algorithmic predictions
- To become familiar with an expanded scope of bioethics to include information technologies in healthcare through a framework for ethical analysis
- To make ethically-informed judgements involving information technologies in healthcare
- To incorporate ethical, legal, and social issues into practice

Introduction

Precision and personalized medicine[1] present exciting possibilities for improving
health and healthcare by tailoring treatment to each individual based on that person's genetic make-up, physiological measures, lifestyle, and other personal characteristics. Prestigious healthcare organizations promote precision medicine for
conditions ranging from genetic diseases to sepsis risk to cancer care (Permanente
Medicine 2017; Intermountain Healthcare 2021; United States Government
Department of Health and Human Services National Institutes of Health, National
Cancer Institute 2020; Mayo Clinic 2021). Based on analyzing data from a vast pool
of patients by using various forms of artificial intelligence, attributes of the individual to be treated are matched to like individuals to predict health issues and to
recommend treatments that were beneficial for other people with those
characteristics.

Large-scale projects are under way to improve health through precision medicine by undertaking research to develop customized care recommendations based
on data from each patient's health records and data concerning that person's living
environment, lifestyle, and family history, so as to match the right care to the right
treatment for people of different backgrounds, ages, and regions (United States

---

[1] Some use the terms "precision medicine" and "personalized medicine" interchangeably. Others
may differentiate them, so that precision medicine is taken to focus on genomics or molecular
bases of disease. Personalized medicine combines this with digital health, with its focus on data
generated by patients' devices, together with more traditional sources of patient information. I
generally use the terms interchangeably.

Government Department of Health and Human Services National Institutes of Health 2020a, b). In addition, tool development is being encouraged for the kind of data analysis on which precision medicine will depend (United States Government Department of Health and Human Services National Institutes of Health 2020c). Digital health tools—mobile health apps, wearables, telehealth and telemedicine, social networks, internet applications—are seen as enhancing diagnostic accuracy, therapeutics, and healthcare delivery by giving providers a more holistic view of patient health and patients more control over their health. Access to data is expected to improve outcomes as well as efficiency, provide new opportunities for disease prevention and management, improve access, reduce costs, increase quality, and make medicine more personalized (United States Government Department of Health and Human Services Food and Drug Administration 2021a, b). Digital phenotyping, for example, is promoted so that data collected by wearables and social media can be used to detect and develop improved treatments for cardiometabolic disease, insomnia, and various psychiatric, neurologic, and cognitive disorders (Jain et al. 2015; Onnela and Rauch 2016; Kaplan and Ranchordás 2019).

These trends are the latest in a series of developments that changed how the body and disease are conceptualized and treated. Over recent centuries, treatment moved from home to hospital, and now, back again to home. Meanwhile, as modern information technologies were becoming more common for patient care, the locus of clinical decision-making moved away from the patient's bedside as decisions were made based on data, measures, and images, thereby diverting attention to representations of a patient's condition and away from focusing on the actual patient (Bosk and Frader 1980; Kaplan 1995; Sandelowski 2002; Kaplan et al. 2007; Verghese 2009). Trends toward digitalization and virtualization burgeoned with the advent of the COVID-19 pandemic as in-person was replaced by on-line interaction; telemedicine and telehealth, another way representations of patients are treated, became the preferred means of healthcare, making ethical, legal, and social issues all the more apparent (Kaplan 2020a).

Personalized medicine, it seems to me, is the latest manifestation conflating an actual patient with an encoded and quantified version, part of a larger trend towards digitalizing healthcare and replacing a living person with a virtual representation. Something is gained, something is lost.

Because the benefits are more obvious, this chapter outlines some of what may be lost in the hopes of minimizing those losses and realizing the promise of personalized medicine in ethical ways. An ELSI (Ethical, Legal, and Social Issues) framework shown in Table 23.1 includes a wide range of considerations: what constitutes quality of care and the relationship between clinician and patient; access and effects on various populations and patients; consent and autonomy; privacy protections and a variety of other legal and regulatory issues; commercialization of healthcare, commodification of data; issues pertaining to algorithms, data, technology design, and the obvious role of information technologies in healthcare; and both institutional and governmental policy (Kaplan 2020a, 2022). In line with the emphases of this

Table 23.1 Health information technologies ELSI framework

Assess what are, and should be, effects regarding each category in the framework, by considering:

- Are people treated humanely, well, and fairly? Who? How? By what standard?
- Are people acting ethically? What will facilitate their doing so?
- What values are embedded in different models and means of care? In data and algorithms? What values should be promoted?
- What can be learned from experience so that the promises of better health and healthcare are ethically realized?
- Quality of care
  - Clinician-patient relationship, including whether same as face-to-face; depersonalization and the importance of human contact and touch, empathy, and non-verbal cues
  - All are treated equally, without disparities, but tailored to person and situation instead of in a uniform one-size-fits-all way
- Consent and autonomy
  - Who consents
  - How meaningful is the consent, including lack of choice and required end-user agreements (EULAs)
- Access, including to care and to technology
  - Clinician access
  - Patient access, including suitability and usability (vulnerabilities, disabilities, age, etc.), location infrastructure, digital divide, underserved and unserved populations
- Legal and regulatory
  - Privacy, confidentiality, cybersecurity, data protection
  - Licensure/authorization and credentialing, state rules
  - Liability, malpractice
  - Device regulation/certification/functioning
  - Conflicting jurisdictions and rules
  - Data sharing and ownership
- Clinician responsibilities
  - Knowledge of limitations and consequences, and informing patients
  - Data protection for devices, storage, transmission
  - Quality of received data
  - New skills, training curriculum
  - Cultural/language sensitivity
- Patient responsibilities
  - Active participation/shared decision making
  - Usability, including negotiating vulnerabilities, disabilities, age, etc.
  - Self-monitoring and disease management
- Changed relationships
  - Clinician-patient, clinician-clinician, clinician-community (including sensitivity to locale)
  - Patient-family-community
  - Care coordination
  - Trust, information provision, patient advocacy/fiduciary responsibility
- Commercialization of healthcare
  - Conflicts of interest

Table 23.1 (continued)

– Mission transparency
– Trading off of values, e.g., rationality, efficiency, cost-cutting vs caregiving; improve health vs create market needs; market needs/vendors' interests prioritized
• Policy – Institutional and governmental
– Guidelines and policies
– Other uses of resources
– New care models
– Underlying values and priorities
– Reimbursement and coding
– Overwhelming emergencies
• Information needs
– Available for and from patient encounters and from individuals at large
– Automated guidelines and disease management
– Data integrity
– AI and algorithms, including transparency, explainability, fairness
• Evaluation and assessment – Beforehand and on-going
– Quality and satisfaction
– Unintended consequences
– Information linkages
– Guidelines needed
– How and what to roll out, appropriate clinical and medical conditions, suitability of technologies
– Usability
Cybersecurity and privacy
– Changes in care priorities
– End-user agreements
– Patient, family, community, clinician acceptability

Based on (Kaplan (2020a, 2022)

volume on technology and healthcare, of these many possible areas for ELSI analysis, I have chosen to focus ELSI discussion according to themes of this book section: ethics, privacy, bias, and fairness. I especially consider how personalized medicine and the digitalization and virtualization of care and of the patient pertain to quality of care. I start with quality of care in general, followed by briefer discussions of privacy, bias, and fairness in relation to quality of care.

Quality of Care

What constitutes quality of care is not only a medical concern, but also an ethical one. Virtualization comes with many benefits, and also many ELSI considerations. I argue that:

- virtualization reduces distinctions between illness and health, and between individuals; and that
- virtualization reduces knowledge of the patient and patient's body.

Therefore, virtualization results in:

- changing relationships, and
- shifting the locus of care away from the patient while decontextualizing data.

Further:

- data, algorithms, and proxies lack transparency; and
- predictions influence care.

All of these

- can compromise care and
- threaten personhood and autonomy.

Instead

- make personalization personal.

Benefits of Virtualization

Virtualization has improved both care and access to it in many ways. Budding clinicians practice on simulated patients that may be embodied life-like manikins or virtual three-dimensional images. This is obviously far safer than practicing on people and a good way to begin developing clinical technique and knowledge. Trying out therapies, developing predictions, and testing hypotheses on synthetic patients rather than real ones also can protect privacy and provide both research and treatment opportunities beyond what would be possible with real people (Purnell 2020). Telemedicine and telehealth services are godsends for people who otherwise might have no care or would need to undertake inconvenient travel for it. Remote monitoring using data from implantable, ingestible, or wearable devices not only is convenient, but may forestall or catch problems. People are able to take more control over disease management or keep track of their health, whether ill or well. Commercial smart-phone applications have vastly expanded these capabilities. The quantified self has become popular both in clinics and homes. Even mundane patient records are no longer quite as mundane as they become electronic; integrate patient-generated data, data from monitoring devices, and from mobile apps; and interface with algorithms to provide alerts, prognoses, and treatment advice.

Virtualization Reduces Distinctions Between Illness and Health, and Between Individuals

Personalized medicine provides means for measuring just where along a spectrum of health and illness each individual is by comparison with others, for assessing where a person is in terms of disease trajectories and etiologies, and for predictions that, it is hoped, will forestall negative health events and outcomes. Though distinguishing between illness and health has always been challenging, one effect of personalized medicine is to reduce sharp distinctions between health and illness. No longer, too, are individuals distinct. More and more, each individual is seen as a disembodied autonomous stable self in terms of others considered similar. This trend moves healthcare away from caring for a patient as an individual to caring for patients as members of groups represented by data. It transforms how individual bodies are conceptualized, managed, and visually displayed. Reconfiguring the body changes how bodies, personal identity, and health and illness are understood (Armstrong 1995; Lupton 2013). Healthcare changes and becomes more depersonalized.

Virtualization Reduces Knowledge of the Patient and Patient's Body

Quality of care depends not only on clinical knowledge and acumen, but also on the relationship between clinician and patient, knowledge of what each patient considers important in terms of health and lifestyle, cultural and social norms, visual and sensory cues, empathy, expectations of patients' and clinicians' responsibilities, and professionalism and autonomy appropriate for both patient and clinician, i.e., quality depends on treating patients and clinicians as individual people. The loss of clinicians' sensory and intuitive capabilities that are part of in-person encounters and the technological burdens on both clinician and patient require a significant shift in professional practices and attitudes and in clinician-patient relationships. Professional codes of ethics therefore recommend training (Kaplan 2020a; Lupton 2013; Kaplan and Litewka 2008; Botrugno 2019), and a new specialty of "medical virtualists," in light of digital advances in healthcare, telehealth, and mHealth, has been proposed (Nochomovitz and Sharma 2018). Patients, too, must take on additional responsibilities for their health and healthcare, learn the technologies and how to use them effectively, and learn how to adjust to new clinical practices and power relationships (Kaplan 2020a).

But training is not enough. When technologies mediate interaction, the meanings attributed to a clinical consultation change. The explosion of on-line interaction due to the COVID pandemic has taught us that, in addition to the many benefits and opportunities it allows, "zoom fatigue" has become commonplace, and on-line classes can reduce learning. It is reasonable to assume there will be similar effects for healthcare at a distance. If, as in telemedicine, there are images, image size and perceived distance can affect each person's sense of power. When patients appear only in terms of images and data, aspects of quality shift. Relationships become reduced to encounters, transactions, trackable actions, and scores (Klugman 2018). As mentioned above, concepts of patients' bodies and patients' identities are changed in the process, and consequently, relationships related to care are changed. If a clinician knows only what data or images indicate about a patient, the clinician does not know about the person *per se* and lacks the visual and sensory cues that are part of an examination, such as palpation for diagnostic purposes or detecting odors associated with some conditions. Bodily findings are not all that is missing. Context, too, is absent.

Virtualization Shifts Locus of Care, Decontextualizes Data, Compromises Care

Without knowing the circumstances of data collection, i.e., the activities that generated the data or the cultural norms and practices that surround those activities, it is difficult to interpret them correctly for that patient. Shifting the locus of care away from the actual person means the data being collected and the care given both lack context. Without knowing the person, it is difficult to collaborate in healthcare and achieve goals important to the patient. It is hard to assess what is normal, or at least acceptable, for that patient and what to make of where the patient fits with other supposedly similar patients. Similar, that is, according only to similar data, but perhaps not in other significant respects.

As clinicians are presented voluminous streams of data—vital signs, behavioral and lifestyle data, environmental hazard exposure, health status—from various monitoring devices, they may miss the forest for the trees. The equivalent of zoom fatigue may set in. Removed from the context in which data are generated, and unable to notice sensory and emotional cues or provide the therapeutic value of physical presence, care becomes depersonalized and perhaps compromised, especially if what is missing leads to missed diagnoses (Kaplan and Litewka 2008; Botrugno 2021). Telecare, when patient and clinician are physically distant, may lead to over-treatment or an excess of procedures related to the desire to collate and act on more data; missing patient information that is not reflected in existing data can increase the potential for unnecessary screening (Adams and Petersen 2016). There already is evidence that telemedicine may involve antibiotic over-prescribing and other inappropriate prescriptions (Jain et al. 2019; Hoffman 2020).

Inappropriate decisions based on data can be exacerbated if the digital version of a person is a frozen snapshot instead of being updated by changing conditions, and if the algorithms acting on the digital version of the person are not updated with that individual's changing data, data changes of all others in the dataset, and the latest clinical and research knowledge. Clinicians may be influenced in diagnosis and treatment by prior data no longer applicable, or that the patient may have wanted to withhold in order to get a fresh clinical view (Zubrzycki 2021).

Virtualization Threatens Personhood and Autonomy

Making it impossible to "forget" part of a record threatens the role memory has as part of identity and self-presentation. Treating data as a true, or at least a sufficient, representation of a person, also threatens personhood by separating the person from the data (Suter 2004). If patients are represented by data, that data may not present them as they would present themselves. Patients who wish some control over their self-presentation by withholding data or providing it in a particular way can lose that opportunity (Zubrzycki 2021). Stigma can result from identifying a set of characteristics as indicative of a fault or disadvantage. It may lead to exclusion or discrimination, or to recrimination and blame for not behaving more responsibly in regards to one's health. Yet resisting these consequences by falsifying or withholding data can compromise the data on which algorithms are trained or deployed, causing potential harm to all patients.

Lack of Transparency About Data, Algorithms, and Proxies Threatens Quality of Care

Lack of knowing the patient is compounded by lack of knowing about data sources and algorithms. Without knowing the technologies of data generation and collection, including their limitations and potential inaccuracies, it is difficult to know what should be made of the data or of the patient's or the technology's reliability. Current artificial intelligence methods make it difficult, if not impossible, to know much about either the data or how the resultant algorithms work.

When algorithms are proprietary, intellectual property protections can prevent public knowledge of significant aspects of algorithm development, testing, and verification. Without confidence in an algorithm and enough understanding of the basis for whatever it recommends, clinicians are more reluctant to use it (Kaplan 2020b). That can be unfortunate, as some algorithms perform exceedingly well.

It can be unfortunate, too, if an algorithm has unknown limitations. For example, secrecy would prevent discoveries such as that a widely-used algorithm resulted in black patients not receiving needed care. Only when it was studied was it realized that the algorithm used health costs as a proxy for health needs, and so falsely concluded that black patients were healthier than equally sick white ones (Obermeyer et al. 2019). Proxies present additional problems. A person's health status and predictions of future status are based on associations found in datasets, on functions of sets of characteristics represented in the data and the way potential outcomes are defined. They are proxies rather than causes, and reflect what those creating and training the algorithms consider important or measurable (Barocas and Selbst 2016). That changes definitions of disease and when interventions occur, and so changes care (Adams and Petersen 2016).

Predictions Affect Quality of Care

Data can be indicators and suggestive of appropriate care decisions, but clinical judgement along with knowledge of the patient and of the technology also are necessary. One-size-fits-all may not fit that patient, or the circumstances. To ensure that all are treated equally, according to their individual conditions, literally equal treatment may not mitigate against disparities or missing crucial differences between patients with profiles that may be similar only because contextual information and personal knowledge are lacking.

A further quality of care consideration is avoiding self-fulfilling prophecies. In the extreme, if predictive algorithms indicate a high chance of developing a fatal condition, the person so "condemned" may simply not see the point of behaving in a healthy manner. At the other extreme, too many risks may be taken if no future health issues are expected. For some patients, symptoms of anxiety, paranoia, or obsessiveness may be exacerbated by giving them feedback from monitoring them (Onnela and Rauch 2016). Though such possibilities are illustrative, it is easier to imagine a person (clinician or patient) becoming depressed, unduly optimistic, more or less apt to take preventive measures, or of acting in wiser or misguided ways than would have occurred without the predictions. On the plus side, it is also easier to imagine taking precautions and preventive actions that forestall a negative predicted outcome. In either case, both the individual patient's and clinician's judgment and values are important in considering whether the prediction and actions based on it are right for that clinical relationship.

Make Personalization Personal

An overarching question is how changes in care relate to understandings of whether personalized medicine depersonalizes care and dehumanizes both clinicians and patients, and of what is humane and ethical treatment. We risk prioritizing data, devices, and measures over our bodies, individuality, personhood, and patients' and clinicians' sense of these (Lupton 2013; Klugman 2013). Different people will have different preferences, values, and needs, and, therefore, different priorities for their health and healthcare. Some patients may prefer making their own decisions in collaboration with the clinicians treating them, others might not. Increasing collaboration and engagement may be intimidating to some, empowering to others (Kaplan and Litewka 2008). Self-care may be enhanced for some, while for others agency is reduced and dependency increased (Mort et al. 2013). To promote health and healthcare, personalization based on data can be of potential benefit, but only if we keep in the foreground that people, and health, are more than data; human experience cannot be reduced to data points and algorithmic predictions. Personalization needs to be personal.

Privacy

Privacy has taken center stage in discussions of ELSI. It intersects with other concerns. Some of those intersections are foreshadowed above. Privacy also is a paramount legal issue. Discussions of privacy recognize the need for regulation and the difficulty of enabling data collection and use for beneficent purposes while preventing maleficent ones. Although there may be disagreement over just how to do that, the legal and medical literatures generally agree that this is a problematic area.

Making images and data related to a patient available to anyone who might treat the patient means patients will have less control over what they wish to disclose, how they wish to disclose it, and to whom (Zubrzycki 2021). A number of additional privacy concerns arise if much of the data come from outside the healthcare system or leave the system. With the Big Data needed for personalized medicine, privacy risks are higher because of the repeated uses and combinations of multiple datasets, and the impossibility of predicting what those datasets will be, how the data will be used, and what they will yield. That makes assessing resulting risks very difficult *a priori* (Vayena 2018). Nevertheless, some are predictable.

I discuss ELSI regarding privacy, Big Data, and virtualized representations of patients, again with a focus on quality of care. Here I argue that:

- trust in confidentiality is part of the patient-clinician relationship, and so a basis for quality of care; however
- anonymity is impossible, making consent for data sharing and use also impossible, and therefore possibly leading to
- undermining trust in ways that can compromise care.
- Trust is a basis for care.

Confidentiality has been part of the medical tradition at least since the Hippocratic Oath. Maintaining confidentiality is seen as a physician's professional duty around the world (Kaplan 2016). As the World Medical Association put it in 2002: "Confidentiality is at the heart of medical practice and is essential for maintaining trust and integrity in the patient-physician relationship. Knowing that their privacy will be respected gives patients the freedom to share sensitive personal information with their physician" (World Medical Association 2002). The free exchange of sensitive information, then, forms a foundation on which clinical decisions are made and affects quality of care. However, personalized medicine and basing care on virtual representations of patients necessarily compromises privacy and poses potential harms that could well compromise quality of care.

Anonymity Is Impossible

One of the issues is to what extent de-identification or anonymization protects individuals, and how a sense of privacy is related to care. Re-identification techniques are improving; as has been known for some while, the more data that is combined, the better the chance of re-identification (Ohm 2010). Genomes are unique, so identifiable. In some states, it is legal to include genomic information in research databases without that person's permission. Re-identification is possible by comparing such information with other data, such as that held by law enforcement or commercial genetic testing companies. Privacy is compromised, for that individual and for everyone who is genetically related to an individual and is identifiable, leading some to wonder if privacy is the price of precision medicine (Kulynych and Greely 2018).

Lack of Consent

For personalized medicine, data about any person must be identified in some way so as to be linked in order to create profiles of and target care to each person. That, then, gets into numerous issues related to consent for data collection and use as well as to privacy. In a research environment, consent is governed by The Common Rule in the US and similar protections for human subject research elsewhere. Clinical data is similarly protected by data protection regulations such as the Health Information Portability and Accountability Act (HIPAA) in the US, and the General Data Protection Regulation (GDPR) in the European Union. For healthcare research and clinical care, the bioethics literature amply explores issues of consent, who may consent, how informed they may be, how to enhance understanding, and like issues. However, specific apps and platforms collect, encrypt, and handle data differently, making consenting more confusing (Onnela and Rauch 2016). Moreover, in the US, privacy protection safeguards and considerations are limited for data collected commercially through mobile health apps, social media websites, wearables, and medical devices that are not regulated by the Food and Drug Administration or by HIPAA, but instead by click-through non-negotiable end-user agreements (EULAs). Regardless of data source and even with privacy protections in place, when data become part of a database mined for digital medicine and personalized healthcare, the person associated with that data has become part of what the person may consider a research project to which that person possibly would not have consented. Unlike in the US, the GDPR and related regulations cover all personal data, including commercially-collected data (Kaplan 2020b, 2021). Still, potential privacy threats remain. Despite years of security issues, including malware, lack of encryption, and insecure data storage and transmission (Kaplan and Ranchordás 2019), mobile apps remain vulnerable to hacking and data leakage (Horowitz 2021). EULAs themselves are opaque and may not be honored by vendors; their problematic basis in notice-and-consent is well recognized in legal scholarship (Kaplan 2020b, 2021).

Moreover, with expansive data collection needed for precision and personalized medicine, all data can become health data (Kaplan 2020b). Because many things may serve as health predictors or indicators, a person's daily activities, behaviors, lifestyle, social engagements, messages about everything from what one ate to one's mood to what times someone dozed off, all are grist for monitoring for health and predictive purposes. There is, then, little distinction (other than legal) between research data, clinical data, or any other source of data.

It is not surprising, then, that most of the 60 thought leaders—scholars of ethics, genomics, health law, government, and disadvantaged populations interviewed for a study of precision medicine research data—considered general approaches to confidentiality, such as technical security measures and US data protection rules (including HIPAA, the Common Rule, and data access restrictions), as necessary, but not sufficient (Hammack et al. 2019). Whether a person gives permission for data collection or sharing through any of these mechanisms, it is impossible to predict every possible way data may be shared, combined, or used as it is packaged, transmitted, aggregated with other data, distributed to others, and becomes part of other databases, in never-ending combinations and future potential uses. No one can anticipate all future uses or attendant risks. Being informed and consenting are both impossible.

Potential Harms

Potential harms of re-identification and misuse of electronic health record, genomic, social media, and digital device data include physical, dignitary, group, economic, psychological, and legal harms, with consequences ranging from embarrassment to stigmatization to discrimination to criminalization. Moreover, because these harms could result from predictions instead of actual medical conditions, the uncertainties can unsettle people and lead to consequences based on speculative events that may never happen (Beskow et al. 2021).

Because algorithms create ad hoc groups using various criteria pre-defined to be of interest, group harms become more significant. These harms can both undermine patients' trust in confidentiality and also compromise their well-being at both individual and group levels. Among these harms are bias, discrimination, and disparities, with implications for fairness.

Bias and Fairness

Considerations of fairness and bias concern individuals and also the groups in which they are placed by algorithms used for precision medicine, based on data that supposedly represents them. The laudable intent of introducing recommendation generated by these algorithms is the expectation that divorcing the patient from the patient's body will result in clinicians not being influenced by stereotypes and preconceived notions concerning irrelevant aspects of the body's appearance. Basing care on data can reduce discrimination and unintentional bias in treatment decisions. At least, that is the hope. Nevertheless, relying on data and algorithms may be problematic. Data quality, on which all else rests, for example, can be questionable (Lun 2018). Each step, from data collection and algorithm development on, is prone to biases (Barocas and Selbst 2016). It is difficult to overcome numerous sources of bias or to adjust data and treatment to account for them (Hoffman and Podgurski 2020). I argue that these difficulties are endemic because:

- encoded bias replicates social biases,
- disparities in access lead to care disparities,
- care disparities can lead to biases in data, and this
- lack of representativeness in data reinforces and further exacerbates biases and disparities in care for individuals and groups.

Basing care on algorithmic outputs, then, decenters the person by replacing each patient with a data profile based on how the person is categorized. That, in turn, treats each patient according to the group into which the algorithm sorts the patient. Care presumed suitable for members of that group may not be suited to that individual patient.

Encoding Bias

Commentators, critics, and scholars have identified ways in which data and algorithms encode biases. Racism, for example, is encoded by considering "healthy skin" to be white or by being less accurate in detecting skin lesions when skin is dark (Pasquale 2019; Raji 2020). The kind of sorting algorithms do also can lead to increasing disparities and biases by reinforcing them. They can result in people being denied various services because they are identified as "disabled" or "mentally ill" or of a group thought undesirable or less treatable for racial, ethnic, age, or gender reasons based on the genes or health conditions characteristic of groups identified by predetermined criteria (Hoffman 2018; Taylor et al. 2017). Groupings through the use of data may channel people into particular kinds of services they may not find suitable, or fair, or effective. Equity is hardly served if algorithmic sorting places someone in a particular category that stems from or results in discrimination, negative profiling, stigma, or disparate services and quality of care. These algorithms may then result in further data that simply amplify or reinforce the initial biases.

Access Disparities Lead to Care Disparities

The COVID-19 pandemic brought biases and fairness, addressed here in terms of disparities, in health and healthcare to the forefront. Before the pandemic, telemedicine was little used despite high expectations that it could equalize access for underserved, rural, and remote areas. With fears of COVID contagion, regulatory and reimbursement restrictions were relaxed and usage skyrocketed (Kaplan 2020a), but the hopes were not completely realized. In densely-populated New York City, hard hit at the outset of the pandemic, telemedicine visits at New York University Langone Health sharply increased. More patients, both black and white, used the service than during the same period the previous year. That improved access. Yet the uptake of telemedicine by white patients was higher than by black patients (Chunara et al. 2020). More generally, telehealth increased more in US urban areas and in counties with low poverty levels than in other locations (Rand Corporation 2021a). The upshot: "The COVID-19 pandemic has affected telehealth utilization disproportionately based on patient age, and both county-level poverty rate and urbanicity" (Cantor et al. 2021). Moreover, among lower income patients, telehealth services overwhelmingly were telephone only (Rand Corporation 2021b). Similar patterns also have been evident in more varied locations in the US where "[i]ncreasing age, rural status, Asian or Black/African American race, Hispanic ethnicity, and self-pay/uninsured status were significantly negatively associated with having a video visit" (Hsiao et al. 2021).

Infrastructure is one of multiple factors that can affect access to digital health technologies (Chunara et al. 2020). Lower-income patients may lack the technological means to access video visits. Depressed areas may not have infrastructure for high-bandwidth transmissions. About one third of rural Americans do not have the broadband services to support video telehealth and so are limited to voice. These are the very areas with higher prevalence of chronic disease (Hirko et al. 2020). Voice-only visits necessarily cannot provide service equivalent to in-person visits, widely recognized as the standard of care for telemedicine (Kaplan 2020a). Similar concerns could plague care for those with disabilities because technologies are often neither designed nor deployed with their needs in mind. Voice-only care would hardly serve those with difficulties hearing or speaking. Telephone visits can result in unnecessary or lower quality care. They also may be more prone to fraud and abuse. Nevertheless, they may be better than previous levels of service and the ability to meet patient needs (Uscher-Pines et al. 2021). They also allow patients more options for accessing care and controlling how, or if, they are seen.

Telehealth and mHealth may reduce access barriers, but attention is needed to training in their use for both patients and clinicians. Design, implementation, and policy should take account of those with low technological or health literacy, little education, poor access to care and support, difficulties hearing or seeing, lack of mobility or dexterity, mental illness or cognitive impairment, frailties, language barriers, and other impediments to use (Kaplan and Ranchordás 2019; Valdez et al. 2020). These individuals may not be well-equipped to take advantage of digital health initiatives or assume responsibility for managing their health and healthcare.

Disparities are increased if these differences are ignored. Instead of trying to fit patients to the system, technologies and care need to be fitted to patients (Botin et al. 2020).

Biases in Data

Personalized medicine and digital health depend on massive stores of data, algorithms to analyze the data, and data about the individual to be treated. This, in turn, depends on assumptions of accurate, well-documented, representative, comprehensive, appropriate, timely, and unbiased data collection and training, evaluation, interpretation, and development and use of algorithms. Each of these criteria may not be met. Biases can be hard to detect in very large databases, which tend to represent people from places with good internet access or greater wealth, and who engage in "standard" behavior, language, appearance, and practices. The high cost of developing datasets and of creating, training, testing, and sustaining algorithms also will tend toward their use by wealthier organizations (Hao 2020). Data from research studies limited to one gender, to particular age groups, or to lack of co-morbidities necessarily are biased. The studies may be well-designed, but the data are hardly representative.

Combining data from multiple sources can help produce more representative data; this increases privacy threats and may not address a variety of other reasons why data may not be representative. The location and circumstances of data collection can affect the data (for example, if blood pressure is measured at home or in the emergency room) and what data are collected. Data, such as from electronic patient records, will not include those who have not been treated within the healthcare system for reasons ranging from lack of access, to fear of stigma or law enforcement, to lack of ability to pay, to lack of trust, to preferences for alternative forms of treatment, or simply to the patient's having been referred from one setting to another or to data being collected at different locations or health systems (Phelan et al. 2017). Under-coding, under-reporting, and lack of adequate biomarkers add to the skewing (Walsh et al. 2020). People who adjust behaviors due to monitoring and data collection also generate data impossible to distinguish from data that was not adjusted due to feedback or simply to knowing one is being monitored (Onnela and Rauch 2016). Consequently, some kinds of people and conditions will be over-represented, others, absent. Ensuring inclusion of all kinds of people, regardless of race, location, education level, disability, age, or any other factor would improve the quality of the data on which decisions are based. Without representative and inclusive data, the algorithmic sorting of people into categories, indeed, the creation of categories themselves, may be compromised. Health predictors may not apply to people not well-represented in data.

Additionally, care must be taken beyond representativeness in data and in assumptions built into algorithms. Mixing data from multiple sources can create its own problems (Phelan et al. 2017). More inclusive data, though potentially beneficial, also could lead to less representative data or worse, such as more abuse of data and the people represented by the data. Sorting people into categories based on various health indicators can affect groups as well as individuals. Just as privacy violations may harm the person concerned, everyone identified in the same category may be compromised, embarrassed, stigmatized, or subject to discrimination. Past practices exacerbate these concerns. Tribal leaders barred university researchers in 2003 (and by 2010 had sued and reached a settlement) because blood samples from the Havasupai Native American tribe were collected for diabetes research but then also unexpectedly used to study schizophrenia. The Navajo Nation confirmed their 2002 moratorium on genetic research because they would not have oversight in how the All of Us Research Program would use data from their members, and were outraged when they learned tribal members were recruited without consulting the leaders (Resnik 2021).

Of course, everyone in the group may benefit from what is learned about the group. The point, though, is that the decisions based on data affect the group as well as the individual. Each individual, then, is no longer central. That leads to another concern: it displaces the individual patient focus on which care was traditionally based. It "challenges the very foundations of most currently existing legal, ethical and social practices and theories" (Taylor et al. 2017). It reinforces trends towards categorizing and objectifying people based on data profiles as "bundles of symptoms" (Botin et al. 2020). Individual patients themselves are not as visible and heard.

Remedies and Frameworks

Some remedies to problems of ethics, privacy, bias, and fairness are suggested in the preceding discussion, such as better training and education, improving understanding of the advantages and limitations of the technologies, and treating each patient as a person. Another remedy is to be more inclusive, both in data and in design so that all kinds of people are represented (Kaplan 2020a; Valdez et al. 2020; Botin et al. 2020). Here I propose three more general remedies:

- evaluation and ethical analysis informed by an ELSI framework, which expands the scope of bioethics for information technologies in healthcare;
- expanding the scope of bioethics through multidisciplinarity; and
- placing individuals and their bodies at the center of care.

ELSI Framework for Evaluation and Ethical Analysis

ELSI analysis can be shaped by an ELSI framework. Several have been proposed for telecare and its evaluation (e.g (Kaplan 2020a; Mort et al. 2013; Kidholm et al. 2017)). They can be useful for examining considerations of increasing virtualization of healthcare, especially if combining several to serve as suggestions for issues to be addressed. Table 23.1 is based on a recent framework—generated in examining telecare in light of the COVID pandemic—of issues that characterize all use of health information technologies in patient care (Kaplan 2020a, 2022). Although this chapter addresses only those aspects of the framework related to quality of care, privacy, biases, and fairness, the entire framework can be helpful for considering other aspects of personalized medicine, virtualization of patients, Big Data, and algorithms. Key questions for ELSI analysis include:

- Are people treated humanely, well, and fairly? Who? How? By what standard?
- Are people acting ethically? What will facilitate their doing so?
- What values are embedded in different models and means of care? in data and algorithms? What values should be promoted?
- What can be learned from experience so that the promises of better health and healthcare are ethically realized?

Many, though not all, of these questions are addressed above in discussing privacy, biases, and fairness, in terms of quality of care. They can and should be examined further from different perspectives.

Multidisciplinarity

There is much to be learned from scholars working in a variety of areas, including law, surveillance studies, sociology, philosophy, computer science, anthropology, geography, human rights, and, of course, informatics (Kaplan 2020b; Taylor et al. 2017; Cohen 2015; Aarts et al. 2016; Novak et al. 2018). Multidisciplinary cross-fertilization can further an additional goal, that of broadening ELSI discussions beyond the common bioethics framework of beneficence, autonomy, and justice, so that the areas evident from the rapid expansion of delivering care mediated by information technologies are taken into account. Table 23.1 indicates areas for this expansion of the scope of bioethics (Kaplan 2022).

Conclusion

Healthcare is About Different People, with Bodies

The value of data pertaining to a patient's condition that includes measurements of bodily functions, laboratory values, scores and calculations, and the like, is indisputable. Such data enables not only comparisons of a patient's condition over time, but comparisons with norms and common measures. Such data are crucial, not only for each individual patient, but for the entire process of care and clinical research. Personalized medicine, telemedicine, digital phenotyping, and what has come to be called digital health all hold great promise.

But important, too, is that patients are people, with bodies. They are far more than data representations. Clinicians, too, are people, with bodies, far more than any screen images or notes in patient records. Good care requires everyone to relate to each other as people, not solely as representations. What counts as "quality of care," or "fairness" or even "ethical" can vary with people, their values, and situations. What information they wish to share and under what circumstances they wish to share it also will vary. Allowing for this variety would further meaningful choice, empowerment, and participation for patients—and clinicians. Care that takes into consideration differences as well as similarities among people also needs to take into consideration the roles of data and algorithms in that care.

A laudable goal of personalized medicine and personal health informatics is to use data, including real-world evidence, for informing care tailored to each individual. Artificial intelligence techniques and resultant algorithms generated from these data are envisioned to improve clinical practice, patient engagement, health, and healthcare. There already have been impressive results based on this approach. To more fully realize the promise, ethical considerations should inform developments so as to reduce potential harms.

This chapter has highlighted some possible harms stemming from replacing real individual patients and clinicians with disembodied virtual representations based on data and images. Moving care away from actual bodies changes care. These changes can affect quality of care, raising issues not only of health but also of ethics. As this promising field develops, ELSI should be considered along with health outcomes. Healthcare is about individual people, with bodies. Each person shares characteristics with others in ways that should inform care, but each is unique. Rather than personalized medicine, how about personalized care?

Key Points that Readers Can Use In Their Daily Clinical Informatics Practice
- Take into account both the strengths and limitations of technologies, algorithms, and data for delivering healthcare and doing research.
- Be mindful of the ethical, legal, and social considerations that computer-mediated care entails.
- Treat the person, not data or representations of the person.

Chapter Review Questions
- There has been increasing concern about bias in predictive algorithms. For example, algorithms may miscategorize pathologies of the skin for people with dark skin. Social media and various apps are generating alerts for people considered suicidal. Which of the following is most likely to bias results produced by an algorithms' predictions of suicide risk that are based on large data sets?

  (a) underreported suicide rates
  (b) the algorithm is developed commercially for sale to doctors' offices
  (c) whether the reason for the prediction is given
  (d) lack of a psychiatrist's participation in developing the algorithm

Answer

a. If the data on which the algorithm is trained or validated do not accurately reflect suicide rates, cases like the ones not reported will not be as likely to be predicted.

- A patient consults a doctor who writes a prescription and transmits it electronically to the pharmacy. The patient covers the cost of the prescription using a
  credit card or through insurance. Most pharmacies sell prescription data to a data
  aggregator for further combination with other data and sell that data to pharmaceutical companies, insurance companies, credit rating agencies, and others. The
  diagnosis and prescription become part of the patient's record. The prescription
  and credit card data are sold, aggregated and the patient re-identified. The credit
  card information, diagnosis, and prescription data become part of a database
  used for training predictive algorithms. The algorithms connect this information
  and bases prognoses on others with similar credit card transactions, diagnoses,
  and prescriptions. What likely may result from this transaction?

  (a) The patient's family sees the credit card statement and becomes concerned
      about expenses.
  (b) The predicted prognosis may influence treatment for any person with similar
      credit card transactions and prescriptions, thereby affecting their healthcare,
      their credit rating, and other aspects of their lives.
  (c) The pharmacy refuses to accept credit card payment when the patient refills
      the prescription because they are concerned the prognosis means the patient
      will be unable to pay the credit card bill.
  (d) The pharmacy may be fined for violating the patient's privacy.

Answer:

b. It is unknown exactly what data is used for credit scoring, but credit card information is involved. Credit scores as well as health-related data are used for decisions regarding insurance, employment, and finance.

- A clinician and patient have a telemedicine visit concerning a urological problem. The patient is delighted not to have to make a lengthy trip to the clinician's
  office but instead to have the visit while at home. The patient and clinician never
  met each other in person because the problem is new and each is avoiding contact
  as much as possible due to the COVID pandemic. However, the clinician has
  good record information about the patient and also has data from the patient's
  fitness tracker and diet apps. The clinician is able to compare this patient's data
  with data from other, similar patients. What should the clinician be particularly
  concerned about in terms of making an accurate diagnosis when being consulted
  by a patient in this way?

  (a) The telemedicine connection is spotty, interfering with connection quality. It
      also may be insecure and the patient's privacy therefore compromised.
  (b) The patient and doctor are not in the same state and far enough away from
      each other that it is unlikely they ever will meet in person. They may not be
      able to continue the relationship even via telemedicine because the clinician
      works for a telehealth company and may not be on duty when the patient
      needs follow-up.

(c) The clinician is not able to examine the patient well because no palpation is possible, skin condition is not easily visible (or, if the visit is only by telephone, not visible at all), and the possible presence of the patient's family makes a frank discussion difficult.

(d) The patient may be using the consultation as a way to get attention and reduce loneliness during COVID isolation.

Answer:

c. Although all should be of concern, most relevant *to making a diagnosis* is the ability to conduct a thorough physical exam. Without being able to physically examine the patient, important findings may be missed.

References

Aarts J, Adams S, Kaplan B, DeMuro PR, Solomonides T. Protecting patient privacy in cyber environments. AMIA Annual Symp Proc. 2016.

Adams SA, Petersen C. Precision medicine: opportunities, possibilities, and challenges for patients and providers. J Am Med Inf Assoc. 2016;23(4):787–90. https://doi.org/10.1093/jamia/ocv215.

Armstrong D. The rise of surveillance medicine. Sociol Health Illn. 1995;17(3):393–404.

Barocas S, Selbst AD. Big data's disparate impact. Calif Law Rev. 2016;104(3):671–732.

Beskow LM, Hammack-Avaran CM, Brelsford KM. Thought leader comparisons of risks in precision medicine research. Ethics Hum Res. 2021;42(6):35–40. https://doi.org/10.1002/eahr.500059.

Bosk C, Frader J. The impact of place of decision-making on medical decisions. Proc SCAMC. 1980;2:1326–9.

Botin L, Bertelsen PS, Kayser L, Turner P, Villumsen S, Nøhr C. People centeredness, chronic conditions and diversity sensitive ehealth: exploring emancipation of the 'health care system' and the 'patient' in health informatics. Life (Basel, Switzerland). 2020;10(12):329. https://doi.org/10.3390/life10120329.

Botrugno C. Towards an ethics for telehealth. Nurs Ethics. 2019;26(2):357–67. https://doi.org/10.1177/0969733017705004.

Botrugno C. Information technologies in healthcare: Enhancing or dehumanising doctor–patient interaction? Health (London). 2021;25(4-July):475–93. https://doi.org/10.1177/1363459319891213.

Cantor J, McBain RK, Pera MF, Bravata DM, Whaley C. Who is (and isn't) receiving telemedicine care during the COVID-19 pandemic. Am J Prev Med. 2021. https://doi.org/10.1016/j.amepre.2021.01.030.

Chunara R, Zhao Y, Chen J, Lawrence K, Testa PA, Nov O, et al. Telemedicine and healthcare disparities: a cohort study in a large healthcare system in New York City during COVID-19. J Am Med Inf Assoc. 2020;28(1):33–41. https://doi.org/10.1093/jamia/ocaa217.

Cohen J. Studying law studying surveillance. Surveillance & Soc'y. 2015;91:91–101.

Hammack CM, Brelsford KM, Beskow LM. Thought leader perspectives on participant protections in precision medicine research. J Law Med Ethics. 2019;47(1):134–48. https://doi.org/10.1177/1073110519840493.

Hao K. We read the paper that forced Timnit Gebru out of Google. Here's what it says. Technol Rev. 2020. https://www.technologyreview.com/2020/12/04/1013294/google-ai-ethics-research-paper-forced-out-timnit-gebru/. Accessed February 7, 2021.

Hirko KA, Kerver JM, Ford S, Szafranski C, Beckett J, Kitchen C, et al. Telehealth in response to the COVID-19 pandemic: implications for rural health disparities. J Am Med Inf Assoc. 2020;27(11):1816–8. https://doi.org/10.1093/jamia/ocaa156.

Hoffman LC. Shedding light on telemedicine & online prescribing: the need to balance access to health care and quality of care. Am J Law Med. 2020;46(2–3):237–51. https://doi.org/10.1177/0098858820933497.

Hoffman S. Big data's new discrimination threats: amending the Americans with Disabilities Act to cover discrimination based on data-driven predictions of future diseases. In: Cohen IG, Lynch HF, Vayena E, Gasser U, editors. Big data, health law, and bioethics. Cambridge: Cambridge University Press; 2018. p. 85–97.

Hoffman S, Podgurski A. Artificial intelligence and discrimination in health care. Yale J Health Policy Law Ethics. 2020;19(3):50.

Horowitz BT. Mobile health apps leak sensitive data through APIs, report finds. Fierce Healthcare; 2021 [updated February 24, 2021]. https://www.fiercehealthcare.com/tech/mobile-health-apps-leak-sensitive-data-through-apis-report-finds. Accessed February 25, 2021.

Hsiao V, Chandereng T, Lankton RL, Huebner JA, Baltus JJ, Flood GE, et al. Disparities in telemedicine access: a cross-sectional study of a newly established infrastructure during the COVID-19 pandemic. Appl Clin Inform. 2021;12(03):445–58.

Intermountain Healthcare. Precision genomics: For patients. [updated 2021]. https://intermountainhealthcare.org/services/genomics/patients/. Accessed March 29, 2021.

Jain SH, Powers BW, Hawkins JB, Brownstein JS. The digital phenotype. Nat Biotechnol. 2015;33(5):462–3. https://doi.org/10.1038/nbt.3223.

Jain T, Lu RJ, Mehrotra A. Prescriptions on demand: the growth of direct-to-consumer telemedicine companies. JAMA. 2019;322(10):925–6. https://doi.org/10.1001/jama.2019.9889.

Kaplan B. Objectification and negotiation in interpreting clinical images: Implications for computer-based patient records. Artif Intell Med. 1995;280(October):439–54.

Kaplan B. How should health data be used? Privacy, secondary use, and big data sales. Camb Q Healthc Ethics. 2016;25(2):312–29. https://www.cambridge.org/core/journals/cambridge-quarterly-of-healthcare-ethics/article/how-should-health-data-be-used/D3762C502A4C38EA79F1B516AD3665D2.

Kaplan B. Revisiting health information technology ethical, legal, and social issues and evaluation: telehealth/telemedicine and COVID-19. Int J Med Inf. 2020a;143(November):104239. https://doi.org/10.1016/j.ijmedinf.2020.104239.

Kaplan B. Seeing through health information technology: the need for transparency in software, algorithms, data privacy, and regulation. J Law Biosci. 2020b;7:Isaa062. https://doi.org/10.1093/jlb/lsaa062.

Kaplan B, with appendix by Monteiro APL. PHI protection under HIPAA: An overall analysis. In: Dallari AB, Monaco GFdC, editors. LGPD na saúde (LGPD applicable to health). São Paulo: Editora Revista dos Tribunais (Thomsom Reuters); 2021. pp. 61–88.

Kaplan B. Ethics, guidelines, standards, and policy: telemedicine, COVID-19, and broadening the ethical scope. Camb Q Healthc Ethics. 2022;31(1):105–18. https://doi.org/10.1017/S0963180121000852.

Kaplan B, Elkin PL, Gorman PN, Koppel R, Sites F, Talmon J. Virtual patients. In: Crowston K, Sieber S, Wynn E, editors. Virtuality and virtualization, IFIP International Federation for Information Processing, vol. 236. Boston: Springer; 2007. p. 397–401.

Kaplan B, Litewka S. Ethical challenges of telemedicine and telehealth. Camb Q Healthc Ethics. 2008;17(4):401–16. https://www.cambridge.org/core/journals/cambridge-quarterly-of-healthcare-ethics/article/ethical-challenges-of-telemedicine-and-telehealth/5D777B4EDE6E97934FB4B442F9CE0B33.

Kaplan B, Ranchordás S. Alzheimer's and m-health: regulatory, privacy, and ethical considerations. In: Hayre CM, Muller D, Scherer M, editors. Everyday technologies in healthcare. Boca Raton, London, New York: CRC Press; 2019. p. 31–52.

Kidholm K, Clemensen J, Caffery LJ, Smith AC. The Model for Assessment of Telemedicine (MAST): a scoping review of empirical studies. J Telemed Telecare. 2017;29(9):803–13. https://doi.org/10.1177/1357633X17721815.

Klugman C. Quantified self: your life in data. 2013. http://www.bioethics.net/2015/06/quantified-self-your-life-in-data/. Accessed November 30, 2020.

Klugman C. I, my love, and apps. AJOB. 2018;18(2):1–2. https://doi.org/10.1080/15265161.2018.1423793.

Kulynych J, Greely HT. Clinical genomics, big data, and electronic medical records: reconciling patient rights with research when privacy and science collide. J Law Biosci. 2018;4(1):94–132. https://doi.org/10.1093/jlb/lsw061.

Lun K-C. The datafication of everything - even toilets. Yearb Med Inform. 2018;27(1):234–6. https://doi.org/10.1055/s-0038-1641199.

Lupton D. The digitally engaged patient: self-monitoring and self-care in the digital health era. Soc Theory Health. 2013;11(3):256–70. https://doi.org/10.1057/sth.2013.10.

Mayo Clinic. Precision medicine for breast cancer. 2021. https://www.mayoclinic.org/tests-procedures/precision-medicine-breast-cancer/about/pac-20385240. Accessed March 29, 2021.

Mort M, Roberts C, Pols J, Domenech M, Moser I. On behalf of the EFORTT investigators. Ethical implications of home telecare for older people: a framework derived from a multisited participative study. Health Expect. 2013;18:438–49. https://doi.org/10.1111/hex.12109.

Nochomovitz M, Sharma R. Is it time for a new medical specialty?: the medical virtualist. JAMA. 2018;319(5):437–8. https://doi.org/10.1001/jama.2017.17094.

Novak L, Kuziemsky C, Kaplan B. Festschrift for Dr. Samantha Adams: Sam Adams and the social construction of technology and health: implications for biomedical informatics. Appl Clin Inform. 2018;9(3):496–88. https://www.thieme-connect.com/products/ejournals/abstract/10.1055/s-0038-1656524.

Obermeyer Z, Powers B, Vogeli C, Mullainathan S. Dissecting racial bias in an algorithm used to manage the health of populations. Science. 2019;366(6464):447–53. https://doi.org/10.1126/science.aax2342.

Ohm P. Broken promises of privacy: responding to the surprising failure of anonymization. UCLA Law Rev. 2010;57:1701–77.

Onnela J-P, Rauch SL. Harnessing smartphone-based digital phenotyping to enhance behavioral and mental health. Neuropsychopharmacology. 2016;41(7):1691–6. https://doi.org/10.1038/np.2016.7.

Pasquale F. Data-informed duties in AI development. Columbia Law Rev. 2019;119(7):1917–40.

Permanente Medicine. Stephen Parodi, MD, discusses Kaiser Permanente's use of predictive analytics to improve care. Kaiser Permanente; 2017 [updated December 5, 2017]. https://permanente.org/stephen-parodi-md-discusses-kaiser-permanentes-use-predictive-analytics-improve-care/. Accessed March 29, 2021.

Phelan M, Bhavsar NA, Goldstein BA. Illustrating informed presence bias in electronic health records data: how patient interactions with a health system can impact inference. EGEMS (Washington, DC). 2017;5(1):1–14. https://doi.org/10.5334/egems.243.

Purnell A. How synthetic data will improve veteran health and care. United States Department of Veterans Affairs; 2020 [updated December 7, 2020]. https://blogs.va.gov/VAntage/81908/synthetic-data-improve-veteran-care/. Accessed April 8, 2021.

Raji D. How our data encodes systematic racism. Technol Rev. 2020;123(6). https://www.technologyreview.com/2020/12/10/1013617/racism-data-science-artificial-intelligence-ai-opinion/. Accessed February 8, 2021.

Rand Corporation. Growth of telehealth during pandemic occurred mostly in more affluent and in metropolitan areas. Rand Corporation; 2021a [updated March 15, 2021]. https://www.rand.org/news/press/2021/03/15.html. Accessed March 16, 2021.

Rand Corporation. Nearly all telehealth appointments at clinics for lower-income Americans were audio-only, raising questions about quality and equity. Rand Corporation; 2021b [updated February 2, 2021]. https://www.rand.org/news/press/2021/02/02.html. Accessed March 16, 2021.

Resnik D. Treat human subjects with more humanity. Am Sci. 2021;109(4):232–37. https://doi.org/10.1511/2021.109.4.232.

Sandelowski M. Visible humans, vanishing bodies, and virtual nursing: complications of life, presence, place, and identity. Adv Nurs Sci. 2002;24(3):58–70.

Suter S. Disentangling privacy from property: toward a deeper understanding of genetic privacy. George Washington Law Rev. 2004;72(4):737–814.

Taylor L, Floridi L, van der Sloot B. Introduction: A new perspective on privacy. In: Taylor L, Floridi L, van der Sloot B, editors. Group privacy: new challenges of data technologies. Philosophical studies series. Dordrecht: Springer International Publishing; 2017. p. 1–12.

United States Government Department of Health and Human Services Food and Drug Administration. Digital Health Center of Excellence. 2021a [updated January 12, 2021]. https://www.fda.gov/medical-devices/digital-health-center-excellence. Accessed March 12, 2021.

United States Government Department of Health and Human Services Food and Drug Administration. What is digital health? 2021b [updated September 22, 2020]. https://www.fda.gov/medical-devices/digital-health-center-excellence/what-digital-health. Accessed March 12, 2021.

United States Government Department of Health and Human Services National Institutes of Health. All of Us: About. 2020a. https://allofus.nih.gov/about. Accessed March 27, 2020.

United States Government Department of Health and Human Services National Institutes of Health. All of Us research program overview. 2020b. https://allofus.nih.gov/about/all-us-research-program-overview. Accessed December 28, 2020.

United States Government Department of Health and Human Services National Institutes of Health. Big data to knowledge. 2020c [updated July 23, 2020]. https://commonfund.nih.gov/bd2k. Accessed December 28, 2020.

United States Government Department of Health and Human Services National Institutes of Health, National Cancer Institute. Targeted therapy to treat cancer. 2020 [updated March 11, 2020]. https://www.cancer.gov/about-cancer/treatment/types/targeted-therapies. Accessed March 29, 2021.

Uscher-Pines L, Sousa J, Jones M, Whaley C, Perrone C, McCullough C, et al. Telehealth use among safety-net organizations in California during the COVID-19 pandemic. JAMA. 2021;325(11):1106–7. https://doi.org/10.1001/jama.2021.0282.

Valdez RS, Rogers CC, Claypool H, Trieshmann L, Frye O, Wellbeloved-Stone C, et al. Ensuring full participation of people with disabilities in an era of telehealth. J Am Med Inf Assoc. 2020;28(2):389–92. https://doi.org/10.1093/jamia/ocaa297.

Vayena E. Protecting health privacy in the world of big data. In: Cohen IG, Lynch HF, Vayena E, Gasser U, editors. Big data, health law, and bioethics. Cambridge: Cambridge University Press; 2018. p. 157–9.

Verghese A. If we can't measure it, it doesn't exist. The Atlantic. September 22, 2009. https://www.theatlantic.com/technology/archive/2009/09/if-we-cant-measure-it-it-doesnt-exist/26988/. Accessed December 14, 2020.

Walsh CG, Chaudhry B, Dua P, Goodman KW, Kaplan B, Kavuluru R, et al. Stigma, biomarkers, and algorithmic bias: recommendations for precision behavioral health with artificial intelligence. JAMIA Open. 2020;3(1-April):9–15. https://doi.org/10.1093/jamiaopen/ooz054.

World Medical Association. Declaration on ethical considerations regarding health databases. 2002. www.wma.net/en/30publications/10policies/d1/. Accessed May 2, 2014.

Zubrzycki CM. Privacy from doctors. Yale Law Policy Rev. 2021;39(2):526–92.

Index

Printed in the United States
by Baker & Taylor Publisher Services